The Orbitofrontal Cortex

The Orbitofrontal Cortex

Edmund T. Rolls
Oxford Centre for Computational Neuroscience
Oxford, England

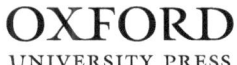

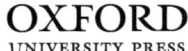

Great Clarendon Street, Oxford, OX2 6DP,
United Kingdom

Oxford University Press is a department of the University of Oxford.
It furthers the University's objective of excellence in research, scholarship,
and education by publishing worldwide. Oxford is a registered trade mark of
Oxford University Press in the UK and in certain other countries

© Oxford University Press 2019

The moral rights of the authors have been asserted

First Edition published in 2019

All rights reserved. No part of this publication may be reproduced, stored in
a retrieval system, or transmitted, in any form or by any means, without the
prior permission in writing of Oxford University Press, or as expressly permitted
by law, by licence or under terms agreed with the appropriate reprographics
rights organization. Enquiries concerning reproduction outside the scope of the
above should be sent to the Rights Department, Oxford University Press, at the
address above

You must not circulate this work in any other form
and you must impose this same condition on any acquirer

Published in the United States of America by Oxford University Press
198 Madison Avenue, New York, NY 10016, United States of America

British Library Cataloguing in Publication Data

Data available

Library of Congress Control Number: 2019938269

ISBN 978–0–19–884599–7

Links to third party websites are provided by Oxford in good faith and
for information only. Oxford disclaims any responsibility for the materials
contained in any third party website referenced in this work.

Preface

This book describes the orbitofrontal cortex. This is a part of the brain that is important in human emotion, pleasure, decision-making, valuation, and personality. The analysis of the orbitofrontal cortex includes its connections; how it relates to the previous and succeeding areas in brain processing; its neuron level neurophysiology which is essential for understanding what information is represented in the orbitofrontal cortex; functional neuroimaging of the orbitofrontal cortex; the effects of damage to the orbitofrontal cortex which provide important evidence about its functions; how the orbitofrontal cortex is involved in psychiatric disorders including depression, bipolar disorder, and autism; and how and what the orbitofrontal cortex computes.

The book aims to describe current understanding of the orbitofrontal cortex, and to provide a foundation for future research.

The orbitofrontal cortex develops greatly in humans and other primates, and for this reason the focus is on the orbitofrontal cortex in humans and other primates, though a Chapter on the rodent orbitofrontal cortex is included, as this can be explored with optogenetics.

A treatment of emotion, and how the orbitofrontal cortex is involved in Emotion, is provided in Emotion and Decision-Making Explained (Rolls 2014a), with an updated brief version that is suitable also for non-specialists and which incorporates a focus on depression in *The Brain, Emotion, and Depression* (Rolls 2018b). More detailed information is available too in the papers available as .pdfs on my website https://www.oxcns.org.

To understand how the brain works, including how it functions in emotion and decision-making, it is necessary to combine different approaches, including neural computation. Neurophysiology at the single neuron level is needed because this is the level at which information is exchanged between the computing elements of the brain, the neurons (Rolls 2016c). Evidence from the effects of brain damage, including that available from neuropsychology, is needed to help understand what different parts of the system do, and indeed what each part is necessary for. Neuroimaging is useful to indicate where in the human brain different processes take place, and to show which functions can be dissociated from each other. Knowledge of the biophysical and synaptic properties of neurons is essential to understand how the computing elements of the brain work, and therefore what the building blocks of biologically realistic computational models should be. Knowledge of the anatomical and functional architecture of the cortex is needed to show what types of neuronal network actually perform the computation. And finally the approach of neural computation is needed, as this is required to link together all the empirical evidence to produce an understanding of how the system actually works (Rolls 2016c). This book utilizes evidence from all these disciplines to develop an understanding of how emotion and decision-making are implemented by processing in the brain, and in particular the roles of the orbitofrontal cortex.

In this book, I show how it is now possible to follow processing in the brain from the sensory representation and perception of objects including visual and taste objects that are independent of reward value; to brain regions where reward value (both outcome value and expected value) are represented, which are crucial components of decision-making; to brain mechanisms that actually implement the choice part of the decision-making, with a mechanism that is common to categorization and decision-making in other brain systems and cortical areas. I believe that this represents a major advance in neuroscience that we are able to understand at the level of mechanisms all of these processes, and to see how they are linked together in the brain to implement much of our behaviour. Moreover, all of this neural understanding is linked to an understanding of the adaptive value of this organization of behaviour, how emotion is a key component, and even how the subjective feeling of pleasure may arise and be related to these processes.

My book *Cerebral Cortex: Principles of Operation* (Rolls 2016c) shows how some of the neural mechanisms described in this book, and a number of others, provide a unifying computational neuroscience approach to understanding many aspects of brain function, including short-term memory, long-term memory, top-down attention, visual object recognition, and information representation in the brain, as well as decision-making. *Cerebral Cortex: Principles of Operation* (Rolls 2016c) includes Appendices that may be useful for those wishing an introduction to the computational neuroscience mechanisms involved in many aspects of brain function, including the operation of the orbitofrontal cortex. The Appendices to that book are available online at www.oxcns.org, and include descriptions of the operation of pattern association and attractor networks, which are important as a basis for understanding some of the functions of the orbitofrontal cortex. The book also describes computer programs written in Matlab available from my website to illustrate the properties of these networks.

The Noisy Brain: Stochastic Dynamics as a Principle of Brain Function (Rolls & Deco 2010) describes in detail stochastic dynamics in the brain, how it can be understood with the techniques of theoretical physics, how it contributes to many aspects of brain function and behaviour, including the probabilistic decision-making about rewards and how this is implemented in the orbitofrontal cortex and the brain regions to which it projects.

The overall plan of this book is described in Chapter 1.

The material in this text is the copyright of Edmund T. Rolls. Part of the material described in the book reflects research performed over many years in collaboration with many colleagues, whose tremendous contributions are warmly appreciated. The contributions of many will be evident from the references cited in the text. In addition, I have benefited enormously from the discussions I have had with a large number of colleagues and friends, many of whom I hope will see areas of the text that they have been able to illuminate. Particular thanks are due to Fabian Grabenhorst and Sylvia Wirth to whom this book is dedicated who have discussed this project very helpfully. Much of the work described would not have been possible without financial support from a number of sources, particularly the Medical Research Council of the UK, the Human Frontier Science Program, the Wellcome Trust, the McDonnell-Pew Foundation, and the European Union.

The book was typeset by the author in LATEX using the WinEdt editor and MiKTeX.

The cover shows a schematic diagram of some of the connections of the orbitofrontal cortex modified from Fig. 2.2; and the human orbitofrontal cortex (left) and macaque orbitofrontal cortex (right) modified from Fig. 1.3. The images on the back cover and spine are from 'Adam and Eve' painted in c. 1528 by Lucas Cranach the Elder (Uffizi Gallery, Florence), which provides an early interpretation of early human emotions, and emotion-related decision-making. This book provides a scientific approach to the orbitofrontal cortex, which implements inter alia many aspects of emotion and emotion-related decision-making.

Updates to the publications cited in this book and .pdf files of many papers and some of my books are available at https://www.oxcns.org. Matlab software (which will run with the freeware Octave) to provide simple demonstrations of the operation of some of the neuronal networks described in Chapter 9 are available at my website in connection with my book *Cerebral Cortex: Principles of Operation* (Rolls 2016c), the Appendices of which describing the software are also online at https://www.oxcns.org.

Edmund T. Rolls dedicates this work to the overlapping group: his family, friends, and colleagues: *in salutem praesentium, in memoriam absentium*.

Contents

1 Introduction to the orbitofrontal cortex — 1
 1.1 Introduction — 1
  1.1.1 Historical background — 1
  1.1.2 Topology — 2
 1.2 The importance of understanding the primate, including human, brain — 4
 1.3 Functional neuroimaging in humans, neuronal encoding, and brain computation — 7
 1.4 The orbitofrontal cortex: the plan of the book — 8

2 Orbitofrontal cortex: anatomy and connections — 10
 2.1 Connections — 10
 2.2 Output pathways from the orbitofrontal cortex to the dopamine and serotonin brainstem systems — 14

3 Orbitofrontal cortex processing: neurophysiology and neuroimaging — 17
 3.1 An overall framework for the role of the orbitofrontal cortex in the processing of reward in the brain — 17
 3.2 Taste and oral texture: outcome value — 20
  3.2.1 Taste pathways to the orbitofrontal cortex — 20
  3.2.2 Taste representations in the orbitofrontal cortex — 20
  3.2.3 Taste value is represented in the orbitofrontal cortex — 24
  3.2.4 Oral texture in the orbitofrontal cortex — 27
  3.2.5 Taste and oral texture in the insular primary taste cortex — 32
  3.2.6 Taste in an output region of the orbitofrontal cortex, the anterior cingulate cortex — 34
 3.3 An olfactory representation in the orbitofrontal cortex of expected value — 36
  3.3.1 Olfactory pathways to and responses in the primate orbitofrontal cortex — 36
  3.3.2 Learning and reversal of olfactory-taste associations in the orbitofrontal cortex — 37
  3.3.3 Olfactory reward value and pleasantness are represented in the orbitofrontal cortex — 39
  3.3.4 Encoding of olfactory information in the orbitofrontal cortex — 42
 3.4 Convergence of taste and olfactory inputs in the orbitofrontal cortex: the representation of flavour — 43
 3.5 Somatosensory and temperature inputs to the orbitofrontal cortex, and affective value — 44
 3.6 Expected value of visual stimuli — 45
  3.6.1 The representation of the expected value of visual stimuli — 45

	3.6.2	Visual reversal to compute expected value can be rapid and rule-based in primates including humans	47
	3.6.3	Visual stimulus-selective expected value neurons	48
	3.6.4	Devaluation shows that orbitofrontal cortex visual neurons represent expected value	50
	3.6.5	A representation of faces and social stimuli in the orbitofrontal cortex	52
	3.6.6	Visual inputs to the orbitofrontal cortex from the temporal lobe visual cortical areas	56
3.7		Monetary reward value, and many other types of reward, are represented in the orbitofrontal cortex	73
3.8		Negative reward prediction error neurons in the orbitofrontal cortex	75
3.9		Cognitive influences on the orbitofrontal cortex	80
3.10		Attentional modulation of affective vs sensory processing	83
3.11		The topology of the functional neuroimaging activations in the orbitofrontal cortex	87
3.12		Value representations in the orbitofrontal cortex and neuroeconomic decision-making	92
	3.12.1	Choosing between rewards with different value	92
	3.12.2	A common scale of value for different goods in the orbitofrontal cortex, but no conversion to a common currency	98
	3.12.3	Absolute value and relative value are both represented in the orbitofrontal cortex	101
	3.12.4	The representation of expected reward value, uncertainty, and risk	105
	3.12.5	Delay of reward, emotional choice, and rational choice	106
3.13		Decision-making mechanisms in the orbitofrontal cortex and elsewhere in the brain	108
	3.13.1	Introduction	108
	3.13.2	Decision-making in an attractor network	109
	3.13.3	Analyses of reward-related decision-making mechanisms in the orbitofrontal cortex	113
	3.13.4	Neuroimaging investigations of decision-making in the orbitofrontal cortex	118
3.14		A representation of novel visual stimuli, and memory-related effects, in the orbitofrontal cortex	123
3.15		Deep brain stimulation of the orbitofrontal cortex	125
3.16		The orbitofrontal cortex and addiction	128
4		**Orbitofrontal cortex damage effects in humans and other primates**	**130**
4.1		Non-human primates	130
	4.1.1	Emotion and reward-related learning impairments	130
	4.1.2	Impairment of reward value as altered by selective satiation, reward size, and delay of reward	131
	4.1.3	Credit assignment vs the comparison of choices	131
	4.1.4	Rapid reversal learning	132
4.2		Humans	134
	4.2.1	Introduction	134
	4.2.2	Reward valuation, and reversal learning	135

	4.2.3	Social behaviour, subjective emotional change, and personality	139
	4.2.4	Face and voice expression identification	141
	4.2.5	Orbitofrontal cortex lesions and impulsiveness: some similarities with Borderline Personality Disorder	143
	4.2.6	Frontotemporal dementia	144

5 Orbitofrontal cortex output pathways: cingulate cortex, basal ganglia, and dopamine 145

- 5.1 The cingulate cortex 145
  - 5.1.1 Introduction to and overview of the cingulate cortex 145
  - 5.1.2 Anterior cingulate cortex anatomy and connections 146
  - 5.1.3 Anterior cingulate cortex functional neuroimaging and neuronal activity 148
  - 5.1.4 A framework 148
  - 5.1.5 Pregenual representations of reward value, and supracallosal representations of punishers and non-reward 150
  - 5.1.6 Anterior cingulate cortex and action-outcome representations 151
  - 5.1.7 Anterior cingulate cortex lesion effects 152
  - 5.1.8 Subgenual cingulate cortex 152
  - 5.1.9 Mid-cingulate cortex, the cingulate motor area, and action–outcome learning 153
  - 5.1.10 The posterior cingulate cortex 154
  - 5.1.11 The cingulate cortex: synthesis 155
- 5.2 Dopamine systems in the brain and reward prediction errors 155
  - 5.2.1 Dopamine pathways 156
  - 5.2.2 Self-administration of dopaminergic substances, and addiction 157
  - 5.2.3 Behaviours associated with the release of dopamine 158
  - 5.2.4 Dopamine neurons and reward prediction error 159
- 5.3 The basal ganglia 160
  - 5.3.1 Overview of the basal ganglia 160
  - 5.3.2 Systems-level architecture of the basal ganglia 160
  - 5.3.3 Neuronal activity in the striatum 162
  - 5.3.4 How do the basal ganglia perform their computations? 164

6 The orbitofrontal cortex and emotion 165

- 6.1 An introduction to emotion 165
- 6.2 Rewards and punishers 169
- 6.3 Individual differences in emotion, personality, and the orbitofrontal cortex 172
- 6.4 Emotional orbitofrontal vs rational routes to action 173
  - 6.4.1 Some of the different routes to action produced by emotion-related stimuli 173
  - 6.4.2 Examples of some complex behaviours that may be performed implicitly 174
  - 6.4.3 A reasoning, rational, route to action 175
  - 6.4.4 The Selfish Gene vs The Selfish Phenotype 176
  - 6.4.5 Decision-making between the implicit and explicit systems 178

6.5　Comparison between the functions of the orbitofrontal cortex and amygdala in emotion　179
   6.5.1　Overview of the functions of the amygdala in emotion　180
   6.5.2　The amygdala and the associative processes involved in emotion-related learning　181
   6.5.3　Connections of the amygdala　181
   6.5.4　Effects of amygdala lesions　182
   6.5.5　Neuronal activity in the primate amygdala to reinforcing stimuli　184
   6.5.6　Responses of primate amygdala neurons to novel stimuli that are reinforcing　187
   6.5.7　Neuronal responses in the amygdala to faces　187
   6.5.8　Evidence from humans　189

7　The orbitofrontal cortex, depression, and other mental disorders　191
7.1　Depression　191
   7.1.1　The economic and social cost of depression　191
   7.1.2　The triggers and causes of depression: non-reward systems　191
   7.1.3　Brain systems that underlie depression　194
7.2　A non-reward attractor theory of depression　195
7.3　Evidence consistent with the non-reward attractor theory of depression　197
7.4　Advances in understanding the functions of the orbitofrontal cortex in depression　199
   7.4.1　Overview　199
   7.4.2　Orbitofrontal cortex　203
   7.4.3　Anterior cingulate cortex　206
   7.4.4　Posterior cingulate cortex　207
   7.4.5　Amygdala　209
   7.4.6　Precuneus　211
   7.4.7　Effective connectivity in depression　213
   7.4.8　Depression and poor sleep quality　215
7.5　Possible subtypes of depression　216
7.6　Implications for treatments for depression　217
   7.6.1　Brain-based treatments　217
   7.6.2　Behavioural treatments and cognitive therapy　218
7.7　Pharmacological treatments for depression　220
   7.7.1　Serotonin (5HT)　220
   7.7.2　Ketamine　221
7.8　Mania and bipolar disorder　222
   7.8.1　Mania, increased responsiveness to reward, and decreased responsiveness to non-reward　223
   7.8.2　Attractor networks, mania, increased responsiveness to reward, and decreased responsiveness to non-reward　224
   7.8.3　Other aspects of bipolar disorder　224
7.9　Autism　225
7.10　Attention-deficit / hyperactivity disorder　226
7.11　Compulsivity　226

8　The rodent orbitofrontal cortex　228

8.1	Evolutionary trends	228
	8.1.1 Evolution of the taste and flavour system	228
	8.1.2 Evolution of the temporal lobe cortex	231
8.2	Divisions and functions of the rodent orbitofrontal cortex	231
8.3	Neuronal activity in the rodent orbitofrontal cortex	233
8.4	A state space representation in the rodent orbitofrontal cortex?	234
8.5	Synthesis	235

9 Orbitofrontal cortex computations in a systems-level perspective — 237

9.1	Pattern association memory	237
	9.1.1 Architecture and operation	237
	9.1.2 Properties	240
9.2	Autoassociation or attractor memory	240
	9.2.1 Architecture and operation	241
	9.2.2 Introduction to the analysis of the operation of autoassociation networks	242
	9.2.3 Properties	244
	9.2.4 Use of autoassociation networks in the brain	248
9.3	An integrate-and-fire implementation of an attractor network for decision-making	248
9.4	A model for reversal learning in the orbitofrontal cortex	251
9.5	A theory and model of non-reward neural mechanisms in the orbitofrontal cortex	255

10 Synthesis: the Roles of the Orbitofrontal Cortex — 257

10.1	Synthesis	257
	10.1.1 The orbitofrontal cortex is the first stage of processing to represent reward value	257
	10.1.2 The orbitofrontal cortex represents the reward value of particular stimuli with different neuronal populations	257
	10.1.3 The orbitofrontal cortex represents expected value, outcome value, and negative reward prediction error	257
	10.1.4 The orbitofrontal cortex represents neuroeconomic value	258
	10.1.5 Activations in the orbitofrontal cortex are often linearly related to the conscious subjective pleasantness (or unpleasantness) of stimuli	258
	10.1.6 Face expression and face identity are both represented in the orbitofrontal cortex, and both are important for social interactions	258
	10.1.7 The orbitofrontal cortex implements one-trial rule-based reward reversal	258
	10.1.8 A common scale of reward value, but not a common currency	258
	10.1.9 Relative and absolute value may both be represented in the orbitofrontal cortex	259
	10.1.10 Top-down cognition and attention, even from the level of language, exert effects on the orbitofrontal cortex, and bias it	259
	10.1.11 Decision-making in the ventromedial prefrontal cortex, VMPFC	259
	10.1.12 Decision confidence is represented in the ventromedial prefrontal cortex, VMPFC	259

10.1.13 Decision-making in the orbitofrontal cortex reflects noise introduced by the Poisson nature of neuronal firing   259
10.1.14 Net value needs to be provided as the input to an attractor decision-making network   259
10.1.15 The orbitofrontal cortex is a key brain area in emotion   259
10.1.16 The orbitofrontal cortex does not represent actions or behavioural responses   260
10.1.17 The orbitofrontal cortex projects value information to several brain systems   260
10.1.18 The orbitofrontal cortex develops greatly during evolution in primates and humans, and appears to overshadow the amygdala in emotion in primates including humans   261
10.1.19 The rodent orbitofrontal cortex is much less developed than the primate including human orbitofrontal cortex   261
10.1.20 In addition to the orbitofrontal cortex reward value-based system for taking decisions, there is also a rational, reasoning route   261
10.1.21 The orbitofrontal cortex is a key brain area in depression   261
10.1.22 The orbitofrontal cortex and addiction   261
10.2 The orbitofrontal cortex: future directions   262

A Glossary   **265**
A.1 General   265
A.2 Learning theory terms   266

References   **269**

Index   **302**

1 Introduction to the orbitofrontal cortex

1.1 Introduction

1.1.1 Historical background

The prefrontal cortex has for long been implicated in emotion, though it is only relatively recently that there has been a firm scientific foundation for understanding how it functions. Let us look first at some of the background.

1.1.1.1 Phineas Gage

One of the first indications that the prefrontal cortex is involved in emotion came from the remarkable case of Phineas Gage, who was working as a foreman for a railway development in Vermont in the USA (Harlow 1848). In 1848, he was tamping down explosives with a tamping iron when unexpectedly the tamping detonated the explosive. The tamping iron, a long bar like a crowbar approximately 3 ft 7 inches long, shot into the air and passed upwards through the front of Phineas Gage's brain (Damasio, Grabowski, Frank, Galaburda & Damasio 1994). Gage survived but from that time on became a changed person. Formerly he had held responsibility as a foreman, but after the operation he became less reliable, and did not appear to be so concerned about the consequences of his actions. Moreover, in his personal life, he was described as being a changed person ("No longer Gage", short-tempered, capricious and profane). However, these personality and emotional changes took place without other general changes in Phineas Gage's intellectual abilities and intelligence. Hannah and Antonio Damasio and colleagues have reconstructed the site of the brain damage from the fractures found in the skull, and have shown that there would have been considerable damage to the lower (or ventral) part of the frontal cortex, which is where the orbitofrontal cortex is located (Damasio et al. 1994, Damasio 1994)). (It is so-called because it is just above the orbit of the eye.) The case of Phineas Gage suggested that the prefrontal cortex is involved in some way in emotion and personality, and that these functions are dissociable in the brain from many other types of function.

1.1.1.2 Prefrontal leucotomy

Another historical line of evidence implicates the frontal lobes in emotion. During an investigation of the effects of frontal lobe lesions in non-human primates on a short-term spatial memory task, Jacobsen (1936) noted that after the operation one of his animals became calmer and showed less frustration when reward was not given. Hearing of this emotional change, Moniz, a Portuguese neurosurgeon, argued that anxiety, irrational fears, and emotional hyperexcitability in humans might be treated by damage to the frontal lobes. He operated on twenty patients and published an enthusiastic report of his findings (Moniz 1936) (see Fulton (1951)). This rapidly led to the widespread use of this surgical procedure, and more than 20,000 patients were subjected to prefrontal 'lobotomies' (in which a part of the frontal lobe was removed) or 'leucotomies' (in which some of the white matter connections of the frontal lobe were cut) of varying extent during the next 15 years. Although irrational anxiety or emotional outbursts were sometimes controlled, it was not clear that the surgery treated effectively the symptoms for which it was intended, side-effects were often apparent, and the effects were

2 | Introduction to the orbitofrontal cortex

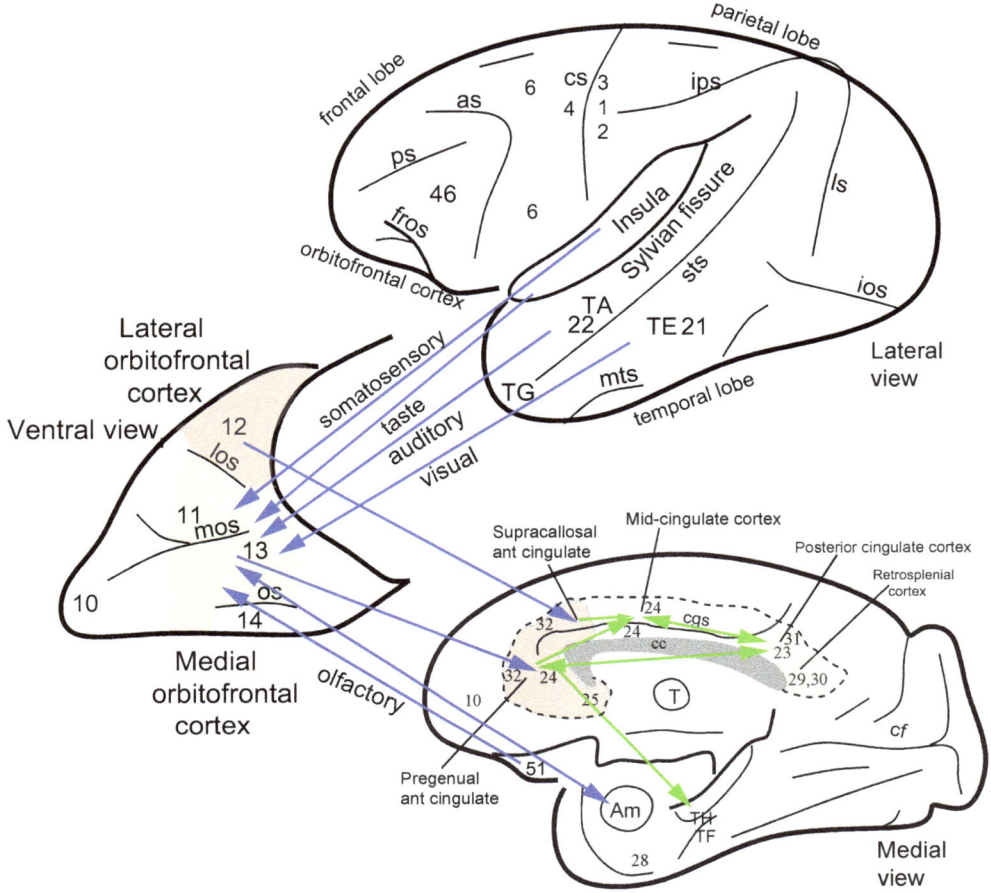

Fig. 1.1 The orbitofrontal cortex forms the ventral (lower) part of the frontal lobes of the primate (illustrated) including human brain. This diagram shows some of the gustatory, olfactory, visual, and auditory pathways to the orbitofrontal cortex, and some of the outputs of the orbitofrontal cortex. The secondary taste cortex and the secondary olfactory cortex are within the orbitofrontal cortex. The medial orbitofrontal cortex (areas 13 and 11) is shaded green, and the lateral orbitofrontal cortex (area 12) is shaded red. V1, primary visual cortex. V4, visual cortical area V4. Abbreviations: as, arcuate sulcus; cc, corpus callosum; cf, calcarine fissure; cgs, cingulate sulcus; cs, central sulcus; ls, lunate sulcus; ios, inferior occipital sulcus; mos, medial orbital sulcus; os, orbital sulcus; ots, occipito-temporal sulcus; ps, principal sulcus; rhs, rhinal sulcus; sts, superior temporal sulcus; the Sylvian (or lateral) fissure has been opened to reveal the insula; Am, amygdala; ant cingulate, anterior cingulate cortex (shaded red); T, thalamus; TE (21), inferior temporal visual cortex; TA (22), superior temporal auditory association cortex; TF and TH, parahippocampal cortex; TG, temporal pole cortex; 3,1,2, somatosensory cortex; 4, motor cortex; 6, premotor cortex; 14, gyrus rectus; 28, entorhinal cortex; 51, olfactory (prepyriform and periamygdaloid) cortex.

irreversible (Rylander 1948, Valenstein 1974). For these reasons these operations have been essentially discontinued. A lesson is that very careful and full assessment and follow-up of patients should be performed when a new neurosurgical (or any medical) procedure is being developed, before it is ever considered for widespread use. In relation to pain, patients who underwent a frontal lobotomy sometimes reported that after the operation they still had pain but that it no longer bothered them affectively (Freeman & Watts 1950, Melzack & Wall 1996).

1.1.2 Topology

Given this historical background, we now turn to a more systematic and fundamental consideration of how some parts of the frontal lobes are involved in emotion. The prefrontal cortex is the region of cortex that receives projections from the mediodorsal nucleus of the thalamus and is situated in front of the motor and premotor cortices (Areas 4 and 6) in the frontal lobe (see Fig. 1.1).

Based on the divisions of the mediodorsal nucleus, the prefrontal cortex may be divided into three main regions (Fuster 2015). First, the magnocellular, medial (meaning towards the midline), part of the mediodorsal nucleus projects to the orbital (ventral) surface of the prefrontal cortex (which includes Areas 13, 11, and 12) (see Figs. 1.1, 1.2 and 1.3). It is called the orbitofrontal cortex, and is the part of the primate prefrontal cortex that appears to be primarily involved in emotion. The orbitofrontal cortex receives information from the part of the visual system concerned with forming representations of objects (the inferior temporal visual cortex), and taste, olfactory, touch (somatosensory, body sensory), and auuditory inputs (see Figs. 1.1, 2.1 and 2.2).

Second, the parvocellular, lateral, part of the mediodorsal nucleus of the thalamus projects to the dorsolateral prefrontal cortex. This part of the prefrontal cortex receives inputs from the parietal cortex, and is involved in tasks such as spatial short-term memory tasks, attention, and, in humans, functions such as planning (Fuster 2015, Passingham & Wise 2012, Rolls 2016c, Shallice & Cipolotti 2018, Deco & Rolls 2003). Third, the pars paralamellaris (most lateral) part of the mediodorsal nucleus projects to the frontal eye fields (Area 8) in the anterior bank of the arcuate sulcus.

The orbitofrontal cortex is considered in the rest of this chapter. The cortex on the orbital surface of the frontal lobe includes Area 13 caudally, Area 11 anteriorly, and Area 14 medially, and the cortex on the inferior convexity includes Area 12 (see Figs. 1.1, 1.2, 1.3, and 2.4 and (Carmichael & Price 1994, Petrides & Pandya 1994, Ongur & Price 2000, Ongur, Ferry & Price 2003, Mackey & Petrides 2014, Henssen, Zilles, Palomero-Gallagher, Schleicher, Mohlberg, Gerboga, Eickhoff, Bludau & Amunts 2016, Kringelbach & Rolls 2004). The orbitofrontal cortex is poorly developed in rodents, but well developed in primates including humans. To understand the function of this brain region in humans, the majority of the studies described here have therefore been performed with macaque monkeys or with humans. There is some variability in the sulcal patterns in the human orbitofrontal cortex (Mackey & Petrides 2014, Henssen et al. 2016), and it is useful to take this into account in imaging studies (Kringelbach & Rolls 2004).

The automated anatomical labelling atlas 2 (AAL2) (Rolls, Joliot & Tzourio-Mazoyer 2015a) does parcellate the orbitofrontal cortex into different gyri. In resting state functional magnetic resonance imaging (fMRI) studies using the AAL2 (see e.g. Chapter 7), a group of areas can be grouped together as medial orbitofrontal cortex because of their high correlations (OFCmed, OFCant, OFCpost, and rectus), and a group can similarly be termed lateral orbitofrontal cortex (OFClat and IGForb), and these two groups have low correlations with each other (Rolls, Cheng, Gilson, Qiu, Hu, Li, Huang, Yang, Tsai, Zhang, Zhuang, Lin, Deco, Xie & Feng 2018a).

In this book, the term **medial orbitofrontal cortex refers to areas 13 and 11** shown in Figs. 1.1, 1.2, 1.3, and 2.4; and **lateral orbitofrontal cortex refers to area 12 (12/47 in humans)**. A connectional network of mainly cingulate areas has been termed a medial prefrontal network; and a connectional network involving mainly the orbitofrontal cortex has been termed an orbital prefrontal network, and is of course lateral to the 'medial prefrontal network' (Carmichael & Price 1996) (see Chapter 2). It is important to understand that the terms medial and lateral orbitofrontal cortex refer to well defined anatomical areas, and not to medial prefrontal or orbital/lateral prefrontal networks, and this needs to be borne in mind very fully when interpreting some studies (Rudebeck, Saunders, Lundgren & Murray 2017, Murray & Rudebeck 2018, Rao, Sellers, Wallace, Lee, Bijanzadeh, Sani, Yang, Shanechi, Dawes & Chang 2018) (see further Section 4.1.4).

4 | Introduction to the orbitofrontal cortex

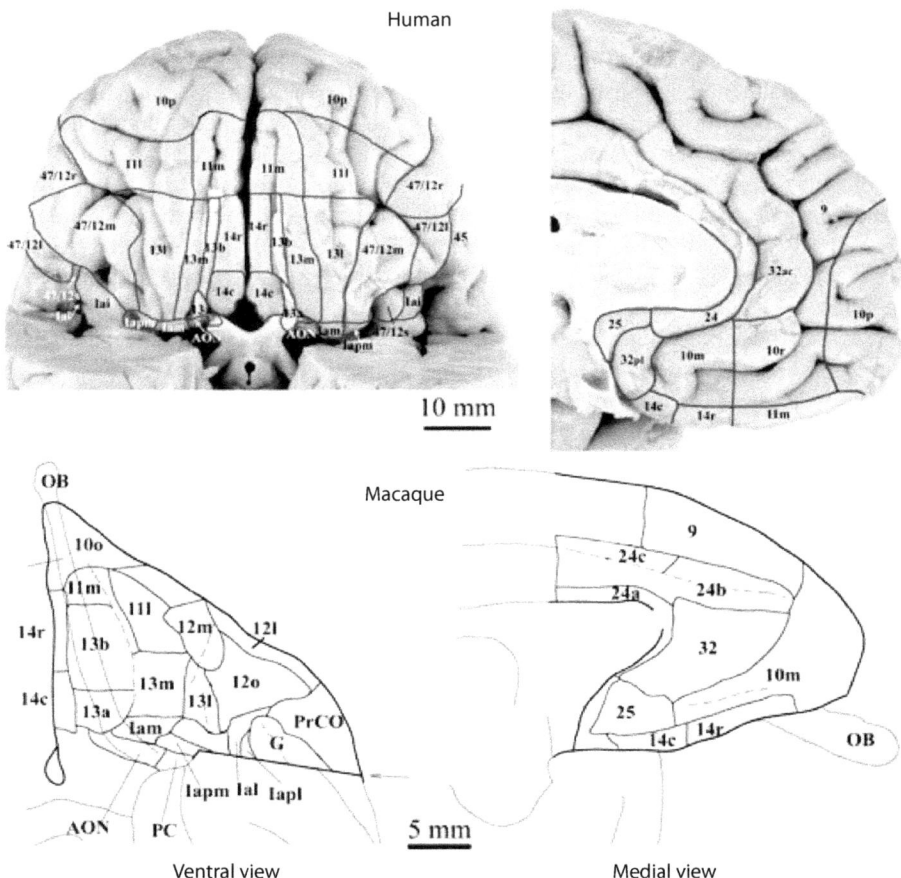

Fig. 1.2 Maps of architectonic areas in the orbitofrontal cortex (left) and medial prefrontal cortex (right) of humans (above) and monkeys (below). Left: ventral view. Right: medial view. The orbitofrontal cortex includes **areas 13 and 11 (termed medial orbitofrontal cortex in this book)** and **area 12 (47/12 in humans) (termed lateral orbitofrontal cortex in this book)**. The anterior cingulate cortex includes area 32 and the parts of area 24 shown, with area 25 named the subgenual cingulate cortex. Medial prefrontal cortex area 10 refers to the parts of area 10 shown on the medial views of the brains. The ventromedial prefrontal cortex (VMPFC) refers to ventral parts of this medial region. AON - anterior olfactory nucleus; G - primary gustatory cortex; Iai, Ial, Iam, Iapm - subdivisions of the agranular insular cortex; OB - olfactory bulb; PC - pyriform cortex; PrCO - precentral opercular area. (Above: Adapted from Dost Ongur, Amon T. Ferry, and Joseph L. Price, Architectonic subdivision of the human orbital and medial prefrontal cortex, Journal of Comparative Neurology, 460 (3), pp. 425–449, Copyright © 2003, Wiley-Liss, Inc. Below: Adapted from S. T. Carmichael and J. L. Price, Architectonic subdivision of the orbital and medial prefrontal cortex in the macaque monkey, Journal of Comparative Neurology, 346 (3), pp. 366–402, Copyright © 1994, Wiley-Liss, Inc.)

1.2 The importance of understanding the primate, including human, brain

It is because of the intended relevance to understanding the human orbitofrontal cortex, and human emotion and its disorders, that emphasis is placed in this book on findings from research in non-human primates, including monkeys, as well as in humans. This is important, for the orbitofrontal cortex and many of the brain systems that are involved in emotion and motivation have undergone considerable development in primates (e.g. monkeys and humans) compared to non-primates (for example rats and mice).

For example, the temporal lobe has undergone great development in primates, and several systems in the temporal lobe are either involved in emotion (e.g. the amygdala), or provide some of the main sensory inputs to brain systems involved in emotion and motivation. In particular, the amygdala and the orbitofrontal cortex, key brain structures in emotion, both receive inputs from the highly developed temporal lobe cortical areas, including those involved in invariant visual object recognition and face identity and expression processing.

Another example is that the orbitofrontal cortex has undergone great development in primates, and is very little developed in rodents, yet is one of the major brain areas involved in emotion and motivation in primates including humans. Indeed, it has been argued that the granular prefrontal cortex is a primate innovation, and the implication of the argument is that any areas that might be termed orbitofrontal cortex in rats (Schoenbaum, Roesch, Stalnaker & Takahashi 2009) are homologous only to the agranular parts of the primate orbitofrontal cortex (shaded mid grey in Fig. 1.3), that is to areas 13a, 14c, and the agranular insular areas labelled Ia in Fig. 1.3 (Wise 2008, Passingham & Wise 2012). It follows from that argument that for most areas of the orbitofrontal and medial prefrontal cortex in humans and macaques (those shaded light grey in Fig. 1.3), special consideration must be given to research in macaques and humans. As shown in Fig. 1.3, there may be no cortical area in rodents that is homologous to most of the primate including human orbitofrontal cortex (Preuss 1995, Wise 2008, Passingham & Wise 2012).

The development of some cortical areas has been so great in primates that even evolutionarily old systems such as the taste system appear to be differently connected, compared with that of rodents, to place much more emphasis on cortical processing, taking place in areas such as the orbitofrontal cortex (Rolls & Scott 2003, Scott & Small 2009, Small & Scott 2009, Rolls 2016b, Rolls 2016f) (Section 8.1.1.2) (Figs. 2.2 and 8.1). In primates, the reward value of the taste is represented in the orbitofrontal cortex in that the responses of orbitofrontal taste neurons are modulated by hunger in just the same way as is the reward value or palatability of a taste. In particular, it has been shown that orbitofrontal cortex taste neurons stop responding to the taste of a food with which a monkey is fed to satiety, and that this parallels the decline in the acceptability of the food (see Fig. 3.25) (Rolls, Sienkiewicz & Yaxley 1989). In contrast, the representation of taste in the insular primary taste cortex of primates (Scott, Yaxley, Sienkiewicz & Rolls 1986, Yaxley, Rolls & Sienkiewicz 1990) is not modulated by hunger (Rolls, Scott, Sienkiewicz & Yaxley 1988, Yaxley, Rolls & Sienkiewicz 1988, Rolls 2016b). Thus in the primary taste cortex of primates (and at earlier stages of taste processing including the nucleus of the solitary tract), the reward value of taste is not represented, and instead the identity of the taste is represented (see Section 3.2.5). The importance of cortical processing of taste in primates, first for identity and intensity in the primary taste cortex, and then for reward value in the orbitofrontal cortex, is that both types of representation need to be interfaced to visual and other processing that requires cortical computation. For example, it may have adaptive value to be able to represent exactly what taste is present, and to link it by learning to the sight and location of the source of the taste, even when hunger and reward is not being produced, so that the source of that taste can be found in future, when it may have reward value. In line with cortical processing to dominate the processing of taste in primates, there is no modulation of taste responsiveness at or before the primary taste cortex, and the pathways for taste are directly from the nucleus of the solitary tract in the brainstem to the taste thalamus and then to the taste cortex (Figs. 2.2 and 8.1). In contrast, in rodents such as the rat, the nucleus of the solitary tract connects to a pontine taste area, the parabrachial nucleus, that is not present in primates (Rolls & Scott 2003, Scott & Small 2009, Small & Scott 2009, Rolls 2016b, Rolls 2016f). The rodent pontine taste area then not only has connections to the thalamus and thus to the cortex, but also has direct connections to many subcortical areas important in appetite control, including the amygdala and hypothalamus (Section 8.1.1.2 and Fig. 8.1). Moreover, in rodents, satiety reduces the responsiveness

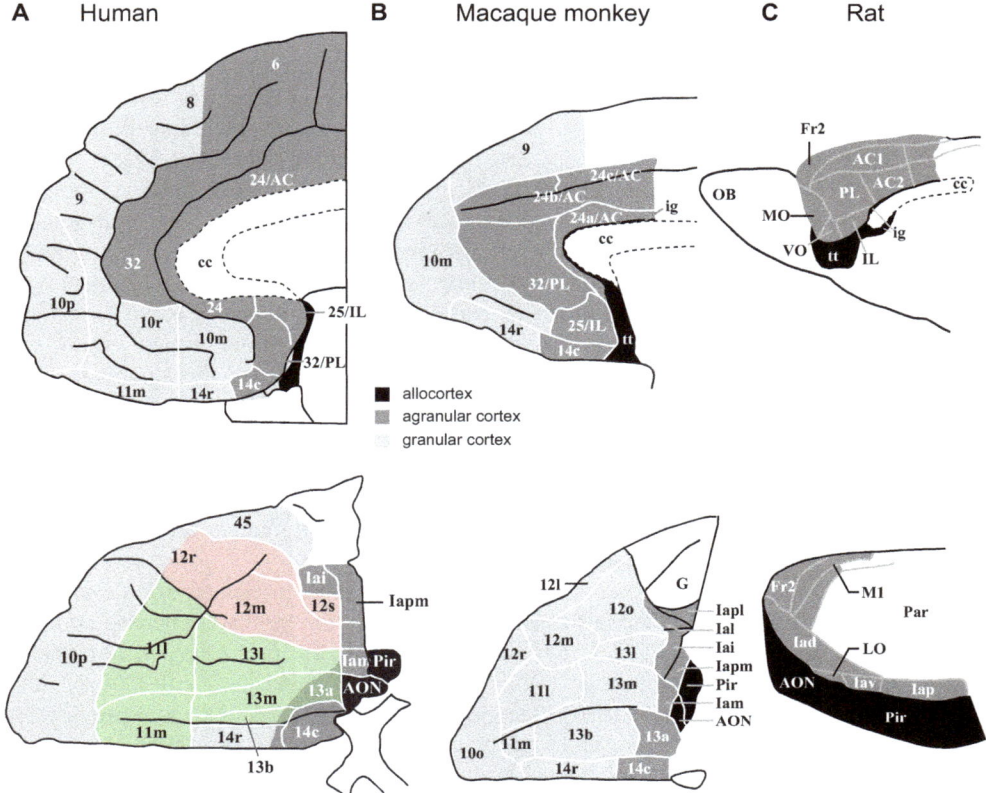

Fig. 1.3 Comparison of the orbitofrontal (below) and medial prefrontal (above) cortical areas in humans, macaque monkeys, and rats. (A) Medial (top) and orbital (bottom) areas of the human frontal codex (Ongur et al. 2003). The medial orbitofrontal cortex is shown in green (areas 13 and 11), and the lateral orbitofrontal cortex in red (area 12). Almost all of the human orbitofrontal cortex except area 13a is granular. Agranular cortex is shown in dark grey. The part of area 45 shown is the orbital part of the inferior frontal gyrus pars triangularis. (B) Medial (top) and orbital (bottom) areas of the macaque frontal cortex (Carmichael and Price 1994). (C) Medial (top) and lateral (bottom) areas of rat frontal cortex (Palomero-Gallagher and Zilles 2004). Rostral is to the left in all drawings. Top row: dorsal is up in all drawings. Bottom row: in (A) and (B), lateral is up; in (C), dorsal is up. Not to scale. Abbreviations: AC, anterior cingulate cortex; AON, anterior olfactory 'nucleus'; cc, corpus callosum; Fr2 second frontal area; Ia, agranular insular cortex; ig, induseum griseum; IL, infralimbic cortex; LO, lateral orbital cortex; MO, medial orbital cortex; OB, olfactory bulb; Pr, piriform (olfactory) cortex; PL, prelimbic cortex; tt, tenia tecta; VO, ventral orbital cortex; Subdivisions of areas are labelled caudal (c); inferior (i), lateral (l), medial (m); orbital (o), posterior or polar (p), rostral(r), or by arbitrary designation (a, b). (Modified from Passingham and Wise (2012). (a) Adapted from Dost Ongur, Amon T. Ferry, and Joseph L. Price, Architectonic subdivision of the human orbital and medial prefrontal cortex, Journal of Comparative Neurology, 460 (3), pp. 425–49. doi.org/10.1002/cne.10609. Copyright © 2003 John Wiley and Sons. (b) Adapted from S. T. Carmichael and J. L. Price, Architectonic subdivision of the orbital and medial prefrontal cortex in the macaque monkey, Journal of Comparative Neurology, 346 (3), pp. 366–402 Copyright © 1994 John Wiley and Sons. (c) Adapted from Nicola Palomero-Gallagher and Karl Zilles, 'Isocortex', in Paxinos, George ed., The Rat Nervous System, 3e, pp. 729–757, doi.org/10.1016/B978-012547638-6/50024-9. Copyright © 2004 Elsevier Inc. All rights reserved.)

of neurons in the nucleus of the solitary tract to the taste of food by approximately 30%, so that taste processing in rodents is from the first synapse in the brain confounded by reward value, by hedonics. That makes the taste (and reward) system of rodents very difficult to understand functionally for different functions are not separated (taste identity and intensity vs hedonics), and makes the taste system of rodents a poor one with which to understand primate including human taste reward processing (Rolls 2016b, Rolls 2016f, Rolls 2016c). This evidence emphasizes the importance of understanding the evidence from primates including humans, even in a system such as the taste system that one might think is evolutionarily so old (Section 8.1.1.2).

Another reason for focusing interest on the primate brain is that there has been great development of the visual system in primates (Section 8.1.2), and this itself has had important implications for the types of sensory stimuli that are processed by brain systems involved in emotion and motivation (Rolls 2014a, Rolls 2016c, Rolls 2018b), and also in memory systems (Rolls & Wirth 2018). One example is the importance of face identity and face expression decoding, which are both important in primate emotional behaviour, and indeed provide an important part of the foundation for much primate social behaviour. These are among the reasons why emphasis is placed on brain systems in primates, including humans, in the approach taken here.

The overall medically relevant aim of the research described in this book is to provide a foundation for understanding in humans the orbitofrontal cortex, and its involvement in many processes including emotion, motivation, and decision-making, and thus their disorders, including depression, anxiety, addiction, sociopathy, borderline personality disorder, schizophrenia, eating disorders, and decision-making disorders including pathological gambling.

1.3 Functional neuroimaging in humans, neuronal encoding, and understanding the brain computationally

When considering brain mechanisms involved in emotion and decision-making, findings with human brain imaging are described. These approaches include functional magnetic resonance imaging (fMRI) to measure changes in brain oxygenation level locally (using a signal from deoxyhaemoglobin) to provide an index of local brain activity, as well as positron emission tomography (PET) studies to estimate local regional cerebral blood flow, again to provide an index of local brain activity. It is, however, important to note that these functional neuroimaging approaches provide rather coarse approaches to brain function, in that the spatial resolution is seldom better than 3 mm, so that the picture given is one of 'blobs on the brain', which give some indication of what is happening where in the brain, and what types of dissociation of functions are possible.

However, because there are millions of neurons in each of the areas that are typically resolved with functional neuroimaging, such imaging techniques give rather little evidence on how the brain works. For this, one needs to know what information is represented in each brain area at the level at which information is exchanged between the computing elements of the brain, the neurons (brain cells) (Rolls 2016c). One also needs to know how the representation of information (for example about stimuli or events in the world) changes from stage to stage of the processing in the brain, to understand how the brain works as a system. It turns out that one can 'read' or decode this information from the brain by recording the activity of single neurons, or groups of single neurons (Rolls & Treves 2011, Rolls 2016c). The reason that this is an effective procedure for understanding what is represented is that each neuron has one information output channel, the firing of its action potentials, so that one can measure the full richness of the information being represented in a region by measuring the firing of its neurons. This can reveal fundamental evidence crucial for understanding how the brain operates (Rolls 2016c). For example, neuronal recording can reveal all the information represented in an area even if parts of it are encoded by relatively small numbers, perhaps a few percent, of its neurons. (This is impossible with brain-imaging techniques, which also are susceptible to the interpretation problem that whatever causes the largest activation is interpreted as 'what' is being encoded in a region.)

Neuronal recording also provides evidence for the level at which it is appropriate to build computational models of brain function, the neuronal network level. Such neuronal network computational models consider how populations of neurons with the connections found in a given brain area, and with biologically plausible properties such as learning rules for altering the strengths of synaptic connections between neurons, actually could perform useful computation to implement the functions being performed by that brain area (Rolls 2016c). This approach should not really be considered as a metaphor for brain operation, but as a theory of how each part of the brain operates. The neuronal network computational theory, and any model or simulation based on it, may of course be simplified to some extent to make it tractable, but nevertheless the point is that the neuron-level approach, coupled with neuronal network models that analyse the functions of populations of neurons, together provide some of the fundamental elements for understanding how the brain actually works (Rolls 2016c). For this reason, emphasis is also placed in this book on what is known about what is being processed in each brain area as shown by recordings from neurons. Such evidence, in terms of building theories and models of how the brain functions, can never be replaced by brain imaging evidence, although these approaches do complement each other very effectively.

The approach to brain function in terms of computations performed by neuronal networks in different brain areas is the subject of the books *Neural Networks and Brain Function* by Rolls & Treves (1998), *Computational Neuroscience of Vision* by Rolls & Deco (2002), *Memory, Attention, and Decision-Making: A Unifying Computational Neuroscience Approach* by Rolls (2016c), *The Noisy Brain: Stochastic Dynamics as a Principle of Brain Function* by Rolls & Deco (2010), and *Cerebral Cortex: Principles of Operation* by Rolls (2016c). The reader is referred to these books for more comprehensive accounts of this biologically plausible approach to brain function. It can be described as a mechanistic approach to understanding brain function, in that the underlying computational processes that underlie behaviour and thought must be explicitly understood (and are the 'proximate' causes of behaviour), and must be placed in the context of the evolutionary adaptive value of those mechanisms, the 'ultimate' causes of the behaviour (Rolls 2014a, Rolls 2016c). In this book, some of the neurophysiological evidence and its computational implications for understanding how our brains work to produce emotion and motivation, and the nature of their adaptive value, are described.

1.4 The orbitofrontal cortex: the plan of the book

After this introductory Chapter (1), the anatomy and connections of the orbitofrontal cortex are described (Chapter 2). In Chapter 3, evidence on the neurophysiology and functional neuroimaging of the orbitofrontal cortex is described, leading to a foundation for understanding the functions of the orbitofrontal cortex. This understanding is enhanced by providing evidence on the information processing in the preceding and succeeding stages to the orbitofrontal cortex, both in Chapter 3, and in key output regions of the orbitofrontal cortex, the cingulate cortex and basal ganglia including the dopamine systems (Chapter 5). Chapter 4 considers the effects of damage to the orbitofrontal cortex, which provides important evidence on the causal roles of the orbitofrontal cortex in brain processing and behaviour, and conscious emotional feelings. Chapter 5 provides evidence on the processing in a key output region of the orbitofrontal cortex, the anterior cingulate cortex, and helps to show that value and not actions are represented in the orbitofrontal cortex; and that actions are learned to maximize the reward outcome or value in the anterior cingulate cortex. In Chapter 6 I consider how the orbitofrontal is fundamental to understanding emotion in humans and other primates, and overshadows the amygdala as a result of the great development in evolution of the orbitofrontal cortex in humans. A very interesting point here is that evidence is emerging that although the amygdala may be involved in some emotional responses, it may not be primarily involved in emotional feelings (LeDoux & Pine 2016, LeDoux, Brown, Pine & Hofmann 2018). In contrast, evidence is described in Chapter 4 that the orbitofrontal cortex is involved in conscious, subjective, emotional feelings. This highlights the important point that there are multiple output routes for the brain systems being considered (Section 6.4), and these routes have different connectivity and are involved in different functions, some of which can take place without conscious processing.

Chapter 7 develops a theory of how the orbitofrontal cortex is important in understanding depression, because of the importance of the orbitofrontal cortex in processing rewards, punishers, and in particular non-rewards (obtaining less reward than expected, which might lead to sadness). Chapter 7 also describes evidence about how the orbitofrontal cortex is involved in other mental disorders, including bipolar disorder, autism, and attention deficit hyperactivity disorder (ADHD).

Chapter 8 considers evidence on the rodent orbitofrontal cortex, which has its own Chapter, because of the great differences between the rodent and primate including human orbitofrontal cortex due to the great development of the primate including human orbitofrontal cortex (Fig. 1.3).

Chapter 9 provides insight into formal computational analyses of how the neural networks in the orbitofrontal cortex perform their functions.

Chapter 10 provides a synthesis on the orbitofrontal cortex, and a discussion of some areas for further research.

2 Orbitofrontal cortex: anatomy and connections

2.1 Connections

The topology of the orbitofrontal cortex is described in Section 1.1.2. Some of the connections of the orbitofrontal cortex (Price 2006, Ongur & Price 2000) are shown schematically in Figs. 1.1, 2.1, 2.2, and 2.4, and are described in this Chapter. The three tiers of processing shown in the schematic Fig. 2.2 are described in Section 3.1 on page 17.

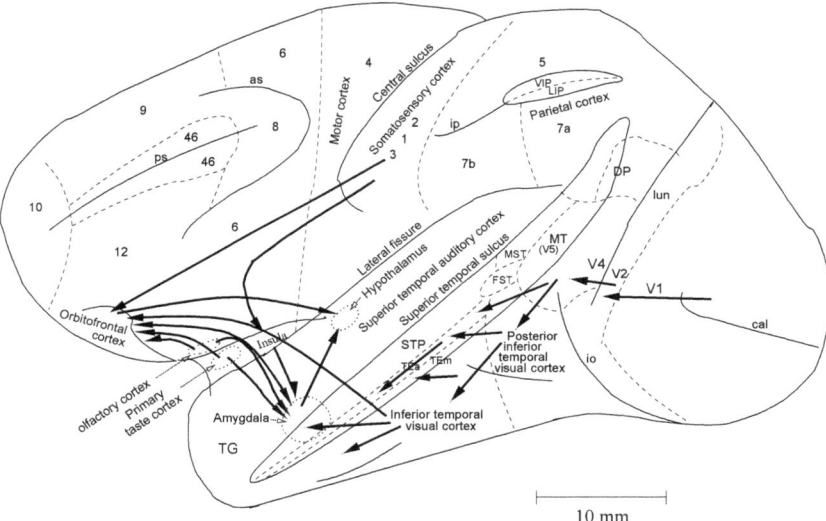

Fig. 2.1 Some of the connections of the primate orbitofrontal cortex shown on this lateral view of the brain of the macaque monkey. Connections from the primary taste and olfactory cortices to the orbitofrontal cortex and amygdala are shown. Connections are also shown in the 'ventral visual system' from V1 to V2, V4, the inferior temporal visual cortex, etc., with some connections reaching the amygdala and orbitofrontal cortex. In addition, connections from the somatosensory cortical areas 1, 2, and 3 that reach the orbitofrontal cortex directly and via the insular cortex, and that reach the amygdala via the insular cortex, are shown. as, arcuate sulcus; cal, calcarine sulcus; cs, central sulcus; lf, lateral (or Sylvian) fissure; lun, lunate sulcus; ps, principal sulcus; io, inferior occipital sulcus; ip, intraparietal sulcus (which has been opened to reveal some of the areas it contains); sts, superior temporal sulcus (which has been opened to reveal some of the areas it contains). AIT, anterior inferior temporal cortex; FST, visual motion processing area; LIP, lateral intraparietal area; MST, visual motion processing area; MT, visual motion processing area (also called V5); PIT, posterior inferior temporal cortex; STP, superior temporal plane; TA, architectonic area including auditory association cortex; TE, architectonic area including high order visual association cortex, and some of its subareas TEa and TEm; TG, architectonic area in the temporal pole; V1–V4, visual areas V1–V4; VIP, ventral intraparietal area; TEO, architectonic area including posterior visual association cortex. The numerals refer to architectonic areas, and have the following approximate functional equivalence: 1,2,3, somatosensory cortex (posterior to the central sulcus); 4, motor cortex; 5, superior parietal lobule; 7a, inferior parietal lobule, visual part; 7b, inferior parietal lobule, somatosensory part; 6, lateral premotor cortex; 8, frontal eye field; 12, part of orbitofrontal cortex; 46, dorsolateral prefrontal cortex.

Rolls, Yaxley & Sienkiewicz (1990) discovered a taste area in the primate orbitofrontal cortex by showing that neurons in it respond to taste placed into the mouth, and showed that this was the secondary taste cortex in that it receives a major projection from the primary taste

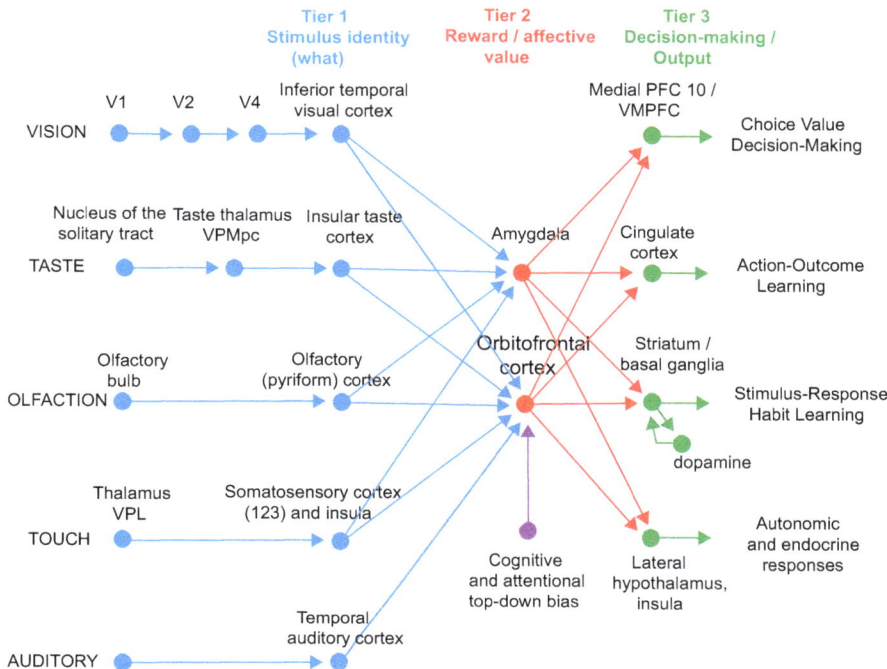

Fig. 2.2 Schematic diagram showing some of the connections of the taste, olfactory, somatosensory, visual and auditory pathways to the orbitofrontal cortex and amygdala in primates. V1, primary visual (striate) cortex; V2 and V4, further cortical visual areas. PFC, prefrontal cortex. The Medial PFC area 10 is part of the ventromedial prefrontal cortex (VMPFC). VPL, ventro-postero-lateral nucleus of the thalamus, which conveys somatosensory information to the primary somatosensory cortex (areas 1, 2 and 3). VPMpc, ventro-postero-medial nucleus pars parvocellularis of the thalamus, which conveys taste information to the primary taste cortex. Pregen Cing, pregenual cingulate cortex. For purposes of description, the stages can be described as Tier 1, representing what object is present independently of reward value; Tier 2 in which reward value is represented; and Tier 3 in which decisions between stimuli of different value are taken, and in which value is interfaced to behavioural output systems. A pathway for top-down attentional and cognitive modulation of emotion is shown in purple. Auditory inputs also reach the amygdala.

cortex as shown by retrograde anatomical tracing (Baylis, Rolls & Baylis 1994) (Fig. 2.3).

More medially, there is an olfactory area (Rolls & Baylis 1994). Anatomically, there are direct connections from the primary olfactory cortex, pyriform cortex, to area 13a of the posterior orbitofrontal cortex, which in turn has onward projections to a middle part of the orbitofrontal cortex (area 11) (Price, Carmichael, Carnes, Clugnet & Kuroda 1991, Morecraft, Geula & Mesulam 1992, Barbas 1993, Carmichael, Clugnet & Price 1994) (see Figs. 2.4 and 1.1).

Visceral inputs may reach the posteromedial and lateral areas of the orbitofrontal cortex from the ventral part of the parvicellular division of the ventroposteromedial nucleus of the thalamus (VPMpc) (Carmichael & Price 1995b). Visceral inputs may also reach the orbitofrontal cortex from the antero-ventral insula (just below the primary taste cortex) (Baylis, Rolls & Baylis 1994), from which neurons project to the orbitofrontal cortex (Fig. 2.3), and which is probably an area of visceral cortex (Rolls 2016b, Critchley & Harrison 2013, Hassanpour, Simmons, Feinstein, Luo, Lapidus, Bodurka, Paulus & Khalsa 2018). (In humans, there is also a mid-insular region that has activity related to visceral effects (Hassanpour et al. 2018).)

Visual inputs reach the orbitofrontal cortex directly from the inferior temporal visual cortex, the cortex in the superior temporal sulcus, and the temporal pole, especially from areas TEav and the fundus and ventral bank of the superior temporal sulcus (Jones & Powell 1970, Barbas 1988, Barbas 1993, Barbas 1995, Petrides & Pandya 1988, Barbas & Pandya 1989, Seltzer & Pandya 1978, Seltzer & Pandya 1989, Morecraft et al. 1992, Carmichael &

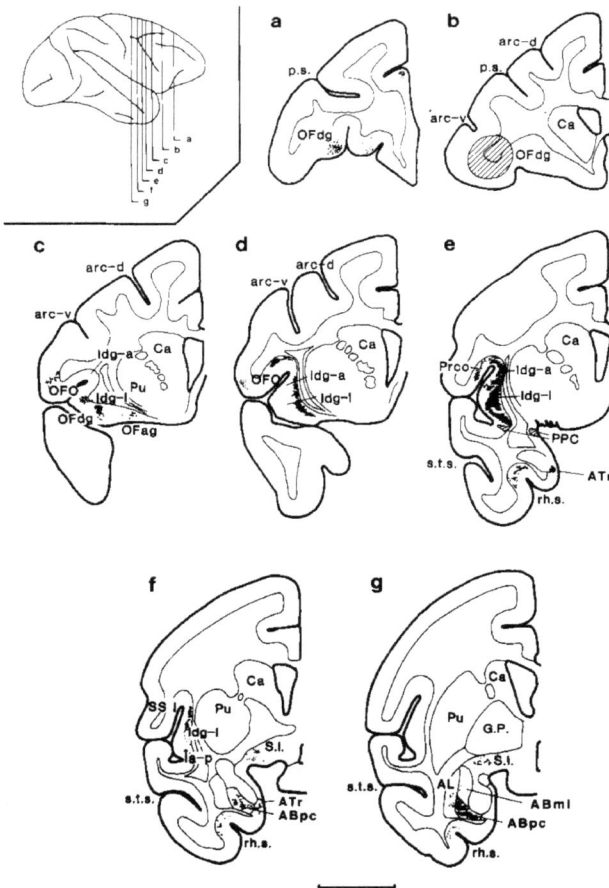

Fig. 2.3 Projections from the primary taste cortex in the upper part of the dysgranular insula and frontal operculum to the orbitofrontal cortex. The horseradish peroxidase injection site into the lateral orbitofrontal cortex where taste neurons were recorded is shown shaded in (b). Filled neurons are shown in e.g.(e) as black circles in the primary taste cortex in the upper part of areas Idg-a (Insula dysgranular area, anterior part: the insular primary taste cortex) and the area labelled Prco in (e) the frontal opercular taste cortex. The visceral region of the anterior insula may be the cells in the lower half of the anterior insula (Idg-l) which is also shown here to project to the orbitofrontal cortex. Abbreviations: AB: basal nucleus of the amygdala with mc magnocellular and pc parvocellular parts; AL: lateral nucleus of the amygdala; arc-d: dorsal limb of the arcuate sulcus; arc-v: ventral limb of the arcuate sulcus; Ca: caudate nucleus; GP: globus pallidus; Idg-l: liminal part of the dysgranular field of the insula; OF: orbitofrontal cortex (with ag agranular and dg dysgranular fields); OFO: orbitofrontal opercular area; PPC: prepyriform cortex (olfactory); Prco: precentral operculum; ps: principal sulcus; Pu: putamen; rh s: rhinal sulcus; SI: substantia innominata; SS 1: primary somaesthetic cortex; sts: superior temporal sulcus. (Reprinted from *Neuroscience*, 64 (3), L. L. Baylis, E. T. Rolls, and G. C. Baylis, Afferent connections of the caudolateral orbitofrontal cortex taste area of the primate, pp. 801–12, Copyright, 1995, with permission from Elsevier.)

Price 1995b, Saleem, Kondo & Price 2008).

There are corresponding auditory inputs, which reach the lateral orbitofrontal cortex area 12 and the adjacent inferior temporal gyrus areas BA45 and BA44 from temporal cortical auditory areas (Barbas 1988, Barbas 1993, Plakke & Romanski 2014). Somatosensory inputs reach the orbitofrontal cortex from somatosensory cortical areas 1, 2 and SII in the frontal and pericentral operculum, and from the dysgranular insula area (Id) (Barbas 1988, Preuss & Goldman-Rakic 1989, Carmichael & Price 1995b, Saleem et al. 2008).

The lateral orbitofrontal cortex area 12 receives inputs from other parts of the orbitofrontal cortex, from temporal lobe visual cortical areas, and from a dorsal part of the anterior cingulate cortex (Saleem, Miller & Price 2014b). (As will be shown in Chapter 3, the lateral orbitofrontal

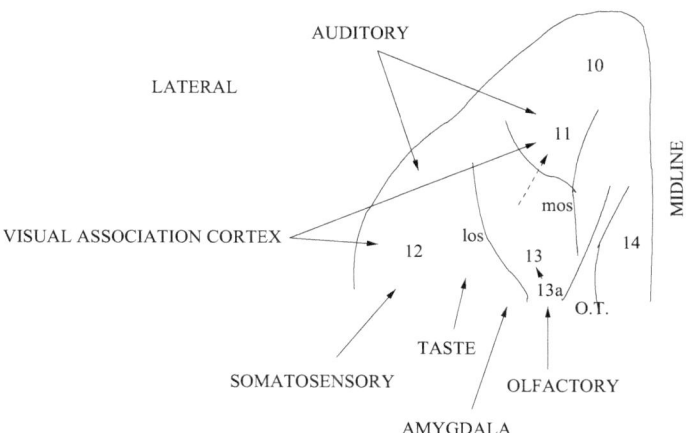

Fig. 2.4 Ventral view of the macaque orbitofrontal cortex. The midline is on the right of the diagram, and the inferior convexity is laterally, on the left. Subdivisions, and some afferents to the orbitofrontal cortex, are shown. mos, medial orbital sulcus; los, lateral orbital sulcus. (Adapted from H. Barbas and D. N. Pandya, Architecture and intrinsic connections of the prefrontal cortex in the rhesus monkey, Journal of Comparative Neurology, 286 (3), pp. 353–375, Copyright © 1989, Alan R. Liss, Inc.)

cortex area 12 and the dorsal anterior cingulate cortex are both involved in punishment and non-reward.) Area 12 is included terminologically in what is described as ventrolateral prefrontal cortex (VLPFC). The VLPFC also includes areas BA45 and BA44 of the inferior frontal gyrus, which receive major auditory inputs (Saleem et al. 2014b) (and which in humans on the left are Broca's area (Amunts & Zilles 2012)).

The caudal orbitofrontal cortex (area 13) has strong reciprocal connections with the amygdala (Price et al. 1991, Carmichael & Price 1995a, Barbas 2007, Garcia-Cabezas & Barbas 2017) and with the pregenual anterior cingulate cortex area 32 (Garcia-Cabezas & Barbas 2017). (As will be shown in Chapter 3, the caudal orbitofrontal cortex and the pregenual cingulate cortex are both involved in reward.)

The orbitofrontal cortex also receives inputs via the mediodorsal nucleus of the thalamus, pars magnocellularis, which itself receives afferents from temporal lobe structures such as the prepyriform (olfactory) cortex, amygdala, and inferior temporal cortex (Nauta 1972, Krettek & Price 1974, Krettek & Price 1977).

This orbital network just described is somewhat separate from a 'medial prefrontal network' that includes cingulate cortex areas 24, 32 and 24 and medial prefrontal cortex areas 10 and 14 (Saleem et al. 2008, Carmichael & Price 1995a, Carmichael & Price 1996) (see Section 5.1). This medial prefrontal system is connected with the rostral superior temporal gyrus (STGr) and the dorsal bank of the superior temporal sulcus (STSd), and with the entorhinal, parahippocampal, and cingulate/retrosplenial cortex (Saleem et al. 2008, Insausti, Amaral & Cowan 1987). In more detail, in macaques a 'medial prefrontal network' (mainly anterior cingulate cortex) selectively involved medial areas 14r, 14c, 24, 25, 32, and 10m, rostral orbital areas 10o and 11m, and agranular insular area Iai in the posterior orbital cortex in macaques (Carmichael & Price 1996). An 'orbital prefrontal network' (mainly the orbitofrontal cortex) linked most of the areas within the orbital cortex, including areas Iam, Iapm, Ial, 12l,12m, and 12r in the caudal and lateral parts of the orbital cortex, with areas 13l, 13m, and 13b in the central orbital cortex, with further onward connections to the rostral orbital area 11l (Carmichael & Price 1996). Two orbital areas, 13a and 12o, had connections to both the medial and orbital networks. Many of these areas are shown in Figs. 1.2, 1.3 and 5.1.

The orbitofrontal cortex projects back to temporal lobe areas such as the inferior temporal visual cortex (Saleem et al. 2008), to the amygdala (Barbas 2007) and to the anterior cingulate cortex (Carmichael & Price 1995a, Morecraft & Tanji 2009, Vogt 2009).

The orbitofrontal cortex also projects to the preoptic region, lateral hypothalamus and brainstem autonomic areas such as the dorsal motor nucleus of the vagus and the nucleus of the solitary tract, to the ventral tegmental area (Van der Kooy, Koda, McGinty, Gerfen & Bloom 1984, Rempel-Clower & Barbas 1998, Price 2006), and to the head of the caudate nucleus (Kemp & Powell 1970).

Further details on the cytoarchitecture and connections of the orbitofrontal cortex including routes via the entorhinal and perirhinal cortex for reward information to reach the hippocampal memory system are available (Petrides & Pandya 1994, Pandya 1996, Carmichael & Price 1994, Carmichael & Price 1995a, Carmichael & Price 1995b, Barbas 1995, Ongur & Price 2000, Ongur et al. 2003, Price 2006, Barbas 2007, Saleem et al. 2008, Mackey & Petrides 2010, Barbas, Zikopoulos & Timbie 2011, Petrides, Tomaiuolo, Yeterian & Pandya 2012, Yeterian, Pandya, Tomaiuolo & Petrides 2012, Saleem et al. 2014b, Henssen et al. 2016, Rolls 2019d).

2.2 Output pathways from the orbitofrontal cortex to the dopamine and serotonin brainstem systems

In this section, some of the output pathways of the orbitofrontal cortex (and amygdala) reward processing systems to the subcortical systems that utilize dopamine and serotonin (5-hydroxytryptamine) as neurotransmitters are considered. The operation of the dopamine systems is considered further in Section 5.2.

A somewhat unaddressed issue is how the dopamine neurons in the brainstem, implicated in positive reward prediction error signalling to brain regions such as the striatum (Schultz 2013, Schultz 2016a) (Section 5.2), and in addiction (Koob & Volkow 2016), receive their information about rewards. In this context, it has now been suggested that reward and non-reward areas of the brain such as the orbitofrontal cortex and amygdala do provide a source of relevant inputs to the dopamine neurons (Rolls 2017a). Pathways that provide a route for reward and emotion-related information to reach the dopamine neurons in the midbrain are shown in Fig. 2.5. These connections are shown in the context of some of the pathways involved in reward-related processes and emotion shown on the lateral view of the brain of the macaque monkey in the upper part of Fig. 2.5 (Rolls 2017a). Connections from the primary taste and olfactory cortices to the orbitofrontal cortex and amygdala are shown. Connections are also shown in the 'ventral visual system' from the visual cortical areas V1 to V2, V4, the inferior temporal visual cortex, etc., with some connections reaching the amygdala and orbitofrontal cortex. In addition, connections from the somatosensory cortical areas BA 1, 2, and 3 that reach the orbitofrontal cortex directly and via the insular cortex, and that reach the amygdala via the insular cortex, are shown.

The orbitofrontal cortex, amygdala (and probably anterior cingulate cortex and subgenual cingulate cortex) systems involved in reward and non-reward can operate via a basal ganglia route (striatum, ventral pallidum, and globus pallidus / bed nucleus of the stria terminalis) to influence the Lateral Habenula, lateral part, which in turn via the GABAergic Rostromedial Tegmental nucleus can influence dopamine neurons in the Substantia Nigra pars compacta and ventral Tegmental Area (SNc and VTA). This provides a route for reward, non-reward, and reward prediction error signals of largely cortical origin to influence the dopamine neurons. Details of some of these anatomical connections are provided elsewhere (Haber 2014, Proulx, Hikosaka & Malinow 2014, Loonen & Ivanova 2016). In particular, as shown in Section 3.1, reward outcome value, reward expectation value, and neurons that respond when less reward

Output pathways from the orbitofrontal cortex to the dopamine and serotonin brainstem systems | 15

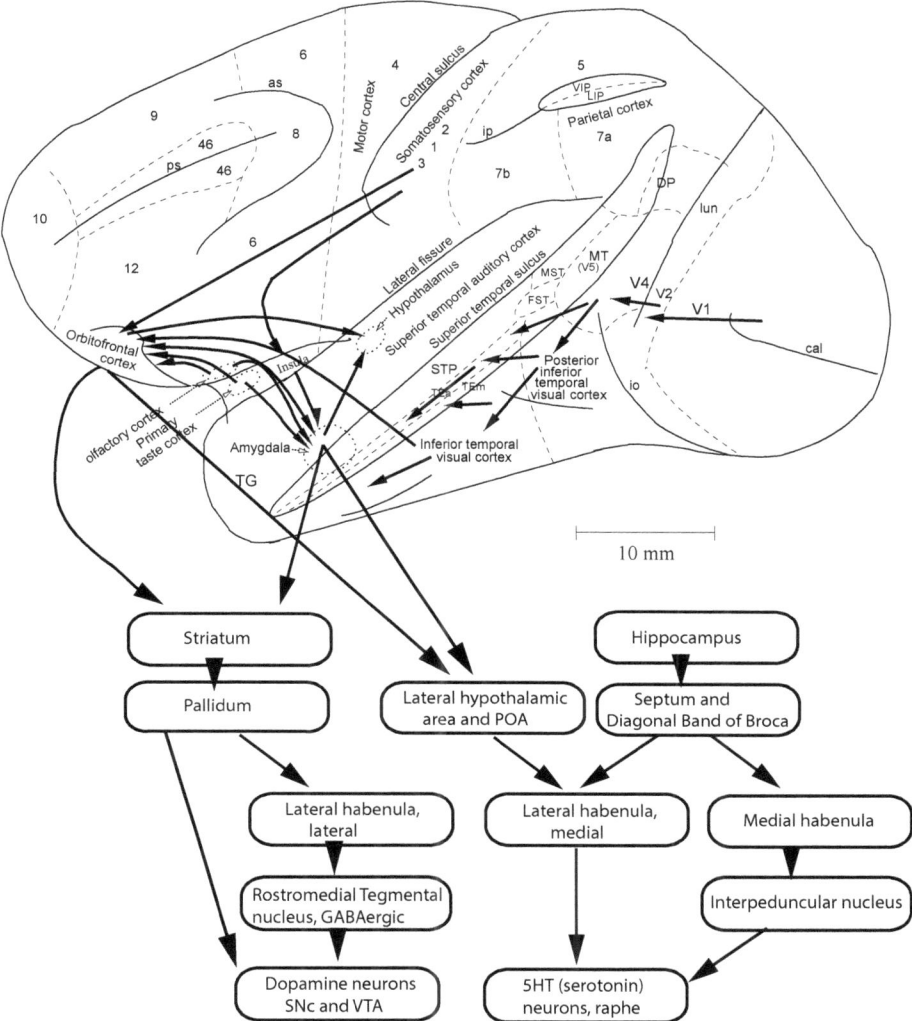

Fig. 2.5 Possible routes for reward and non-reward related information from the orbitofrontal cortex and amygdala to reach the brainstem dopamine and serotonin (5-HT) neurons (see text). One route is via the ventral striatum and ventral pallidum. A second route is via the ventral striatum, ventral pallidum, lateral habenula, and rostromedial tegmental nucleus. as, arcuate sulcus; cal, calcarine sulcus; cs, central sulcus; lf, lateral (or Sylvian) fissure; lun, lunate sulcus; ps, principal sulcus; io, inferior occipital sulcus; ip, intraparietal sulcus (which has been opened to reveal some of the areas it contains); sts, superior temporal sulcus (which has been opened to reveal some of the areas it contains). AIT, anterior inferior temporal cortex; FST, visual motion processing area; LIP, lateral intraparietal area; MST, visual motion processing area; MT, visual motion processing area (also called V5); PIT, posterior inferior temporal cortex; POA, preoptic area; SNc, substantia nigra pars compacta; STP, superior temporal plane; TA, architectonic area including auditory association cortex; TE, architectonic area including high order visual association cortex, and some of its subareas TEa and TEm; TG, architectonic area in the temporal pole; V1–V4, visual areas V1–V4; VIP, ventral intraparietal area; TEO, architectonic area including posterior visual association cortex; VTA, ventral tegmental area. The numerals refer to architectonic areas, and have the following approximate functional equivalence: 1,2,3, somatosensory cortex (posterior to the central sulcus); 4, motor cortex; 5, superior parietal lobule; 7a, inferior parietal lobule, visual part; 7b, inferior parietal lobule, somatosensory part; 6, lateral premotor cortex; 8, frontal eye field; 12, part of orbitofrontal cortex; 46, dorsolateral prefrontal cortex. (Modified from Rolls 2017a.)

than expected is obtained (negative reward prediction error neurons) are all present in the orbitofrontal cortex, and can provide much evidence about rewards to subcortical structures. Positive reward prediction error neurons have not been described in the primate orbitofrontal cortex, but signals of this type are in the ventral striatum (at least as shown by fMRI in humans (Hare, O'Doherty, Camerer, Schultz & Rangel 2008) but see Section 10.2), and may be computed in the striatum from the inputs received from the orbitofrontal cortex. Indeed, in an fMRI investigation it was found that goal values are correlated with activity in the medial orbitofrontal cortex, and positive reward prediction errors are correlated with activity in the ventral striatum (Hare et al. 2008). In addition to the habenula route, there are also connections from the ventral striatum to the region of the dopamine neurons in the substantia nigra pars compacta (Haber 2014) (see Fig. 2.5).

Consistent with these points (Rolls 2017a), in the lateral habenula, neurons that respond to signaled low reward value or to punishment have been described (Matsumoto & Hikosaka 2009b), and so have neurons that reflect negative reward prediction error (Bromberg-Martin & Hikosaka 2011). Similar neurons are found in the globus pallidus glutamatergic excitatory habenula-projecting neurons, providing evidence that the necessary computations are not performed in the lateral habenula (Stephenson-Jones, Yu, Ahrens, Tucciarone, van Huijstee, Mejia, Penzo, Tai, Wilbrecht & Li 2016).

Serotonin neurons, whose cell bodies are in the raphe nucleus in the brainstem, also have widespread projections throughout the brain, and serotonin is implicated in the effects of some antidepressants (Rolls 2018b). The origin of the relevant inputs to the serotonin neurons is also a somewhat unaddressed question: how do the serotonin neurons in the raphe nucleus in the midbrain receive inputs might influence depression in the first place. In this context, it has now been suggested that reward and non-reward areas of the brain such as the orbitofrontal cortex and amygdala do provide a source of relevant inputs to the 5-HT neurons, via brain regions such as the habenula and ventral striatum (Rolls 2017a) (Fig. 2.5). The suggestion is that the orbitofrontal cortex and amygdala systems involved in reward and non-reward can operate via a lateral hypothalamic area / lateral preoptic area (POA) to influence the Lateral Habenula, medial part, which in turn can influence the 5-HT (serotonin) neurons in the raphe nuclei. Many antidepressant drugs may influence this cortical to brainstem pathway by influencing the effects of the 5-HT neurons, which terminate in many brain areas. The hippocampal influence via the septal nuclei and diagonal band of Broca may enable reward context to access the same Lateral Habenula, medial part, to 5-HT-neuron system (de Araujo, Ferreira, Tellez, Ren & Yeckel 2012, Rolls 2015a). The medial habenula also receives septal inputs, and projects to the interpeduncular nucleus, and thereby to 5-HT neurons (and probably dopamine neurons) (Fig. 2.5) (Proulx et al. 2014, Loonen & Ivanova 2016).

3 Orbitofrontal cortex processing: neurophysiology and neuroimaging

In this Chapter, evidence on the functions of the orbitofrontal cortex from neurophysiology and functional neuroimaging is considered, starting with a framework.

3.1 An overall framework for the role of the orbitofrontal cortex in the processing of reward in the brain

The hypothesis that the orbitofrontal cortex is involved in representing reward value and rapidly updating these representations (Rolls 1975, Rolls 1999a, Rolls 2000a, Rolls 2005, Rolls 2014a, Rolls 2017c, Rolls 2018b) has been investigated by making recordings from single neurons in the orbitofrontal cortex while monkeys performed tasks known to be impaired by damage to the orbitofrontal cortex. It has been shown that some neurons respond to primary reinforcers such as taste and touch, and represent **outcome value**; that others respond to learned secondary reinforcers, such as the sight of a rewarded visual stimulus, and thus encode **expected value**; and that the rapid learning of associations between previously neutral visual stimuli and primary reinforcers to encode expected value is reflected in the responses of orbitofrontal cortex neurons in primates (Rolls 2000a, Rolls 2004b, Rolls 2006a, Rolls & Grabenhorst 2008, Rolls 2014a, Rolls 2017c, Rolls 2018b). These types of neuron, and extensions of these concepts using functional neuroimaging in humans, are described in this Chapter.

The plan of the Chapter is that for each topic, for example taste processing, neuronal activity in macaques and human functional neuroimaging are considered together, so that knowledge of the neuronal responses can complement what fMRI studies in humans show, which necessarily involve the averaged activity of many tens of thousands of neurons so that much information is lost, because each neuron conveys somewhat different information (Rolls & Treves 2011, Rolls 2016c). In addition, for each topic, activity in the orbitofrontal cortex is compared with that in preceding and succeeding stages of processing, for that provides a rigorous approach to what operation or computation is performed by each brain area, as described in the Preface and by Rolls (2016c).

An overall framework for helping to understand the functions of the orbitofrontal cortex is shown in Fig. 2.2 on page 11, which shows three tiers of processing, with the orbitofrontal cortex in Tier 2.

1. In Tier 1 (Fig. 2.2), information is processed to a level at which the neurons represent 'what' the stimulus is, independently of the reward or punishment and hence emotional value of the stimulus.

   For example, neurons in the primary taste cortex represent what the taste is, and its intensity; but not its reward value (including how pleasant or unpleasant the taste is).

   In the inferior temporal visual cortex, the representation is of objects and faces, invariantly with respect to the exact position on the retina, size, and even view. Forming invariant representations involves a great deal of cortical computation in the hierarchy

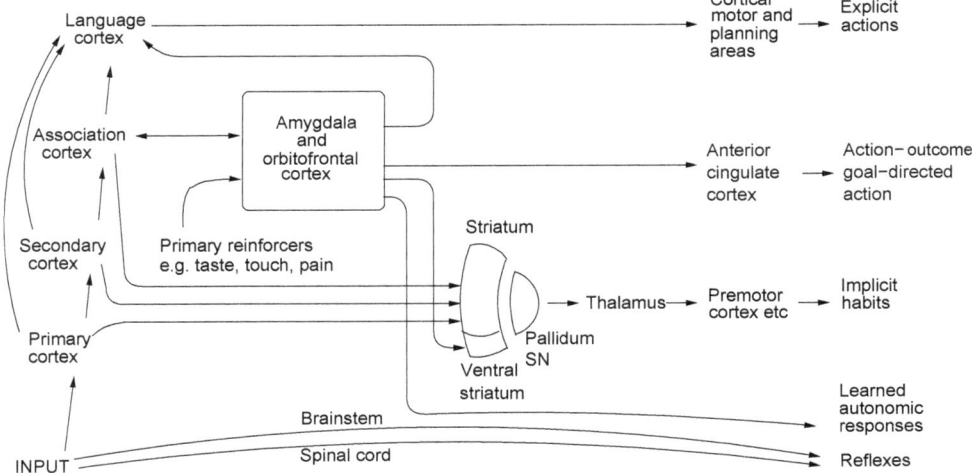

Fig. 3.1 Multiple routes to the initiation of actions and responses to rewarding and punishing stimuli. The inputs from different sensory systems to brain structures such as the orbitofrontal cortex and amygdala allow these brain structures to evaluate the reward- or punishment-related value of incoming stimuli, or of remembered stimuli. One type of route is via the language systems of the brain, which allow explicit (verbalizable) decisions involving multistep syntactic planning to be implemented. The other type of route may be implicit, and includes the anterior cingulate cortex for action–outcome, goal-dependent, learning; and the striatum and rest of the basal ganglia for stimulus–response habits. Pallidum / SN – the globus pallidus and substantia nigra. Outputs for autonomic responses can also be produced using outputs from the orbitofrontal cortex and anterior cingulate cortex (some of which are routed via the ventral, visceral, part of the anterior insular cortex) and amygdala.

of visual cortical areas from the primary visual cortex V1 to the inferior temporal visual cortex (Rolls 2016c, Rolls 2012d). The fundamental advantage of this separation of 'what' processing in Tier 1 from reward value processing in Tier 2 is that any learning in Tier 2 of the value of an object or face seen in one location on the retina, size, and view will generalize to other views etc, because the representation provided by Tier 1 is invariant.

Evidence that there is no such clear separation of 'what' from 'value' representations in rodents, for example in the taste system, is described in Sections 1.2 and 8.1.1.2, and this property makes the processing in rodents not only different from that in primates including humans, but also much more difficult to analyse.

2. There are brain mechanisms in Tier 2 that are involved in computing the reward value of primary (unlearned) reinforcers. Because reward value is represented in Tier 2, the orbitofrontal cortex becomes involved in emotional processing (Chapter 6).

   The primary (unlearned) reinforcers include taste, touch (both pleasant touch and pain), and to some extent smell, and perhaps certain visual stimuli, such as face expression.

   There is a representation of the (reward/punishment) value of very many primary reinforcers in the orbitofrontal cortex, including taste, positive touch and pain, face expression, face beauty, and auditory consonance/dissonance.

3. Brain regions in Tier 2 are also concerned with learning associations between previously neutral stimuli (such as the sight of objects or of individuals' faces), and primary reinforcers. The representations thus include the 'expected value' of stimuli. An example might be the expected value produced when we see our favourite food being prepared, which may soon lead to the primary reward of the taste of the food.

   These expected value signals in Tier 2 are sent to Tier 3 where they provide the goals for action systems.

   Because reward-related signals are being represented by these expected value neurons, Tier 2 is further involved in emotions.

These Tier 2 brain regions include the orbitofrontal cortex and amygdala.

4. In the orbitofrontal cortex in Tier 2, the representation is of the value of stimuli, and actions are not represented.

   The value of very many different types of stimuli, events or goals are represented separately at the neuronal level, providing the basis for choice between stimuli, and the selection at later stages of processing of appropriate actions to obtain the chosen goal.

5. Rewards and subjective pleasure tend to be reflected in neural activity in the medial (towards the midline) and middle orbitofrontal cortex, areas 13 and 11 (which are shown in Fig. 1.3), as shown in Fig. 3.54.

   Not obtaining rewards, punishers, and subjective unpleasantness tend to be reflected in neural activity in the lateral orbitofrontal cortex, areas 12/47 and the adjacent part of the inferior frontal gyrus (which are shown in Fig. 1.3), as shown in Fig. 3.54. It is the lateral orbitofrontal cortex that therefore may be related directly to depression, which can be produced by no longer receiving expected or hoped-for rewards.

6. Whereas the orbitofrontal cortex in Tier 2 represents the value of stimuli (potential goals for action) on a continuous scale, an area anterior to this, medial prefrontal cortex area 10 (sometimes called ventromedial prefrontal cortex, VMPFC) (in Tier 3), is implicated in decision-making between stimuli, in which a selection must be made, moving beyond representation of value on a continuous scale towards a decision between goods based on their value.

7. The brain regions in which the reinforcing, and hence emotional, value of stimuli are represented interface to four main types of output system in Tier 3 (Figs. 2.2 and 3.1):

The first is the autonomic and endocrine system, for producing such changes as increased heart rate and release of adrenaline (the Greek form is epinephrine), which prepare the body for action.

The second type of output is to brain systems concerned with performing habit-related responses. Such a brain system is the basal ganglia, which include the striatum (caudate, putamen, and ventral striatum), and then globus pallidus and substantia nigra (Section 5.3). These are for 'stimulus-response' behaviour, which can occur when a behaviour has been overlearned, and which may not be associated with much emotion when the behaviour is highly learned and automatic.

The third type of output is to brain systems concerned with performing actions in order to obtain the goals of rewards or of avoiding punishers. These brain systems include the anterior cingulate cortex for action–outcome, that is, goal-directed, learning. (The 'outcome' is the reward or punisher that is or is not obtained when the action is performed.) The learning of the correct action typically occurs by trial and error. In contrast to the orbitofrontal cortex, the cingulate cortex has representations of actions (indeed the mid-cingulate cortex is termed the cingulate motor area), and hence is in terms of its connections appropriate for learning action-outcome associations (Section 5.1).

The fourth type of output is to a system capable of planning many steps ahead, and for example deferring short-term rewards in order to execute a multiple-step long-term plan (Section 6.4). This system may use syntactic processing to perform the multiple-step planning, and is therefore part of a linguistic system. Such a system can perform explicit (conscious) processing and reasoning, as described more fully elsewhere (Rolls 2012c, Rolls 2014a, Rolls 2018b).

3.2 Taste and oral texture: outcome value

The evidence described in this section shows that within even the domain of taste and oral texture, many different primary reinforcers are represented in terms of reward or punishment value in the primate including human orbitofrontal cortex.

3.2.1 Taste pathways to the orbitofrontal cortex

We discovered a taste representation in the macaque orbitofrontal cortex (Rolls, Yaxley & Sienkiewicz 1990, Thorpe, Rolls & Maddison 1983). We proved that the orbitofrontal cortex includes a secondary taste cortical area, in a retrograde neuronal tracing study with horseradish peroxidase administered to an orbitofrontal cortex region containing taste neurons which backfilled neurons in the primary taste cortex in the insula and adjoining frontal operculum (see Fig. 2.3 and Baylis, Rolls & Baylis (1994)). (The location of the macaque primary taste cortex was shown anatomically by Pritchard, Hamilton, Morse & Norgren (1986), and neurophysiologically by Scott, Yaxley, Sienkiewicz & Rolls (1986) and Yaxley, Rolls & Sienkiewicz (1990).) More medial orbitofrontal cortex areas may also receive inputs directly from the insular and frontal opercular primary taste cortical areas, for, as illustrated in Fig. 3.18, taste neurons are also common in this more medial part of the orbitofrontal cortex (see further Rolls & Baylis (1994) and Critchley & Rolls (1996a)). The same anatomical paper (Baylis, Rolls & Baylis 1994) also showed that a more anterior part of the orbitofrontal cortex is a tertiary taste cortical area, for it receives inputs from the secondary, orbitofrontal, taste cortex, but not from the primary taste cortex. The more middle / medial part of the orbitofrontal cortex (close to the region indicated in Fig. 3.18) also has neurons that decrease their taste responses in relation to sensory-specific satiety (in a taste devaluation experiment), and a few that do not (Critchley & Rolls 1996c). The presence of taste neurons in the middle / medial part of the macaque orbitofrontal cortex, and their modulation by satiety, has been confirmed (Pritchard, Schwartz & Scott 2007). Thus the macaque posterior orbitofrontal cortex contains taste, and also olfactory and visual, neurons throughout its mediolateral extent, apart from the most medial 3–4 mm (Rolls 2008d). In contrast, the taste and olfactory reward areas in humans appear to reach to the midline (see e.g. Figs. 3.16, 3.17, 3.20 and 3.50).

3.2.2 Taste representations in the orbitofrontal cortex

One of the discoveries that has helped us to understand the functions of the orbitofrontal cortex in behaviour is that it contains a major cortical representation of taste (Rolls, Yaxley & Sienkiewicz 1990, Kadohisa, Rolls & Verhagen 2005b, Rolls 2008d, Rolls 2009b, Rolls 2014a, Rolls 2015c, Rolls 2015b, Rolls 2016f) (cf. Fig. 2.2). Given that taste can act as a primary reinforcer, that is without learning as a reward or punisher, we now have the start for a fundamental understanding of the functions of the orbitofrontal cortex in stimulus–reinforcer association learning. We now know how one class of primary reinforcer reaches and is represented in the orbitofrontal cortex in terms of its value. Moreover, it is clear that many different primary reinforcers are represented, because different neurons respond to different combinations of different tastes and different oral textures, and as we will see below, also of different odours. A representation of primary reinforcers is essential for a system that is involved in learning associations between previously neutral stimuli and primary reinforcers, e.g. between the sight of an object, and its taste.

3.2.2.1 Sweet, salt, bitter, and sour tastes

The most direct and precise evidence that taste is represented in the primate orbitofrontal cortex comes from recording the activity of single neurons in the macaque orbitofrontal cortex. It

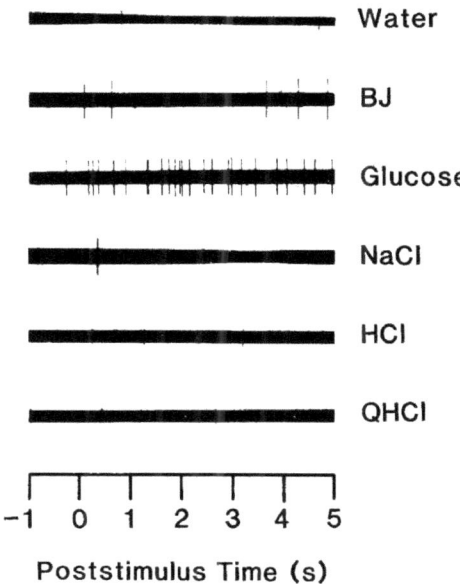

Fig. 3.2 Examples of the responses recorded from one caudolateral orbitofrontal taste cortex neuron to the six taste stimuli, water, 20% blackcurrant juice (BJ), 1 M glucose, 1 M NaCl, 0.01 M HCl, and 0.001 M quinine HCl (QHCl). The stimuli were placed in the mouth at time 0. (Reproduced from Journal of Neurophysiology, 64 (4), Gustatory responses of single neurons in the caudolateral orbitofrontal cortex of the macaque monkey, E. T. Rolls, S. Yaxley, Z. J. Sienkiewicz, © 1990, The American Physiological Society.)

has been shown that different single neurons respond differently to the prototypical tastes sweet, salt, bitter, and sour (Rolls, Yaxley & Sienkiewicz 1990), to the 'taste' of water (Rolls, Yaxley & Sienkiewicz 1990), and to the taste of protein or umami (Rolls 2001a, Rolls 2009b) as exemplified by monosodium glutamate (Baylis & Rolls 1991) and inosine monophosphate (Rolls, Critchley, Wakeman & Mason 1996c). Each neuron typically responds to more than one taste, as shown in Figs. 3.2 and 3.3, but each taste can be clearly identified by considering the activity of a population of taste cells (Rolls, Critchley, Verhagen & Kadohisa 2010a). This is called population encoding, and it has many very useful properties that are described by Rolls & Treves (2011) and Rolls (2016c). The properties include generalisation to similar stimuli, graceful degradation of function if some of the neurons or synapses are lost, and high memory capacity because it is a sparse distributed representation and because the neurons convey information that is somewhat independent (Rolls et al. 2010a, Rolls 2016c).

In addition to representations of the 'prototypical' taste stimuli sweet, salt, bitter, and sour, different neurons in this region respond to other taste and taste-related stimuli that provide information about the reward value of a potential food (Rolls 2008a, Rolls 2006b, Kadohisa, Rolls & Verhagen 2005b). One example of this additional taste information is the set of neurons that respond to umami taste, as described next.

3.2.2.2 Umami taste

An important food taste which appears to be different from that produced by sweet, salt, bitter, or sour is the taste of protein. At least part of this taste is captured by the Japanese word 'umami', which is a taste common to a diversity of food sources including fish, meats, mushrooms, cheese, some vegetables such as tomatoes, and human mothers' milk. Within these food sources, it is glutamates and 5′ nucleotides, sometimes in a synergistic combination, that

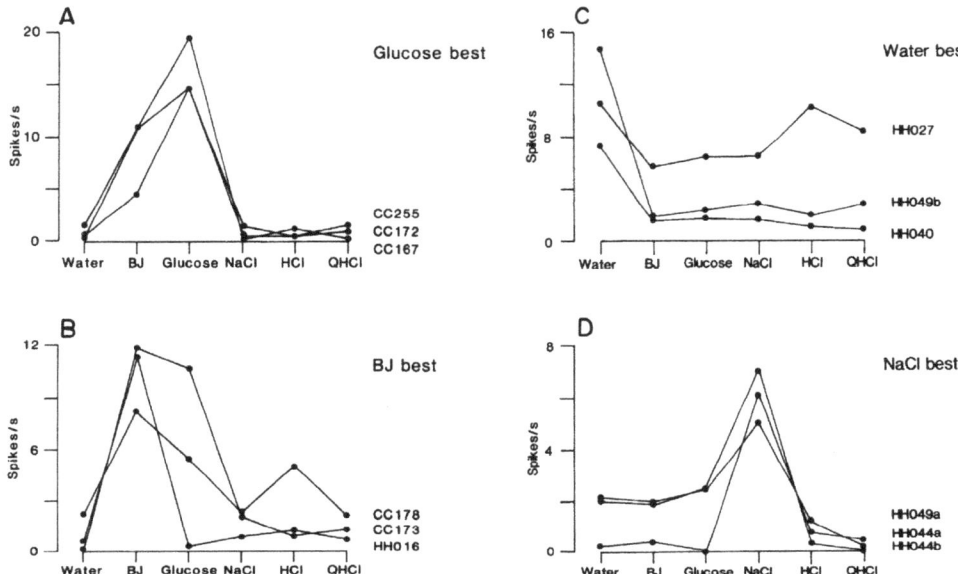

Fig. 3.3 Typical response profiles to different tastes of different orbitofrontal cortex taste neurons. Some responded best to the taste of 1 M glucose (a), to blackcurrant fruit juice (BJ) (b), to water (c), and to 0.1 M sodium chloride (NaCl) (d). HCl, 0.01 M HCl, sour; QHCl, 0.001 M quinine hydrochloride (bitter). (Reproduced from Journal of Neurophysiology, 64 (4), Gustatory responses of single neurons in the caudolateral orbitofrontal cortex of the macaque monkey, E. T. Rolls, S. Yaxley, Z. J. Sienkiewicz, © 1990, The American Physiological Society.)

create the umami taste (Kurihara 2015, Ikeda 1909, Kawamura & Kare 1992). Monosodium L-glutamate (MSG), and the 5′ nucleotides guanosine 5′-monophosphate (GMP), and inosine 5′-monophosphate (IMP), are examples of umami stimuli.

These findings raise the question of whether umami taste operates through information channels in the primate taste system which are separable from those for the 'prototypical' tastes sweet, salt, bitter, and sour. To investigate the neural encoding of glutamate in the primate, Baylis & Rolls (1991) made recordings from 190 taste-responsive neurons in the primary taste cortex and adjoining orbitofrontal cortex taste area in macaques. Single neurons were found that were tuned to respond best to monosodium glutamate (umami taste), just as other cells were found with best responses to glucose (sweet), sodium chloride (salty), HCl (sour), and quinine HCl (bitter). Across the population of neurons, the responsiveness to glutamate was poorly correlated with the responsiveness to NaCl, so that the representation of glutamate was clearly different from that of NaCl. Further, the representation of glutamate was shown to be approximately as different from each of the other four tastants as they are from each other, as shown by multidimensional scaling and cluster analysis. Moreover, it was found that glutamate is approximately as well represented in terms of mean evoked neural activity and the number of cells with best responses to it as the other four stimuli glucose, NaCl, HCl and quinine. It was concluded that in primate taste cortical areas, glutamate, which produces umami taste in humans, is approximately as well represented as are the tastes produced by: glucose (sweet), NaCl (salty), HCl (sour) and quinine HCl (bitter) (Baylis & Rolls 1991).

In a further investigation, these findings have been extended beyond the sodium salt of glutamate to other umami tastants which have the glutamate ion but which do not introduce sodium ion into the experiment; and to a nucleotide umami tastant (Rolls, Critchley, Wakeman & Mason 1996c). In recordings made mainly from neurons in the orbitofrontal cortex taste area, it was shown that single neurons that had their best responses to sodium glutamate also had good responses to glutamic acid. The correlation between the responses to these two tastants was higher than between any other pair which included in addition a prototypical set including glucose (sweet), sodium chloride (salty), HCl (sour), and quinine HCl (bitter). Moreover, the responsiveness to glutamic acid clustered with the response to monosodium glutamate in a cluster analysis with this set of stimuli, and glutamic acid was close to sodium glutamate in a space created by multidimensional scaling. It was also shown that the responses of these neurons to the nucleotide umami tastant inosine 5'-monophosphate were more correlated with their responses to monosodium glutamate than to any prototypical tastant.

Thus neurophysiological evidence in primates does indicate that there is a representation of umami flavour in the cortical areas which is separable from that to the prototypical tastants sweet, salt, bitter, and sour (see further Rolls, Critchley, Browning & Hernadi (1998a)). This representation is probably important in the taste produced by proteins (Chaudhari & Roper 2010, Haid, Widmayer, Voigt, Chaudhari, Boehm & Breer 2013). These neurons are found not only in the orbitofrontal cortex taste areas, but also in the primary taste cortex (Baylis & Rolls 1991).

There is now clear evidence that there are taste receptors on the tongue specialized for umami taste (Chaudhari, Landin & Roper 2000, Zhao, Zhang, Hoon, Chandrashekar, Erlenbach, Ryba & Zucker 2003, Lin, Ogura & Kinnamon 2003, Chandrashekar, Hoon, Ryba & Zuker 2006, Chaudhari & Roper 2010, Haid, Widmayer, Voigt, Chaudhari, Boehm & Breer 2013, Kurihara 2015, Roper & Chaudhari 2017).

3.2.2.3 Human neuroimaging of taste

There is also evidence from functional neuroimaging that taste can activate the human orbitofrontal cortex. For example, Francis, Rolls, Bowtell, McGlone, O'Doherty, Browning, Clare & Smith (1999) showed that the taste of glucose can activate the human orbitofrontal cortex, and O'Doherty, Rolls, Francis, Bowtell & McGlone (2001b) showed that the taste of glucose and salt activate nearby but separate parts of the human orbitofrontal cortex. De Araujo, Kringelbach, Rolls & Hobden (2003a) showed that umami taste (the taste of protein) as exemplified by monosodium glutamate is represented in the human orbitofrontal cortex as well as in the primary taste cortex as shown by functional magnetic resonance imaging (fMRI) (Fig. 3.4). The taste effect of monosodium glutamate (present in e.g. tomato, green vegetables, fish, and human breast milk) was enhanced in an anterior part of the orbitofrontal cortex in particular by combining it with the nucleotide inosine monophosphate (present in e.g. meat and some fish including tuna), and this provides evidence that the activations found in the orbitofrontal cortex are closely related to subjectively reported taste effects (Rolls 2009b, Rolls & Grabenhorst 2008). Small and colleagues have also described activation of the orbitofrontal cortex by taste (Small, Zald, Jones-Gotman, Zatorre, Petrides & Evans 1999, Small, Bender, Veldhuizen, Rudenga, Nachtigal & Felsted 2007).

In addition to activating the orbitofrontal cortex, the umami tastants monosodium glutamate and inosine monophosphate activate the human primary taste cortex in the insula/operculum, and the cingulate cortex (De Araujo, Kringelbach, Rolls & Hobden 2003a), as shown in Fig. 3.4. This Figure provides a useful guide to some of the different brain regions that are frequently referred to in this book. It is notable that the pregenual cingulate cortex is activated by the pleasant sweet taste of glucose, whereas the more ambivalent taste of monosodium glutamate as a pure taste (which is generally in this form only just on the pleasant side of neutral) activates the supracallosal cingulate cortex, where many unpleasant stimuli are represented.

This evidence shows that umami taste, an indicator of the presence of protein, is implemented by neurons in the primary and secondary taste cortex that are tuned to umami stimuli. Umami is a component of many foods which helps to make them taste pleasant, especially when the umami taste is paired with a consonant savoury odour (Rolls, Critchley, Browning

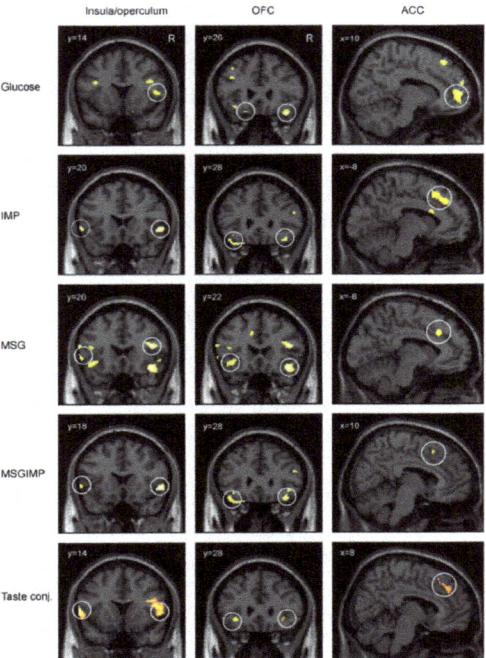

Fig. 3.4 Activation of the human primary taste cortex in the insula/frontal operculum; the orbitofrontal cortex (OFC); and the anterior cingulate cortex (ACC) by taste. The stimuli used included glucose, two umami taste stimuli (monosodium glutamate (MSG) and inosine monophosphate (IMP)), and a mixture of the two umami stimuli. Taste conj. refers to a conjunction analysis over all the taste stimuli. (Reproduced from Journal of Neurophysiology, 90 (1), Representation of umami taste in the human brain, I. E. T. De Araujo, M. L. Kringelbach, E. T. Rolls, and P. Hobden, pp. 313–319 © 2003, The American Physiological Society.)

& Hernadi 1998a, McCabe & Rolls 2007, Rolls 2009b).

3.2.3 Taste value is represented in the orbitofrontal cortex

The nature of the representation of taste in the orbitofrontal cortex is that the reward value of the taste is represented. The evidence for this from devaluation experiments is that the responses of orbitofrontal cortex taste neurons are modulated by hunger in just the same way as is the reward value or palatability of a taste. In particular, it has been shown that orbitofrontal cortex taste neurons stop responding to the taste of a food with which the monkey is fed to satiety, and that this parallels the decline in the acceptability of the food (see Fig. 3.5) (Rolls et al. 1989). In contrast, the representation of taste in the primary taste cortex (Scott, Yaxley, Sienkiewicz & Rolls 1986, Yaxley, Rolls & Sienkiewicz 1990) is not modulated by hunger (Rolls, Scott, Sienkiewicz & Yaxley 1988, Yaxley, Rolls & Sienkiewicz 1988). Thus in the primary taste cortex of primates (and at earlier stages of taste processing), the reward value of taste is not represented, and instead the identity of the taste is represented (Scott, Yan & Rolls 1995, Rolls & Scott 2003, Rolls 2015b).

Additional evidence that the reward value of food is represented in the orbitofrontal cortex is that monkeys work for electrical stimulation of the orbitofrontal cortex if they are hungry, but not if they are satiated (Mora, Avrith, Phillips & Rolls 1979, Rolls 2005). Thus the electrical stimulation of this brain region produces reward that is equivalent to food for a hungry animal. Further evidence implicating the firing of neurons in the orbitofrontal cortex in reward is that neurons in the orbitofrontal cortex are activated from many brain-stimulation reward sites (Rolls, Burton & Mora 1980, Mora, Avrith & Rolls 1980, Rolls 2005) (Section

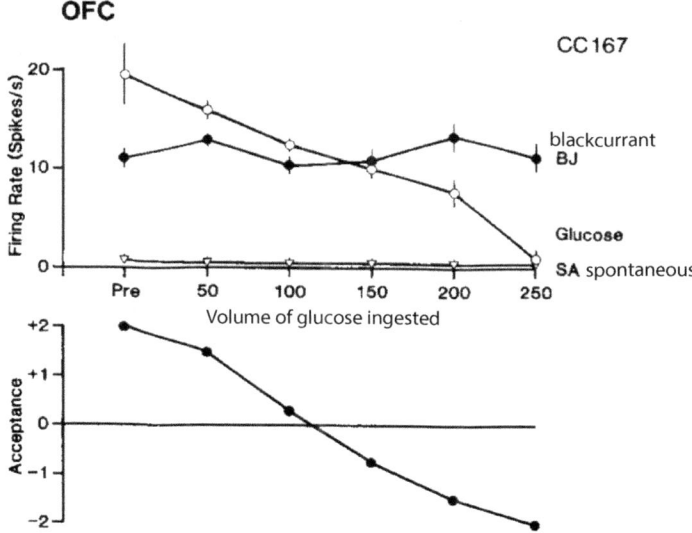

Fig. 3.5 The effect of feeding to satiety with glucose solution on the responses (rate ± s.e.m.) of a neuron in the secondary taste cortex to the taste of glucose (open circles) and of blackcurrant juice (BJ). The spontaneous firing rate is also indicated (SA). Below the neuronal response data, the behavioural measure of the acceptance or rejection of the solution on a scale from +2 (strong acceptance) to −2 (strong rejection) is shown. The solution used to feed to satiety was 20% glucose. The monkey was fed 50 ml of the solution at each stage of the experiment as indicated along the abscissa, until he was satiated as shown by whether he accepted or rejected the solution. Pre is the firing rate of the neuron before the satiety experiment started. (Reproduced from E. T. Rolls, Z. J. Sienkiewicz, and S. Yaxley, Hunger modulates the responses to gustatory stimuli of single neurons in the caudolateral orbitofrontal cortex of the macaque monkey, European Journal of Neuroscience, 1 (1) pp. 53–60, Copyright © 1989 John Wiley and Sons.)

3.15). Thus there is clear evidence that it is the reward value of taste that is represented in the orbitofrontal cortex, as shown by devaluation investigations.

In humans, there is evidence that the reward value, and, what can be directly reported in humans, the subjective pleasantness, of food is represented in the orbitofrontal cortex. The evidence comes from an fMRI study in which humans rated the pleasantness of the flavour of chocolate milk and tomato juice, and then ate one of these foods to satiety. It was found that the pleasantness of the flavour of the food eaten to satiety decreased, and that this decrease in pleasantness was reflected in decreased activation in the orbitofrontal cortex (Kringelbach, O'Doherty, Rolls & Andrews 2003) (see Fig. 3.6). (This was measured in a functional magnetic resonance imaging (fMRI) investigation in which the activation as reflected by the blood oxygenation-level dependent (BOLD) signal was measured, which reflects increased blood flow due to increased neuronal activity (Stephan, Weiskopf, Drysdale, Robinson & Friston 2007, Rolls, Grabenhorst & Franco 2009).) Further evidence that the pleasantness of flavour is represented here is that the pleasantness of the food not eaten to satiety showed very little decrease, and correspondingly the activation of the orbitofrontal cortex to this food not eaten in the meal showed little decrease. The phenomenon itself is called sensory-specific satiety, is an important property of reward systems, and is described in more detail below and by Rolls (2014a). The experiment of Kringelbach, O'Doherty, Rolls & Andrews (2003) was with a whole food, but further evidence that the pleasantness of taste, or at least a stimulus very closely related to a taste, is represented in the human orbitofrontal cortex is that the orbitofrontal cortex is activated by water in the mouth when thirsty but not when satiated (De Araujo, Kringelbach, Rolls & McGlone 2003b). Thus, the neuroimaging findings with a whole food, and with water when thirsty, provide evidence that the activation to taste *per se* in the human orbitofrontal cortex is related to the subjective pleasantness or

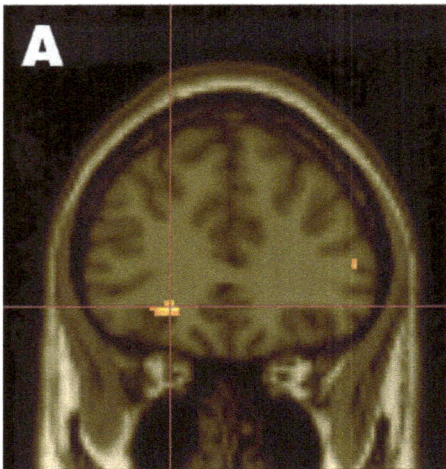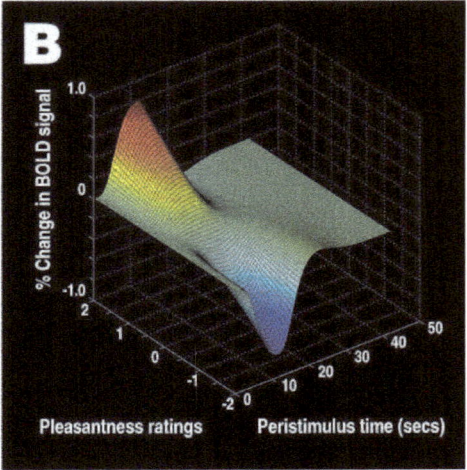

Fig. 3.6 Areas of the human orbitofrontal cortex with activations correlating with pleasantness ratings for food in the mouth. (A) Coronal section through the region of the orbitofrontal cortex from the random effects group analysis showing the peak in the left orbitofrontal cortex (Talairach co-ordinates X,Y,Z=[–22 34 –8], z-score=4.06), in which the BOLD signal in the voxels shown in yellow was significantly correlated with the subjects' subjective pleasantness ratings of the foods throughout an experiment in which the subjects were hungry and found the food pleasant, and were then fed to satiety with the food, after which the pleasantness of the food decreased to neutral or slightly unpleasant. The design was a sensory-specific satiety design, and the pleasantness of the food not eaten in the meal, and the BOLD activation in the orbitofrontal cortex, were not altered by eating the other food to satiety. The two foods were tomato juice and chocolate milk. (B) Plot of the magnitude of the fitted haemodynamic response from a representative single subject against the subjective pleasantness ratings (on a scale from –2 to +2) and peristimulus time in seconds. (Reproduced from Cerebral Cortex, 13 (10) Activation of the Human Orbitofrontal Cortex to a Liquid Food Stimulus is Correlated with its Subjective Pleasantness, M.L. Kringelbach, J. O'Doherty, E.T. Rolls, and C. Andrews, pp. 1064–1071, doi.org/10.1093/cercor/13.10.1064 Copyright © 2003, Oxford University Press.)

affective value of taste and flavour, that is, to *pleasure*. Further evidence on reward value for taste is that in fMRI investigations, activations in the human orbitofrontal cortex are linearly related to the subjective pleasantness of the taste (Grabenhorst & Rolls 2008) (Fig. 3.51).

Sensory-specific satiety is one of the most important factors that affects reward value, and is therefore described briefly here, in the context that it is computed in the orbitofrontal cortex. Sensory-specific satiety is a decrease in the reward value of a stimulus that is at least partly specific to that reward, and is a result of delivering that reward (Rolls 2014a). Sensory-specific satiety was discovered during neurophysiological experiments on brain mechanisms of reward and satiety by Edmund Rolls and colleagues in 1974. They observed that if a lateral hypothalamic neuron had ceased to respond to a food on which the monkey had been fed to satiety (a discovery described in *The Brain and Reward* (Rolls 1975)), then the neuron might still respond to a different food (see Rolls (2014a)). This occurred for neurons with responses associated with the taste (Rolls 1981b, Rolls 1981a, Rolls, Murzi, Yaxley, Thorpe & Simpson 1986) or sight (Rolls 1981b, Rolls & Rolls 1982, Rolls, Murzi, Yaxley, Thorpe & Simpson 1986) of food. Corresponding to this neuronal specificity of the effects of feeding to satiety, the monkey rejected the food on which he had been fed to satiety, but accepted other foods that he had not been fed. The neurophysiological finding was published for example in Rolls (1981b) and Rolls et al. (1986). This is now described as a devaluation procedure, and provides evidence that these, and orbitofrontal cortex neurons that provide inputs to the lateral hypothalamus, encode **value**.

Subsequent research showed that sensory-specific satiety is present (and computed (Rolls 2014a, Rolls 2016c)) in the orbitofrontal cortex (Rolls, Sienkiewicz & Yaxley 1989, Critchley & Rolls 1996c, Kringelbach, O'Doherty, Rolls & Andrews 2003) but not in earlier cortical areas such as the insula (Rolls, Scott, Sienkiewicz & Yaxley 1988, Yaxley, Rolls

& Sienkiewicz 1988). We showed that sensory-specific satiety is one of the most important factors influencing in humans what and how much is ingested in a meal (Rolls & Rolls 1982, Rolls, Rolls, Rowe & Sweeney 1981a, Rolls, Rowe, Rolls, Kingston, Megson & Gunary 1981b, Rolls, Rowe & Rolls 1982a, Rolls, Rowe & Rolls 1982b, Rolls & Rolls 1997, Rolls 1999a, Rolls 2014a), showed that olfactory sensory-specific satiety can be produced in part by merely sniffing a food for as long as it would typically be eaten in a meal (Rolls & Rolls 1997), and showed that there is a long-term form of sensory-specific satiety (Rolls & de Waal 1985). Sensory-specific satiety is not a sensory adaptation, in that it does not occur in primary taste cortical areas, and the inferior temporal visual cortex (Rolls, Judge & Sanghera 1977), and in that there is little decline in the intensity of the stimulus even though the pleasantness declines greatly (Rolls, Rolls & Rowe 1983a). The hypothesis is that sensory-specific satiety is produced by adaptation of active afferent synapses onto neurons in the orbitofrontal cortex that represent reward value (Rolls 2014a). I have argued that it is one of the factors that as a result of variety can overstimulate food intake and be associated with obesity, and is one of many factors that may all need to be taken into account in controlling food intake to prevent or minimize obesity (Rolls 2016f, Rolls 2014a, Rolls 2018b, Rolls 2012b). The evolutionary adaptive value of sensory-specific satiety is that it leads to animals not only eating a variety of food and maintaining good nutrition, but also in performing a whole set of different rewarded behaviours which promote successful reproduction and passing the successful set of genes into the next generation (Rolls 2014a). Moreover, although sensory-specific satiety is a property of all reward systems, for the reason given, it is not a property of any punishment system, in that aversive stimuli such as a thorn on the foot must be the subject of action, for any single punishing event could threaten reproductive success making any sensory-specific reductions that might occur for punishers highly maladaptive (Rolls 2014a).

Further evidence on the nature of the taste-related value representations, analyzed in a neuroeconomic framework, is described in Section 3.12.

Consistent with these anatomical and neurophysiological findings, damage to the orbitofrontal cortex in the monkey produces altered preferences for foods, including a reduced tendency to reject foods such as meat (Butter, Snyder & McDonald 1970, Butter & Snyder 1972, Butter, McDonald & Snyder 1969), a failure to display the normal preference ranking for different foods (Baylis & Gaffan 1991), and disrupts the rapid updating of object value during selective satiation (Rudebeck & Murray 2011). In humans there are few published descriptions of changes of affective reactions to foods after selective damage to the orbitofrontal cortex (when damage to the olfactory tract which runs just under the orbitofrontal cortex is excluded). However, of the patients in the groups with damage in the orbitofrontal cortex that we have studied (Rolls, Hornak, Wade & McGrath 1994a, Hornak, Rolls & Wade 1996, Hornak, Bramham, Rolls, Morris, O'Doherty, Bullock & Polkey 2003, Hornak, O'Doherty, Bramham, Rolls, Morris, Bullock & Polkey 2004) and in similar patients, the most common complaint they make to the physician is about the quality of their taste and smell sensations. There are large changes in their emotional behaviour that will be described below (Section 4.2), but these patients do not usually actually complain about the emotional changes that others observe. Altered food preferences, often including an increased preference for sweet foods, are common in fronto-temporal dementia (Piguet 2011).

3.2.4 Oral texture in the orbitofrontal cortex

The orbitofrontal cortex also contains neurons that represent oral texture, including viscosity, fat texture, grittiness, capsaicin, astringency, and temperature, and some neurons combine this information with taste inputs (Rolls, Critchley, Browning, Hernadi & Lenard 1999,

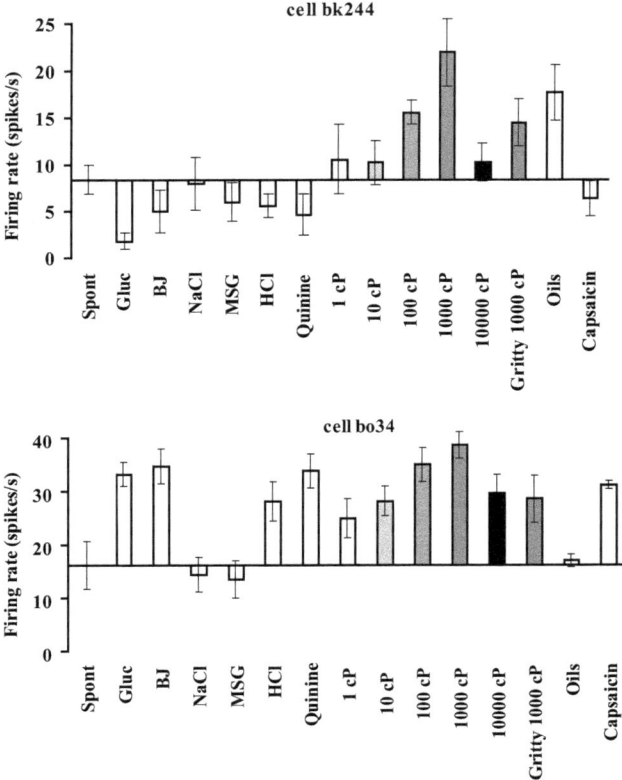

Fig. 3.7 Above. Firing rates (mean ± s.e.m.) of orbitofrontal cortex viscosity-sensitive neuron bk244 which did not have taste responses. The firing rates are shown to the viscosity series (carboxymethylcellulose in the range 1–10,000 centiPoise), to the gritty stimulus (carboxymethylcellulose with Fillite microspheres), to the taste stimuli 1 M glucose (Gluc), 0.1 M NaCl, 0.1 M MSG, 0.01 M HCl and 0.001 M QuinineHCl, and to fruit juice (BJ). Spont = spontaneous firing rate. Below. Firing rates (mean ± s.e.m.) of viscosity-sensitive neuron bo34 which had no response to the oils (mineral oil, vegetable oil, safflower oil and coconut oil, which have viscosities which are all close to 50 cP). The neuron did not respond to the gritty stimulus in a way that was unexpected given the viscosity of the stimulus, was taste tuned, and did respond to capsaicin. (Reproduced from Journal of Neurophysiology, 90 (6), Representations of the texture of food in the primate orbitofrontal cortex: neurons responding to viscosity, grittiness, and capsaicin, E. T. Rolls, J. V. Verhagen, and M. Kadohisa, pp. 3711–3724, © 2003, The American Physiological Society.)

Verhagen, Rolls & Kadohisa 2003, Rolls, Verhagen & Kadohisa 2003e, Kadohisa, Rolls & Verhagen 2004, Kadohisa, Rolls & Verhagen 2005b, Rolls 2011b). By responding to different combinations of these inputs (e.g. Fig. 3.7), and by showing selective effects of reward devaluation by feeding to satiety, these neurons provide evidence about the specific reward outcome value, not about general reward value converted to a common currency, and this is crucial for enabling different actions to be learned to obtain particular goals (outcomes), and for the mechanisms of sensory-specific satiety (Section 3.2.3). Evidence on these oral texture inputs follows.

In one set of experiments, oral texture was shown to be important by the addition of methyl cellulose or gelatine, or by pureeing a semi-solid food (Rolls 2011b).

3.2.4.1 Viscosity, food thickness

We have been able to show that some of these oral texture sensitive neurons respond to the viscosity of the food in the mouth, as altered parametrically using the standard food thickening agent carboxymethylcellulose made up in viscosities of 1–10,000 cPoise (Rolls, Verhagen & Kadohisa 2003e). (10,000 cP is approximately the viscosity of toothpaste.) Some of these

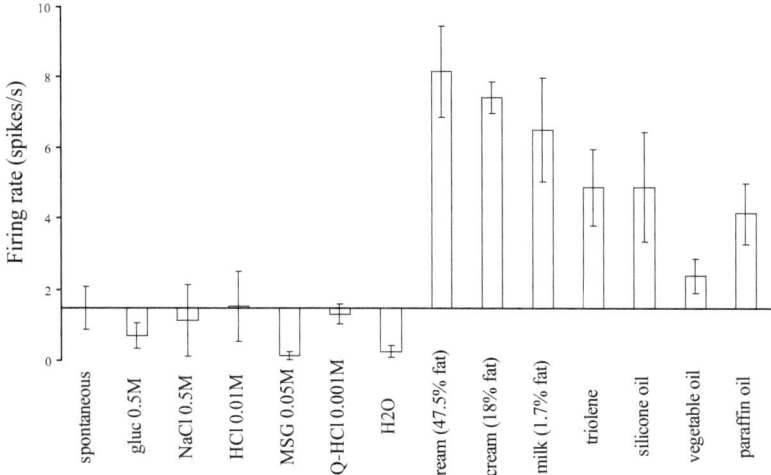

Fig. 3.8 A neuron in the primate orbitofrontal cortex responding to the texture of fat in the mouth. The neuron increased its firing rate to cream (double and single cream, with the fat proportions shown), and responded to texture rather than the chemical structure of the fat in that it also responded to 0.5 ml of silicone oil $(Si(CH_3)_2O)_n)$ or paraffin oil (hydrocarbon). The neuron did not have a taste input. Gluc, glucose; NaCl, salt; HCl, sour; Q-HCl, quinine, bitter. The spontaneous firing rate of the cell is also shown. (Reproduced from Journal of Neuroscience, 19 (4), Responses to the sensory properties of fat of neurons in the primate orbitofrontal cortex, E. T. Rolls, H. D. Critchley, A. S. Browning, A. Hernadi, and L. Lenard, pp. 1532–1540, © 1999, The Society for Neuroscience.)

neurons are unimodal, responding just to texture and not to taste (see Fig. 3.7 upper). The upper neuron had a tuned response to viscosity with the maximum response to 1000 cP, did respond to fatty and other oils, and did not respond to capsaicin (chilli). Other neurons respond to different combinations of texture and taste, as illustrated in Fig. 3.7 (lower). The lower neuron responded to sweet, sour and bitter but not to salt and MSG taste, had a tuned response to viscosity with the maximum response to 1000 cP, did not respond to fatty and other oils, and did respond to capsaicin. These recordings provide unique evidence about the texture channels that convey information from the mouth to the cortex, for they show that the system can potentially have responses to texture separately from the other sensory attributes of food, as well as to particular combinations of taste, texture, and other sensory properties of food.

The somatosensory inputs may reach the orbitofrontal cortex via the primary taste cortex in the rostral insula and adjoining frontal operculum, which we have shown does project into this region (Baylis, Rolls & Baylis 1994), and which also contains a representation of the viscosity of what is in the mouth (Verhagen, Kadohisa & Rolls 2004). A number of parts of the insula are known to receive somatosensory inputs (Mesulam & Mufson 1982a, Mesulam & Mufson 1982b, Mufson & Mesulam 1982). The texture of food is an important cue about the quality of the food, for example about the ripeness of fruit.

These findings have been extended to humans, with the finding with fMRI that the activation of the primary taste cortex is proportional to the logarithm of the viscosity of the stimulus in the mouth (De Araujo & Rolls 2004). Further, the subjective thickness rating is also proportional to the log of the viscosity (Kadohisa, Rolls & Verhagen 2005b). This also shows that the subjective thickness of oral texture is linearly related to the magnitude of the BOLD signal in this brain region.

3.2.4.2 Oral fat texture

Texture in the mouth is also an important indicator of whether fat is present in the food, which is important not only as a high value energy source, but also as a potential source of essential

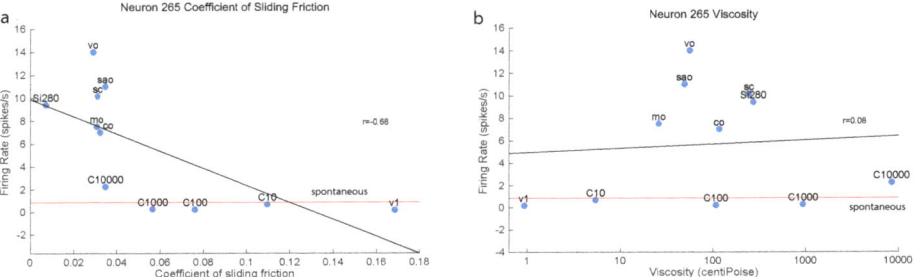

Fig. 3.9 An orbitofrontal cortex neuron with responses non-linearly correlated with decreases in the coefficient of sliding friction (a). The neuron responds almost not at all until the coefficient of sliding friction falls below 0.04. The neuron is thus very selective for fat texture, because of its non-linear response in relation to the coefficient of sliding friction. The linear regression line has a correlation of r = -0.68 (p=0.02). (b): There is a much weaker relation to viscosity (r = 0.08, p=0.82), with the oils producing a larger response than predicted linearly. Further, a regression line through the non-oil stimuli would have a lower slope. C10-C10000: carboxymethyl cellulose with the nominal viscosity of 10, 100, 1000 and 10,000 cP. v1: water (1 cP). co: coconut oil; mo: mineral oil; sao: safflower oil; vo: vegetable oil; sc: single cream. Si280: silicone oil with a nominal viscosity of 280 cP. Li: linoleic acid; La; lauric acid. The horizontal red line indicates the spontaneous firing rate. The Pearson correlation between the firing rate of each neuron and (a) the coefficient of sliding friction, and (b) the viscosity, was calculated to show to what extent the firing of a neuron reflected one or other of these measures. Linear regression lines are shown in the Figure for how the firing rates were related to the coefficient of sliding friction, or to the log of the viscosity. (Reproduced from Edmund T Rolls, Tom Mills, Abigail B Norton, Aris Lazidis, and Ian T Norton, The Neuronal Encoding of Oral Fat by the Coefficient of Sliding Friction in the Cerebral Cortex and Amygdala, Cerebral Cortex, 28 (11), doi.org/10.1093/cercor/bhy213 © 2018 Rolls, Mills, Norton, Lazidis, and Norton. This work is licensed under the Creative Commons Attribution License (CC BY). It is attributed to the authors Rolls, Mills, Norton, Lazidis, and Norton.)

fatty acids. In the orbitofrontal cortex, Rolls, Critchley, Browning, Hernadi & Lenard (1999) discovered a population of neurons that responds when fat is in the mouth. An example of such a neuron is shown in Fig. 3.8. This neuron had no response to taste, but some other neurons had convergence of fat texture and taste inputs. The fat-related responses of these neurons are produced at least in part by the texture of the food rather than by chemical receptors sensitive to certain chemicals, in that such neurons typically respond not only to foods such as cream and milk containing fat, but also to paraffin oil (which is a pure hydrocarbon) and to silicone oil (which contains $(Si(CH_3)_2O)_n$).

To investigate the bases of the responses of fat-sensitive neurons, we measured the correlations between their responses and physical measures of the properties of the set of stimuli, including viscosity and the coefficient of sliding friction (Rolls, Mills, Norton, Lazidis & Norton 2018d). The coefficient of sliding friction is the force required to slide two surfaces divided by the force normal to the surfaces. This is also known as kinetic or dynamic friction. It measures effectively the lubricity or the slipperiness of a substance. We found that some fat-sensitive neurons increased their firing rates linearly as the coefficient of sliding friction of the stimuli became smaller. Another population of neurons had their firing rates non-linearly related to the coefficient of sliding friction, and increased their rates only when the coefficient of sliding friction became less than 0.04, and were thus highly selective to the fats and the non-fat oils (see example in Fig. 3.9) (Rolls et al. 2018d). These neurons were more likely to be found in the orbitofrontal cortex than the primary taste cortex, consistent with the hypothesis of non-linear encoding in hierarchical cortical systems (Rolls 2016c). Another population of neurons had responses that were inhibited by fat: they had responses that increased linearly with the coefficient of sliding friction. The activity of these fat-sensitive neurons was not closely related to viscosity. The responses of these neurons are related to the reward value of fat in the mouth, in that the responses decrease to zero during feeding to satiety (Rolls, Critchley, Browning, Hernadi & Lenard 1999). The fat-sensitive neurons did not have responses to lauric or linoleic acid, so their responses were not related to fatty acid sensing. A separate population of neurons did have responses to linoleic or lauric fatty acids, but not to fat in the mouth. Their responses may be related to "off tastes" of food produced for example by butyric acid, which food manufacturers aim to minimize in foods (Rolls 2019c). Another population of neurons had responses related to the log of viscosity (which correlates with subjective ratings of food thickness (Kadohisa et al. 2005b)), but not with the coefficient of sliding friction (Rolls et al. 2018d).

This new understanding of the representation of oral fat by the coefficient of sliding friction in the cerebral cortex opens the way for the systematic development of foods with the pleasant mouth-feel of fat, together with ideal nutritional content, and has great potential to contribute to healthy eating and a healthy body weight (Rolls et al. 2018d, Rolls 2019c).

Some of the fat-related neurons have multimodal convergent inputs from the chemical senses, in that in addition to taste inputs, some of these neurons respond to the odour associated with a fat, such as the odour of cream (Rolls, Critchley, Browning, Hernadi & Lenard 1999). Similar neurons have been recorded in the pregenual cingulate cortex (Rolls 2008d).

This type of discovery can be made only at the single neuron level, and paves the way for further studies of the transducing mechanism, understanding of which could be important in the design of foods with pleasant textures which do not bring with them high caloric content with its implications for obesity (Rolls 2011b).

These findings have been extended to the human, with the finding with fMRI that activation of the orbitofrontal cortex and perigenual cingulate cortex is produced by the texture of fat in the mouth (De Araujo & Rolls 2004). Moreover, activations in the orbitofrontal cortex and pregenual cingulate cortex are correlated with the pleasantness of fat texture in the mouth (Grabenhorst, Rolls, Parris & D'Souza 2010b).

3.2.4.3 Astringency, tannic acid

Another taste-related stimulus quality that provides important information about the reward value of a potential food source is astringency. In humans, tannic acid elicits a characteristic astringent taste. Oral astringency is perceived as the feeling of long-lasting puckering and drying sensations on the tongue and membranes of the oral cavity. High levels of tannic acid in some potential foods makes them unpalatable without preparative techniques to reduce its presence (Johns & Duquette 1991), yet in small quantities it is commonly used to enhance the flavour of food. In this context tannic acid is a constituent of a large range of spices and condiments, such as ginger, chillies, and black pepper (Uma-Pradeep, Geervani & Eggum 1993). (Tannic acid itself is not present in tea, yet a range of related polyphenol compounds are, particularly in green tea, and also in wine (Graham 1992, Lesschaeve & Noble 2005).) Tannic acid is a natural antioxidant by virtue of its chemical structure (see Critchley & Rolls (1996a)).

The evolutionary adaptive value of the ability to detect astringency may be related to some of the properties of tannic acid. Tannic acid is a member of the class of compounds known as polyphenols, which are present in a wide spectrum of plant matter, particularly in foliage, the skin and husks of fruit and nuts, and the bark of trees. The tannic acid in leaves is produced as a defence against insects. There is less tannic acid in young leaves than in old leaves. Large monkeys cannot obtain the whole of their protein intake from small animals, insects etc., and thus obtain some of their protein from leaves. Tannic acid binds protein (hence its use in tanning) and amino acids, and thus prevents their absorption. Thus it is adaptive for monkeys to be able to taste tannic acid, so that they can select food sources without too much tannic acid (Hladik 1978).

In order to investigate whether astringency is represented in the cortical taste areas concerned with taste, Critchley & Rolls (1996a) recorded from taste-responsive neurons in the orbitofrontal cortex and adjacent insula. Single neurons were found that were tuned to respond to tannic acid (0.001 M), and represented a subpopulation of neurons that was distinct from neurons responsive to the tastes of glucose (sweet), NaCl (salty), HCl (sour), quinine

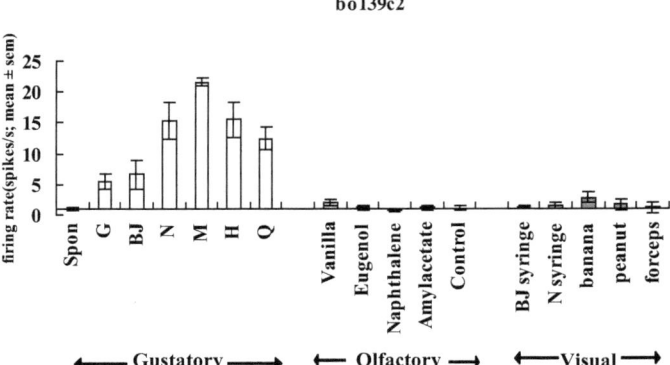

Fig. 3.10 Responses of an insular taste cortex neuron (bo139c2) with taste responses, to show the lack of response to a range of olfactory and visual stimuli. The mean (/pm the standard error of the mean, sem) firing rate responses to each stimulus calculated in a 1 s period over 4–6 trials are shown. The spontaneous (Spon) firing rate is shown by the horizontal line. The taste stimuli were 1 M glucose (G), 0.1 M NaCl (N), 0.1 M MSG (M), 0.01 M HCl (H) and 0.001 M QuinineHCl (Q). The visual stimuli were: BJ syringe: the sight of a syringe containing fruit (blackcurrant) juice; N syringe: the sight of a syringe containing 0.1 N NaCl; forceps: control, showing the feeding forceps alone that were used to show and feed banana or peanut. (Modified from Verhagen, Rolls and Kadohisa, 2004).)

(bitter) and monosodium glutamate (umami). In addition, across the population of taste-responsive neurons, tannic acid was as well represented as the tastes of NaCl, HCl, quinine, or monosodium glutamate. Multidimensional scaling analysis of the neuronal responses to the tastants indicates that tannic acid lies outside the boundaries of the four conventional taste qualities (sweet, sour, bitter, and salty). Taken together these data indicate that the astringent taste of tannic acid should be considered as a distinct 'taste' quality, which receives a separate representation from sweet, salt, bitter, and sour in the primate cortical taste areas. Tannic acid may produce its 'taste' effects not through the taste nerves, but through the somatosensory inputs conveyed through the trigeminal nerve. Astringency is thus strictly not a sixth taste in the sense that umami is a fifth taste. However, what has been shown in these studies is that the orosensory, probably somatosensory, sensations produced by tannic acid do converge with effects produced through taste inputs, to result in neurons in the orbitofrontal cortex responding to both taste stimuli and to astringent stimuli (Critchley & Rolls 1996a).

3.2.5 Taste and oral texture in the insular primary taste cortex

It is important to compare neuronal activity in connected brain regions to understand the operations performed by each brain region. The taste insula and taste opercular cortex, the primary taste cortex, projects into the orbitofrontal cortex. In contrast to the orbitofrontal cortex, the insular cortex does not represent taste value, but instead what the taste is independently of value (Rolls 2016b). The location of the macaque primary taste cortex in the macaque anterior insula and adjoining frontal operculum was described by Pritchard et al. (1986) based on anatomically defined inputs from the taste thalamus.

To investigate whether there are neurons in the primary gustatory cortex that are more closely tuned to respond to foods as compared to non-foods, and whether hunger modulates the responsiveness of these neurons, we recorded the activity of single neurons in the primary gustatory cortex during feeding in the monkey. In the primary gustatory cortex in the insula and adjoining frontal operculum, neurons are more sharply tuned to gustatory stimuli than in the nucleus of the solitary tract, with some neurons responding primarily, for example, to sweet, and much less to salt, bitter, or sour stimuli (Scott, Yaxley, Sienkiewicz & Rolls 1986, Yaxley,

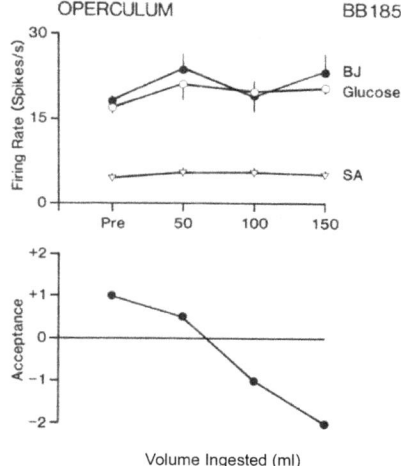

Fig. 3.11 No effect of feeding to satiety with glucose solution on the responses (firing rate /pm s.e.m.) of a neuron in the primary taste cortex in the insular/frontal opercular area to the taste of glucose (open circles) and of blackcurrant fruit juice (BJ). The spontaneous firing rate is also indicated (SA). Below the neuronal response data, the behavioral measure of the acceptance or rejection of the solution on a scale from +2 (strong acceptance) to -2 (strong rejection) is shown. The solution used to feed to satiety was 20% glucose. The monkey was fed 50 ml of the solution at each stage of the experiment as indicated along the abscissa, until he was satiated as shown by whether he accepted or rejected the solution. Pre is the firing rate of the neuron before the satiety experiment started. (Modified from Yaxley, Rolls and Sienkiewicz (1988) and Rolls, Scott, Sienkiewicz and Yaxley (1988).)

Rolls & Sienkiewicz 1990, Scott & Plata-Salaman 1999). The responses of an insular taste cortex neuron with significantly different responses to different tastes are illustrated in Fig. 3.10. This neuron had no significant responses to oral viscosity, fat, or temperature. The neuron also had no significant responses to any of the olfactory and visual stimuli tested (see Fig. 3.10). None of the insular taste cortex neurons had responses to olfactory stimuli, and none could be shown to have responses to visual stimuli that were clearly not just related to mouth movements and the accompanying somatosensory input (Verhagen et al. 2004), in contrast to the orbitofrontal cortex where responses to olfactory and visual stimuli associated with food are common (see Sections 3.3 and 3.6).

Neurons in the macaque primary taste cortex do not represent the reward value of taste, that is the appetite for a food, in that their firing is not decreased to zero by feeding the taste to satiety (Rolls, Scott, Sienkiewicz & Yaxley 1988, Yaxley, Rolls & Sienkiewicz 1988) (see example in Fig. 3.11). This was confirmed in 17 separate experiments on neurons in the insular and frontal opercular primary taste cortex, using anatomical confirmation that these neurons were in the primary taste cortex by the use of X-ray localization and then histological reconstruction. The neurons showed no reduction in their firing to the taste (typically glucose) after it had been fed to satiety (Rolls, Scott, Sienkiewicz & Yaxley 1988, Yaxley, Rolls & Sienkiewicz 1988). Consistent with this, activations in the human insular primary taste cortex are linearly related to the subjective intensity of the taste and not to the pleasantness rating (Fig. 3.51 (Grabenhorst & Rolls 2008)). Further, activations in the human insular primary taste cortex are related to the concentration of the tastant, for example monosodium glutamate (Grabenhorst, Rolls & Bilderbeck 2008a).

Single neurons in the insular primary taste cortex also represent the viscosity (measured with carboxymethylcellulose) and temperature of stimuli in the mouth, and fat texture (Verhagen, Kadohisa & Rolls 2004, Kadohisa, Rolls & Verhagen 2005b, Rolls, Mills, Norton, Lazidis & Norton 2018d).

In humans, the insular primary taste cortex is activated not only by taste (Francis, Rolls,

Bowtell, McGlone, O'Doherty, Browning, Clare & Smith 1999, Small, Zald, Jones-Gotman, Zatorre, Petrides & Evans 1999, De Araujo, Kringelbach, Rolls & Hobden 2003a, De Araujo & Rolls 2004, De Araujo, Kringelbach, Rolls & McGlone 2003b, Grabenhorst & Rolls 2008, Grabenhorst, Rolls & Bilderbeck 2008a), but also by oral texture including viscosity (with the activation linearly related to the log of the viscosity) and fat texture (De Araujo & Rolls 2004), and temperature (Guest, Grabenhorst, Essick, Chen, Young, McGlone, de Araujo & Rolls 2007). These investigations in humans indicate that there is a taste-related area in the anterior taste insula, in a region typically between Y=10 and Y=20 (see examples in Figs. 3.4 and 3.52), and that activations here are not related to pleasantness, but to intensity (see Fig. 3.52). This is probably the primary taste cortex[1]. Activations posterior to this towards the mid-insula can be produced by oral stimuli including oral texture, chocolate, etc (De Araujo & Rolls 2004, Small 2010, Rolls, Kellerhals & Nichols 2015b); and by any taste where a tasteless control is not subtracted. This latter is because introducing a tastant into the mouth inevitably produces somatosensory and related effects (Francis, Rolls, Bowtell, McGlone, O'Doherty, Browning, Clare & Smith 1999, De Araujo, Kringelbach, Rolls & Hobden 2003a), and can not be relied on as a pure taste stimulus without subtraction of a tasteless control (Rolls 2015b).

Ventral to the taste insula is a region that is probably visceral cortex. Both the anterior insula and the anterior cingulate cortex are activated by visceral / autonomic signals (Al Omran & Aziz 2014, Critchley & Harrison 2013, Quadt, Critchley & Garfinkel 2018). For example, the right anterior insular cortex reactivity predicts interoceptive accuracy on a heartbeat discrimination task and its volume predicts interoceptive sensibility (Quadt et al. 2018). The insula receives inputs from cortical areas such as the orbitofrontal cortex and anterior cingulate cortex that are involved in reward and punishment related processing, and the anterior ventral insula may be part of a route by which such stimuli can elicit autonomic and related responses to such stimuli (Rolls 2015b) (see also Chapter 2).

3.2.6 Taste in an output region of the orbitofrontal cortex, the anterior cingulate cortex

Taste value representations have been found in the pregenual part of the anterior cingulate cortex in single neuron recording studies in monkeys (Rolls 2008d, Rolls 2009c). For example, Gabbott, Verhagen, Kadohisa and Rolls found neurons in the pregenual cingulate cortex that respond to taste (see example in Fig. 3.12), and it was demonstrated that the representation is of reward value, for devaluation by feeding to satiety selectively decreased neuronal responses to the food with which the animal was satiated (Rolls 2008d). The neuron illustrated in Fig. 3.12 also responded to cream in the mouth. Such neurons may be part of the representation of reward outcome, that are needed for action-outcome learning by the anterior cingulate cortex (Rolls 2014a, Rolls 2018b, Rolls 2019d) (Section 5.1).

In fMRI studies in humans, pleasant tastes activate the pregenual cingulate cortex, and less pleasant or unpleasant taste the supracallosal anterior cingulate cortex. For example, pleasant sweet taste activates the most anterior part of the anterior cingulate cortex (De Araujo & Rolls 2004, De Araujo, Kringelbach, Rolls & Hobden 2003a) (Fig. 3.4) where attention to pleasantness (Grabenhorst & Rolls 2008) and cognition (Grabenhorst, Rolls & Bilderbeck 2008a) also enhance activations. Oral somatosensory stimuli such as viscosity and the pleasantness of fat texture also activate this most anterior part of the anterior cingulate

---

[1] In some different investigations, the MNI [X Y Z] coordinates of the taste cortex in the anterior part of the insular taste cortex were as follows: flavour - rinse [30 18 8] (Grabenhorst & Rolls 2014); [30 12 0] and [32 22 0] (Rolls & McCabe 2007); [34 24 6] (McCabe & Rolls 2007); conjunction of taste - rinse and MSG 0.4M - MSG 0.1 M [34 16 4] (Grabenhorst, Rolls & Bilderbeck 2008a); conjunction of texture - rinse and glucose - rinse [-36 12 6] (De Araujo & Rolls 2004).

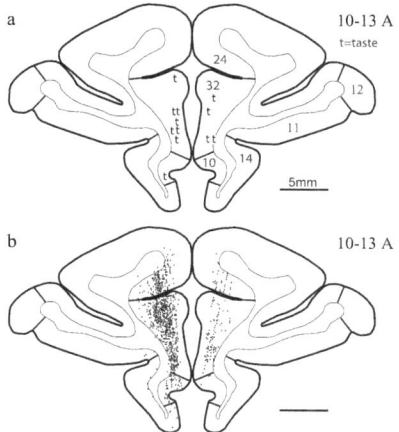
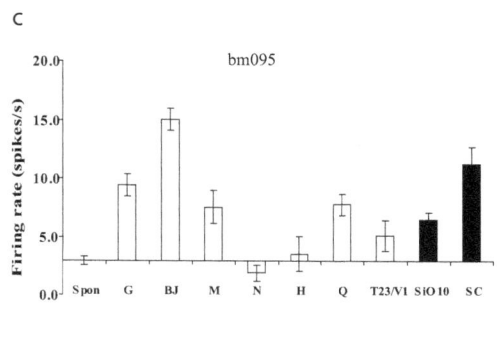

Fig. 3.12 Pregenual cortex taste neurons. The reconstructed positions of the anterior cingulate neurons with taste (t) responses, together with the cytoarchitectonic boundaries determined by Carmichael and Price (1994). Most (11/12) of the taste neurons were in the pregenual cingulate cortex (area 32), as shown. The neurons are shown on a coronal section at 12 mm anterior (A) to the sphenoid reference point. b. The locations of all the 749 neurons recorded in the anterior cingulate region in this study are indicated to show the regions sampled. c. Responses of a pregenual cingulate cortex neuron (bm095) with differential responses to tastes and oral fat texture stimuli. The mean ($\pm$ sem) firing rate responses to each stimulus calculated in a 5 s period over several trials are shown. The spontaneous (Spon) firing rate of 3 spikes/s is shown by the horizontal line, with the responses indicated relative to this line. The taste stimuli were 1 M glucose (G), blackcurrant fruit juice (BJ), 0.1 M NaCl (N), 0.1 M MSG (M), 0.01 M HCl (H) and 0.001 M QuinineHCl (Q); water (T23/V1); single cream (SC); and silicone oil with a viscosity of 10 cP (SiO10). The neuron had significantly different responses to the different stimuli as shown by a one-way ANOVA (F[9,46]=17.7, $p < 10^{10}$). (Data from Rolls, Gabbott, Verhagen, and Kadohisa.) (Reproduced from E. T. Rolls, Functions of the orbitofrontal and pregenual cingulate cortex in taste, olfaction, appetite and emotion, Acta Physiologica Hungarica, 95 pp. 131–164, © 2008, Akademiai Kiado, Budapest.)

cortex (De Araujo & Rolls 2004, Grabenhorst, Rolls, Parris & D'Souza 2010b). Activations in the pregenual anterior cingulate cortex are also produced by the taste of water when it is rewarding because of thirst (De Araujo, Kringelbach, Rolls & McGlone 2003b), and by the flavour of food (Kringelbach, O'Doherty, Rolls & Andrews 2003).

In these studies, the anterior cingulate activations were linearly related to the subjective pleasantness or unpleasantness of the stimuli, providing evidence that the anterior cingulate cortex provides a representation of value on a continuous scale. Moreover, evidence was found that there was a common scale of value in the pregenual cingulate cortex, with the affective pleasantness of taste stimuli and of thermal stimuli applied to the hand producing identically scaled BOLD activations (Grabenhorst, D'Souza, Parris, Rolls & Passingham 2010a). The implication is that the anterior cingulate cortex contains a value representation used in decision-making, but that the decision itself may be made elsewhere. Decisions about actions that reflect the outcomes represented in the anterior cingulate cortex may be made further posterior towards the mid-cingulate cortex (Section 5.1). Decisions about the value of stimuli may be made in the medial prefrontal cortex area 10 (see Section 3.13), which does receive inputs from the orbitofrontal cortex and anterior cingulate cortex.

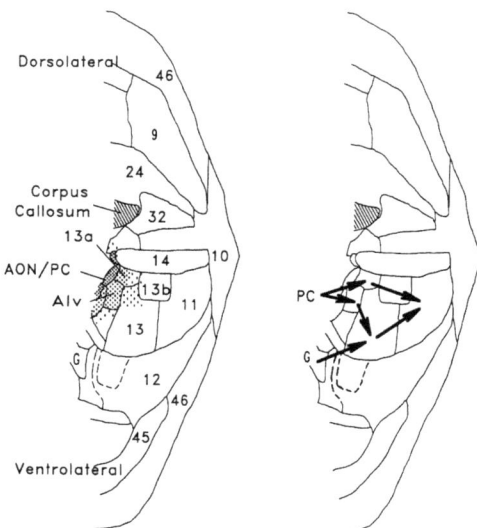

Fig. 3.13 The progression of olfactory inputs to the orbitofrontal cortex in the monkey, drawn on unfolded maps of the frontal lobe. The cortex was unfolded by splitting it along the principal sulcus, which is therefore located at the top and bottom of each map. (Reference to Figs. 2.1 and 2.2 may help to show how the map was constructed.) Left: inputs from the primary olfactory (pyriform) cortex (PC) terminate in the shaded region, that is in the caudal medial part of area 13, i.e. 13a, and in the ventral agranular insular cortex (AIv), which could therefore be termed secondary olfactory cortex. Right: the secondary olfactory cortices then project into the caudolateral orbitofrontal cortex, that is into the secondary taste cortex in that it receives from the primary taste cortex (G); and there are further projections into more anterior and medial parts of the orbitofrontal cortex. (Reproduced from Price, Carmichael, Carnes, Clugnet, and Kuroda, 'Olfactory input to the prefrontal cortex', in Davis, Joel L., and Howard Eichenbaum, eds., Olfaction: A Model System for Computational Neuroscience, Figure 4.10, © 1991 Massachusetts Institute of Technology, by permission of The MIT Press.)

3.3 An olfactory representation in the orbitofrontal cortex of expected value

3.3.1 Olfactory pathways to and responses in the primate orbitofrontal cortex

A schematic diagram of the olfactory pathways in primates is shown in Fig. 2.2 on page 11. There are direct connections from the olfactory bulb to the primary olfactory cortex, pyriform cortex, and from there a connection to a caudal part of the mid (in terms of medial and lateral) orbitofrontal cortex, area 13a, which in turn has onward projections to more rostral parts of the orbitofrontal cortex (area 11) (Price et al. 1991, Carmichael & Price 1994, Carmichael et al. 1994, Ongur & Price 2000, Price 2006) (see Figs. 3.13 and 2.2).

There is evidence that in the rodent olfactory bulb, a coding principle is that in many cases each glomerulus (of which there are approximately 1000) is tuned to respond to its own characteristic hydrocarbon chain length of odourant (Mori, Mataga & Imamura 1992, Imamura, Mataga & Mori 1992, Mori, Nagao & Yoshihara 1999, Mori & Sakano 2011). Evidence for this is that each mitral/tufted cell in the olfactory bulb can be quite sharply tuned, responding for example best to a 5-C length aliphatic odourant (e.g. acid or aldehyde), and being inhibited by nearby hydrocarbon chain-length aliphatic odourants. An effect of this coding might appear to be to spread out (orthogonalize) the olfactory stimulus space in this early part of the olfactory system, based on the stereochemical structure of the odourant. The code would be spread out in that different parts of chemical space would be relatively evenly represented, in that each part would be represented independently of the presence of other odourants, and in that the code would be relatively sparse, leading to low correlations between the representations of different odours. (Such a coding principle might be facilitated by the presence of in the order of 1000 different genes to code for different olfactory receptor molecules (Buck & Axel 1991, Buck & Bargmann 2013, Mombaerts 2006, Mori & Sakano 2011, Zapiec & Mombaerts 2015, Horowitz, Saraiva, Kuang, Yoon & Buck 2014).)

Is this same coding principle, based on simple physico-chemical properties, used later on in the (primate) olfactory system, or do other principles operate? One example of another coding principle is that representations may be built, for example by competitive learning (Rolls 2016c), that represent the co-occurrence of pairs or groups of odourants, so that particular smells in the environment, which typically are produced by combinations of chemical stimuli, are reflected in the responses of neurons (Wilson & Sullivan 2011, Barbaro & Shackelford 2015, Courtiol & Wilson 2017). Another coding principle is that olfactory coding might represent in some sense the biological significance of an odour, for example whether it is a food odour that is normally associated with a particular taste. Another principle is that at some stage of olfactory processing the reward or hedonic value of the odourant is represented (whether the odourant smells good), rather than purely the identity of the odourant. For example, whether a food-related odour smells good and encodes expected value depends on hunger, and this hedonic representation of odours must be represented in some part of the olfactory system. To elucidate these issues, and thus to provide principles by which the primate olfactory system may operate, the following investigations were performed.

Takagi, Tanabe and colleagues (see Takagi (1991)) had described single neurons in the macaque orbitofrontal cortex that were activated by odours. A ventral frontal region had been implicated in olfactory processing in humans in PET[2] and fMRI studies (Jones-Gotman & Zatorre 1988, Zatorre & Jones-Gotman 1991, Zatorre, Jones-Gotman, Evans & Meyer 1992, Rolls, Kringelbach & De Araujo 2003c).

Rolls and colleagues have analysed the rules by which orbitofrontal olfactory representations are formed and operate in primates (Rolls 2001b, Rolls & Grabenhorst 2008, Rolls 2011c). For 65% of neurons in the orbitofrontal olfactory areas, Critchley & Rolls (1996b) showed that the representation of the olfactory stimulus was independent of its association with taste reward (analysed in an olfactory discrimination task with taste reward, as some orbitofrontal cortex olfactory neurons are bimodal, with responses also to taste stimuli (Rolls & Baylis 1994)). For the remaining 35% of the neurons, the odours to which a neuron responded were influenced by the taste (glucose or saline) with which the odour was associated (Critchley & Rolls 1996b). Thus the odour representation for 35% of orbitofrontal neurons appeared to be built by olfactory-to-taste association learning, and thus by learning the neurons come to encode the *expected value* of olfactory stimuli.

3.3.2 Learning and reversal of olfactory-taste associations in the orbitofrontal cortex

This possibility that the odour representation of some primate orbitofrontal cortex olfactory neurons is built by olfactory-to-taste association learning to encode *expected value* was confirmed by reversing the taste with which an odour was associated in the reversal of an olfactory discrimination task. It was found that 73% of the sample of neurons analysed altered the way in which they responded to odour when the taste reinforcer association of the odour was reversed (Rolls, Critchley, Mason & Wakeman 1996a). Reversal was shown by 25% of the neurons (see, for example, Fig. 3.14), and 48% altered their activity in that they no longer discriminated after the reversal. These latter neurons thus respond to a particular odour only if it is associated with a taste reward, and not when it is associated with the taste of salt, a

---

[2]Positron emission tomography is a method of functional neuroimaging that uses radioactively labelled compounds to measure for example altered blood flow in an area to provide a measure of changing activity.

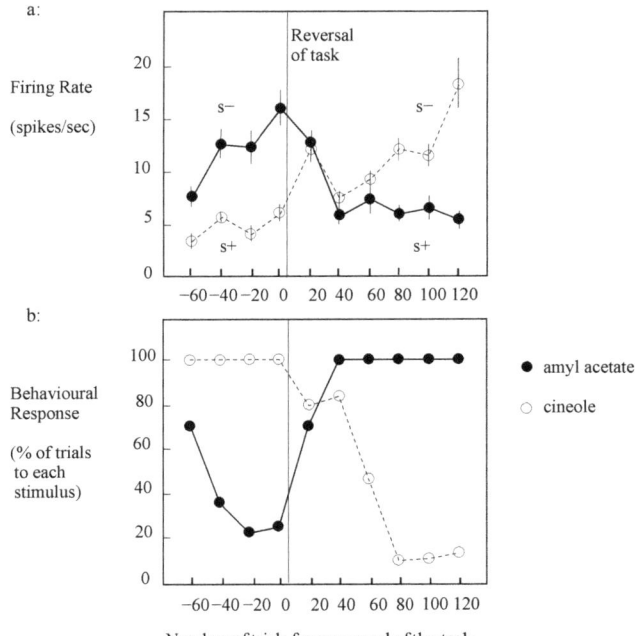

Fig. 3.14 Orbitofrontal cortex: olfactory to taste association reversal. (a) The activity of a single orbitofrontal olfactory neuron during the performance of a two-odour olfactory discrimination task and its reversal is shown. Each point represents the mean poststimulus activity of the neuron in a 500-ms period on approximately 10 trials of the different odourants. The standard errors of these responses are shown. The odourants were amyl acetate (closed circle) (initially S−) and cineole (o) (initially S+). After 80 trials of the task the reward associations of the stimuli were reversed. This neuron reversed its responses to the odourants following the task reversal. (b) The behavioural responses of the monkey during the performance of the olfactory discrimination task. The number of lick responses to each odourant is plotted as a percentage of the number of trials to that odourant in a block of 20 trials of the task. (Reproduced from Journal of Neurophysiology, 75 (5), Orbitofrontal cortex neurons: role in olfactory and visual association learning, E. T. Rolls, H. D. Critchley, R. Mason, E. A. Wakeman, pp. 1970–1981, © 1996, The American Physiological Society.)

punisher. They do not respond to the other odour in the task when it is associated with reward. Thus they respond to a particular combination of an odour, and its being associated with taste reward and not a taste punisher. They may be described as *conditional olfactory-reward neurons*, and may be important in the mechanism by which stimulus–reinforcer (in this case olfactory-to-taste) reversal learning occurs (Deco & Rolls 2005a), as described in Section 9.4.

The olfactory to taste reversal was quite slow, both neurophysiologically and behaviourally, often requiring 20–80 trials, consistent with the need for some stability of flavour (i.e. olfactory and taste combination) representations. The relatively high proportion of olfactory neurons with modification of responsiveness by taste association in the set of neurons in this experiment was probably related to the fact that the neurons were preselected to show differential responses to the odours associated with different tastes in the olfactory discrimination task. Thus the rule according to which the orbitofrontal olfactory representation was formed was for some neurons by association learning with taste.

Consistent findings were found in a human fMRI classical conditioning experiment in which odours were paired with a monetary cue, and representations in the orbitofrontal cortex and one of its subregions the ventromedial prefrontal cortex were influenced by this conditioning (Howard, Gottfried, Tobler & Kahnt 2015, Howard, Kahnt & Gottfried 2016).

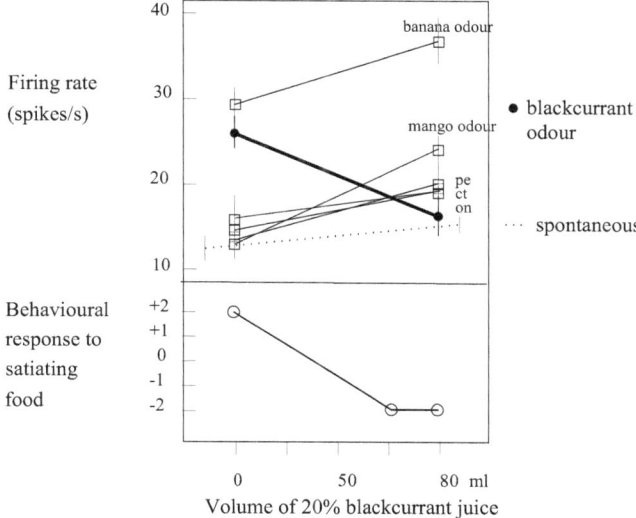

Fig. 3.15 The effect of feeding to satiety on the responses of an olfactory neuron in the orbitofrontal cortex. The monkey was fed to satiety with blackcurrant juice, and the neuronal response to the odour of blackcurrant juice, but not to other odours, decreased as the monkey was being fed to satiety. The neuronal responses reflected the monkey's preference for the blackcurrant juice, as shown in the lower graph. (Reproduced from Journal of Neurophysiology, 75 (4), Hunger and satiety modify the responses of olfactory and visual neurons in the primate orbitofrontal cortex, H. D. Critchley and E. T. Rolls pp. 1673–1686, © 1996, The American Physiological Society.)

3.3.3 Olfactory reward value and pleasantness are represented in the orbitofrontal cortex

The orbitofrontal cortex is likely to be the first stage of processing in humans at which olfactory responses represented expected (reward) value and subjective pleasantness, as activations in primary olfactory cortical areas such as the pyriform cortex are related to the intensity but not the pleasantness of odours (Rolls, Grabenhorst, Margot, da Silva & Velazco 2008a). (In rodents the encoding may be different, in that an influence of reward-association learning on olfactory neuronal responses in the pyriform cortex (a primary olfactory cortical area) has been reported (Schoenbaum & Eichenbaum 1995)). In contrast to rodents, the fact that humans can still report accurately the intensity of an odour even when its reward value and pleasantness as influenced by feeding to satiety are decreased to zero (Rolls & Rolls 1997) suggests that modulation of processing to reflect reward value is not a general property of olfactory processing implemented at early stages in primates including humans (Rolls 2014a, Rolls 2016f, Rolls 2018b).

The olfactory neurons that do not reverse in the reversal of the olfactory–taste reversal task may be carrying information that is in some cases independent of the reinforcer association (i.e. is about olfactory identity). In other cases, the olfactory representation in the orbitofrontal cortex may reflect associations of odours with other primary reinforcers (for example whether sickness has occurred in association with some smells), or may reflect primary reinforcer value provided by some olfactory stimuli. (For example, the smell of flowers may be innately pleasant and attractive and some other odours may be innately unpleasant – see Chapter 6.) In this situation, the olfactory input to some orbitofrontal cortex neurons may represent an unconditioned stimulus input with which other (for example visual) inputs may become associated.

To analyse the nature of the olfactory representation in the orbitofrontal cortex, Critchley & Rolls (1996c) measured the responses of olfactory neurons that responded to food while they fed the monkey to satiety in a reward devaluation experiment. They found that the

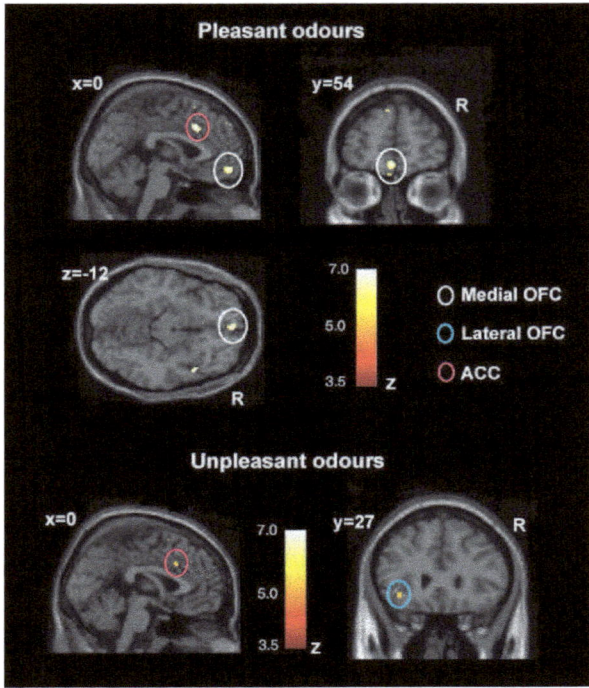

Fig. 3.16 The representation of pleasant and unpleasant odours in the human brain. Above : Group conjunction results for the 3 pleasant odours. Sagittal, horizontal and coronal views are shown at the levels indicated, all including the same activation in the medial orbitofrontal cortex, OFC [0 54 –12] z=5.23). Also shown is activation for the 3 pleasant odours in the anterior cingulate cortex, ACC [2 20 32] z=5.44). These activations were significant at p<0.05 fully corrected for multiple comparisons. Below : Group conjunction results for the 3 unpleasant odours. The sagittal view (left) shows an activated region of the anterior cingulate cortex [0 18 36] z=4.42, p<0.05, svc). The coronal view (right) shows an activated region of the lateral orbitofrontal cortex [–36 27 –8] z=4.23, p<0.05 svc). All the activations were thresholded at p<0.00001 to show the extent of the activations. (Reproduced from Edmund T. Rolls, Morten L. Kringelbach, and Ivan E. T. De Araujo, Different representations of pleasant and unpleasant odours in the human brain, European Journal of Neuroscience, 18 (3) pp. 695–703, Copyright © 2003, John Wiley and Sons.)

majority of orbitofrontal olfactory neurons reduced their responses to the odour of the food with which the monkey was fed to satiety (see Fig. 3.15). Thus for these neurons, the *expected reward value* of the odour is what is represented in the orbitofrontal cortex. This provides a basis for the olfactory sensory-specific satiety that is found in humans (Rolls & Rolls 1997).

Consistent with this finding at the neuronal level in non-human primates, activation of a part of the human orbitofrontal cortex is related to the pleasantness and expected value of food odour, in that the activation measured with fMRI produced by one food odour, banana, decreased after banana was eaten for lunch to satiety, but remained strong to another food odour, vanilla, not eaten in the meal (O'Doherty, Rolls, Francis, Bowtell, McGlone, Kobal, Renner & Ahne 2000). Consistent findings have been reported (Gottfried, O'Doherty & Dolan 2003, Howard & Gottfried 2014, Howard, Gottfried, Tobler & Kahnt 2015).

Signals that reflect satiety must reach the orbitofrontal cortex to decrease the responsiveness of taste, olfactory and flavor neurons in the orbitofrontal cortex. These satiety signals include gastric distension, gut sensing of nutrients (de Araujo, Lin, Veldhuizen & Small 2013), and the concentration of glucose and other indicators, including hormonal, of hunger/satiety in the systemic circulation which must influence the orbitofrontal cortex, either directly or via the hypothalamus and brainstem (Karadi, Oomura, Nishino, Scott, Lenard & Aou 1990, Karadi, Oomura, Nishino, Scott, Lenard & Aou 1992, Oomura, Nishino, Karadi, Aou & Scott 1991, Rolls 2014a). There is clear evidence that the reward value of food is produced by sensory inputs including its sight, taste, texture and smell, whereas satiety is

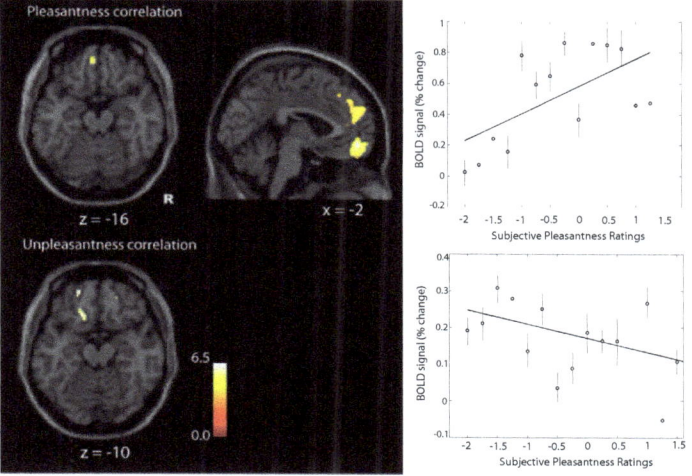

Fig. 3.17 The representation of pleasant and unpleasant odours in the human brain. Random effects group analysis correlation analysis of the BOLD signal with the subjective pleasantness ratings. On the top left is shown the region of the medio-rostral orbitofrontal (peak at [–2 52 –10] z=4.28) correlating positively with pleasantness ratings, as well as the region of the anterior cingulate cortex in the top middle. On the far top-right of the figure is shown the relation between the subjective pleasantness ratings and the BOLD signal from this cluster (in the medial orbitofrontal cortex at Y=52), together with the regression line. The means and s.e.m. across subjects are shown. At the bottom of the figure are shown the regions of left more lateral orbitofrontal cortex (peaks at [–20 54 –14] z=4.26 and [–16 28 –18] z=4.08) correlating negatively with pleasantness ratings. On the far bottom-right of the figure is shown the relation between the subjective pleasantness ratings and the BOLD signal from the first cluster (in the lateral orbitofrontal cortex at Y=54), together with the regression line. The means and s.e.m. across subjects are shown. The activations were thresholded at p<0.0001 for extent. (Reproduced from Edmund T. Rolls, Morten L. Kringelbach, and Ivan E. T. De Araujo, Different representations of pleasant and unpleasant odours in the human brain, European Journal of Neuroscience, 18 (3) pp. 695–703, Copyright © 2003, John Wiley and Sons.)

produced by gut and post-gastric signals (Rolls 2014a). Part of the evidence comes from sham feeding, in that feeding continues even when food does not reach the stomach, and that very small quantities of food tasted and smelled are rewarding, but that direct delivery of food to the gut is not very rewarding (Rolls 2014a). In this context, effects of food in the gut can become conditioned to oral stimuli to reflect energy or nutritional content (Booth 1985, Han, Tellez, Perkins, Perez, Qu, Ferreira, Ferreira, Quinn, Liu, Gao, Kaelberer, Bohorquez, Shammah-Lagnado, de Lartigue & de Araujo 2018), but do not reflect what normally produces the reward value of food, and its pleasantness (Rolls 2014a). Further, dopamine cannot be the primary mediator of reward (Tellez, Han, Zhang, Ferreira, Perez, Shammah-Lagnado, van den Pol & de Araujo 2016), in that specific rewards code for different goals in order for goal-directed behavior to be selective (Rolls 2014a).

Further evidence that pleasant odours are represented in the orbitofrontal cortex is that 3 pleasant odours (linalyl acetate [floral, sweet], geranyl acetate [floral], and alpha-ionone [woody, slightly food-related]) had overlapping activations in the medial orbitofrontal cortex in a region not activated by three unpleasant odours (hexanoic acid, octanol, and isovaleric acid) (Rolls, Kringelbach & De Araujo 2003c) (see Fig. 3.16). Moreover, activation of the medial orbitofrontal cortex was correlated with the subjective pleasantness ratings of the odours, and activation of the lateral orbitofrontal cortex with the subjective unpleasantness ratings of the odours (see Fig. 3.17). Other studies have also shown activation of the human orbitofrontal cortex by odour (Zatorre, Jones-Gotman, Evans & Meyer 1992, Zatorre, Jones-Gotman & Rouby 2000, Royet, Zald, Versace, Costes, Lavenne, Koenig, Gervais, Routtenberg, Gardner & Huang 2000, Anderson, Christoff, Stappen, Panitz, Ghahremani, Glover, Gabrieli & Sobel 2003, Grabenhorst, Rolls, Margot, da Silva & Velazco 2007, Rolls, Grabenhorst, Margot, da Silva & Velazco 2008a).

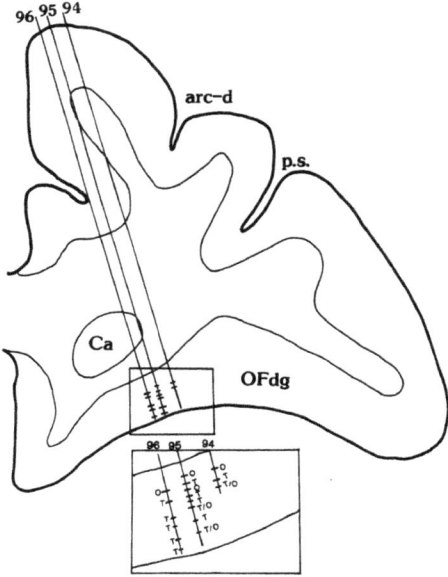

Fig. 3.18 Examples of tracks made into the orbitofrontal cortex in which taste (T) and olfactory (O) neurons were recorded close to each other in the same tracks. Some of the neurons were bimodal (T/O). arc-d, arcuate sulcus; Ca, head of Caudate nucleus; Ofdg, dysgranular part of the Orbitofrontal Cortex; p.s., principal sulcus. (Reproduced from E. T. Rolls and L. L. Baylis, Gustatory, olfactory and visual convergence within the primate orbitofrontal cortex, Journal of Neuroscience 14, pp. 5437–5452 © 1994, Society for Neuroscience.)

3.3.4 Encoding of olfactory information in the orbitofrontal cortex

Although individual neurons do not encode large amounts of information about which of 7–9 odours has been presented, we have shown that the information does increase linearly with the number of neurons in the sample (Rolls, Critchley & Treves 1996b, Rolls, Critchley, Verhagen & Kadohisa 2010a). This ensemble encoding does result in useful amounts of information about which odour has been presented being provided by orbitofrontal olfactory neurons.

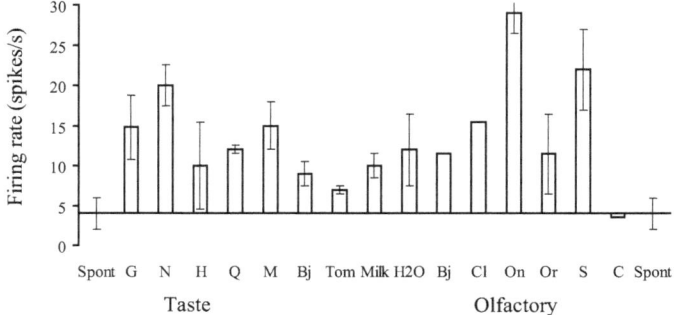

Fig. 3.19 The responses of a bimodal neuron with taste and olfactory responses recorded in the caudolateral orbitofrontal cortex. G, 1 M glucose; N, 0.1 M NaCl; H, 0.01 M HCl; Q, 0.001 M Quinine HCl; M, 0.1 M monosodium glutamate; Bj, 20% blackcurrant juice; Tom, tomato juice; B, banana odour; Cl, clove oil odour; On, onion odour; Or, orange odour; S, salmon odour; C, control no-odour presentation. The mean responses ± s.e.m. are shown. The neuron responded best to the savoury tastes of NaCl and monosodium glutamate and to the consonant odours of onion and salmon. (Reproduced from E. T. Rolls and L. L. Baylis, Gustatory, olfactory and visual convergence within the primate orbitofrontal cortex, Journal of Neuroscience 14, pp. 5437–5452 © 1994, Society for Neuroscience.)

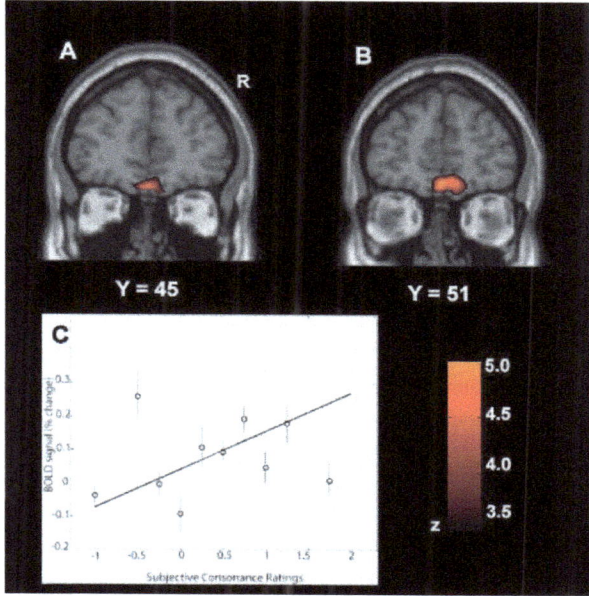

Fig. 3.20 Flavour formation in the human brain, shown by cross-modal olfactory–taste convergence. Brain areas where activations were correlated with the subjective ratings for stimulus (taste–odour) consonance and pleasantness. (A) A second-level, random effects analysis based on individual contrasts (the consonance ratings being the only effect of interest) revealed a significant activation in a medial part of the anterior orbitofrontal cortex. (B) Random effects analysis based on the pleasantness ratings showed a significant cluster of activation located in a (nearby) medial part of the anterior orbitofrontal cortex. The images were thresholded at p<0.0001 for illustration. (C) The relation between the BOLD signal from the cluster of voxels in the medial orbitofrontal cortex shown in (A) and the subjective consonance ratings. The analyses shown included all the stimuli included in this investigation. The means and standard errors of the mean across subjects are shown, together with the regression line, for which r=0.52. (Reproduced from Ivan E. T. De Araujo, Edmund T. Rolls, Morten L. Kringelbach, Francis McGlone, and Nicola Phillips, Taste-olfactory convergence, and the representation of the pleasantness of flavour, in the human brain, European Journal of Neuroscience, 18 (7) pp. 2059–2068 Copyright © 2003, John Wiley and Sons.)

The evidence described in this section shows that the positive and negative value of odour is represented in the orbitofrontal cortex on a continuous scale. Further evidence for this is described in Section 3.13, where it is also shown that in contrast a more anterior region in Tier 3 in Fig. 2.2, the medial prefrontal cortex area 10, is involved in the mechanisms that implement a choice or decision between odours of different value.

3.4 Convergence of taste and olfactory inputs in the orbitofrontal cortex: the representation of flavour

In the more medial and anterior parts of the orbitofrontal cortex, not only unimodal taste neurons, but also unimodal olfactory neurons are found (see Fig. 3.18). In addition some single neurons respond to both gustatory and olfactory stimuli, often with correspondence between the two modalities (Rolls & Baylis 1994) (see Fig. 3.19; cf. Fig. 2.2). It is probably here in the orbitofrontal cortex of primates that these two modalities converge to produce the representation of flavour (Rolls & Baylis 1994), and, consistent with this, neurons in the macaque primary taste cortex do not have olfactory responses (Verhagen, Kadohisa & Rolls 2004, Rolls 2016b).

Consistently, in a human fMRI investigation of olfactory and taste convergence in the brain, it was shown that there is a part of the human taste insula that is not activated by odour (De Araujo, Rolls, Kringelbach, McGlone & Phillips 2003c), though if a taste is recalled by an

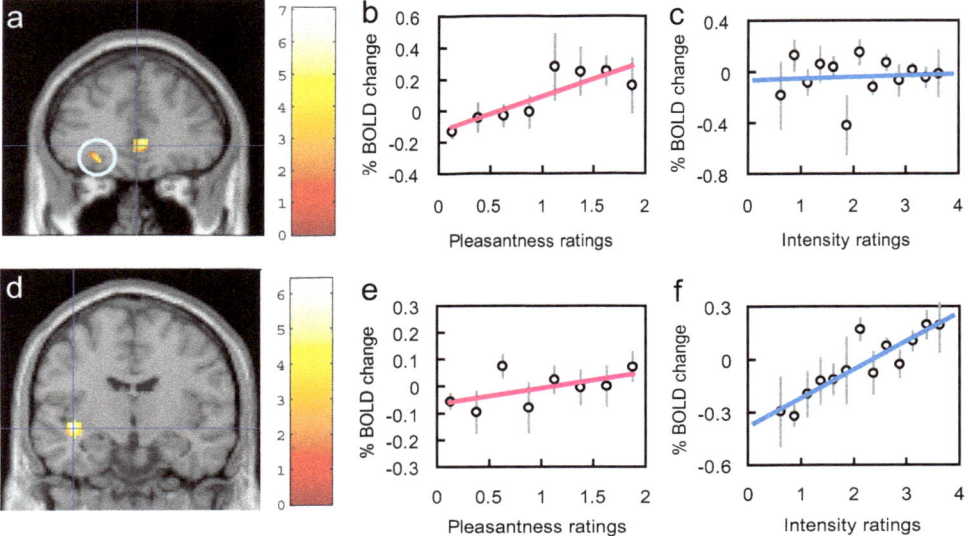

Fig. 3.21 Representation of the pleasantness but not intensity of thermal stimuli in the orbitofrontal cortex (top), and of the intensity but not the pleasantness in the mid ventral (somatosensory) insular cortex (bottom). a. SPM analysis showing a correlation in the mid orbitofrontal cortex (blue circle) at [-26 38 -10] between the BOLD signal and the pleasantness ratings of four thermal stimuli. Correlations are also shown in the pregenual cingulate cortex. For this mid orbitofrontal cortex region, (b) shows the positive correlation between the subjective pleasantness ratings and the BOLD signal (r=0.84, df=7, p<0.01), and (c) shows that there is no correlation between the subjective intensity ratings and the BOLD signal (r=0.07, df=12, p=0.8). d. SPM analysis showing a correlation with intensity in the posterior ventral insula with peak at [-40 -10 -8] between the BOLD signal and the intensity ratings for the four thermal stimuli. For this ventral insula cortex region, (e) shows no correlation between the subjective pleasantness ratings and the BOLD signal (r=0.56, df=7, p=0.15), and (f) shows a positive correlation between the subjective intensity ratings and the BOLD signal (r=0.89, df=12, p<0.001). (Reprinted from NeuroImage 41, Edmund T. Rolls, Fabian Grabenhorst and Benjamin A. Parris, Warm pleasant feelings in the brain, pp. 1504–1513, Copyright, 2008 with permission from Elsevier.)

odour the situation could be different because of the role of cortico-cortical backprojections in recall (Rolls 2016c, Rolls 2016b). The evidence described above (Section 3.3) indicates that these bimodal representations are built by olfactory–gustatory association learning, an example of stimulus–reinforcer association learning.

The human orbitofrontal cortex also reflects the convergence of taste and olfactory inputs, as shown for example by the fact that activations in the human medial orbitofrontal cortex are correlated with both the cross-modal consonance of combined taste and olfactory stimuli (high for example for sweet taste and strawberry odour), as well as for the pleasantness of the combinations, as shown in Fig. 3.20 (De Araujo, Rolls, Kringelbach, McGlone & Phillips 2003c). In addition, the combination of monosodium glutamate taste and a consonant savoury odour produced a supralinear effect in the medial orbitofrontal cortex to produce the rich delicious flavour of umami that makes many foods pleasant that are rich in protein (McCabe & Rolls 2007, Rolls 2009b).

3.5 Somatosensory and temperature inputs to the orbitofrontal cortex, and affective value

In addition to the oral somatosensory and temperature inputs to the orbitofrontal cortex, there are also somatosensory inputs from other parts of the body, and indeed an fMRI investigation we have performed in humans indicates that pleasant and painful touch stimuli to the hand produce greater activation of the orbitofrontal cortex relative to the somatosensory cortex than do affectively neutral stimuli (Francis et al. 1999, Rolls, O'Doherty, Kringelbach, Francis, Bowtell & McGlone 2003d). The activation of parts of the orbitofrontal cortex by painful stimuli is likely to have great clinical relevance, for orbitofrontal cortex damage results in individuals knowing that a painful stimulus is being applied, but not feeling the strong negative affective component, of subjective pain, as described in Chapter 1. The clinical relevance of these discoveries in relation to pain pathways and pain treatment appears to be under-appreciated at present.

Non-glabrous skin such as that on the forearm contains C fibre tactile afferents that respond to light moving touch (Olausson, Wessberg & McGlone 2016). The orbitofrontal cortex is implicated in some of the affectively pleasant aspects of touch that may be mediated through C fibre tactile afferents, in that it is activated more by light touch to the forearm than by light touch to the glabrous skin (palm) of the hand (McCabe, Rolls, Bilderbeck & McGlone 2008, Rolls 2010b, Rolls 2016a).

Warm and cold stimuli have affective components such as feeling pleasant or unpleasant, and these components may have survival value, for approach to warmth and avoidance of cold may be reinforcers or goals for action built into us during evolution to direct our behaviour to stimuli that are appropriate for survival. Understanding the brain processing that underlies these prototypical reinforcers provides a direct approach to understanding the brain mechanisms of emotion. In an fMRI investigation in humans, it was found that the mid-orbitofrontal and pregenual cingulate cortex and the ventral striatum have activations that are correlated with the subjective pleasantness ratings made to warm (41C) and cold (12C) stimuli, and combinations of warm and cold stimuli, applied to the hand (Rolls, Grabenhorst & Parris 2008b) (see Fig. 3.21a-c). Activations in the lateral and some more anterior parts of the orbitofrontal cortex were correlated with the unpleasantness of the stimuli. In contrast, activations in the somatosensory cortex and ventral posterior insula were correlated with the intensity but not the pleasantness of the thermal stimuli (see Fig. 3.21d-f).

A principle thus is that processing related to the affective value and associated subjective emotional experience of thermal stimuli that are important for survival is performed in different brain areas to those where activations are related to sensory properties of the stimuli such as their intensity. This conclusion appears to be the case for processing in a number of sensory modalities, including taste and olfaction (see above), and the finding with such prototypical stimuli as warm and cold (Rolls et al. 2008b) provides strong support for this principle (Rolls 2014a, Rolls 2017c, Rolls 2018b).

3.6 Visual inputs to the orbitofrontal cortex, and visual stimulus–reinforcer association learning and reversal to compute expected value

3.6.1 The representation of the expected value of visual stimuli

We have been able to show that there is a major visual input to many neurons in the orbitofrontal cortex, and that what is represented by these neurons is in many cases the reinforcer (reward or punisher) association of visual stimuli. Many of these neurons reflect the relative preference or reward value of different visual stimuli, in that their responses decrease to zero to the sight of one food on which the monkey is being fed to satiety, but remain unchanged to the sight of other food stimuli. In this sense the visual reinforcement-related neurons predict the reward value that is available from the primary reinforcer, the taste. The visual input is from the ventral, temporal lobe, visual stream concerned with 'what' object is being seen, in that orbitofrontal visual neurons frequently respond differentially to objects or images (but

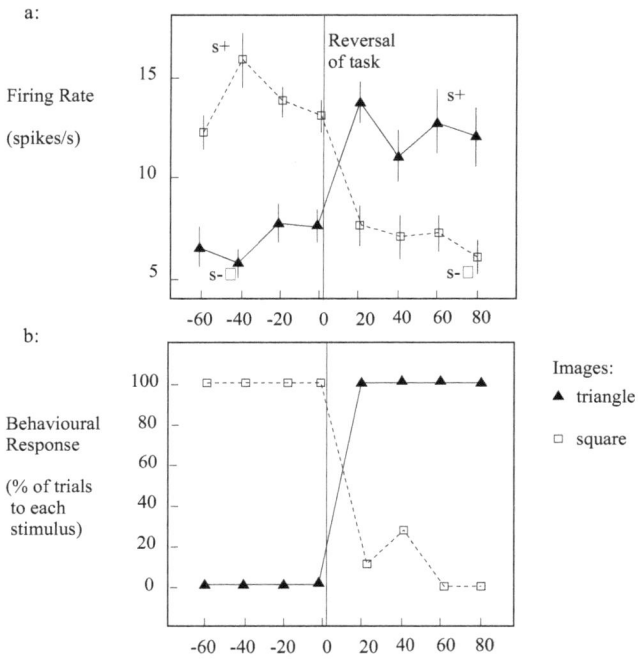

Fig. 3.22 Orbitofrontal cortex: visual discrimination reversal. The activity of an orbitofrontal visual neuron during performance of a visual discrimination task and its reversal. The stimuli were a triangle and a square presented on a video monitor. (a) Each point represents the mean poststimulus activity in a 500 ms period of the neuron based on approximately 10 trials of the different visual stimuli. The standard errors of these responses are shown. After 60 trials of the task the reward associations of the visual stimuli were reversed. s+ indicates that a lick response to that visual stimulus produces fruit juice reward; s− indicates that a lick response to that visual stimulus results in a small drop of aversive tasting saline. This neuron reversed its responses to the visual stimuli following the task reversal. (b) The behavioural response of the monkey to the task. It is shown that the monkey performs well, in that he rapidly learns to lick only to the visual stimulus associated with fruit juice reward. (Reproduced from Journal of Neurophysiology, 75 (5), Orbitofrontal cortex neurons: role in olfactory and visual association learning, E. T. Rolls, H. D. Critchley, R. Mason, and E. A. Wakeman, pp. 1970–1981, © 1996, The American Physiological Society.)

depending on their reward association) (Thorpe, Rolls & Maddison 1983, Rolls, Critchley, Mason & Wakeman 1996a). The primary reinforcer that has been used is taste.

The fact that these neurons represent the reinforcer associations of visual stimuli and hence the expected value has been shown to be the case in formal investigations of the activity of orbitofrontal cortex visual neurons, which in many cases reverse their responses to visual stimuli when the taste with which the visual stimulus is associated is reversed by the experimenter (Thorpe, Rolls & Maddison 1983, Rolls, Critchley, Mason & Wakeman 1996a). An example of the responses of an orbitofrontal cortex neuron that reversed the visual stimulus to which it responded during reward reversal is shown in Fig. 3.22.

This reversal by orbitofrontal visual neurons can be very fast, in as little as one trial, that is a few seconds (see for example Fig. 3.23). The significance of the visual stimulus, a syringe from which the monkey was fed, was altered during the trials. On trials 1–5, no response of the neuron occurred to the sight of the syringe from which the monkey had been given glucose solution to drink from the syringe on the preceding trials. On trials 6–9, the neuron responded to the sight of the same syringe from which he had been given aversive hypertonic saline drink on the preceding trial. Two more reversals (trials 10–15, and 16–17) were performed. The reversal of the neuron's response when the significance of the visual stimulus was reversed shows that the responses of the neuron only occurred to the stimulus when it was associated with aversive saline and not when it was associated with glucose reward.

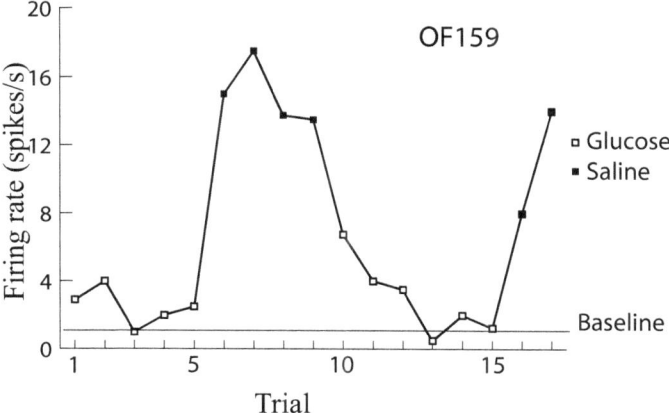

Fig. 3.23 Orbitofrontal cortex: one-trial visual discrimination reversal by a neuron. On trials 1–5, no response of the neuron occurred to the sight of a 2 ml syringe from which the monkey had been given orally glucose solution to drink on the previous trial. On trials 6–9, the neuron responded to the sight of the same syringe from which he had been given aversive hypertonic saline to drink on the previous trial. Two more reversals (trials 10–15, and 16–17) were performed. The reversal of the neuron's response when the significance of the same visual stimulus was reversed shows that the responses of the neuron only occurred to the sight of the visual stimulus when it was associated with a positively reinforcing and not with a negatively reinforcing taste. Moreover, it is shown that the neuronal reversal took only one trial. (Reproduced from Experimental Brain Research, 49 (1) pp. 93–115, The orbitofrontal cortex: Neuronal activity in the behaving monkey, S. J. Thorpe, E. T. Rolls, and S. Maddison (c) 1983, Springer Science and Business Media. With kind permission from Springer Science and Business Media.)

3.6.2 Visual reversal to compute expected value can be rapid and rule-based in primates including humans

It is of great importance for understanding the functions of the primate including human orbitofrontal cortex that this reward reversal learning can be very fast, in one trial. This is shown by the fact that after an expected reward was not obtained due to a reversal contingency being applied, on the very next trial the macaque selected the previously non-rewarded stimulus. This occurred despite the fact that the stimulus now chosen had been previously associated with punishment. This shows that rapid reversal can be performed by a non-associative process, and must be rule-based. The primate must learn the rule that if one stimulus is not longer reward, then the other stimulus will be rewarded on the next trial. More generally, if a stimulus is no longer rewarded, then behaviour should change to another stimulus. This is of great adaptive value for many aspects of primate (including human) behaviour, including social behaviour, in which it may be appropriate to adjust behaviour after even a subtle change in reinforcing feedback (outcome) is received. An example of this demonstrated in an fMRI study is shown in Fig. 3.47. A model for this rule-based reversal is the subject of Section 9.4. This rapid stimulus-reward learning and reversal, so important in primate behaviour, has not been demonstrated in rodents as far as I know, and may be one of the fundamental advances provided for by the great evolution of the primate including human orbitofrontal cortex, especially in the context of the representations of social reinforcers that are described in Section 3.6.5.

These neurons thus reflect the information about which stimulus is currently associated with reward during reversals of visual discrimination tasks – they are reward predicting neurons, that is, they represent *expected value*. If a reversal occurs, then the taste cells provide the outcome information that an unexpected taste reinforcer has been obtained, another group of cells shows a vigorous discharge that reflects the error between the expected reward value and the reward outcome actually obtained (see below), and the visual cells with reinforcer association-related responses reverse the stimulus to which they are responsive. These neurophysiological changes take place rapidly, in as little as 5 s, and are part of the neuronal learning mechanism that enables primates to alter their knowledge of the reinforcer association of visual stimuli so rapidly. This capacity is important whenever behaviour must be corrected when expected reinforcers are not obtained, in, for example, feeding, emotional, and social situations (see Chapter 6) (Rolls 2014a, Rolls 2018b, Kringelbach & Rolls 2003). In that these neurons reflect whether a visual stimulus is associated with reward or a punisher, they reflect the relative preference for different stimuli, i.e. the value (Thorpe, Rolls & Maddison 1983, Rolls, Critchley, Mason & Wakeman 1996a) (as found also by Tremblay & Schultz (1999)). Consistent with this evidence that the responses of some orbitofrontal cortex neurons reflect the learned predictive reward value of visual stimuli, Thorpe, Rolls & Maddison (1983) and Tremblay & Schultz (2000) found that orbitofrontal cortex neurons learned to respond differently to new stimuli that did or did not predict reward. Different neurons in the orbitofrontal cortex are tuned to different learned or conditioned reinforcers, with for example approximately 5% responding to visual stimuli associated with taste reward, and 3% to visual stimuli associated with taste punishment (see Table 3.3 on page 77) (Thorpe, Rolls & Maddison 1983, Rolls, Critchley, Mason & Wakeman 1996a).

Although using a somewhat different test situation, classical conditioning, Saez, Saez, Paton, Lau & Salzman (2017) found consistent evidence: they found that neuronal responses to reward-predictive cues update more rapidly in the macaque orbitofrontal cortex than amygdala, and activity in the orbitofrontal cortex but not the amygdala was modulated by recent reward history.

3.6.3 Visual stimulus-selective expected value neurons

In the visual discrimination reversal task, a second class of neuron was found that codes for particular stimuli only if they are associated with reward, and not if they are associated with punishment. Such a neuron might respond to a green stimulus associated with reward; after reversal not respond to the green stimulus when it was associated with punishment; and not respond to a blue stimulus irrespective of whether it was associated with reward or punishment (Thorpe, Rolls & Maddison 1983) (see example in Fig. 3.24). They may be described as *conditional visual stimulus-to-taste reward neurons* or *conditional expected value neurons* (Rolls et al. 1996a), and are analogous to their olfactory counterparts described above in Section 3.3 (Rolls et al. 1996a). These neurons are probably important in the mechanisms that implement rapid reversal, as described in Section 9.4. More generally, they are part of a mechanism that enables the orbitofrontal cortex to specify individual objects or individuals who may be currently associated with reward, or not.

In addition to selectivity for which stimulus or class of stimulus is currently associated with reward, the fact that many different types of primary reinforcer are present in the orbitofrontal cortex enables it to represent the expected value of many different types of primary reinforcer.

The proportions of neurons showing reversal, or conditional visual stimulus–reinforcer related responses, are shown in Table 3.1. Most visual neurons showed full or conditional reversal, while the proportion of olfactory neurons (see Section 3.3) was lower (Rolls, Critchley, Mason & Wakeman 1996a).

This reversal learning found in orbitofrontal cortex neurons probably is implemented in the orbitofrontal cortex, for it does not occur one synapse earlier in the visual inferior temporal cortex (Rolls, Judge & Sanghera 1977), and it is in the orbitofrontal cortex that there is convergence of visual and taste pathways on to the same neurons (Thorpe, Rolls & Maddison 1983, Rolls, Critchley, Mason & Wakeman 1996a).

A possible mechanism for this learning is Hebbian modification of synapses conveying visual input on to taste-responsive neurons, implementing a pattern-association network (Rolls 2016c) (Section 9.1). In this model the unconditioned stimulus forcing the output neurons to

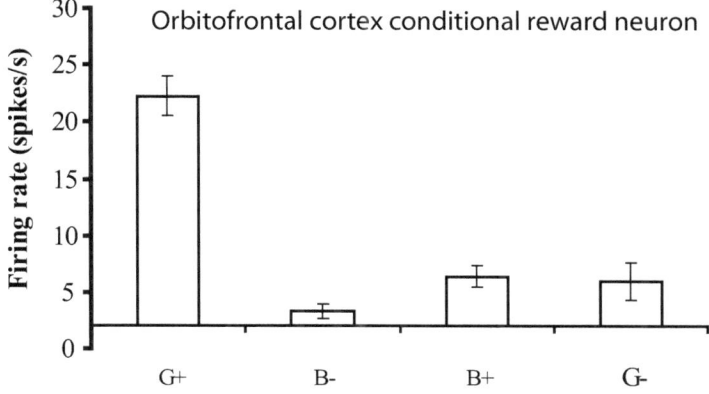

Fig. 3.24 A conditional reward neuron recorded in the orbitofrontal cortex which responded only to the Green stimulus when it was associated with reward (G+), and not to the Blue stimulus when it was associated with Reward (B+), or to either stimuli when they were associated with a punisher, the taste of salt (G– and B–). The mean firing rate ± the s.e.m. is shown. (Reproduced from Experimental Brain Research, 49 (1) pp. 93–115, The orbitofrontal cortex: Neuronal activity in the behaving monkey, S. J. Thorpe, E. T. Rolls, and S. Maddison, (c) 1983, Springer Science and Business Media. With kind permission from Springer Science and Business Media.)

Table 3.1 Proportion of neurons in the primate orbitofrontal cortex showing reversal, or conditional reversal (ceasing to discriminate or ceasing to respond after the reversal), or no change of responses, during visual or olfactory discrimination reversal. (Reproduced from Journal of Neurophysiology, 75 (5), Orbitofrontal cortex neurons: role in olfactory and visual association learning, E. T. Rolls, H. D. Critchley, R. Mason, E. A. Wakeman, pp. 1970–81 © 1996, The American Physiological Society.)

	Olfactory cells Number	%	Visual cells Number	%
Reversal	7	25.0	12	70.6
Conditional reversal	12	42.9	4	23.5
No change	9	32.1	1	5.9
Total	28	100.0	17	100.0

respond is the (taste) primary reinforcer, and the (visual or olfactory) conditioned stimulus becomes associated with this by associatively modifiable synapses) (Rolls & Treves 1998, Rolls 1999a, Rolls 2016c). Such a pattern association network could in principle unlearn the association by using associative synapses that incorporate long-term depression (Rolls & Treves 1998, Rolls 2016c). Although reversal might be implemented by having long-term synaptic depression (LTD) for synapses that represented the reward-associated stimulus before the reversal, and long-term potentiation (LTP) of the synapses activated by the new stimulus that after reversal is associated with reward, this would require one-trial LTP and one-trial heterosynaptic LTD to account for one-trial stimulus–reward reversal (Thorpe, Rolls & Maddison 1983, Rolls, Critchley, Mason & Wakeman 1996a, Rolls 2000a). To implement the reversal learning very rapidly, in as little as one trial after a number of reversals when reversal learning set has been acquired, a special switching network that uses a rule in the orbitofrontal cortex may be required, and a model of this (Deco & Rolls 2005a) is described in Section 9.4.

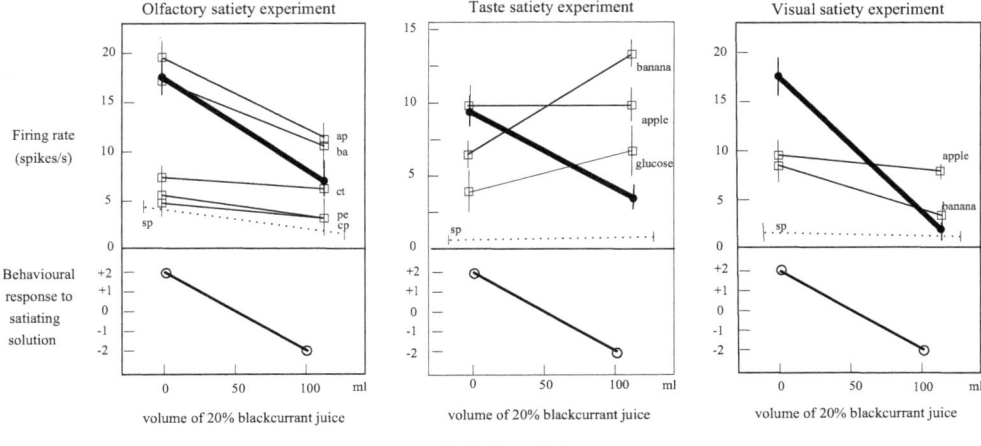

Fig. 3.25 Orbitofrontal cortex neuron with visual, olfactory and taste responses, showing the responses before and after feeding to satiety with blackcurrant juice. The solid circles show the responses to blackcurrant juice. The olfactory stimuli included apple (ap), banana (ba), citral (ct), phenylethanol (pe), and caprylic acid (cp). The spontaneous firing rate of the neuron is shown (sp). (Reproduced from Journal of Neurophysiology, 75 (4), Hunger and satiety modify the responses of olfactory and visual neurons in the primate orbitofrontal cortex, H. D. Critchley and E. T. Rolls pp. 1673–1886, © 1996, The American Physiological Society.)

3.6.4 Devaluation shows that orbitofrontal cortex visual neurons represent expected value

Another way in which it has been shown that the visual neurons in the orbitofrontal cortex reflect the expected value predicted by visual stimuli is by reducing the reward value by feeding to satiety in devaluation experiments. With this sensory-specific satiety (or reward devaluation) paradigm, it has been shown that the visual (as well as the olfactory and taste) responses of orbitofrontal cortex neurons in the macaque decrease to zero as the monkey is fed to satiety with one food, but remain unchanged to another food not eaten in the meal (Critchley & Rolls 1996c) (see example in Fig. 3.25). In that these neurons parallel the changing preference of the monkey for the food being eaten to satiety vs the food not being eaten to satiety, they reflect the relative preference for different visual stimuli, that is the expected value (Thorpe, Rolls & Maddison 1983, Rolls, Critchley, Mason & Wakeman 1996a) (as found also by Tremblay & Schultz (1999) and Wallis & Miller (2003)).

Further evidence that these orbitofrontal cortex neurons encode expected value is that they represent choices made when the 'offers' (the visual stimuli) are different amounts or different qualities of the 'goods' (for example the type of fruit juice that is the reward outcome of the choice) and different probabilities of obtaining reward), as described in Section 3.12 (Padoa-Schioppa & Assad 2006, Padoa-Schioppa 2011, Nymberg, Jia, Lubbe, Ruggeri, Desrivieres, Barker, Buchel, Fauth-Buehler, Cattrell, Conrod, Flor, Gallinat, Garavan, Heinz, Ittermann, Lawrence, Mann, Nees, Salatino-Oliveira, Paillere Martinot, Paus, Rietschel, Robbins, Smolka, Banaschewski, Rubia, Loth, Schumann & Consortium 2013, Padoa-Schioppa & Conen 2017).

All this evidence shows that the great majority of neurons in the orbitofrontal cortex encode stimuli, frequently in terms of the (outcome) value or expected value, and do not reflect the actions or responses or spatial responses being performed by the macaques (Thorpe, Rolls & Maddison 1983, Rolls, Critchley, Mason & Wakeman 1996a, Critchley & Rolls 1996c, Rolls & Baylis 1994, Rolls 2014a, Wallis & Miller 2003, Padoa-Schioppa & Assad 2006, Grattan & Glimcher 2014). Indeed, most orbitofrontal cortex neurons that we have recorded do not respond in relation to movements or action (such as the lick instrumental responses made in a visual discrimination task), and in this sense reflect the value of sensory stimuli, though some do respond to oral or perioral somatosensory stimuli (Thorpe et al. 1983, Rolls et al. 1996a, Critchley & Rolls 1996c, Rolls & Baylis 1994, Rolls 2014a). Consistent with this, orbitofrontal cortex neurons were found to respond to rewards but not to the eye movements being made to obtain the rewards (Grattan & Glimcher 2014). These findings are consistent with the hypothesis that expected reward value is represented in the orbitofrontal cortex, reflects stimulus–reinforcer (sensory–sensory) association learning, and that this information is projected to other structures such as the cingulate cortex for action–outcome learning (Section 5.1), or to the basal ganglia for stimulus-response habit learning (Section 5.2). Outputs of the orbitofrontal cortex to the dorsolateral prefrontal cortex may be used in tasks requiring planning, for example where rewarding stimuli must be flexibly linked to particular responses, and where delays may be involved, in ways that have been modelled by Deco & Rolls (2003) and Deco & Rolls (2005a).

Given that reward value and not action is implemented in the orbitofrontal cortex, it is an interesting further question about whether the reward value represented in the orbitofrontal cortex is influenced by the costs of actions. Some evidence for this was that in the macaque orbitofrontal cortex, some (but not other) neurons responded less to an expected reward if the cost involved in obtaining it was high (Cai & Padoa-Schioppa 2019). The neurons that represent value independently of cost are important, for in a sense they represent the absolute value of the good, which is necessary for long-term economic choice. The neurons that have their value representation affected by the cost of the action to obtain the reward correspond more to relative value representations, which may be useful to guide choice in the current session especially when the costs for different rewards are altered (see further Section 3.12.3).

In summary, different orbitofrontal cortex neurons are tuned to respond to different stimuli that are primary reinforcers and encode *outcome value*, such as different tastes, different viscosities, oral fat texture (Thorpe et al. 1983, Rolls et al. 1999, Rolls et al. 1990, Verhagen et al. 2003, Rolls et al. 2003e, Kadohisa et al. 2005b, Rolls et al. 2018d), different somatosensory stimuli (Thorpe et al. 1983, Kadohisa et al. 2004) (including in human fMRI studies pleasant and painful touch (Rolls et al. 2003d, McCabe et al. 2008)), different combinations of these with odours to form flavours (Critchley & Rolls 1996b, Rolls et al. 1996a) (cf. (McCabe & Rolls 2007)), and, as shown below, to face expression and identity (Rolls, Critchley, Browning & Inoue 2006a) (important in social contexts), and to novel visual stimuli (Rolls, Browning, Inoue & Hernadi 2005a) (which can be rewarding). The majority of these (and visual and olfactory) neurons reflect value, in that devaluation, for example by feeding to satiety, decreases their responses to zero (Rolls et al. 1989, Critchley & Rolls 1996c, Rolls et al. 1999). Some neurons in the orbitofrontal cortex can perform very rapid learning of associations between visual stimuli and reinforcers, in one trial (Thorpe et al. 1983). These visual neurons can reverse these reinforcer associations in one trial in what must be a rule-based reversal, in that the neurons and the macaques after a reward has not been delivered to a previously rewarded stimulus switch their encoding so that the previously punished stimulus becomes treated as a reward on the very next trial before that visual stimulus has been followed by a reward outcome (Thorpe et al. 1983). These visual and olfactory neurons encode *expected value*. This very rapid, rule-based, learning, is likely to be very important in human social behaviour and cooperation, in which great sensitivity to the reinforcers being received, and an ability to adjust the reward value of incoming stimuli, for example in social interactions, is very important and adaptive.

Similar results have been described by others (Tremblay & Schultz 1999). Different orbitofrontal cortex neurons increased their firing in relation to reward expectation, and after the receipt of rewards (presumably taste / oral texture reward outcome neurons). Many of

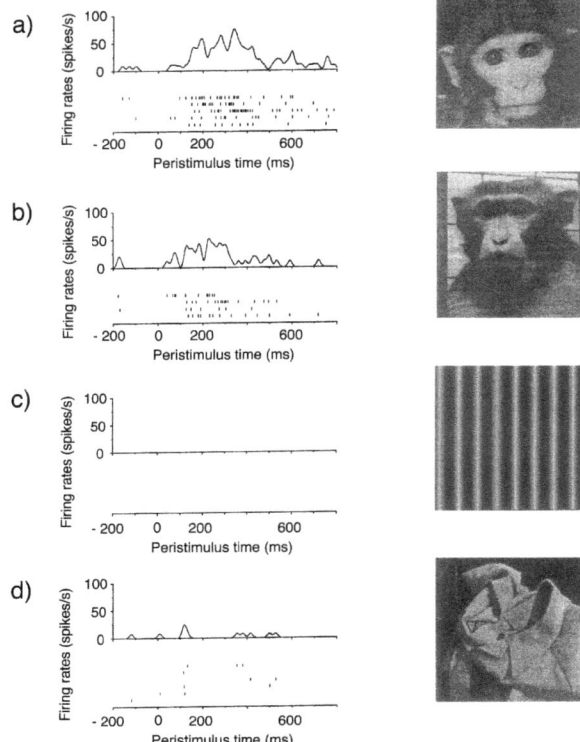

Fig. 3.26 Orbitofrontal cortex face-selective neuron as found in macaques. Peristimulus rastergrams and time histograms are shown. Each trial is a row in the rastergram. Several trials for each stimulus are shown. The ordinate is in spikes/s. The neuron responded best to face (a), also responded, though less to face (b), had different responses to other faces (not shown), and did not respond to non-face stimuli (e.g. (c) and (d)). The stimulus appeared at time 0 on a video monitor. (Reproduced from Experimental Brain Research, 170 (1) pp. 743–87, Face-selective and auditory neurons in the primate orbitofrontal cortex, Rolls, E. T., Critchley, H. D., Browning, A. S. and Inoue, K., (c) 2006, Springer Science and Business Media. With kind permission from Springer Science and Business Media.)

the neurons responded in relation to more preferred rewards (which of course is shown during sensory-specific satiety reward devaluation), and not in relation to movements. Visual stimulus to reward outcome learning by orbitofrontal cortex neurons has also been confirmed (Tremblay & Schultz 2000).

3.6.5 A representation of faces and social stimuli in the orbitofrontal cortex

Another type of information represented in the orbitofrontal cortex is information about faces (Rolls, Critchley, Browning & Inoue 2006a). There is a population of orbitofrontal cortex face-selective neurons that respond in many ways similarly to those in the temporal cortical visual areas (Rolls 1984, Rolls 1992b, Rolls 2000b, Rolls 2007a, Rolls 2008c, Rolls 2011a, Rolls 2012d, Rolls 2016c). The orbitofrontal face-responsive neurons, first observed by Thorpe, Rolls & Maddison (1983), then by Rolls, Critchley, Browning & Inoue (2006a), tend to respond with longer latencies than temporal lobe neurons (140–200 ms typically, compared with 80–100 ms); they also convey information about which face is being seen, by having different responses to different faces (see Fig. 3.26); and are typically rather harder to activate strongly than temporal cortical face-selective neurons, in that many of them respond much better to real faces than to two-dimensional images of faces on a video monitor (cf.

Expected value of visual stimuli | 53

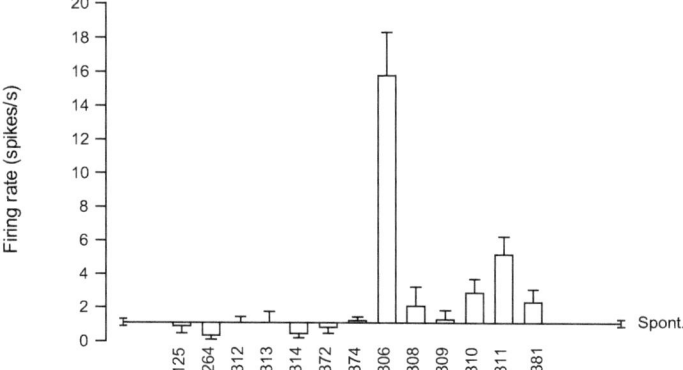

Fig. 3.27 Orbitofrontal cortex face-selective neuron tuned to face identity in the macaque. Firing rate histogram of cell be009 to different face stimuli (306-311 and 381) and different non-face stimuli (125, 264, 312, 313, 314, 372 and 374). Stimuli 305–308 and 381 were macaque faces with different identities, 309-311 were human face stimuli with different identities, and the other stimuli were different non-face stimuli (25=hand, 372=triangle, 374=saline-associated square, 312 - Fourier boundary curvature descriptor, 313 grating, 314 shirt). The means and standard error of the mean (sem) of the responses in spikes/s are shown as changes from the spontaneous rate (Spont).) (Reproduced from Experimental Brain Research, 170 (1) pp. 743–87, Face-selective and auditory neurons in the primate orbitofrontal cortex, Rolls, E. T., Critchley, H. D., Browning, A. S. and Inoue, K., (c) 2006, Springer Science and Business Media. With kind permission from Springer Science and Business Media.)

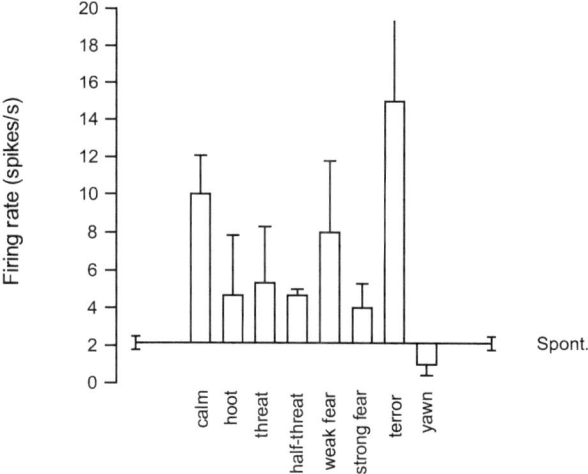

Fig. 3.28 Orbitofrontal cortex face-selective neuron tuned to face expression in the macaque. A firing rate histogram of cell aq045 to different face expressions is shown. The means and standard error of the mean (sem) of the responses in spikes/s are shown as changes from the spontaneous rate (Spont).) (Reproduced from Experimental Brain Research, 170 (1) pp. 743–87, Face-selective and auditory neurons in the primate orbitofrontal cortex, Rolls, E. T., Critchley, H. D., Browning, A. S. and Inoue, K., (c) 2006, Springer Science and Business Media. With kind permission from Springer Science and Business Media.)

Rolls & Baylis (1986)). As shown in Fig 3.27, some orbitofrontal cortex neurons respond to face identity.

Other orbitofrontal cortex face-selective neurons are tuned to the emotional expression of a face, as illustrated in Fig. 3.28.

We hypothesized that both face identity and face expression information is represented in the macaque orbitofrontal cortex because it is important to take into account both the identity of the individual and the expression on a face in order to produce an appropriate emotional response to a face (Rolls et al. 2006a).

Information about the category of the individual, such as whether the individual is juvenile, as well as face expression and identity, may also be useful to determine the appropriate responses to a face. This type of information about category is also present in the orbitofrontal cortex. This was shown in an investigation in which face stimuli of young, male, female etc macaques were shown while recording from orbitofrontal cortex neurons. Using a method described by Rolls, Lu, Wan, Yan, Wang, Yang, Tan, Li, Group, Yu, Liddle, Palaniyappan, Zhang, Yue & Feng (2017), k-means analysis was performed on the neuronal responses to the set of stimuli to determine how the orbitofrontal cortex neurons categorised the set of stimuli, and then a correlation matrix was formed to show the categories (Barat, Wirth & Duhamel 2018). The results are shown in Fig. 3.29 (Barat, Wirth & Duhamel 2018). Cluster 1 comprised seven pictures of young monkeys. Cluster 2 was almost exclusively composed of threat and grin face expressions (five threats, six grins). Cluster 3 was composed of lip smack face expressions, and cluster 4 contained several mouth expressions (three lip smack, three threats, and one grin). These results confirm the results of Rolls et al. (2006a) that face expressions are represented by some orbitofrontal cortex neurons, but add that categories such as young faces are also represented (Barat, Wirth & Duhamel 2018). In another study, it was reported that some orbitofrontal cortex face-selective neurons are sensitive to the rank of the individual being viewed in the social hierarchy, with neurons also reflecting social hierarchy in the amygdala and anterior cingulate cortex (Munuera, Rigotti & Salzman 2018).

Some of the orbitofrontal cortex face-selective neurons are responsive to face gesture or movement, as illustrated in Fig. 3.30 (Rolls et al. 2006a). Such neurons are very likely to be involved in social situations, when for example the turn of a head towards or away from the viewer may have great social significance.

The discovery of face-selective neurons in the primate orbitofrontal cortex is consistent with the likelihood that these neurons are activated via the inputs from the temporal cortical visual areas in which face-selective neurons are found (see Fig. 2.2). The significance of the neurons is likely to be related to the fact that faces convey information that is important in social reinforcement, both by conveying face expression (cf. Hasselmo, Rolls & Baylis (1989a)), which can indicate reinforcement, and by encoding information about which individual is present, also important in evaluating and utilizing reinforcing inputs in social situations (Rolls, Critchley, Browning & Inoue 2006a, Rolls 2011a).

Consistent with these findings in macaques, and as described above, in humans, activation of the lateral orbitofrontal cortex occurs when a rewarding smile expression is expected, but an angry face expression is obtained, in a visual discrimination reversal task (Kringelbach & Rolls 2003). This is an example of the operation of a social reinforcer, and, consistent with these results, Farrow, Zheng, Wilkinson, Spence, Deakin, Tarrier, Griffiths & Woodruff (2001) have found that activation of the orbitofrontal cortex is found when humans are making social judgements. In addition, activation of the medial orbitofrontal cortex is correlated with face attractiveness (O'Doherty, Winston, Critchley, Perrett, Burt & Dolan 2003).

These orbitofrontal cortex face-selective neurons are frequently found close to the lateral orbitofrontal sulcus (Rolls, Critchley, Browning & Inoue 2006a), and are visible, as expected, with fMRI (area PO) (D'Urso, Dell'Osso, Rossi, Brunoni, Bortolomasi, Ferrucci, Priori, de Bartolomeis & Altamura 2017). Face selective neurons have also been found in the inferior prefrontal cortex below the principal sulcus (O'Scalaidhe, Wilson & Goldman-Rakic 1997, Romanski & Diehl 2011, Diehl & Romanski 2014) (area PL), and in the anterior bank of the arcuate sulcus (O'Scalaidhe et al. 1997) (area PA).

We also discovered that some orbitofrontal cortex neurons are activated by auditory stimuli, such as vocalization (Fig. 3.31 (Rolls, Critchley, Browning & Inoue 2006a). This has been confirmed (Plakke & Romanski 2014), and indeed in the ventrolateral prefrontal cortex (which includes areas 12, 45, and 44) neurons may be tuned to the type of call or to the identity of the caller (Plakke, Diltz & Romanski 2013, Plakke & Romanski 2014).

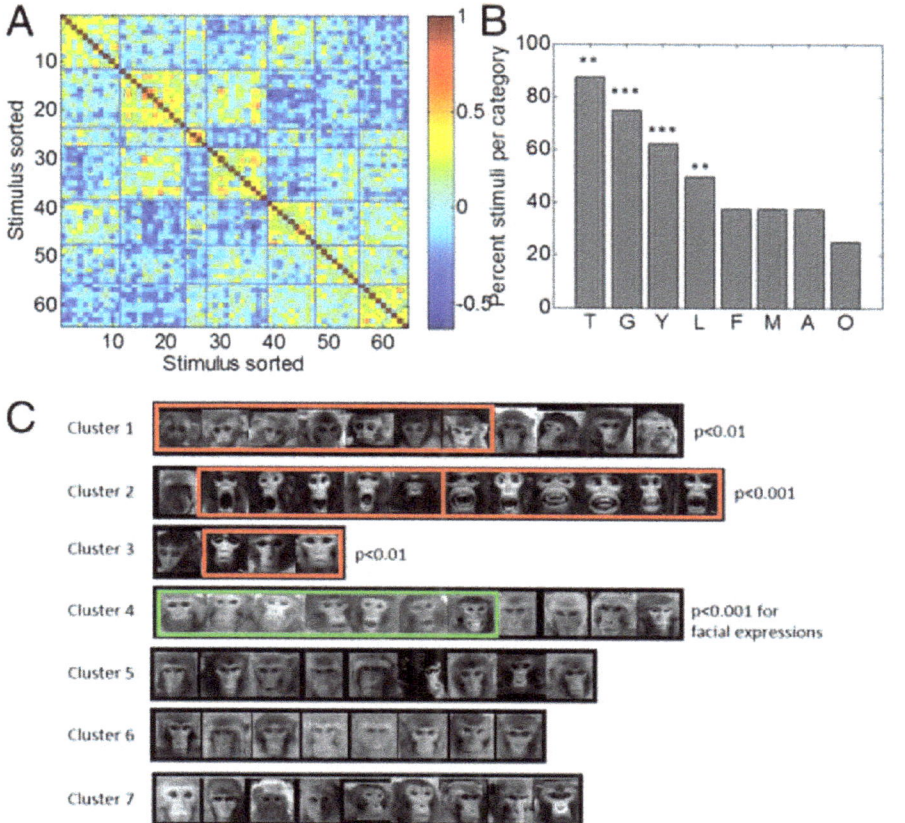

Fig. 3.29 Orbitofrontal cortex neuron tuned to different categories of faces. Unsupervised cluster analysis on the face stimuli. (A) Cross-correlation matrix with stimuli sorted with respect to stimuli cluster assignment. (B) Percent of stimuli for each prelabeled category that were grouped together in the unsupervised cluster analysis. The prelabeled categories included T–threat, G–grin, Y–young, L–lip smack, F–female, M–male, A–averted, O–old. (C) Actual photos corresponding to the stimuli (1-64) for each cluster shown in A. The red rectangles highlight the stimulus groupings that are above chance with eight categories of eight stimuli. The green rectangle highlights the stimulus grouping above chance when all facial expressions are grouped. Black rectangles surround images whose cluster was not significant. (Reproduced from Elodie Barat, Sylvia Wirth, and Jean-Rene Duhamel, Face cells in orbitofrontal cortex represent social categories, Proceedings of the National Academy of Sciences, 115 (47), E11158–E11167, doi.org/10.1073/pnas.1806165115 /copyright 2018 Barat, Wirth, and Duhamel. This work is licensed under the Creative Commons Attribution License (CC BY). It is attributed to the authors Barat, Wirth, and Duhamel.)

Neurons in this ventrolateral prefrontal cortex region can also be influenced by the sight or the sound of a vocalization, and by mismatches between these (Diehl & Romanski 2014). Auditory stimuli may have similar representations in the orbitofrontal cortex related to their affective value. For example, Blood, Zatorre, Bermudez & Evans (1999) found a correlation between subjective ratings of dissonance and consonance of musical chords and the activations produced in the orbitofrontal cortex (see also Blood & Zatorre (2001) and Frey, Kostopoulos & Petrides (2000)). The transition of harmony towards a pleasant resolution also activates the orbitofrontal cortex (Fujisawa & Cook 2011).

In one study in a social situation it was found that neurons in the macaque orbitofrontal cortex predominantly encoded rewards that were delivered to the self (Chang, Gariepy & Platt 2013). But in a social situation in which rewards were given to the self and to another monkey, some orbitofrontal cortex neurons reflected not only the value of the reward, but also the identity and social status of the other monkey (Azzi, Sirigu & Duhamel 2012).

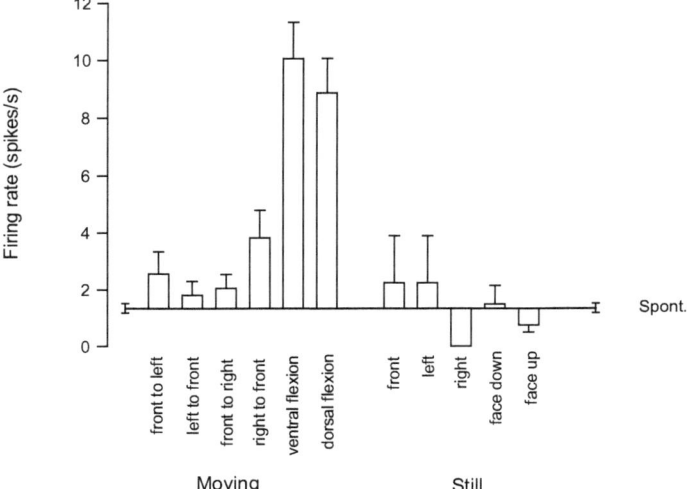

Fig. 3.30 Orbitofrontal cortex face-selective neuron tuned to some movements of a head, but with no response when the head was still. (Reproduced from Experimental Brain Research, 170 (1) pp. 743–87, Face-selective and auditory neurons in the primate orbitofrontal cortex, Rolls, E. T., Critchley, H. D., Browning, A. S. and Inoue, K., (c) 2006, Springer Science and Business Media. With kind permission from Springer Science and Business Media.)

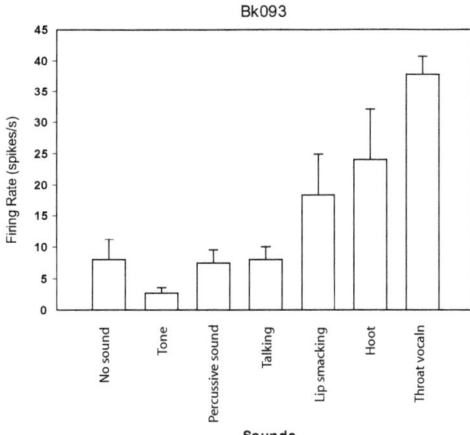

Fig. 3.31 Orbitofrontal cortex neuron in a macaque tuned to some vocalizations. (Reproduced from Experimental Brain Research, 170 (1) pp. 743–87, Face-selective and auditory neurons in the primate orbitofrontal cortex, Rolls, E. T., Critchley, H. D., Browning, A. S. and Inoue, K., (c) 2006, Springer Science and Business Media. With kind permission from Springer Science and Business Media.)

3.6.6 Visual inputs to the orbitofrontal cortex from the temporal lobe visual cortical areas

To understand what is special about processing in the orbitofrontal cortex, it is helpful to understand what is being provided to the orbitofrontal cortex by its input regions, and how processing in those input regions may differ from that in the orbitofrontal cortex. We do this now in this subsection for the visual inputs to the orbitofrontal cortex, which come largely from temporal cortical visual areas (see Chapter 2).

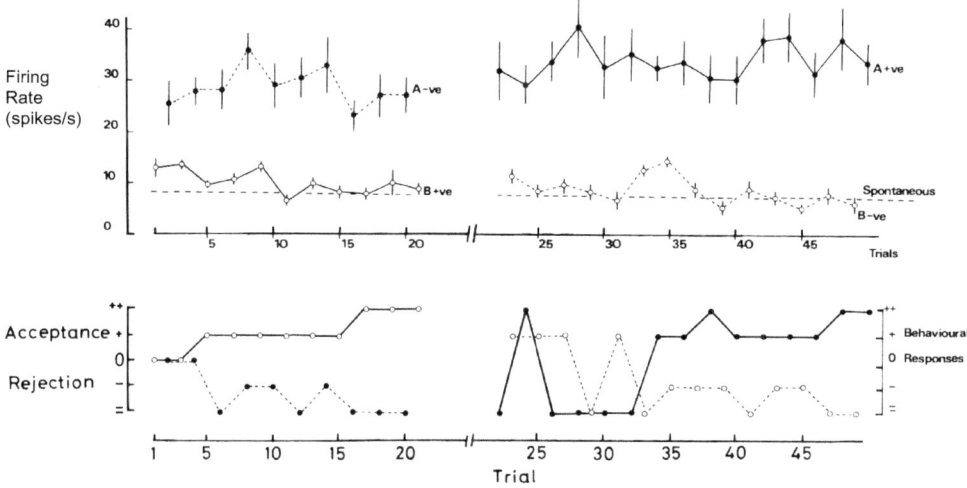

Fig. 3.32 Examples of the responses of a neuron in the inferior temporal visual cortex, showing that its responses (firing rate in spikes/s, upper panel) do not reverse when the reward association of the visual stimuli reverses. For the first 21 trials of the visual discrimination task, visual stimulus A was aversive (–ve, because if the monkey licked he obtained saline), and visual stimulus B was associated with reward (+ve, because if the monkey licked when he saw this stimulus, he obtained fruit juice). The neuron responded more to stimulus A than to stimulus B. After trial 21, the contingencies reversed (so that A was now +ve, and B –ve). The monkey learned the reversal correctly by about trial 35 (lower panel). However, the inferior temporal cortex neuron did not reverse when the reinforcement contingency reversed – it continued to respond to stimulus A after the reversal, even though the stimulus was now +ve. Thus this, and other inferior temporal cortex neurons, respond to the physical aspects of the visual stimuli, and not to the stimuli based on their reinforcement association or the reinforcement contingency. (Reprinted from Brain Research, 130 (2), E. T. Rolls, S. J. Judge, and M. K. Sanghera, Activity of neurones in the inferotemporal cortex of the alert monkey, pp. 229–38, Copyright, 1997, with permission from Elsevier.)

3.6.6.1 Objects, and not their reward and punishment associations or value, are represented in the inferior temporal visual cortex

We now consider whether associations between visual stimuli and reinforcers are learned, and stored, in the visual cortical areas that proceed from the primary visual cortex, V1, through V2, V4, and the inferior temporal visual cortex (see Figs. 2.1 and 2.2). Is the emotional or motivational valence of visual stimuli represented in these regions?

One way to answer the issue just raised is to test monkeys in a learning paradigm in which one visual stimulus is associated with reward (for example glucose taste, or fruit juice taste), and another visual stimulus is associated with an aversive taste, such as strong saline. Rolls, Judge & Sanghera (1977) performed just such an experiment and found that single neurons in the inferior temporal visual cortex did not respond differently to objects based on their reward association. To test whether a neuron might be influenced by the reward association, the monkey performed a visual discrimination task in which the reinforcement contingency could be reversed during the experiment. (That is, the visual stimulus, for example a triangle, to which the monkey had to lick to obtain a taste of fruit juice, was after the reversal associated with saline – if the monkey licked to the triangle after the reversal, he obtained mildly aversive salt solution.) An example of such an experiment is shown in Fig. 3.32. The neuron responded more to the triangle, both before reversal when it was associated with fruit juice, and after reversal, when the triangle was associated with saline. Thus the reinforcement association of the visual stimuli did not alter the response to the visual stimuli, which was based on the physical properties of the stimuli (for example their shape, colour, or texture). The same was true for the other neurons recorded in this study.

This conclusion, that the responses of inferior temporal neurons during visual discriminations do not code for whether a visual stimulus is associated with reward or punishment, is also consistent with further findings (Ridley, Hester & Ettlinger 1977, Jarvis & Mishkin 1977, Gross, Bender & Gerstein 1979, Sato, Kawamura & Iwai 1980), including an investigation in which macaques search for food-related stimuli in complex visual scenes (Rolls, Aggelopoulos & Zheng 2003a). In the visual food reward search task the monkeys searched a complex natural visual scene to find and touch one of two objects in order to obtain fruit juice reward. If the wrong object was touched, the monkeys obtained mildly aversive hypertonic saline. The neurons responded to one of the selected stimuli in this experiment, and when the reward/punisher was reversed between the stimuli, the neuron continued to respond independently of whether the stimulus was associated with reward or with the punisher (Rolls, Aggelopoulos & Zheng 2003a). This independence from reward association seems to be characteristic of neurons right through the temporal visual cortical areas, and must be true in earlier cortical areas too, in that they provide the inputs to the inferior temporal visual cortex (Rolls & Deco 2002, Rolls 2016c, Rolls 2012d).

I need to make it clear that these conclusions relate to whether neurons in temporal cortical visual areas encode the *valence* of visual stimuli, that is, whether the visual stimuli are currently associated with reward or punishment. That is quite different from for example the effects of top-down attention or interest, which may modulate neuronal responses if one stimulus is for example more rewarding than another (Rolls 2016c). For example, if two visual stimuli are associated with different probabilities of water reward, any modulation of neural processing (Kaskan, Costa, Eaton, Zemskova, Mitz, Leopold, Ungerleider & Murray 2017) may be due only to different interest or attention. Unless valence has been reversed with one stimulus related to reward, and the other to punishment, and a neuron reverses, we cannot conclude that the reward/punishment valence of the stimulus is being represented. The evidence thus remains, as shown by investigations of reversal, that reward/punishment valence is not represented in the inferior temporal visual cortex (Rolls, Judge & Sanghera 1977, Rolls, Aggelopoulos & Zheng 2003a), but is represented in the orbitofrontal cortex (Thorpe, Rolls & Maddison 1983, Rolls, Critchley, Mason & Wakeman 1996a). Moreover, devaluation by feeding to satiety reduces neuronal responses to food-related visual stimuli to zero in the orbitofrontal cortex (Critchley & Rolls 1996c), but not in the inferior temporal visual cortex (Rolls, Judge & Sanghera 1977). Similar points hold for the primary auditory cortex (Brosch, Selezneva & Scheich 2011).

3.6.6.2 Why reward and punishment associations of objects are not represented early in information processing in the primate brain

The processing stream that has just been considered is that concerned with objects and faces, that is with what is being looked at. Two fundamental points about pattern association networks for stimulus–reinforcer association learning can be made from what we have considered.

The first point is that sensory processing in the primate brain proceeds as far as the invariant representation of objects (invariant with respect to, for example, size, position on the retina, and even view), independently of reward vs punisher association. Why should this be, in terms of systems-level brain organization? The suggestion that is made is that the visual properties of the world about which reward associations must be learned are generally objects (for example the sight of a banana, or of an orange), and are not just raw pixels or edges, with no invariant properties, which is what is represented in the retina and the primary visual cortex (V1). The implication and principle is that usually the sensory processing must proceed to the stage of the invariant representation of objects before it is appropriate to learn reinforcer associations (Rolls 2016c, Rolls 2014a). The invariance aspect is important too, for if we had different representations for an object at different places in our visual field, then if we learned when an object was at one point on the retina that it was rewarding, we would not generalize correctly to it when presented at another position on the retina. If it had previously been punishing at that retinal position, we might find the same object rewarding when at one point on the retina, and punishing when at another. This is inappropriate given the world in which we live, and in which our brain evolved, in that the most appropriate assumption is that objects have the same reinforcer association wherever they are on the retina.

The same systems-level principle of brain organization is also likely to be true in other sensory systems, such as those for touch and hearing. For example, we do not generally want to learn that a particular pure tone is associated with a reward or punisher. Instead, it might be a particular complex pattern of sounds such as a vocalization that carries a reinforcement signal, and this may be independent of the exact pitch at which it is uttered. Thus, cases in which some modulation of neuronal responses to pure tones in parts of the brain such as the medial geniculate (the thalamic relay for hearing) (LeDoux 1994, LeDoux 2012) where tonotopic tuning is found, may be rather special model systems (that is simplified systems on which to perform experiments), and may not reflect the way in which auditory-to-reinforcer pattern associations are normally learned. Indeed, the auditory cortex is the normal route for the processing of complex sounds (Ahveninen, Huang, Nummenmaa, Belliveau, Hung, Jaaskelainen, Rauschecker, Rossi, Tiitinen & Raij 2013, Rauschecker & Scott 2009).

Similar arguments against the normal relevance of subcortical to amygdala processing for emotional stimuli, the so-called 'low-road', apply to emotional blindsight, the ability of blindsight patients with striate cortex damage to respond above chance to emotional expressions even when having no subjective experience of seeing the face (Tamietto, Pullens, de Gelder, Weiskrantz & Goebel 2012). The same may be true for touch in so far as one considers associations between objects identified by somatosensory input, and primary reinforcers. An example might be selecting a food object from a whole collection of objects in the dark.

The second point, which complements the first, is that the visual system is not provided with the appropriate primary reinforcers for such pattern-association learning, in that visual processing in the primate brain is mainly unimodal to and through the inferior temporal visual cortex (see Fig. 2.2) (Rolls 2016c, Rolls 2012d). It is only after the inferior temporal visual cortex, when it projects to structures such as the amygdala and orbitofrontal cortex, that the appropriate convergence between visual processing pathways and pathways conveying information about primary reinforcers such as taste and touch/pain occurs (Fig. 2.2).

3.6.6.3 Processing to the inferior temporal cortex in the primate visual system to form invariant representations of faces and objects

A schematic diagram to indicate some aspects of the processing involved in object and face identification from the primary visual cortex, V1, through V2 and V4 to the posterior inferior temporal cortex (TEO) and the anterior inferior temporal cortex (TE) is shown in Fig. 3.33 (Rolls 2016c, Blumberg & Kreiman 2010, Orban 2011, Rolls 2011a, Rolls 2012d). Their approximate location on the brain of a macaque monkey is shown in Fig. 3.34, which also shows that TE has a number of different subdivisions. The different TE areas all contain visually responsive neurons, as do many of the areas within the cortex in the superior temporal sulcus (Baylis, Rolls & Leonard 1987). For the purposes of this summary, these areas will be grouped together as the anterior inferior temporal cortex (IT), except where otherwise stated.

There is a host of visual areas in the inferior temporal visual cortex, with those especially relevant in providing inputs to the orbitofrontal cortex which we have studied found approximately 11 to 15 mm anterior to the interaural plane (Baylis, Rolls & Leonard 1987, Rolls 2007a, Rolls 2007b, Rolls 2016c, Rolls 2012d). For comparison, the 'middle face patch' of Tsao, Freiwald, Tootell & Livingstone (2006) was at A6, which is probably part of the posterior inferior temporal cortex (Tsao & Livingstone 2008, Rolls 2011a) (see Fig. 3.35). Similarly, in humans there are a number of separate visual representations of faces, other body parts, and objects (Spiridon, Fischl & Kanwisher 2006, Weiner & Grill-Spector 2013, Vul, Lashkari,

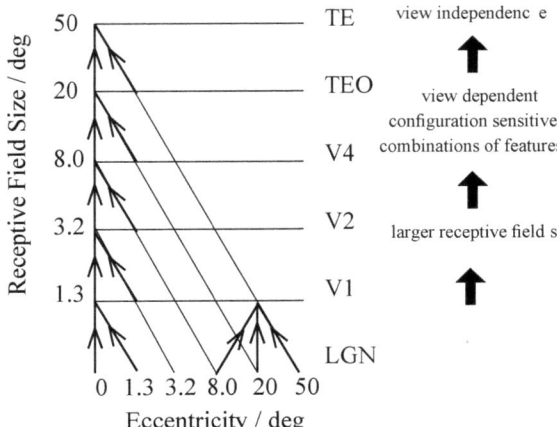

Fig. 3.33 Schematic diagram showing convergence achieved by the forward projections in the visual system, and the types of representation that may be built by competitive networks operating at each stage of the system from the primary visual cortex (V1) to the inferior temporal visual cortex (area TE) (see text). LGN, lateral geniculate nucleus. Area TEO forms the posterior inferior temporal cortex. The receptive fields in the inferior temporal visual cortex (for example in the TE areas) cross the vertical midline (not shown). (For details, see Rolls 2016c.)

Hsieh, Golland & Kanwisher 2012, Weiner & Grill-Spector 2015), with the clustering together of neurons with similar responses influenced by the self-organizing map processes that are a result of cortical design (Rolls 2016c). Many of the studies on neurons in the inferior temporal cortex and cortex in the superior temporal sulcus have been performed with neurons that respond particularly to faces, because such neurons can be found regularly in recordings in this region, and therefore provide a good population for systematic studies (Rolls 2000b, Rolls & Deco 2002, Rolls 2004a, Rolls 2007a, Rolls 2011a, Rolls 2012d, Rolls 2016c).

The somewhat patchy organisation of groups of neurons in the macaque temporal cortex is shown with fMRI. For example, Fig. 3.35 shows patches of face cells (Tsao & Livingstone 2008, Freiwald & Tsao 2010, Shepherd & Freiwald 2018). The neurons discovered and analyzed by Rolls and colleagues described here in the inferior temporal cortex area TE that respond with invariance to face identity (e.g. Rolls (1984), Hasselmo, Rolls, Baylis & Nalwa (1989b), Tovee, Rolls, Treves & Bellis (1993), Rolls (2000b), Rolls (2012d), and Rolls (2016c)) would be in or close to AL, and the neurons discovered and analyzed by Rolls and colleagues that respond to face expression and face movement in the cortex in the superior temporal sulcus (STS) (e.g. Hasselmo, Rolls & Baylis (1989a) and Hasselmo, Rolls, Baylis & Nalwa (1989b)) would be in or close to AF.

3.6.6.4 Receptive field size and translation invariance

There is convergence from each small part of a region to the succeeding region (or layer in the hierarchy) in such a way that the receptive field sizes of neurons (for example 1 degree near the fovea in V1) become larger by a factor of approximately 2.5 with each succeeding stage. [The typical parafoveal receptive field sizes found would not be inconsistent with the calculated approximations of, for example, 8 deg in V4, 20 deg in TEO, and 50 deg in inferior temporal cortex (Boussaoud, Desimone & Ungerleider 1991) (see Fig. 3.33)]. Such zones of convergence would overlap continuously with each other (see Fig. 3.33). This connectivity provides part of the basis for the fact that many neurons in the temporal cortical visual areas respond to a stimulus relatively independently of where it is in their receptive field, and moreover maintain their stimulus selectivity when the stimulus appears in different parts of the visual field (Gross, Desimone, Albright & Schwartz 1985, Tovee, Rolls & Azzopardi 1994, Rolls, Aggelopoulos & Zheng 2003a). This is called translation or shift

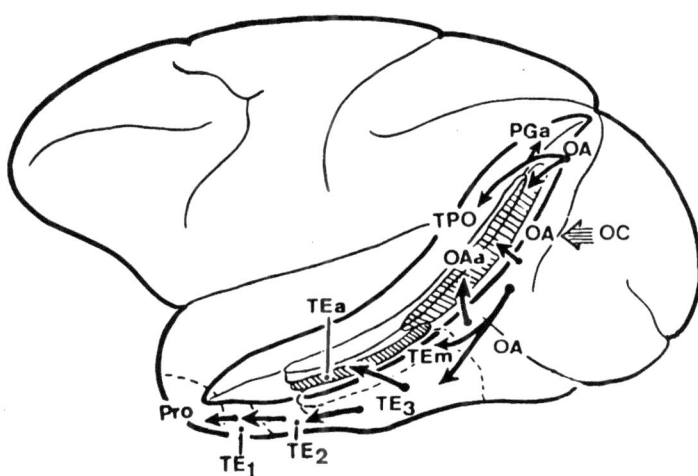

Fig. 3.34 Lateral view of the macaque brain (left hemisphere) showing the different architectonic areas (e.g. TEm, TPO) in and bordering the anterior part of the superior temporal sulcus (STS) of the macaque (see text; after Seltzer and Pandya 1978).

invariance. We found that this type of invariance is greater in the anterior inferior temporal cortex (area TE, in or close to AL in Fig. 3.35) than in the posterior inferior temporal cortex (area TEO, in or close to ML in Fig. 3.35). We therefore focussed on neurons in the anterior part of the temporal lobe in most of our investigations of the properties of temporal cortex visual neurons.

In addition to having topologically appropriate connections, it is necessary for the connections to have the appropriate synaptic weights to perform the mapping of each set of features, or object, to the same set of neurons in the inferior temporal visual cortex. How this could be achieved is addressed in the computational neuroscience models that we have developed (Rolls 2016c, Rolls 2012d, Wallis & Rolls 1997, Rolls & Deco 2002, Rolls & Webb 2014, Webb & Rolls 2014, Robinson & Rolls 2015, Rolls & Mills 2018) which learn by making use of the spatio-temporal continuity that characterizes objects when they are viewed.

3.6.6.5 Reduced translation invariance in natural scenes, and the selection of a rewarded object

Until relatively recently, research on translation invariance considered the case in which there is only one object in the visual field. What happens in a cluttered, natural, environment? Do all objects that can activate an inferior temporal neuron do so whenever they are anywhere within the large receptive fields of inferior temporal neurons? If so, the output of the visual system might be confusing for structures that receive inputs from the temporal cortical visual areas, such as the orbitofrontal cortex (see Fig. 3.36). If one of the objects in the visual field was associated with reward, and another with punishment, would the output of the inferior temporal visual cortex to emotion-related brain systems be an amalgam of both stimuli? If so, how would we be able to choose between the stimuli, and have an emotional response to one but not perhaps the other, and select one for action and not the other?

To investigate how information is passed from the inferior temporal visual cortex (IT) to other brain regions such as the orbitofrontal cortex to enable stimuli to be selected from natural scenes for valuation, emotion, and action, Rolls, Aggelopoulos & Zheng (2003a) analysed the responses of single and simultaneously recorded IT neurons to stimuli presented in complex natural backgrounds. In one situation, a visual fixation task was performed in which the

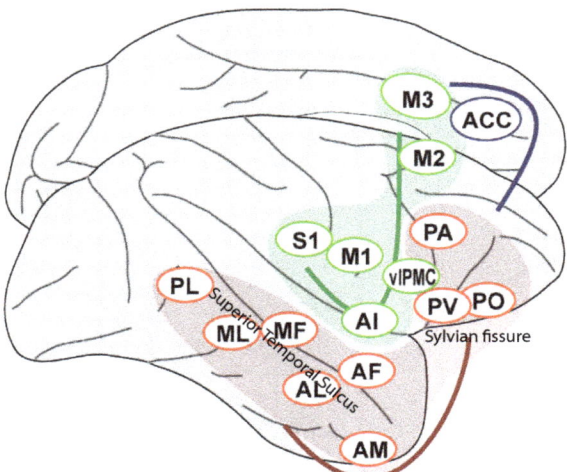

Fig. 3.35 View of the macaque brain with face patch areas shown with fMRI in the temporal lobe cortex. A signifies anterior, M signifies middle, and P posterior. L signifies lateral (i.e. on the inferior temporal gyrus), and F signifies fundus, i.e. in the cortex in the superior temporal sulcus (STS). The neurons discovered and analyzed by Rolls and colleagues in the inferior temporal cortex area TE that respond with invariance to face identity would be in or close to AL, and the neurons discovered and analyzed by Rolls and colleagues that respond to face expression and face movement in the cortex in the STS would be in or close to AF. Neurons in ML and MF show less invariance. The areas above the lateral or Sylvian fissure in the lateral frontal cortex are more involved in movements, including movements made to social stimuli. (Adapted from Neuron, 99 (2), Stephen V. Shepherd and Winrich A. Freiwald, Functional Networks for Social Communication in the Macaque Monkey, pp. 250–253, doi.org/10.1016/j.neuron.2018.06.027 © 2018 Elsevier Inc., with permission from Elsevier.)

monkey fixated at different distances from the effective stimulus. In another situation the monkey had to search for two objects on a screen, and a touch of one object was rewarded with juice, and of another object was punished with saline (see Fig. 3.36). In both situations neuronal responses to the effective stimuli for the neurons were compared when the objects were presented in the natural scene or on a plain background. It was found that the overall response of the neuron to objects was sometimes somewhat reduced when they were presented in natural scenes, though the selectivity of the neurons remained. However, the main finding was that the magnitudes of the responses of the neurons typically became much less in the real scene the further the monkey fixated in the scene away from the object (see Fig. 3.37). Results that are consistent have been described by Sheinberg & Logothetis (2001). It is proposed that this reduced translation invariance in natural scenes helps an unambiguous representation of an object which may be the target for action to be passed to the brain regions that receive from the primate inferior temporal visual cortex. It helps with the binding problem, by reducing in natural scenes the effective receptive field of inferior temporal cortex neurons to approximately the size of an object in the scene. The computational utility and basis for this is considered by Rolls & Deco (2002), Trappenberg, Rolls & Stringer (2002), Deco & Rolls (2004), Aggelopoulos & Rolls (2005) and Rolls & Deco (2006), and includes an advantage for what is at the fovea because of the large cortical magnification of the fovea, and shunting interactions between representations weighted by how far they are from the fovea (Rolls 2016c).

These findings suggest that the principle of providing strong weight to whatever is close to the fovea is an important principle governing the operation of the inferior temporal visual cortex, and in general of the output of the visual system in natural environments. This principle of operation is very important in interfacing the visual system to action systems, because the effective stimulus in making inferior temporal cortex neurons fire is in natural scenes usually at or close to the fovea. This means that the spatial coordinates of where the object is in the scene do not have to be represented in the inferior temporal visual cortex, nor passed from

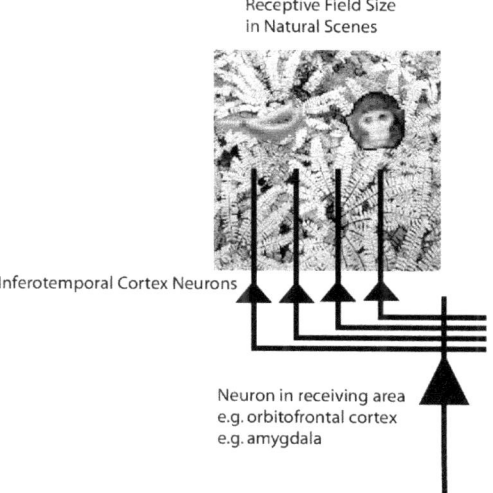

Fig. 3.36 Objects shown in a natural scene, in which the task was to search for and touch one of the stimuli. The objects in the task as run were smaller. The diagram shows that if the receptive fields of inferior temporal cortex neurons are large in natural scenes with multiple objects (in this scene, bananas and a face), then any receiving neuron in structures such as the orbitofrontal cortex and amygdala would receive information from many stimuli in the field of view, and would not be able to provide evidence about each of the stimuli separately.

it to the action selection system, as the latter can assume that the object making IT neurons fire is close to the fovea in natural scenes. Thus the position in visual space being fixated provides part of the interface between sensory representations of objects and their coordinates as targets for actions in the world. The small receptive fields of IT neurons in natural scenes make this possible. Moreover, it is now known that asymmetries in the receptive fields of inferior temporal cortex neurons become evident in complex natural cluttered scenes, and this means that there is some information about where a particular object is with respect to the fovea (Aggelopoulos & Rolls 2005, Rolls 2012d, Rolls 2016c). In addition, local, egocentric, processing implemented in the dorsal visual processing stream using e.g. stereodisparity may be used to guide action towards reward-associated objects (Rolls & Deco 2002).

The reduced receptive field size in complex natural scenes also enables emotions to be selective to just what is being fixated, because this is the information that is transmitted by the firing of anterior inferior temporal cortex neurons to structures such as the orbitofrontal cortex and amygdala.

3.6.6.6 Size and spatial frequency invariance

Some neurons in the inferior temporal visual cortex and cortex in the anterior part of the superior temporal sulcus (IT/STS) respond relatively independently of the size of an effective face stimulus, with a mean size invariance (to a half maximal response) of 12 times (3.5 octaves) (Rolls & Baylis 1986). This is not a property of a simple single-layer network (see Fig. 8.1 of Rolls & Deco (2002)), nor of neurons in V1, which respond best to small stimuli, with a typical size-invariance of 1.5 octaves. (Some neurons in IT/STS also respond to face stimuli that are blurred, or that are line drawn, showing that they can also map the different spatial frequencies with which objects can be represented to the same representation in IT/STS, see Rolls, Baylis & Leonard (1985).)

Some neurons in the temporal cortical visual areas actually represent the absolute size of objects such as faces independently of viewing distance (Rolls & Baylis 1986). The utility of this representation by a small population of neurons is that the absolute size of an object is a useful feature to use as an input to neurons that perform object recognition. Faces only come

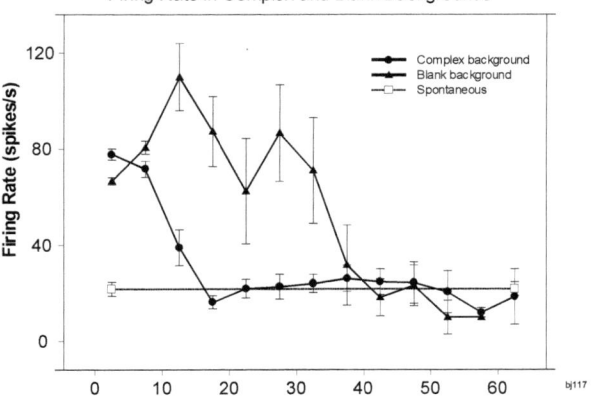

Fig. 3.37 Firing of a temporal cortex neuron to an effective stimulus presented either in a blank background or in a natural scene, as a function of the angle in degrees at which the monkey was fixating away from the effective stimulus. The task was to search for and touch the stimulus. (Reproduced from E. T. Rolls, N. C. Aggelopoulos, and F. Zheng, The receptive fields of inferior temporal cortex neurons in natural scenes, The Journal of Neuroscience 23, pp. 339–348, doi.org/10.1523/JNEUROSCI.23-01-00339.2003 © 2003, Society for Neuroscience.)

in certain sizes.

3.6.6.7 Combinations of features in the correct spatial configuration

Many cells in this processing stream respond to combinations of features (including objects), but not to single features presented alone, and the features must have the correct spatial arrangement. This has been shown, for example, with faces, for which it has been shown by masking out or presenting parts of the face (for example eyes, mouth, or hair) in isolation, or by jumbling the features in faces, that some cells in the cortex in IT/STS respond only if two or more features are present, and are in the correct spatial arrangement (Perrett, Rolls & Caan 1982, Rolls, Tovee, Purcell, Stewart & Azzopardi 1994b, Rolls 2011a, Freiwald, Tsao & Livingstone 2009). Corresponding evidence has been found for non-face cells. For example, Tanaka, Saito, Fukada & Moriya (1990) showed that some posterior inferior temporal cortex neurons might only respond to the combination of an edge and a small circle if they were in the correct spatial relation to each other. Evidence consistent with the suggestion that neurons are responding to combinations of a few variables represented at the preceding stage of cortical processing is that some neurons in V2 and V4 respond to end-stopped lines, to tongues flanked by inhibitory subregions, or to combinations of colours (Rolls & Deco 2002, Rolls 2016c, Rolls 2012d). Neurons that respond to combinations of features but not to single features indicate that the system is non-linear and can operate using competitive learning (Elliffe, Rolls & Stringer 2002, Rolls 2016c, Rolls 2012d).

A rather different approach suggests that neurons code simple metric properties of faces, such as the distance between face features, and that an ensemble of such neurons could be used to encode face identity (Chang & Tsao 2017). In contrast to that approach, the model of Rolls utilizes a feature hierarchy model and competitive learning to form non-linear combinations of features in the correct relative spatial position so that different neurons together span the space, and utilizes slow learning to learn invariant transforms of faces and objects. As it is a self-organizing system, the approach also provides a theory of how the computation is performed by the brain (Rolls 1992b, Wallis & Rolls 1997, Rolls & Deco 2002, Rolls 2008b, Rolls 2012d, Rolls 2016c).

3.6.6.8 A view-invariant representation

For recognizing and learning about objects (including faces), it is important that an output of the visual system should be not only translation- and size-invariant, but also relatively view-invariant. In an investigation of whether there are such neurons, we found that some temporal cortical neurons reliably responded differently to the faces of two different individuals independently of viewing angle (Hasselmo, Rolls, Baylis & Nalwa 1989b), although in most cases (16/18 neurons) the response was not perfectly view-independent. Mixed together in the same cortical regions there are neurons with view-dependent responses (for example Hasselmo, Rolls, Baylis & Nalwa (1989b) and Rolls & Tovee (1995)). Such neurons might respond, for example, to a view of a profile of a monkey but not to a full-face view of the same monkey (Perrett, Smith, Potter, Mistlin, Head, Milner & Jeeves 1985, Hasselmo et al. 1989b).

It is to be expected in a hierarchical face or object recognition system that more invariance is represented the further up the hierarchy one progresses (Rolls 2016c). In line with this, neurons in ML and MF were view-specific for faces; neurons in AL were tuned to identity mirror-symmetrically across views, thus achieving partial view invariance; and neurons in AM, the most anterior face patch, achieved almost full view invariance (Freiwald & Tsao 2010).

These findings, of view-dependent, partially view-independent, and view-independent representations in cortical regions are consistent with the hypothesis discussed below that view-independent representations are being built in the hierarchy by associating together the outputs of neurons that respond to different views of the same individual. These findings also provide evidence that one output of the visual system includes representations of what is being seen, in a view-independent way that would be useful for object recognition and for learning associations about objects; and that another output is a view-based representation that would be useful in social interactions to determine whether another individual is looking at one, and for selecting details of motor responses, for which the orientation of the object with respect to the viewer is required (Rolls 2016c). Both types of information reach the orbitofrontal cortex (Rolls, Critchley, Browning & Inoue 2006a, Rolls 2011a), probably from these temporal cortical visual areas.

Further evidence that some neurons in the temporal cortical visual areas have object-based responses comes from a population of neurons that responds to moving faces, for example to a head undergoing ventral flexion, irrespective of whether the view of the head was full face, of either profile, or even of the back of the head, and even of whether the head was inverted which alters the local motion but not the object-based interpretation of the motion (Hasselmo, Rolls, Baylis & Nalwa 1989b, Rolls & Stringer 2007, Rolls 2011a).

There is also evidence that some neurons in the inferior temporal visual cortex have view-independent responses for objects, and these resulted from self-organizing learning occurring during natural experience of the objects without the need for training with rewards (Booth & Rolls 1998).

3.6.6.9 Distributed encoding for face and object identity

An important question for understanding brain function is whether a particular object (or face) is represented in the brain by the firing of one or a few gnostic (or 'grandmother') cells (Barlow 1972), or whether instead the firing of a group or ensemble of cells each with somewhat different responsiveness provides the representation. Advantages of distributed codes include generalization and graceful degradation (fault tolerance), and a potentially very high capacity in the number of stimuli that can be represented (that is exponential growth of capacity with the number of neurons in the representation) (Rolls & Treves 1998, Rolls 2016c, Rolls & Treves 2011). If the ensemble encoding is sparse, this provides a good input to an associative memory, for then large numbers of stimuli can be stored or associated together

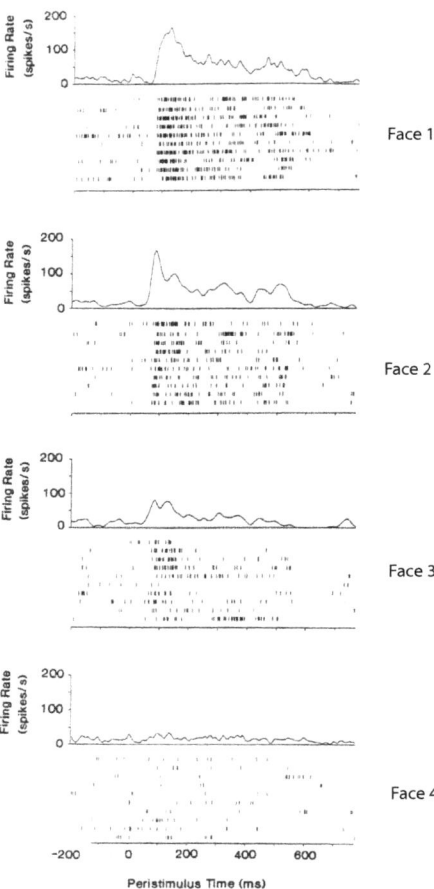

Fig. 3.38 Peristimulus time histograms and rastergrams showing the responses on different trials (originally in random order) of a face-selective neuron in the inferior temporal visual cortex to four different faces. (In the rastergrams each vertical line represents one spike from the neuron, and each row is a separate trial. Each block of the Figure is for a different face.) (Reproduced from Journal of Neurophysiology, 70 (2) 640–654, Information encoding and the responses of single neurons in the primate temporal visual cortex, M. J. Tovee, E. T. Rolls, A. Treves, and R. P. Bellis © 1993, The American Physiological Society.)

(pattern association networks and autoassociation networks are described in Appendix 2 of Rolls (2016c), which is available online at www.oxcns.org). We have shown that in the inferior temporal visual cortex and cortex in the anterior part of the superior temporal sulcus (IT/STS), the responses of a group of neurons, but not of a single neuron, provide evidence on which face was shown. We showed, for example, that these neurons typically respond with a graded set of firing to different faces, with firing rates from 100 spikes/s to the most effective face, to no response at all to a number of the least effective faces (Baylis, Rolls & Leonard 1985, Rolls & Tovee 1995, Rolls 2016c, Rolls & Treves 2011). In fact, the firing rate probability distribution of a single neuron to a set of stimuli is approximately exponential (Rolls & Tovee 1995, Treves, Panzeri, Rolls, Booth & Wakeman 1999, Baddeley, Abbott, Booth, Sengpiel, Freeman, Wakeman & Rolls 1997, Franco, Rolls, Aggelopoulos & Jerez 2007, Rolls 2016c, Rolls & Treves 2011). To provide examples, Fig. 3.38 shows typical firing rate changes of a single neuron on different trials to each of several different faces. This makes it clear that from the firing rate on any one trial, information is available about which stimulus was shown, and that the firing rate is graded, with a different firing rate response of the neuron to each stimulus.

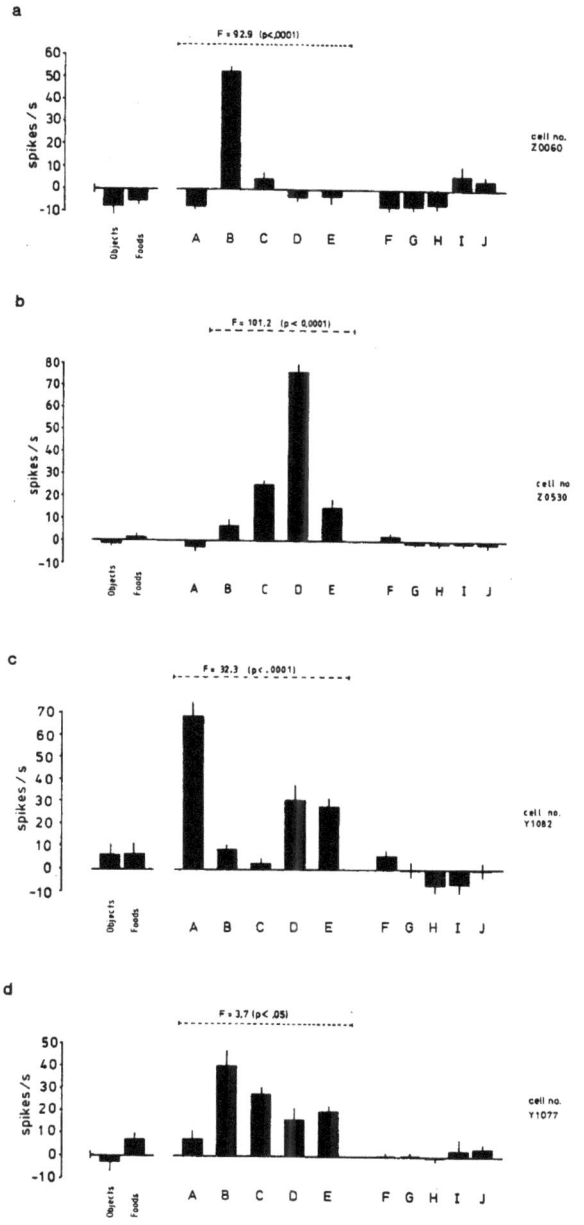

Fig. 3.39 Responses of four different temporal cortex visual neurons to a set of five faces (A–E), and, for comparison, to a wide range of non-face objects and foods. F–J are non-face stimuli. The means and standard errors of the responses computed over 8–10 trials are shown. (Reprinted from Brain Research, 342 (1), G. C. Baylis, E. T. Rolls, and C. M. Leonard, Selectivity between faces in the responses of a population of neurons in the cortex in the superior temporal sulcus of the monkey, pp. 91–102, Copyright, 1985, with permission from Elsevier.)

The distributed nature of the encoding typical for neurons in the inferior temporal visual cortex is illustrated in Fig. 3.39, which shows that temporal cortical neurons typically responded to several members of a set of five faces, with each neuron having a different profile of responses to each face (Baylis, Rolls & Leonard 1985). It would be difficult for most of these single cells to tell which of even five faces, let alone which of hundreds of faces, had been seen. Yet across a population of such neurons, much information about the particular face that has been seen is provided, as shown below.

The single neuron selectivity or sparseness a^S of the activity of inferior temporal cortex neurons was 0.65 over a set of 68 stimuli including 23 faces and 45 non-face natural scenes, and a measure called the response sparseness a_r^S of the representation, in which the spontaneous rate was subtracted from the firing rate to each stimulus so that the responses of the neuron were being assessed, was 0.38 across the same set of stimuli (Rolls & Tovee 1995). [For binary neurons (firing for example either at a high rate or not at all), the single neuron sparseness is the proportion of stimuli that a single neuron responds to. These definitions are described further by Franco, Rolls, Aggelopoulos & Jerez (2007), Rolls & Treves (2011), and by Rolls (2016c) in Appendix 3 also available online at www.oxcns.org.]

It has been possible to apply information theory to show that each IT neuron conveys on average approximately 0.4 bits of information about which face in a set of 20 faces has been seen (Tovee & Rolls 1995, Tovee, Rolls, Treves & Bellis 1993, Rolls, Treves, Tovee & Panzeri 1997b). If a neuron responded to only one of the faces in the set of 20, then it could convey (if noiseless) 4.6 bits of information about one of the faces (when that face was shown). If, at the other extreme, it responded to half the faces in the set, it would convey 1 bit of information about which face had been seen on any one trial. In fact, the average maximum information about the best stimulus was 1.8 bits of information. This provides good evidence not only that the representation is distributed, but also that it is a sufficiently reliable representation that useful information can be obtained from it.

The most impressive result obtained so far is that when the information available from a population of neurons about which of 20 faces has been seen is considered, the information increases approximately linearly as the number of cells in the population increases from 1 to 14 (Rolls, Treves & Tovee 1997c, Abbott, Rolls & Tovee 1996) (see Fig. 3.40). Remembering that the information in bits is a logarithmic measure, this shows that the representational capacity of this population of cells increases exponentially (see Fig. 3.41). This is the case both when an optimal, probability estimation, form of decoding of the activity of the neuronal population is used, and also when the neurally plausible dot product type of decoding is used (Fig. 3.40). (The dot product decoding assumes that what reads out the information from the population activity vector is a neuron or a set of neurons that operates just by forming the dot product of the input population firing rate vector and a neurons' synaptic weight vector – see Rolls, Treves & Tovee (1997c), and Appendix 3 of Rolls (2016c).) By simulation of further neurons and further stimuli, we have shown that the capacity grows very impressively, approximately as shown in Fig. 3.41 (Abbott, Rolls & Tovee 1996). The result has been replicated with simultaneously recorded neurons (Rolls, Franco, Aggelopoulos & Reece 2003b, Rolls, Aggelopoulos, Franco & Treves 2004). (The ability of IT neurons to encode the identity of many faces has also be found by Chang & Tsao (2017), though they propose a metric basis for the representation.) This result is exactly what would be hoped for from a distributed representation. This result is not what would be expected for local encoding, for which the number of stimuli that could be encoded would increase linearly with the number of cells. (Even if the grandmother cells were noisy, adding more replicates to increase reliability would not lead to more than a linear increase in the number of stimuli that can be encoded as a function of the number of cells.) Moreover, the encoding in the inferior temporal visual cortex about objects remains based on the spike count from each neuron, and not on the relative time of firing of each neuron or stimulus-dependent synchronization, when analysed with simultaneous single neuron recording (Franco, Rolls, Aggelopoulos & Treves 2004, Rolls, Franco, Aggelopoulos & Jerez 2006b) even in natural scenes while an attentional task is being performed (Aggelopoulos, Franco & Rolls 2005). Further, much of

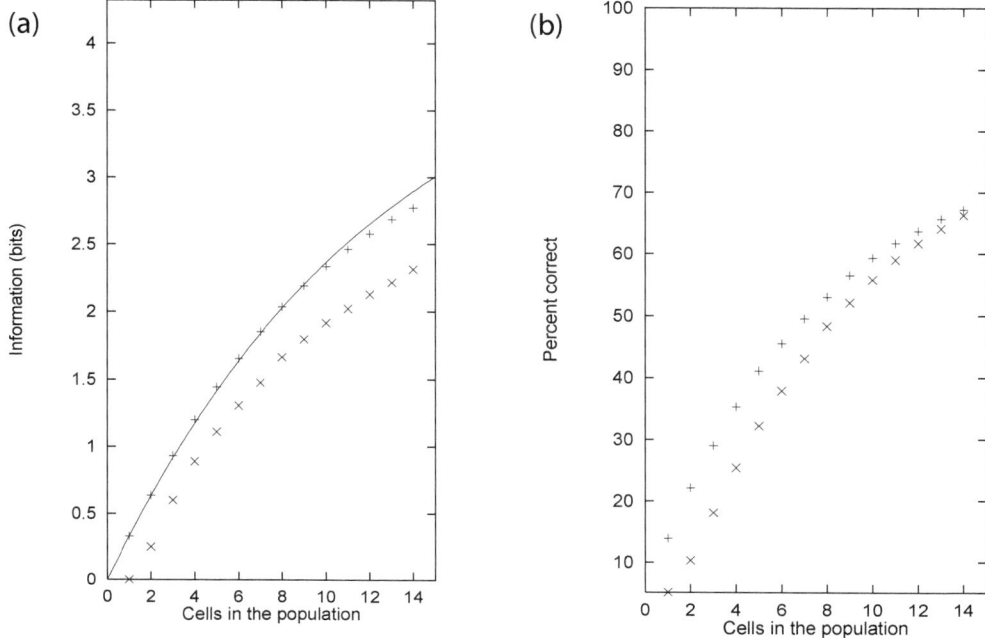

Fig. 3.40 (a) The values for the average information available in the responses of different numbers of these neurons on each trial, about which of a set of 20 face stimuli has been shown. The decoding method was Dot Product (DP, ×) or Probability Estimation (PE, +). The full line indicates the amount of information expected from populations of increasing size, when assuming random correlations within the constraint given by the ceiling (the information in the stimulus set, I = 4.32 bits). (b) The percent correct for the corresponding data to those shown in (a). (Rolls, Treves and Tovee 1997.) (Reproduced from Experimental Brain Research, 114 (1) pp. 149–162, The representational capacity of the distributed encoding of information provided by populations of neurons in primate temporal visual cortex, E. T. Rolls, (c) 1997, Springer Science and Business Media. With kind permission from Springer Science and Business Media.)

the information is available in short times of e.g. 20 or 50 ms (Tovee & Rolls 1995, Rolls, Franco, Aggelopoulos & Jerez 2006b), so that the receiving neuron does not need to integrate over a long time period to estimate a firing rate.

These findings provide very firm evidence that the encoding built at the end of the visual system is distributed, and that part of the power of this representation is that by receiving inputs from relatively small numbers of such neurons, neurons at the next stage of processing (for example in structures such as the orbitofrontal cortex, amygdala, and hippocampus) would obtain information about which of a very great number of stimuli had been shown.

The type of encoding found in the temporal cortex visual areas is thus ideal for providing information about faces and objects to the orbitofrontal cortex. The sparseness provides high capacity and a representation that is easily decoded by neurons (Rolls 2016c). The distributed nature of the code allows for generalization and graceful degradation.

This representational capacity of neuronal populations has fundamental implications for the connectivity of the brain, for it shows that neurons need not have hundreds of thousands or millions of inputs to have available to them information about what is represented in another population of cells, but that instead the real numbers of perhaps 8,000–10,000 synapses per neuron would be adequate for them to receive considerable information from the several different sources between which this set of synapses is allocated (Rolls 2016c).

It may be noted that it is unlikely that there are further processing areas beyond those described where ensemble coding changes into grandmother cell encoding. Anatomically, there does not appear to be a whole further set of visual processing areas present in the brain; and outputs from the temporal lobe visual areas such as those described are taken

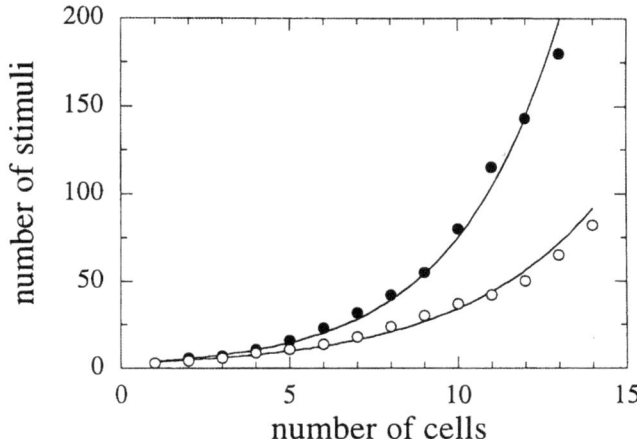

Fig. 3.41 The number of stimuli (in this case from a set of 20 faces) that are encoded in the responses of different numbers of neurons in the temporal lobe visual cortex, based on the results shown in Fig. 3.40. (Data from Experimental Brain Research, 114 (1) pp. 149–162, The representational capacity of the distributed encoding of information provided by populations of neurons in primate temporal visual cortex, E. T. Rolls, 1997 and from L. F. Abbott, E. T. Rolls, and M. J. Tovee, (1996). Representational capacity of face coding in monkeys, Cerebral Cortex, 6, pp. 498–505.)

to the orbitofrontal cortex and to limbic and related regions such as the amygdala and via the entorhinal cortex to the hippocampus (see Rolls (1994), Rolls (2000b), Rolls & Treves (1998), Rolls (2016c) and Rolls & Stringer (2005)). For example, the face-responding neurons in the part of the orbitofrontal cortex that receives from the IT/STS cortex do not have local encoding (Rolls, Critchley, Browning & Inoue 2006a). Further, we have found a population of neurons with face-selective responses in the amygdala, and in the majority of these neurons, different responses occur to different faces, with ensemble (not local) coding still being present (Leonard, Rolls, Wilson & Baylis 1985). The amygdala, in turn, projects to another structure that may be important in other behavioural responses to faces, the ventral striatum, and comparable face-selective neurons have also been found in the ventral striatum (Williams, Rolls, Leonard & Stern 1993).

There are also outputs of the inferior temporal cortex via perirhinal and parahippocampal cortical areas to medial temporal lobe structures such as the hippocampus that are involved in memory and not in emotion. Consistent with the functions of the hippocampus in episodic memory, and the need to maximize the number of memories that can be stored (Rolls 2016c, Rolls 2010a, Rolls 2013b), the representations in the hippocampus are more sparse than in the inferior temporal cortex (Rolls 2016c, Rolls & Treves 2011). In humans, representations in the medial temporal lobe have also been reported to be sparse, with a neuron for example apparently responding to Jennifer Aniston, but here again the representation is sparse distributed rather than like that of a grandmother cell (Quiroga, Kreiman, Koch & Fried 2008, Rolls 2016c, Rolls & Wirth 2018).

3.6.6.10 Face expression, gesture and view represented in a population of neurons in the cortex in the superior temporal sulcus

In the orbitofrontal cortex, there are neurons tuned to face expression (Rolls, Critchley, Browning & Inoue 2006a, Barat, Wirth & Duhamel 2018), as well as other neurons tuned to face identity, and others tuned to head and face motion, all important in social behaviour (Rolls et al. 2006a). What is the likely source of these face expression-related inputs to the orbitofrontal cortex?

In addition to the population of neurons that code for face identity, which tend to have object-based representations and are in areas TEa and TEm on the inferior temporal gyrus and ventral bank of the superior temporal sulcus, there is a separate population in the cortex in the fundus of the superior temporal sulcus (e.g. area TPO) that conveys information about facial expression and face and head movement (Hasselmo, Rolls & Baylis 1989a) (see e.g. Fig. 3.42).

Some of the neurons in this region tend to have view-based representations (so that information is conveyed for example about whether the face is looking at one, or is looking away), and might respond to moving faces, and to facial gesture (Hasselmo, Rolls, Baylis & Nalwa 1989b). For example, some neurons respond to a head turning away from a frontal view, or to closing of the eyes, both of which break social contact (Hasselmo, Rolls, Baylis & Nalwa 1989b). Neurons in this region can also be tuned to small mouth movements, and respond for example to the mouth movements of a TV newsreader even when the sound is turned off. Other neurons respond to head movements in body-centred coordinates, in that they may respond to a head rotating clockwise when it is both upright and inverted, even though the optic flow is opposite in these cases (Hasselmo, Rolls, Baylis & Nalwa 1989b). Face expression and motion of parts of the face frequently occur together and are combined to provide important social signals (Hasselmo, Rolls & Baylis 1989a, Hasselmo, Rolls, Baylis & Nalwa 1989b). This combination of face expression and face motion sensitivity in these cortical areas in the superior temporal sulcus has been confirmed (Furl, Hadj-Bouziane, Liu, Averbeck & Ungerleider 2012). Although face patches that respond to moving faces are visible with fMRI (Fisher & Freiwald 2015), that cannot reveal the exquisite types of tuning actually found to moving face stimuli that is encoded by the responses of single neurons in the cortex in the fundus of the anterior superior temporal sulcus (Hasselmo, Rolls & Baylis 1989a, Hasselmo, Rolls, Baylis & Nalwa 1989b).

In humans, a face expression area has been identified with fMRI in a region that may be homologous to the cortex in the anterior part of the fundus of the superior temporal sulcus, and is in the human middle temporal gyrus (Critchley, Daly, Phillips, Brammer, Bullmore, Williams, Van Amelsvoort, Robertson, David & Murphy 2000). That middle temporal gyrus region, also implicated in theory of mind (Hein & Knight 2008), has decreased functional connectivity with the orbitofrontal cortex in autism in which there is abnormal processing of faces (Cheng, Rolls, Gu, Zhang & Feng 2015). Different parts of the cortex in the superior temporal sulcus in humans are responsive in fMRI studies to theory of mind, faces and voices, and faces and biological motion (Deen, Koldewyn, Kanwisher & Saxe 2015, Isik, Koldewyn, Beeler & Kanwisher 2017).

Thus information in cortical areas that project to the orbitofrontal cortex and amygdala is about face identity, and about face expression and gesture. Both types of information, and information about face motion and face gesture, are present in the orbitofrontal cortex (Rolls et al. 2006a), which receives from these temporal cortical areas. Both types of information are important in social and emotional responses to other primates (including humans), which must be based on who the individual is as well as on the face expression or gesture being made. One output from the orbitofrontal cortex and amygdala face-selective areas (Leonard, Rolls, Wilson & Baylis 1985, Rolls, Critchley, Browning & Inoue 2006a) for this information is probably via the ventral striatum, for a small population of neurons has been found in the ventral striatum with responses selective for faces (Rolls & Williams 1987, Williams, Rolls, Leonard & Stern 1993).

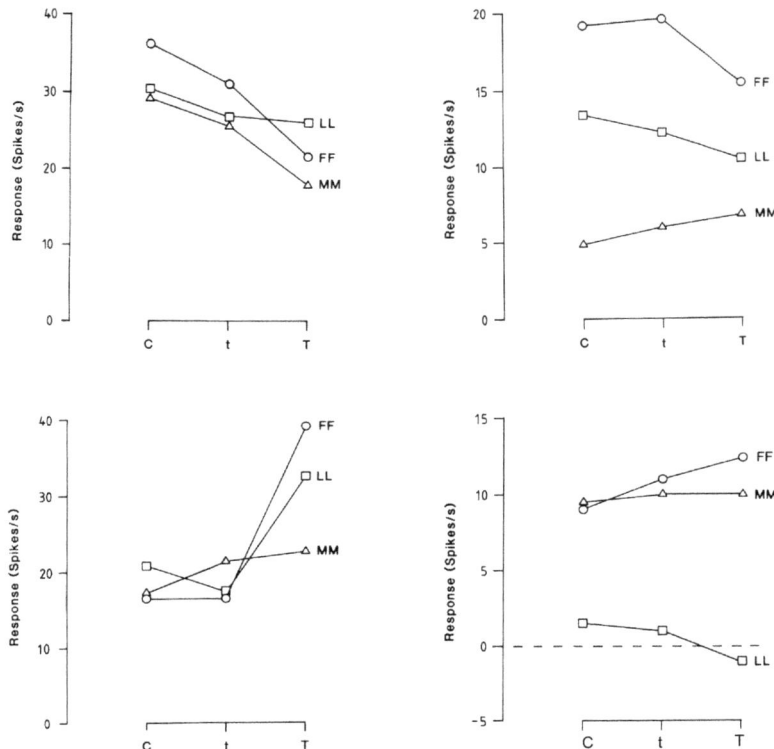

Fig. 3.42 There is a population of neurons in the cortex in the superior temporal sulcus with responses tuned to respond differently to different face expressions. The cells in the two left panels did not discriminate between individuals (faces MM, FF, and MM), but did discriminate between different expressions on the faces of those individuals (C, calm expression; t, mild threat; T, strong threat). In contrast, the cells in the right two panels responded differently to different individuals, and did not discriminate between different expressions. The neurons that discriminated between expressions were found mainly in the cortex in the fundus of the superior temporal sulcus; the neurons that discriminated between identity were in contrast found mainly in the cortex in lateral part of the ventral lip of the superior temporal sulcus (areas TEa and TEm). (Reprinted from Behavioural Brain Research, 32 (3), Michael E. Hasselmo, Edmund T. Rolls, and Gordon C. Baylis, The role of expression and identity in the face-selective responses of neurons in the temporal visual cortex of the monkey, pp. 203–218, Copyright, 1989, with permission from Elsevier.)

3.6.6.11 The brain mechanisms that build the appropriate view-invariant representations of objects required for learning emotional responses to objects, including faces

Some of the ways in which the visual system may produce the invariant distributed representations of objects needed for inputs to the orbitofrontal cortex have been described by Rolls & Treves (1998), Rolls & Deco (2002), Rolls (2016c) and Rolls (2012d), and include a hierarchical feed-forward series of competitive networks using convergence from stage to stage; and the use of a modified Hebb synaptic learning rule that incorporates a short-term memory trace of previous neuronal activity to help learn the invariant properties of objects from the temporo-spatial statistics produced by the normal viewing of objects (Rolls 2016c, Rolls 2012d, Rolls 2004a, Rolls 1992b, Wallis & Rolls 1997, Rolls & Milward 2000, Stringer & Rolls 2000, Rolls & Stringer 2001a, Elliffe, Rolls & Stringer 2002, Stringer & Rolls 2002, Trappenberg, Rolls & Stringer 2002, Deco & Rolls 2004, Stringer, Perry, Rolls & Proske 2006, Perry, Rolls & Stringer 2006, Perry, Rolls & Stringer 2010, Rolls & Stringer 2007, Stringer & Rolls 2008, Stringer, Rolls & Tromans 2007, Rolls & Stringer 2006, Rolls & Webb 2014, Webb & Rolls 2014, Rolls & Mills 2018).

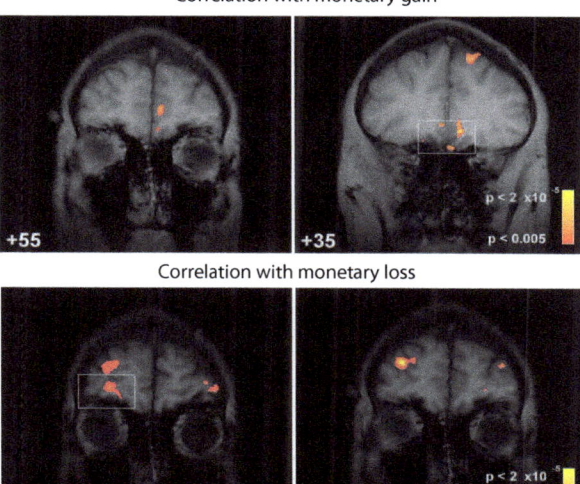

Fig. 3.43 Correlation of brain activations with the amount of money won (upper) or lost (lower) in a visual discrimination reversal task with probabilistic monetary reward and loss. Voxels in the orbitofrontal cortex (upper right, in square box) and pregenual cingulate cortex (upper left) whose activity increased with the amount of money won on each trial. Voxels in an area of left medial orbitofrontal cortex (Talairach coordinates [X,Y,Z] = [−6 34 −28]) correlated positively with Reward Magnitude. Voxels in an area of right lateral orbitofrontal cortex (lower left in square box, Talairach co-ordinates [28 60 −6]) correlated positively with the amount of money lost on each trial. (Reproduced from Nature Neuroscience, 4 (1), J. O'Doherty, M. L. Kringelbach, E. T. Rolls, J. Hornak, and C. Andrews, Abstract reward and punishment representations in the human orbitofrontal cortex, pp. 95–102, Figure 4a, © 2001, Nature Publishing Group.)

3.7 Monetary reward value, and many other types of reward, are represented in the orbitofrontal cortex

The studies in macaques described earlier in this Chapter provide evidence on the details of the neuronal representations in the primate orbitofrontal cortex that are essential for building a computational understanding for exactly what information is represented in it, how it is represented, how these differ from preceding and succeeding stages, and thus how the orbitofrontal cortex operates computationally (see Sections 9.4, 9.5 and Rolls (2016c)). However, the types of visual-reward association that have been studied in primates (and confirmed as applying in humans (O'Doherty, Deichmann, Critchley & Dolan 2002)) include objects associated with taste rewards or punishers. It has therefore been useful not only to confirm that these concepts do indeed apply to humans, but also to extend the types of visual conditioned reinforcers to quite abstract reinforcers such as monetary reward.

In an fMRI study, O'Doherty, Kringelbach, Rolls, Hornak & Andrews (2001a) used a visual discrimination task in which one stimulus was associated with monetary reward, and a different visual stimulus with monetary loss (punishment). The actual amounts of money won on reward trials and lost on punishment trials were probabilistic. This part of the design, and the fact that unexpected visual discrimination reversals occurred so that there were trials on which money was lost, enabled us to show that the magnitude of the activation of the medial orbitofrontal cortex was correlated with the amount of money won on each trial, and the magnitude of the activation of the lateral orbitofrontal cortex was correlated with the amount of money lost on each trial, as shown in Figs. 3.43 and 3.44. These findings have been confirmed in an investigation in 1140 participants, as shown in Fig. 7.5 (Xie, Jia, Rolls, Liu, Banaschewski, Barker, Bodke, Bromberg, C., Quinlan, Desrivieres, Flor, Grigis, Garavan, Gowland, Heinz, Hohmann, Ittermann, Martinot, Martinot, Nees, Papadopoulos Orfanos, Paus, Poustka, Frohner, Smolka, Walter, Whelan, Schumann, Feng & IMAGEN 2019).

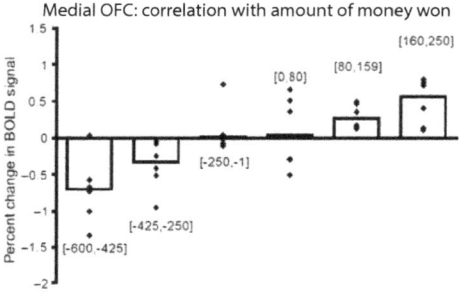
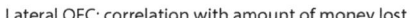
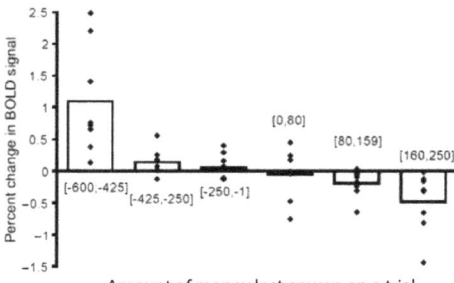

Fig. 3.44 Correlation of brain activations with the amount of money won or lost in a visual discrimination reversal task with probabilistic monetary reward and loss. The mean percent change in the BOLD signal from baseline across subjects for 6 different category ranges of monetary gain or loss plotted along the abscissa. The signal was averaged across a category range within each subject and then the average signal change from each category was averaged across subjects. This is plotted for voxels in the medial OFC that significantly correlated with reward and for voxels in the lateral OFC that significantly correlated with punishment. The ranges of monetary reward and punishment in each category are shown on the chart and were determined by their relative frequencies, which follow from the experimental design. (Reproduced from Nature Neuroscience, 4 (1), J. O'Doherty, M. L. Kringelbach, E. T. Rolls, J. Hornak, and C. Andrews, Abstract reward and punishment representations in the human orbitofrontal cortex, pp. 95–102, Figure 4b © 2001, Nature Publishing Group.)

Consistent with the finding of outcome value and expected value neurons in the same parts of the primate orbitofrontal cortex, the outcome value and the expected value produced activations on the same scale and in the same part of the medial orbitofrontal cortex in humans, when the probability of obtaining the reward was varied to signal different expected values (Rolls, McCabe & Redoute 2008e). This was shown in a probabilistic monetary reward decision task designed to allow variables of interest in neuroeconomics to be measured (Section 3.12). As illustrated in Fig. 3.45a, the subjects could choose either on the right to obtain a large reward outcome with a value of 30 pence, or on the left to obtain a smaller reward outcome with a value of 10 pence with a probability of 0.9. On the right, in different trial blocks, the probability of the large reward was 0.9 (making the expected value which approximates probability × reward value = 27 pence); or the probability was 0.33 making the expected value 10 pence; or the probability was 0.16 making the expected value 5 pence. The expected value on the left was 9 pence (p=0.9 of outcome value of 10 pence). The participants learned in the blocks of 30 trials with the different expected values on the right whether to press on the right or the left to maximize their winnings. They took typically less than 10 trials to adjust to the unsignalled change in expected value every 30 trials, and analysis was performed for the last 20 trials of each block when the expected value had been learned. Fig. 3.45b shows the regions of the orbitofrontal / ventromedial prefrontal cortex where the activations were proportional both to the expected value (measured early in the trial) and the outcome value (measured later in each trial, when the reward outcome was made known)

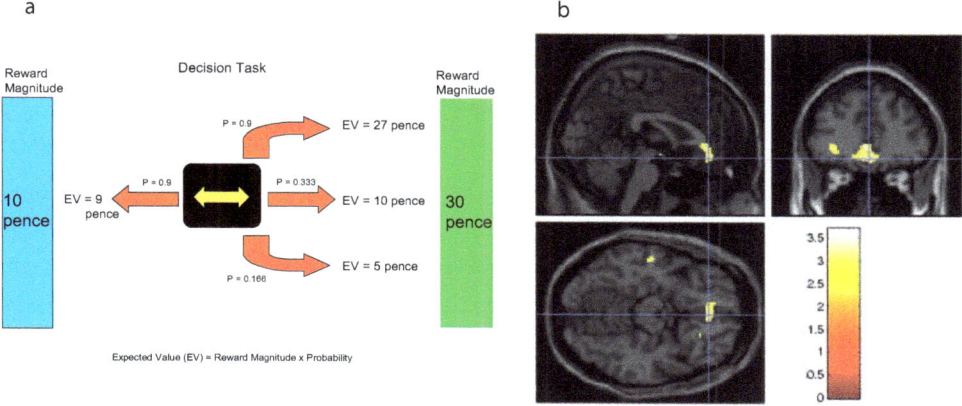

Fig. 3.45 Expected value and outcome value in a probabilistic monetary reward decision task. (a) In the task, subjects could choose either on the right to obtain a large reward with a magnitude of 30 pence, or on the left to obtain a smaller reward with an outcome magnitude of 10 pence with a probability of 0.9 (Expected Value = 9 pence). On the right, in different blocks each 30 trials long, the probability of the large reward was 0.9 (making the Expected Value defined as probability × Reward outcome Magnitude = 27 pence); or the probability was 0.33 (EV=10 pence); or the probability was 0.16 (EV=5 pence). (On the trials on which a reward was not obtained, 0 pence was the Reward outcome Magnitude). (b) Medial orbitofrontal cortex. Conjunction analysis showing brain regions where there were correlations both with Expected Value and with Reward outcome Magnitude (peak MNI coordinates [2 38 -14]). (This material was originally published in Cerebral Cortex, 18 (3), Expected Value, Reward Outcome, and Temporal Difference Error Representations in a Probabilistic Decision Task, Edmund T. Rolls, Ciara McCabe, Jerome Redoute, pp. 652–663, © 2008, Oxford University Press.)

(Rolls, McCabe & Redoute 2008e).

Thus in humans and macaques there is evidence that expected value signalled by for example visual as well as olfactory stimuli is represented in the orbitofrontal cortex. This representation of expected value is important in decision-making, as described further in Section 3.12.

3.8 Negative reward prediction error neurons in the orbitofrontal cortex, and visual stimulus–reinforcer association learning and reversal

In addition to the neurons that encode the reward value of visual stimuli, other neurons (3.5%) in the orbitofrontal cortex detect different types of non-reward, i.e. reward prediction error, the difference between the expected value and the reward outcome value (Thorpe, Rolls & Maddison 1983). For example, some neurons responded in extinction, immediately after a lick had been made to a visual stimulus that had previously been associated with fruit juice reward, but no reward was obtained. Other neurons responded in a reversal task, immediately after the monkey had responded to the previously rewarded visual stimulus, but had obtained the punisher of salt taste rather than reward (see example in Fig. 3.46).

Different populations of such neurons respond to other types of non-reward, including the removal of a formerly approaching taste reward, and the termination of a taste reward (Thorpe, Rolls & Maddison 1983) (see Table 3.2). The fact that different non-reward neurons respond to different types of non-reward (e.g. some to the noise of a switch that indicated that extinction of free licking for fruit juice had occurred, and others to the first presentation of a visual stimulus that was not followed by reward in a visual discrimination task) potentially enables context-specific extinction or reversal to occur. Thus the error neurons can be specific to different tasks, and this could provide a mechanism for reversal in one task to be implemented, while

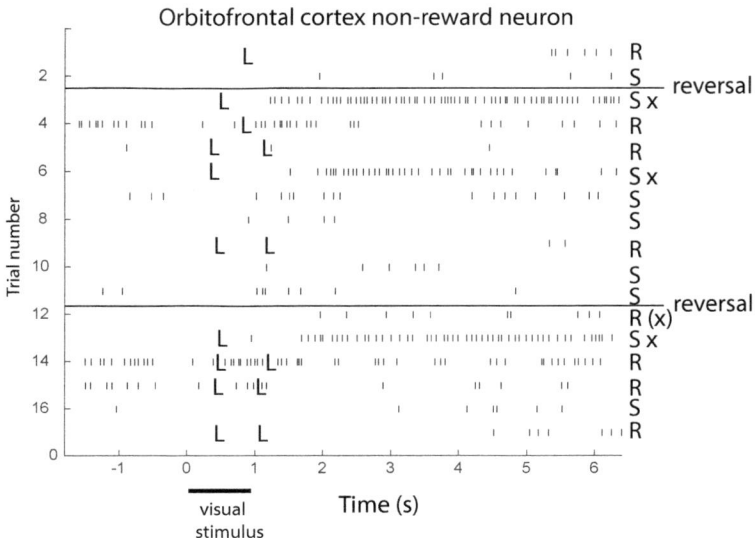

Fig. 3.46 Error neuron: Responses of an orbitofrontal cortex neuron that responded only when the monkey licked to a visual stimulus during reversal, expecting to obtain fruit juice reward, but actually obtaining the taste of aversive saline because it was the first trial of reversal. Each single dot represents an action potential; each vertically arranged double dot represents a lick response. The visual stimulus was shown at time 0 for 1 s. The neuron did not respond on most reward (R) or saline (S) trials, but did respond on the trials marked x, which were the first trials after a reversal of the visual discrimination on which the monkey licked to obtain reward, but actually obtained saline because the task had been reversed. It is notable that after an expected reward was not obtained due to a reversal contingency being applied, on the very next trial the macaque selected the previously non-rewarded stimulus. This shows that rapid reversal can be performed by a non-associative process, and must be rule-based. A model for this is the subject of Section 9.4. (Data from Experimental Brain Research, 49 (1) pp. 93–115, The orbitofrontal cortex: Neuronal activity in the behaving monkey, S. J. Thorpe, E. T. Rolls, and S. Maddison.)

Table 3.2 Numbers of orbitofrontal cortex neurons responding in different types of extinction or reversal. The table shows the tasks (rows) in which individual orbitofrontal neurons responded (1), did not respond (0), or were not tested (blank). (Reproduced from Experimental Brain Research, 49 (1) pp. 93–115, The orbitofrontal cortex: Neuronal activity in the behaving monkey, S. J. Thorpe, E. T. Rolls, and S. Maddison. With kind permission from Springer Science and Business Media.)

Neuron number	1	2	3	4	5	6	7	8	9	10	11	12	13	14	15	16	17	18
Visual discrim: Reversal	1	0	1	0	0	1	1	0						0				
Visual discrim: Extinction	1																	
Ad lib licking: Reversal	1	1		0	0	0		0	1									
Ad lib licking: Extinction	0	0		0	0	0		0	1									
Taste of saline	0		0	0	0	0	0	0	1	0	0	0	0	0	0	0	0	0
Removal of reward	0		1	1	1	0	1	0	1	1	1	1	1	1	1	1	1	1
Visual arousal	1			1	0	0	0	0	1	0	0	0	0	1	0	0	0	

at the same time not reversing behaviour in another task. Also, it provides additional evidence to that in Table 3.2 that these neurons did not respond simply as a function of arousal, or just in relation to a general frustrative non-reward/error signal.

The presence of these orbitofrontal cortex non-reward or negative reward prediction error neurons is fully consistent with the hypothesis that they are part of the mechanism by which the orbitofrontal cortex enables very rapid reversal of behaviour by stimulus–reinforcer association relearning when the association of stimuli with reinforcers is altered or reversed (Rolls 1986a, Rolls 1986b, Rolls 1990a, Rolls 1999a, Rolls 2014a, Rolls 2018b). This information appears to be necessary for primates to rapidly alter behavioural responses when reinforcement contingencies are changed, as shown by the effects of damage to the

Table 3.3 Proportion of different types of neuron recorded in the macaque orbitofrontal cortex during sensory testing and visual discrimination reversal and related tasks. The number of neurons analysed was 463. (Reproduced from Experimental Brain Research, 49 (1) pp. 93-115, The orbitofrontal cortex: Neuronal activity in the behaving monkey, S. J. Thorpe, E. T. Rolls, and S. Maddison. With kind permission from Springer Science and Business Media.)

Sensory testing:
Visual, non-selective	10.7%
Visual, selective (i.e. responding to some objects or images)	13.2%
Visual, food-selective	5.3%
Visual, aversive objects	3.2%
Taste	7.3%
Visual and taste	2.6%
Removal of a food reward	6.3%
Extinction of ad lib licking for juice reward	7.5%

Visual discrimination reversal task:
Visual, reversing in the visual discrimination task	5.3%
Visual, conditional discrimination in the visual discrimination task	2.5%
Visual, stimulus-related (not reversing) in the visual discrimination task	0.8%
Non-reward in the visual discrimination task	0.9%
Auditory tone cue signalling the start of a trial of the visual discrimination task	15.1%

orbitofrontal cortex described in Chapter 4. The existence of neurons in the middle part of the macaque orbitofrontal cortex that respond to non-reward (Thorpe, Rolls & Maddison 1983) (originally described by Thorpe, Maddison & Rolls (1979) and Rolls (1981a)) is confirmed by recordings that revealed 10 such non-reward neurons (of 140 recorded, or approximately 7%) found in delayed match to sample and delayed response tasks by Joaquin Fuster and colleagues (Rosenkilde, Bauer & Fuster 1981).

To the extent that the firing of some dopamine neurons may reflect error signals, one might ask where the error information comes from, given that the dopamine neurons themselves may not receive information about expected rewards (e.g. a visual stimulus associated with the sight of food), obtained rewards (e.g. taste), and would have to compute an error from these signals (Sections 2.2 and 5.2.4). On the other hand, the orbitofrontal cortex does have all three types of neuron and the required neuroanatomically defined inputs, and the orbitofrontal cortex is an important site in the brain for computing error signals.

It is interesting to note the proportions of different types of neuron recorded in the orbitofrontal cortex in relation to what might or might not be seen in a human brain imaging study. The proportions of different types of neuron in the study by Thorpe, Rolls & Maddison (1983) are shown in Table 3.3. It is seen that only a relatively small percentage convey information about, for example, which of two visual stimuli is currently reward-associated in a visual discrimination task. An even smaller proportion (3.5%) responds in relation to non-reward, and in any particular non-reward task, the proportion is very small, that is, just a fraction of the 3.5%. The implication is that an imaging study might not reveal really what is happening in a brain structure such as the orbitofrontal cortex where quite small proportions of neurons respond to any particular condition; and, especially, one would need to be very careful not to place much weight on a failure to find activation in a particular task, as the proportion of neurons responding may be small, and the time period for which they respond may be small too. For example, non-reward neurons typically respond for 2–8 s on the first two non-reward trials of extinction or reversal (Thorpe, Rolls & Maddison 1983).

In that most neurons in the macaque orbitofrontal cortex respond to reinforcers and punishers, or to stimuli associated with rewards and punishers, and do not respond in relation to responses, the orbitofrontal cortex is closely related to stimulus processing, including the stimuli that give rise to affective states. When it computes errors, it computes mismatches between

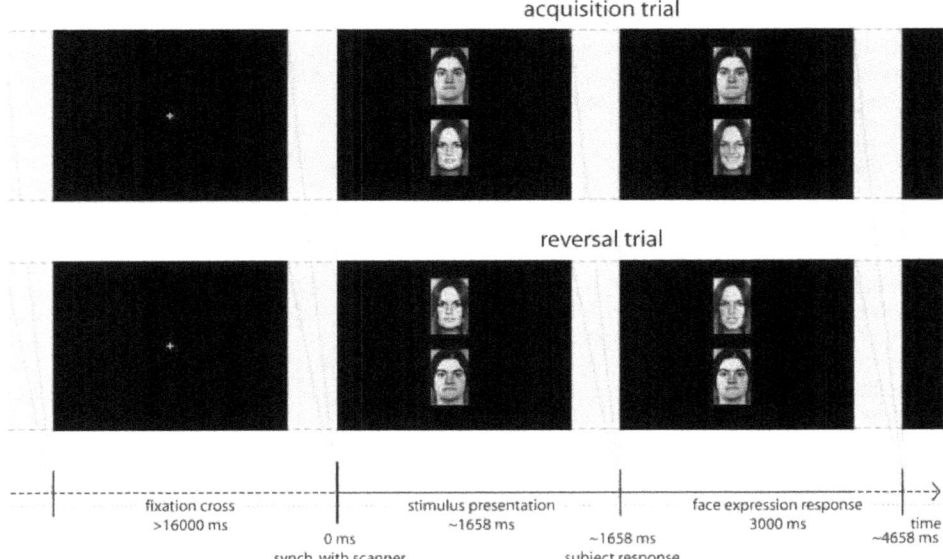

Fig. 3.47 Social reversal task: The trial starts synchronized with the scanner and two people with neutral face expressions are presented to the subject. The subject has to select one of the people by pressing the corresponding button, and the person will then either smile or show an angry face expression for 3000 ms depending on the current mood of the person. The task for the subject is to keep track of the mood of each person and choose the 'happy' person as much as possible (upper row). Over time (after between 4 and 8 correct trials) this will change so that the 'happy' person becomes 'angry' and vice versa, and the subject has to learn to adapt her choices accordingly (bottom row). Randomly intermixed trials with either two men, or two women, were used to control for possible gender and identification effects, and a fixation cross was presented between trials for at least 16000 ms. (Reprinted from NeuroImage 20 (2), Morten L. Kringelbach and Edmund T. Rolls, Neural correlates of rapid reversal learning in a simple model of human social interaction, pp. 1371–83, Copyright, 2003, with permission from Elsevier.)

stimuli that are expected, and stimuli that are obtained, and in this sense the errors are closely related to those required to correct affective states. This type of error representation may thus be different from that represented in the cingulate cortex, in which behavioural responses are represented, where the errors may be more closely related to errors that arise when action–outcome expectations are not met, and where action–outcome rather than stimulus–reinforcer representations need to be corrected (see Section 5.1).

We have also been able to obtain evidence that non-reward used as a signal to reverse behavioural choice is represented in the human orbitofrontal cortex. Kringelbach & Rolls (2003) used the faces of two different people, and if one face was selected then that face smiled, and if the other was selected, the face showed an angry expression. After good performance was acquired, there were repeated reversals of the visual discrimination task (see Fig. 3.47). Kringelbach & Rolls (2003) found that activation of a lateral part of the orbitofrontal cortex in the fMRI study was produced on the error trials, that is when the human chose a face, and did not obtain the expected reward (see Fig. 3.48). Control tasks showed that the response was related to the error, and the mismatch between what was expected and what was obtained, in that just showing an angry face expression did not selectively activate this part of the lateral orbitofrontal cortex. An interesting aspect of this study that makes it relevant to human social behaviour is that the conditioned stimuli were faces of particular individuals, and the unconditioned stimuli were face expressions. Moreover, the study reveals that the human orbitofrontal cortex is very sensitive to social feedback when it must be used to change behaviour (Kringelbach & Rolls 2003, Kringelbach & Rolls 2004).

One behavioural effect of not receiving reward is that it may be important to stop the

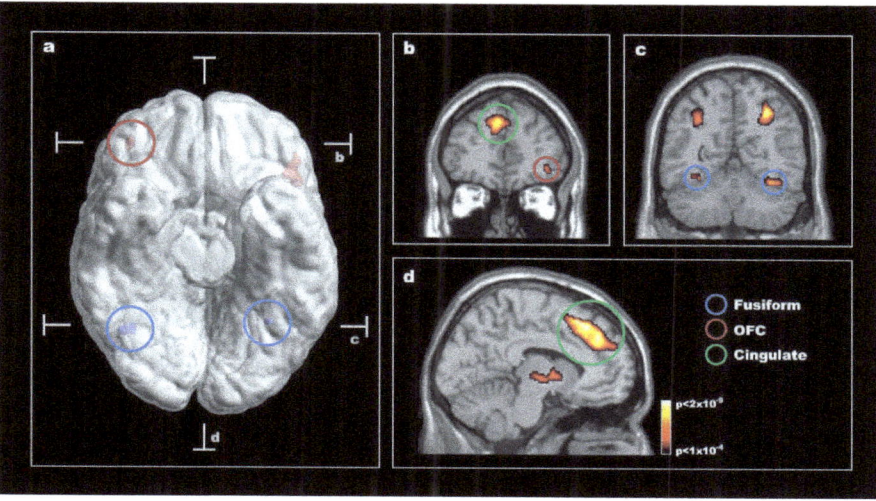

Fig. 3.48 Social reversal: Composite figure showing that changing behaviour based on face expression is correlated with increased brain activity in the human orbitofrontal cortex. a) The figure is based on two different group statistical contrasts from the neuroimaging data which are superimposed on a ventral view of the human brain with the cerebellum removed, and with indication of the location of the two coronal slices (b,c) and the transverse slice (d). The red activations in the orbitofrontal cortex (denoted OFC, maximal activation: z=4.94 [42 42 –8]; and z=5.51 [–46 30 –8]) shown on the rendered brain arise from a comparison of reversal events with stable acquisition events, while the blue activations in the fusiform gyrus (denoted Fusiform, maximal activation: z>8 [36 –60 –20] and z=7.80 [–30 –56 –16]) arise from the main effects of face expression. b) The coronal slice through the frontal part of the brain shows the cluster in the right orbitofrontal cortex across all nine subjects when comparing reversal events with stable acquisition events. Significant activity was also seen in an extended area of the anterior cingulate/paracingulate cortex (denoted Cingulate, maximal activation: z=6.88 [–8 22 52]; green circle). c) The coronal slice through the posterior part of the brain shows the brain response to the main effects of face expression with significant activation in the fusiform gyrus and the cortex in the intraparietal sulcus (maximal activation: z>8 [32 –60 46]; and z>8 [–32 –60 44]). d) The transverse slice shows the extent of the activation in the anterior cingulate/paracingulate cortex when comparing reversal events with stable acquisition events. Group statistical results are superimposed on a ventral view of the human brain with the cerebellum removed, and on coronal and transverse slices of the same template brain (activations are thresholded at p=0.0001 for purposes of illustration to show their extent). (Reprinted from NeuroImage 20 (2), Morten L. Kringelbach and Edmund T. Rolls, Neural correlates of rapid reversal learning in a simple model of human social interaction, pp. 1371–83, Copyright, 2003, with permission from Elsevier.)

behaviour. One way to investigate this is in the stop-signal task, in which a signal is delivered on some trials indicating that the response being made should be stopped. In the stop-signal task, the lateral orbitofrontal cortex and the adjoining inferior frontal gyrus are both activated (Deng, Rolls et al (2017)). Impairments in the performance of the stop-signal task, which measures a type of motor impulsiveness, are associated with damage to the right inferior frontal gyrus (Aron, Robbins & Poldrack 2014). It is proposed that one route by which non-reward can stop behaviour is via the pathway from the lateral orbitofrontal cortex to the right inferior frontal gyrus. Consistent with this proposal, in depression, in which there may be oversensitivity to non-reward, there is increased functional connectivity of the lateral orbitofrontal cortex with the inferior frontal gyrus (see Chapter 7 and Section 7.4.2). In addition, in the context that there are many types of impulsiveness (Dalley & Robbins 2017), we have argued that one mechanism promoting impulsiveness may be under-connectedness of the lateral orbitofrontal cortex non-reward system (Cheng, Rolls, Robbins, Gong, Liu, Lv, Du, Wen, Ma, Quinlan, Garavan, Artiges, Papadopoulos Orfanos, Smolka, Schumann, Kendrick & Feng 2019). Another mechanism that may promote impulsiveness is over-connectedness of the medial orbitofrontal cortex reward system (Cheng et al. 2019). Consistent with this, sensation-seeking is associated with increased functional connectivity of the medial orbitofrontal cortex with the anterior cingulate cortex (Wan, Rolls, Cheng & Feng 2019). Individual differences in the efficacy of these different non-reward and reward mechanisms provides an approach to understanding the neural bases of personality (Rolls 2014a) (see Section 6.3).

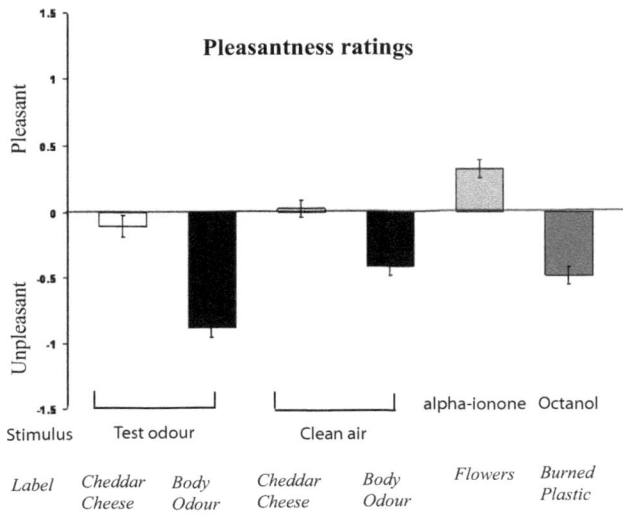

Fig. 3.49 Cognition and emotion. Subjective pleasantness ratings (mean ± s.e.m. across subjects) to odours labelled with words. The corresponding stimulus and label to each bar are listed in the lower part of the figure. The test odour (isovaleric acid) and clean air were paired in different trials with a label of either 'Cheddar cheese' or 'Body odour'. (Reprinted from Neuron, 46 (4), Ivan E. de Araujo, Edmund T. Rolls, Maria Ines Velazco, Christian Margot, and Isabelle Cayeux, Cognitive Modulation of Olfactory Processing, pp. 671–679, Copyright, 2005, with permission from Elsevier.)

3.9 Cognitive influences on the orbitofrontal cortex

Affective states, moods, can influence cognitive processing, including perception and memory (Rolls 2014a, Rolls 2018b). But cognition can also influence emotional states. This is not only in the sense that cognitively processed events, if decoded as being rewarding or punishing, can produce emotional states (Rolls 2014a, Rolls 2018b), but also in the sense described here that a cognitive input can bias emotional states in different directions. The modulation is rather like the top-down effects of attention on perception (Desimone & Duncan 1995, Rolls & Deco 2002, Deco & Rolls 2003, Deco & Rolls 2005c), not only phenomenologically, but also probably computationally. An example of such cognitive influences on the reward/aversive states that are elicited by stimuli was revealed in a study of olfaction described by De Araujo, Rolls, Velazco, Margot & Cayeux (2005).

In this investigation, a standard test odour, isovaleric acid (with a small amount of cheddar cheese odour added to make it more pleasant), was used as the test olfactory stimulus delivered with an olfactometer during functional neuroimaging with fMRI (De Araujo et al. 2005). This odour is somewhat ambiguous, and might be interpreted as the odour emitted by a cheese-like odour (rather like brie), or might be interpreted as a rather pungent and unpleasant body odour. A word was shown during the 8 s odour delivery. On some trials, the test odour was accompanied by the visually presented word 'Cheddar cheese'. On other trials, the test odour was accompanied by the visually presented word 'Body odour'. A word label was used rather than a picture label to make the modulating input very abstract and cognitive. First, it was found (consistent with psychophysical results of Herz & von Clef (2001)) that the word labels influenced the pleasantness ratings of the test odour, as shown in Fig. 3.49.

However, very interestingly, it was found that the word label modulated the activation to the odour in brain regions activated by odours such as the orbitofrontal cortex (secondary olfactory cortex), cingulate cortex, and amygdala (De Araujo et al. 2005). For example, in the

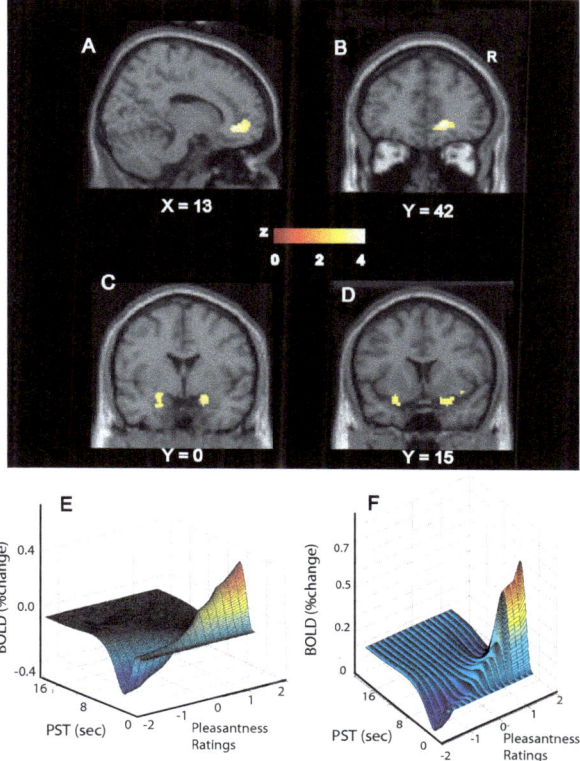

Fig. 3.50 Cognition and emotion. Group (random) effects analysis showing the brain regions where the BOLD signal was correlated with pleasantness ratings given to the test odour. The pleasantness ratings were being modulated by the word labels. (A) Activations in the rostral anterior cingulate cortex, in the region adjoining the medial OFC, shown in a sagittal slice. (B) The same activation shown coronally. (C) Bilateral activations in the amygdala. (D) These activations extended anteriorly to the primary olfactory cortex. The image was thresholded at p<0.0001 uncorrected in order to show the extent of the activation. (E) Parametric plots of the data averaged across all subjects showing that the percentage BOLD change (fitted) correlates with the pleasantness ratings in the region shown in A and B. The parametric plots were very similar for the primary olfactory region shown in D. PST - Post-stimulus time (s). (F) Parametric plots for the amygdala region shown in C. (Reprinted from Neuron, 46 (4), Ivan E. de Araujo, Edmund T. Rolls, Maria Ines Velazco, Christian Margot, and Isabelle Cayeux, Cognitive Modulation of Olfactory Processing, pp. 671–679, Copyright, 2005, with permission from Elsevier.)

medial orbitofrontal cortex the word label 'Cheddar cheese' caused a larger activation to be produced to the test odour than when the word label 'Body odour' was being presented. In these medial orbitofrontal cortex regions and the amygdala, and even possibly in some parts of the primary olfactory cortical areas, the activations were correlated with the pleasantness ratings, as shown in Fig. 3.50. This is consistent with the finding that the pleasantness of odours is represented in the medial orbitofrontal cortex (Rolls, Kringelbach & De Araujo 2003c).

The effects of the word were smaller when clean air was the stimulus, indicating that the effects being imaged were not just effects of a word to influence representations by a top-down recall process, but were instead cognitive top-down effects on states elicited by odours (De Araujo et al. 2005). This type of modulation is typical of a top-down modulatory process such as has been analysed quantitatively in the case of attention (Deco & Rolls 2005c), and indeed no significant effect of the word was found in the amygdala and earlier olfactory cortical areas. A further implication is that the activations in the human amygdala and primary olfactory cortical areas are more closely bound to the eliciting stimulus and are less influenced by cognition than are activations in the orbitofrontal and cingulate cortices.

These findings show that cognition can influence and indeed modulate reward-related (affective) processing as far down the human olfactory system as the secondary olfactory cortex (in the orbitofrontal cortex), and in the amygdala (De Araujo et al. 2005). This emphasizes the importance of cognitive influences on emotion, and shows how, in situations that might range from enjoying food to a romantic evening, the cognitive top-down influences can play an important role in influencing affective representations in the brain. Indeed, these findings lend support to the hypothesis that an interesting role for cognitive systems in emotion is to help set up the optimal conditions in terms of the reinforcers available and contextual surroundings for reinforcers to produce affective states, as treated further in the dual route hypothesis described in Section 6.4.

In an investigation of top-down cognitive modulation of affective processing in another modality, taste, it was found that activations related to the affective value of umami (delicious savoury) taste and flavor (as shown by correlations with pleasantness ratings) in the orbitofrontal cortex were modulated by word-level descriptors (Grabenhorst, Rolls & Bilderbeck 2008a). Affect-related activations to taste were modulated in a region that receives from the orbitofrontal cortex, the pregenual cingulate cortex, and to taste and flavor in another region that receives from the orbitofrontal cortex, the ventral striatum. Affect-related cognitive modulations were not found in the insular taste cortex, where the intensity but not the pleasantness of the taste was represented. Thus top-down language-level cognitive effects reach far down into the earliest cortical areas that represent the appetitive value of taste and flavor, and this type of modulation may be important in appetite control (Rolls 2012b, Rolls 2016f).

Similar cognitive modulation of affective touch is also found. The cognitive modulation was produced by word labels, 'Rich moisturizing cream' or 'Basic cream', while cream was being applied by slow gentle rubbing to the forearm, or was seen being applied to a forearm. The subjective pleasantness and richness were modulated by the word labels, as were the activations to the sight of touch and also the correlations with pleasantness in the pregenual cingulate/orbitofrontal cortex and ventral striatum (McCabe, Rolls, Bilderbeck & McGlone 2008). Further evidence of how the orbitofrontal cortex is involved in affective aspects of touch was that touch to the forearm [which has C fiber Touch (CT) afferents sensitive to light touch] compared with touch to the glabrous skin of the hand (which does not) revealed activation in the mid-orbitofrontal cortex. This is of interest as previous studies have suggested that the CT system is important in affiliative caress-like touch between individuals (McCabe et al. 2008, Rolls 2010b, Rolls 2016a).

Another example of what could be a similar phenomenon is that colour can have a strong influence on olfactory judgements. This was demonstrated when a white wine was artificially coloured red with an odourless dye, and it was found that participants (undergraduates at the Faculty of Oenology of the University of Bordeaux) described the wine using the descriptors normally used for red wine (Morrot, Brochet & Dubourdieu 2001). In this case it is possible that cognitive states elicited by the sight of what was believed to be red wine modulated the olfactory representation. Another possibility is that in a multimodal region such as the orbitofrontal cortex where the sight, smell, taste and texture are brought together onto individual neurons as shown above, the visual input makes a strong contribution to the convergence, and the resulting representation then is available to cognition for verbal description.

The mechanisms by which cognitive states have top-down effects on emotion are probably similar to the biased competition (Desimone & Duncan 1995, Rolls & Deco 2002, Deco & Rolls 2003, Deco & Rolls 2005c, Rolls & Stringer 2001b, Deco & Rolls 2005b) and biased activation (Rolls 2013a, Grabenhorst & Rolls 2010) mechanisms that subserve top-down attentional effects. In such systems, it is important that the top-down influence does not determine the activity in the system, otherwise stimuli and events would be imagined, and would not represent what was happening in the world. But by having a weak influence, facilitated by the fact that the top-down backprojection connections are relatively weak (Rolls 2016c, Rolls 1989a, Rolls & Treves 1998, Renart, Parga & Rolls 1999a, Renart, Parga &

Rolls 1999b, Renart, Moreno, Rocha, Parga & Rolls 2001, Rolls & Stringer 2001b, Rolls & Deco 2002, Deco & Rolls 2005c, Deco & Rolls 2005b, Rolls 2013a), cognition and attention can have beneficial effects in directing sensory and emotional processing towards stimuli and events that the cognitive system has determined are relevant.

Part of the interest and importance of these investigations is that they show that cognitive influences, originating from as high in processing as linguistic representations, can reach down into the first part of the brain in which emotion, affective, hedonic or reward value is made explicit in the representation, the orbitofrontal cortex, to modulate the responses there to affective taste, olfactory, flavour, somatosensory, and visual stimuli. The investigations thus show that linguistic representations can influence how emotional states are represented and thereby experienced. It is in this very direct way that cognition can have a powerful effect on emotional states, emotional behaviour, and emotional experience, because the emotional representations in the first cortical area in which affective value is represented, the orbitofrontal cortex, are altered.

3.10 Attentional modulation of affective vs sensory processing

Attentional instructions at the same, very high, linguistic, level (e.g. 'pay attention to and rate pleasantness' vs 'pay attention to and rate intensity') have a top-down modulatory influence on value representations in the orbitofrontal cortex and anterior cingulate cortex. The attentional instructions can bias processing for a stimulus between a stream through the orbitofrontal and cingulate cortices that processes value and affect, versus a stream involving sensory processing areas such as the insular taste cortex and pyriform primary olfactory cortex.

This modulation of affective processing has been shown for olfactory stimuli (Rolls, Grabenhorst, Margot, da Silva & Velazco 2008a). When subjects were instructed to remember and rate the pleasantness of a jasmin odour, activations in an fMRI investigation were greater in the medial orbitofrontal and pregenual cingulate cortex than when subjects were instructed to remember and rate the intensity of the odour. When the subjects were instructed to remember and rate the intensity, activations were greater in the pyriform primary olfactory cortex and inferior frontal gyrus. Top-down effects of attention occurred not only during odor delivery but started in a preparation period after the instruction before odor delivery, and continued after termination of the odor in a short-term memory period. Thus, depending on the context in which odours are presented and whether affect is relevant, the brain prepares itself, responds to, and remembers an odor differently. These findings show that when attention is paid to affective value, the brain systems engaged to prepare for, represent, and remember a sensory stimulus are different from those engaged when attention is directed to the physical properties of a stimulus such as its intensity.

In an investigation of the effects of selective attention to value and affect vs intensity on taste processing, when subjects were instructed to remember and rate the pleasantness of a savoury taste stimulus, 0.1 M monosodium glutamate, activations were greater in the medial orbitofrontal and pregenual cingulate cortex than when subjects were instructed to remember and rate the intensity of the taste (Grabenhorst & Rolls 2008) (Fig. 3.51). When the subjects were instructed to remember and rate the intensity, activations were greater in the insular taste cortex and a mid-insular cortex region (Fig. 3.52). Thus, depending on the context in which tastes are presented and whether affect is relevant, the brain responds to a taste differently.

The lateral prefrontal cortex, a region implicated in attentional control (Corbetta & Shulman 2002, Bressler, Tang, Sylvester, Shulman & Corbetta 2008, Rolls 2016c), has

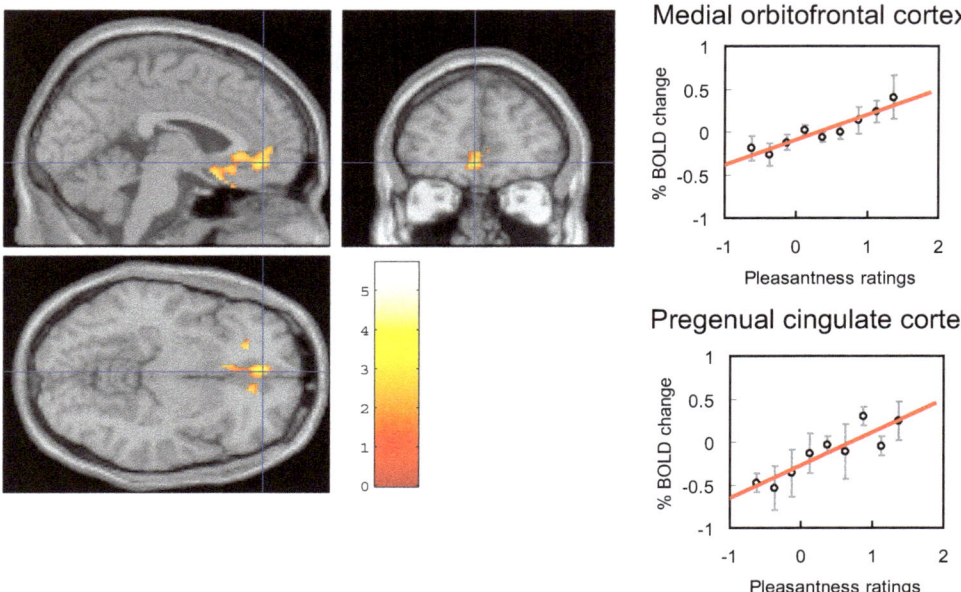

Fig. 3.51 Top-down attention and emotion. Effect of paying attention to the pleasantness of a taste. Left: A significant difference related to the taste period was found in the medial orbitofrontal cortex at [-6 14 -20] z=3.81 p<0.003 (towards the back of the area of activation shown) and in the pregenual cingulate cortex at [-4 46 -8] z=2.90 p<0.04 (at the cursor). Right upper: The correlation between the subjective pleasantness ratings and the activation (% BOLD change) in the orbitofrontal cortex (r=0.94, df=8, p<<0.001). Right lower: The correlation between the pleasantness ratings and the activation (% BOLD change) in the pregenual cingulate cortex r=0.89, df=8, p=0.001). The taste stimulus, monosodium glutamate, was identical on all trials. (Reproduced from Fabian Grabenhorst and Edmund T. Rolls, Selective attention to affective value alters how the brain processes taste stimuli, European Journal of Neuroscience, 27 (3) pp. 723–729 Copyright © 2008, John Wiley and Sons.)

been shown to be a site of origin for these top-down influences of attention on processing to the affective vs physical properties of stimuli. Grabenhorst & Rolls (2010) have shown with fMRI psychophysiological interaction analyses (Friston, Buechel, Fink, Morris, Rolls & Dolan 1997, Dolan, Fink, Rolls, Booth, Holmes, Frackowiak & Friston 1997) that in the anterior lateral prefrontal cortex at Y=53 mm the correlation with activity in the orbitofrontal and pregenual cingulate cortex seed regions was greater when attention was to pleasantness compared with when attention was to intensity. Conversely, in a more posterior region of the lateral prefrontal cortex at Y=34 mm the correlation with activity in the anterior insula seed region was greater when attention was to intensity compared with when attention was to pleasantness. (These seed regions were chosen as they were the regions where attention to affect or to intensity modulated the effects of the taste stimulus.) Grabenhorst & Rolls (2010) also showed that correlations between areas within each of these separate processing streams were dependent on selective attention to affective value versus physical intensity of the stimulus.

Correlations between signals, including signals at the neuronal or at the functional neuroimaging level, do not reveal the direction of the possible influence of one signal on the other. We extended the previous investigation by introducing and using componential Granger causality analysis, which measures the effect of y (for example a timeseries of activations in one brain area) on x (for example a timeseries of activations in another brain area), and allows interaction effects between y and x to be measured (Ge, Feng, Grabenhorst & Rolls 2012). We showed that there is a top-down attentional effect from the anterior dorsolateral prefrontal cortex to the orbitofrontal cortex when attention is paid to the pleasantness of a taste, and that this effect depends on the activity in the orbitofrontal cortex as shown by the interaction

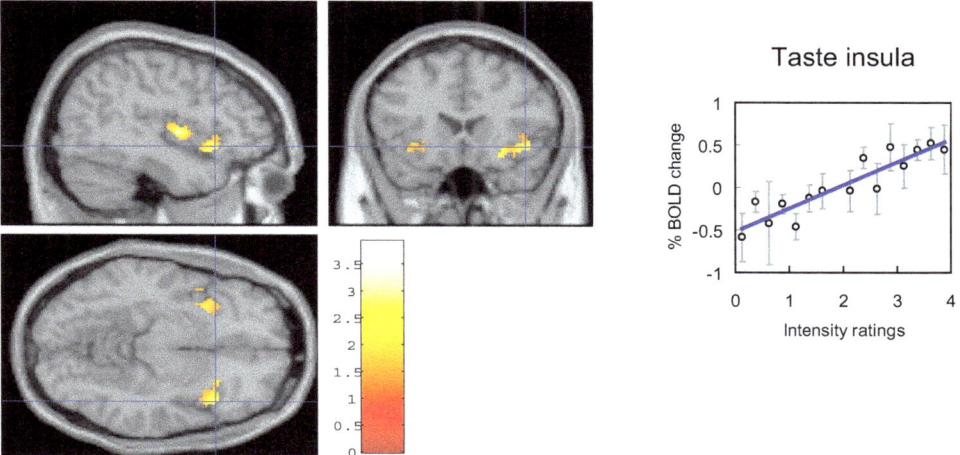

Fig. 3.52 Top-down attention and emotion. Left: Effect of paying attention to the intensity of a taste. Top: A significant difference related to the taste period was found in the taste insula at [42 18 -14] z=2.42 p<0.05 (indicated by the cursor) and in the mid insula at [40 -2 4] z=3.03 p<0.025. Right: The correlation between the intensity ratings and the activation (% BOLD change) in the taste insula (r=0.91, df=14, p<<0.001). The taste stimulus, monosodium glutamate, was identical on all trials. (Reproduced from Fabian Grabenhorst and Edmund T. Rolls, Selective attention to affective value alters how the brain processes taste stimuli, European Journal of Neuroscience, 27 (3) pp. 723–729 Copyright © 2008, John Wiley and Sons.)

term. Correspondingly there is a top-down attentional effect from the posterior dorsolateral prefrontal cortex to the insular primary taste cortex when attention is paid to the intensity of a taste, and this effect depends on the activity of the insular primary taste cortex as shown by the interaction term. These interaction effects reflect the underlying mechanism, that a weak top-down effect can have a large, non-linear, effect on bottom-up inputs when the bottom-up inputs are weak or ambiguous, as shown by an integrate-and-fire neuronal model of the mechanisms of selective attention (Deco & Rolls 2005c), which describes a mechanism for top-down attention (Desimone & Duncan 1995, Rolls 2016c, Rolls 2013a).

The way that one usually thinks of a top-down biased competition mechanism as operating in, for example, visual selective attention (Desimone & Duncan 1995) is that within an area, e.g. a cortical region, some neurons receive a weak top-down input that increases their response to the bottom-up stimuli (Desimone & Duncan 1995), potentially supralinearly if the bottom-up stimuli are weak (Deco & Rolls 2005c, Rolls & Deco 2002, Rolls 2016c). The enhanced firing of the biased neurons then, via the local inhibitory neurons, inhibits the other neurons in the local area from responding to the bottom-up stimuli. This is a local mechanism, in that the inhibition in the neocortex is primarily local, being implemented by cortical inhibitory neurons that typically have inputs and outputs over no more than a few mm (Douglas, Markram & Martin 2004, Rolls 2016c). This model of biased competition is illustrated in Fig. 3.53b.

This type of locally implemented 'biased competition' situation may not apply in the present case, where we have facilitation of processing in a whole cortical area (e.g. orbitofrontal cortex, or pregenual cingulate cortex) or even cortical processing stream (e.g. the linked orbitofrontal and pregenual cingulate cortex) in which any taste neurons may reflect pleasantness and not intensity. So the attentional effect might more accurately be described in this case as biased activation, without local competition being part of the effect. I have therefore proposed a *biased activation theory and model of attention*, illustrated in Fig. 3.53a (Rolls 2013a, Grabenhorst & Rolls 2010), which is a rather different way to implement attention in the brain than biased competition, and each mechanism may apply in different cases, or both mechanisms in some cases. In this case, the short-term memory systems implemented by an attractor network in for example the prefrontal cortex that holds in short-term memory

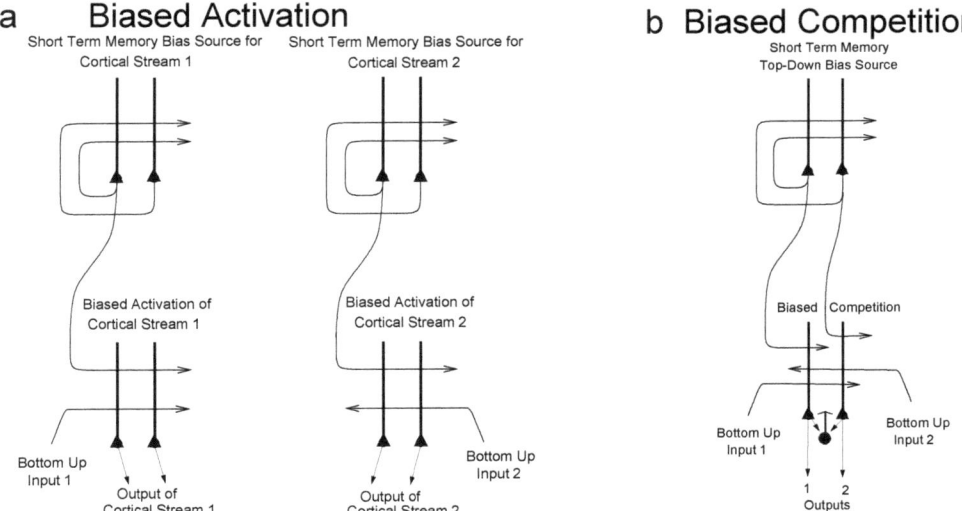

Fig. 3.53 Mechanisms for top-down attention. (a) Biased activation. The short-term memory systems that provide the source of the top-down activations may be separate (as shown), or could be a single network with different attractor states for the different selective attention conditions. The top-down short-term memory systems hold what is being paid attention to active by continuing firing in an attractor state, and bias separately either cortical processing system 1, or cortical processing system 2. This weak top-down bias interacts with the bottom up input to the cortical stream and produces an increase of activity that can be supralinear (Deco and Rolls 2005c). Thus the selective activation of separate cortical processing streams can occur. In the example, stream 1 might process the affective value of a stimulus, and stream 2 might process the intensity and physical properties of the stimulus. The outputs of these separate processing streams then must enter a competition system, which could be for example a cortical attractor decision-making network that makes choices between the two streams, with the choice biased by the activations in the separate streams (see text). (b) Biased competition. There is usually a single attractor network that can enter different attractor states to provide the source of the top-down bias (as shown). If it is a single network, there can be competition within the short-term memory attractor states, implemented through the local GABA inhibitory neurons. The top-down continuing firing of one of the attractor states then biases in a top-down process some of the neurons in a cortical area to respond more to one than the other of the bottom-up inputs, with competition implemented through the GABA inhibitory neurons (symbolized by a filled circle) which make feedback inhibitory connections onto the pyramidal cells (symbolized by a triangle) in the cortical area. The thick vertical lines above the pyramidal cells are the dendrites. The axons are shown with thin lines and the excitatory connections by arrow heads. (Modified from Rolls 2013a.)

the property to which attention should be paid provides top-down inputs which bias the activations in whole processing streams. The short-term memory in the prefrontal cortex could be implemented in a single attractor network with different attractor states (Rolls 2016c) for the different attentional conditions, or, as suggested by the evidence in this case (Grabenhorst & Rolls 2010), the short-term memory networks may be at least partly physically separate, though close to each other in the prefrontal cortex. The systems being modulated could operate as competitive networks, as attractor networks, or, as I have suggested (Rolls 2016c), as networks that can learn mainly by competitive learning, but can maintain activity in memory using associatively modified recurrent collateral connections to implement attractor dynamics.

The outputs of the separate processing streams showing biased activation (Fig. 3.53a) may need to be compared later to lead to a single behaviour. One way in which this comparison could take place is by both outputs entering a single network cortical attractor model of decision-making, in which positive feedback implemented by the excitatory recurrent collateral connections leads through non-linear dynamics to a single winner, which is ensured by competition between the different possible attractor states produced through inhibitory neurons (Deco & Rolls 2006, Rolls & Deco 2010, Wang 2008, Wang 2002). A second way in which the competition could be implemented is by that usually conceptualized as important in biased competition (Deco & Rolls 2005b, Desimone & Duncan 1995, Rolls & Deco 2002), in which a feedforward competitive network using inhibition through local inhibitory neurons provides a way for a weak top-down signal to bias the output especially if the bottom-up inputs are weak (Deco & Rolls 2005b, Rolls & Deco 2002, Rolls 2016c), and this implementation is what is shown at the bottom of Fig. 3.53b. A third way in which the biased activation reflected in the output of the streams shown in Fig. 3.53a could be taken into account is by a mechanism such as that in the basal ganglia, where in the striatum the different excitatory inputs activate GABA (gamma-amino-butyric acid) neurons, which then directly inhibit each other to make the selection (Rolls 2014a, Rolls 2016c) (Section 5.3).

Biased activation as a mechanism for top-down selective attention may be widespread in the brain, and may be engaged when there is segregated processing of different attributes of stimuli. It may apply not only for affective, value-based vs sensory processing, but also to the dorsal vs ventral visual system in vision, and to the 'what' vs 'where' systems for visual processing (Rolls & Deco 2002, Rolls 2016c, Rolls 2013a).

These findings show that, when attention is paid to affective value, the brain systems engaged to represent stimuli are in part different from those engaged when attention is directed to the physical properties of a stimulus such as its intensity. This has many implications for understanding the effects of many stimuli and recalled memories too, and has many implications for sensory testing. These insights have implications for a number of areas related to neuroeconomics and decision-making, including the design of studies in which attentional instructions may influence which brain systems become engaged, as well as situations in which affective processing may be usefully modulated (for example in the control of the effects of the reward value of food and its role in obesity, and in addiction (Rolls 2016c, Rolls 2014a, Rolls 2018b, Rolls 2012b).

Another implication is that paying attention to pleasantness, and also cognitive top-down modulation, may be used to enhance pleasant emotional and aesthetic experiences.

3.11 The topology of the functional neuroimaging activations in the orbitofrontal cortex

We have reviewed evidence that the activations found in functional neuroimaging studies by many types of reward appear to involve relatively medial parts of the human orbitofrontal cortex, and unpleasant stimuli or non-reward more lateral parts of the human orbitofrontal cortex (Grabenhorst & Rolls 2011, Rolls 2014a, Kringelbach & Rolls 2004). For example, we have obtained evidence from an experiment using pleasant, painful and neutral somatosensory stimulation that there is some spatial segregation of the representation of rewards and punishers, where the effects of pleasant somatosensory stimulation are spatially dissociable from the effects of painful stimulation in the human orbitofrontal cortex (Rolls, O'Doherty, Kringelbach, Francis, Bowtell & McGlone 2003d). Further, pleasant odours activate medial, and unpleasant odours lateral, regions of the human orbitofrontal cortex (Rolls, Kringelbach & De Araujo 2003c). Another example comes from the finding that the administration of amphetamine to naive human subjects activates the orbitofrontal cortex and two regions to which it projects the pregenual cingulate cortex and ventral striatum (Voellm, De Araujo, Cowen, Rolls, Kringelbach, Smith, Jezzard, Heal & Matthews 2004). An indication that a rewarding effect is being produced by the amphetamine in part because of an action in the orbitofrontal cortex is that macaques will self-administer amphetamine to the orbitofrontal cortex (Phillips, Mora & Rolls 1981). A clear indication of a differentiation in function between medial versus lateral areas of the human orbitofrontal cortex was found in our study investigating visual discrimination reversal learning, which showed a clear dissociation between the medial orbitofrontal areas correlating with monetary gain, and the lateral areas correlating with monetary loss (O'Doherty, Kringelbach, Rolls, Hornak & Andrews 2001a). This result, and some of

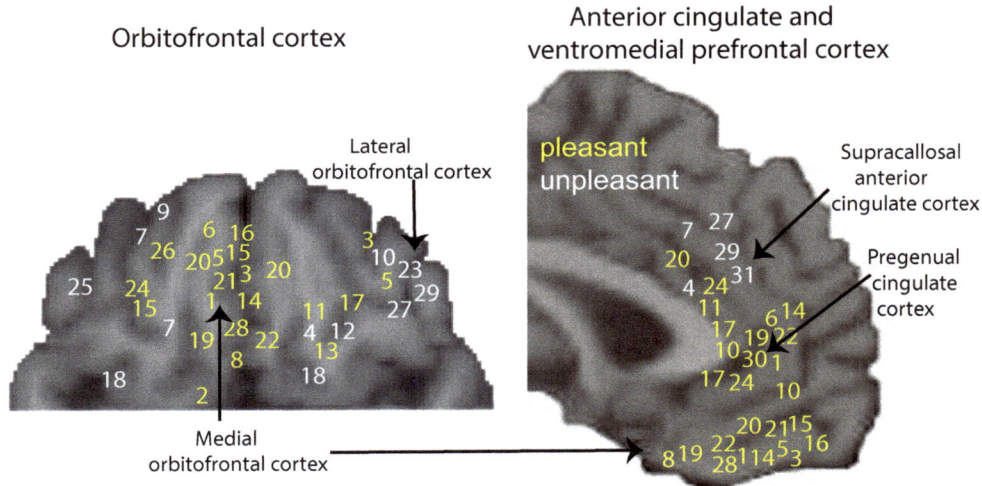

Fig. 3.54 Maps of subjective pleasure in the human orbitofrontal cortex (ventral view) and anterior cingulate and ventromedial prefrontal cortex (sagittal view). Yellow: sites where activations correlate with subjective pleasantness. White: sites where activations correlate with subjective unpleasantness. The numbers refer to effects found in specific studies. Taste: 1, 2; odor: 3-10; flavor: 11-16; oral texture: 17, 18; chocolate: 19; water: 20; wine: 21; oral temperature: 22, 23; somatosensory temperature: 24, 25; the sight of touch: 26, 27; facial attractiveness: 28, 29; erotic pictures: 30; laser-induced pain: 31. (Modified from Trends in Cognitive Sciences, 15 (2), Fabian Grabenhorst and Edmund T. Rolls, Value, pleasure and choice in the ventral prefrontal cortex, pp. 56–67, Copyright, 2011, with permission from Elsevier.)

the other studies included in a meta-analysis (Kringelbach & Rolls 2004), can be interpreted as evidence for a difference in humans between medial orbitofrontal cortex areas involved in decoding and monitoring the reward value of reinforcers, and lateral areas involved in evaluating punishers that when detected may lead to a change in current behaviour. A good example of a study showing the latter involved a visual discrimination reversal task in which face identity was associated with a face expression (Kringelbach & Rolls 2003). When the face expression associated with one of the faces reversed and the face expression was being interpreted as a punisher and indicated that behaviour should change, then lateral parts of the orbitofrontal cortex became activated (Fig. 3.48).

At sites where positive value, produced by a reward, are represented, there are, when they are measured, correlations between the conscious, subjective, state of pleasure and the brain activations, where both are measured on every trial. Similarly, at sites where negative value, produced by a punisher or non-reward, are represented, there are correlations between the subjective state of unpleasantness and the brain activations. Fig. 3.54 shows the peaks of the correlations found in many different investigations related to these subjective states of pleasantness (yellow) and of unpleasantness (white) for both the orbitofrontal and the cingulate and ventromedial prefrontal cortices (see also Section 5.1) (Grabenhorst & Rolls 2011). Reference to Fig. 1.2 on page 4 shows the different cytoarchitectonic areas in these regions.

Although our study on abstract reward found that monetary reward and punishment are correlated with activations in different regions of the orbitofrontal cortex (O'Doherty, Kringelbach, Rolls, Hornak & Andrews 2001a), even this evidence does not show that rewards and punishers have totally separate representations in the human brain. In particular, the medial regions of the orbitofrontal cortex that had activations correlating with the magnitude of monetary reward (area 11) also reflected monetary punishers in the sense that the activations in these medial regions correlated positively with the magnitude of monetary wins and negatively with losses (see Fig. 3.43). Similarly, the more lateral regions (area 10) had activations that correlated negatively with the magnitudes of monetary wins and gains, and positively with monetary loss/punishment. This means that in this experiment the medial and lateral regions were apparently coding for both monetary reward and punishment (albeit in opposite ways). An investigation by Xie, Jia, Rolls et al (2019) with 1140 participants supports this (Fig. 7.5). Further evidence for the same principle, but now for pleasant vs unpleasant odours, is illustrated in Fig. 3.17 (Rolls et al. 2003c).

The neurophysiological evidence suggests that the segregation between rewards and punishers is not purely spatial but rather encoded in the neuronal responses, which the studies in macaques described above show can be exquisitely tuned differently not only to reinforcers in different sensory modalities (taste, smell, touch etc.), but also to combinations of these, and even within any one modality (e.g. with neurons tuned to different tastes). The functional imaging thus provides a very blurred picture of what is really happening at the neuronal and information representation level in the orbitofrontal cortex. Although it is true that similar neurons may tend to cluster together as a result of a self-organizing competitive network with short range excitatory connections (see Rolls & Treves (1998) and Rolls (2016c)), and this may lead to somewhat localized blobs of activity in the cortex, the presence of such blobs should not be taken as more than a gross reflection of the underlying neuronal representations and computations. Integrating over all this heterogeneous neuronal activity is what leads to an fMRI signal.

What account might we give for why so many different types of reward are represented in the human medial orbitofrontal cortex? The types of reward include, as described above, food reward as shown in sensory-specific satiety experiments (Kringelbach, O'Doherty, Rolls & Andrews 2003), pleasant odours (Rolls, Kringelbach & De Araujo 2003c, Grabenhorst, Rolls, Margot, da Silva & Velazco 2007, Rolls, Grabenhorst, Margot, da Silva & Velazco 2008a), pleasant flavours (McCabe & Rolls 2007, Rolls & McCabe 2007, Grabenhorst et al. 2008a, Grabenhorst & Rolls 2008), pleasant touch (Rolls, O'Doherty, Kringelbach, Francis, Bowtell & McGlone 2003d, McCabe, Rolls, Bilderbeck & McGlone 2008, Rolls, Grabenhorst & Parris 2008b), face attractiveness (O'Doherty et al. 2003), monetary reward (O'Doherty, Kringelbach, Rolls, Hornak & Andrews 2001a, Rolls, McCabe & Redoute 2008e), conditioned stimuli associated with drug self-administration in addicts (Childress, Mozley, McElgin, Fitzgerald, Reivich & O'Brien 1999), and also the administration of amphetamine to drug-naive human subjects (Voellm, De Araujo, Cowen, Rolls, Kringelbach, Smith, Jezzard, Heal & Matthews 2004). The neuronal recording studies described above in macaques show clearly that there is an exquisite representation of the detailed properties of these different stimuli, with different neurons by virtue of their different tuning to each of these properties and to combinations of these properties providing information about all the individual properties of each particular stimulus. For example, as a population, different orbitofrontal cortex neurons in macaques have different responses to the following properties of oral stimuli, with some neurons encoding each property independently, and others responding to different combinations of them: taste, fat texture, viscosity, astringency, grittiness, capsaicin content, odour, and sight (see above).

Why are so many of the reward-related properties of stimuli represented in the same medial part of the orbitofrontal cortex? I suggest that part of the functional utility of this is that there can be comparison of the magnitudes of what may be quite different types of reward, implemented by the local lateral inhibition mediated via the inhibitory interneurons.

The architecture required for the implementation is that which is standard for the cerebral cortex (Rolls 2016c): the excitatory pyramidal cells, which are the neurons with the types of often quite selective response just described, connect to inhibitory neurons, which are relatively fewer in number (perhaps 15% of the number of excitatory neurons). The inhibitory neurons receive from random sets of neurons in the vicinity, and project back their summed effects as inhibition to random collections of pyramidal cells. This lateral inhibition system has the effect of controlling the activity of the excitatory neurons, and importantly, the effect of ensuring that the most strongly activated excitatory neurons reduce the activity of less strongly activated excitatory neurons. Contrast enhancement may occur between the competing inputs, and also local scaling of the overall activity of the neurons so that they operate within their working range to reflect in their output firing the inputs being received, in processes that are quantitatively understood and are used in competitive networks (Grossberg 1988, Rolls & Treves 1998, Rolls & Deco 2002, Deco & Rolls 2005c, Rolls 2016c). The result of the mutual inhibition is that the relative magnitude of the different rewards available can be compared, and the most strongly firing neurons after the competition reflect the strongest reward.

This type of comparison would be difficult to implement if each type of reward was represented in a different location in the brain, and may be a useful computational outcome of the fact that different types of reward are represented (by different neurons of course) in the same general brain region, the medial orbitofrontal cortex. This computation would provide scaling of different rewards, both relative to each other when presented simultaneously as in a choice situation, and relative to a fixed maximum if only one reward is present. This would be part of the mechanisms involved in computing relative reward value, and also in adjusting different rewards to be on the same scale of value (see Section 3.12.3).

It may be useful to note that the human medial orbitofrontal cortex region activated by many types of reward may have shifted medially somewhat with respect to its location in macaques. Spurred by the human neuroimaging studies just described, we (Rolls, Kadohisa, Verhagen and Gabbott) have made recordings in the topologically most medial part of the macaque orbitofrontal cortex, and also the nearby anterior cingulate cortex, to determine whether there is a previously undescribed set of reward / taste / olfactory / visual / somatosensory representations in this region (Rolls 2008d). We have not found such neurons in the part of the macaque orbitofrontal cortex that is less than 3–4 mm from the midline (in which area 14 is located). We do find that neurons that respond to the taste, odour, texture, and sight of food start at approximately this laterality, and then extend out laterally from this paramedial orbitofrontal cortex region, through the mid to the far lateral orbitofrontal cortex, at sites shown in Rolls (2008d), which adds to the previous recordings illustrated in a number of other papers (e.g. Rolls & Baylis (1994), Critchley & Rolls (1996a), and Rolls, Critchley, Wakeman & Mason (1996c)). Indeed, some of these more medial sites in which taste neurons are common are illustrated in Fig. 3.18 on page 42 from Rolls & Baylis (1994).

It is quite clear from a retrograde neuronal tracing study with horseradish peroxidase administered to a region containing taste neurons in the macaque lateral orbitofrontal cortex that the lateral part of the orbitofrontal cortex receives direct inputs from the primary taste cortex in the insula (see Fig. 2.3 and Baylis, Rolls & Baylis (1994)). (The location of the macaque primary taste cortex was described by Pritchard et al. (1986).) More medial orbitofrontal cortex areas may also receive inputs directly from the insular and frontal opercular primary taste cortical areas, for, as illustrated in Fig. 3.18, taste neurons are also common in this more medial part of the orbitofrontal cortex (see further Rolls & Baylis (1994) and Critchley & Rolls (1996a)). The same anatomical paper (Baylis, Rolls & Baylis 1994) also showed that a more anterior part of the orbitofrontal cortex is a tertiary taste cortical area, for it receives inputs from the secondary, orbitofrontal, taste cortex, but not from the primary taste cortex. The more middle / medial part of the orbitofrontal cortex (close to the region indicated in Fig. 3.18) also has neurons that decrease their taste responses in relation to sensory-specific satiety, and a few that do not (Critchley & Rolls 1996c). Thus the macaque posterior orbitofrontal cortex contains taste, and also olfactory and visual, neurons throughout its mediolateral extent, apart from the most medial 3–4 mm (Rolls 2008d). In contrast, the taste and olfactory reward areas in humans appear to reach to the midline, and probably do not extend as far lateral as in non-human primates (see e.g. Figs. 3.16, 3.17, 3.20 and 3.50).

I suggest that as the frontal lobes have developed from macaques to humans, more cortex has been added to the dorsolateral prefrontal cortex areas so important in working memory and hence in attention and executive function (Rolls & Deco 2002, Deco & Rolls 2003, Rolls 2016c), thus displacing the inferior convexity prefrontal cortex more medially in humans, and displacing the main orbitofrontal cortex areas of macaques more medially in humans, so that they reach as far as the midline. This would be the same trend that occurs in the temporal lobes of macaques vs humans, in which the enormous development of language areas in the left hemisphere (and corresponding high order processing areas in the right hemisphere) appear to have displaced at least parts of the inferior temporal visual cortex to be much more ventrally and medially represented in for example the human fusiform face and related areas (Rolls & Deco 2002, Baylis, Rolls & Leonard 1987, Dolan, Fink, Rolls, Booth, Holmes, Frackowiak & Friston 1997, Tovee, Rolls & Ramachandran 1996, Kanwisher, McDermott & Chun 1997, Ishai, Ungerleider, Martin & Haxby 2000). The clear mediolateral topology in the orbitofrontal cortex in humans should for this reason not be taken as implying the same topology in monkeys, and this makes comparisons based on topology precarious. Further, from our earliest studies (Thorpe, Rolls & Maddison 1983) we have not seen clear topological segregation of reward, punishment, and error-related neurons in the orbitofrontal cortex of monkeys. However, in a macaque fMRI investigation, activations to non-reward were evident in the lateral orbitofrontal cortex (Chau, Sallet, Papageorgiou, Noonan, Bell, Walton & Rushworth 2015), and further neuronal recording here in non-reward tasks would be of interest. Moreover, it is important to separate the reward areas of the human orbitofrontal cortex proper as visible from a ventral view in Fig. 3.54 from those in the ventromedial prefrontal / cingulate network visible in the sagittal view in Fig. 3.54. The latter, anterior cingulate networks, receive from the orbitofrontal cortex, and perform different functions, as is made clear in Section 5.1.

Another possible topological trend in the human orbitofrontal cortex may be present in the posterior to anterior direction, with the possibility of some hierarchy (Kringelbach & Rolls 2004). Very abstract reinforcers such as loss of money appear to be represented further anterior towards the frontal pole (e.g. O'Doherty, Kringelbach, Rolls, Hornak & Andrews (2001a)) than in posterior areas representing simple reinforcers such as taste (e.g. De Araujo, Kringelbach, Rolls & Hobden (2003a); De Araujo, Kringelbach, Rolls & McGlone (2003b)) or thermal intensity (Craig, Chen, Bandy & Reiman 2000). This posterior–anterior trend is demonstrated in the statistical results from the meta-analysis (Kringelbach & Rolls 2004) and may reflect some kind of hierarchical processing in the orbitofrontal cortex. Relatively far forward in the orbitofrontal cortex, in area 11, another, memory-related, rather than emotion-related, type of representation is present, for here neurons are activated by novel visual stimuli (Rolls, Browning, Inoue & Hernadi 2005a), and activations in humans are produced by novel visual stimuli (Frey & Petrides 2002a).

Another finding is that areas that have supralinear responses to combinations of sensory inputs, for example taste and smell (De Araujo, Rolls, Kringelbach, McGlone & Phillips 2003c), or the umami taste stimuli monosodium glutamate (MSG) and inosine 5'-monophosphate (De Araujo, Kringelbach, Rolls & Hobden 2003a), tend to be more anterior than the areas where the components of the combinations are represented in the orbitofrontal cortex. This could easily reflect hierarchy in the system, with convergence tending to increase from more posterior to more anterior orbitofrontal cortex areas, and thus effects of combinations of inputs becoming more evident anteriorly. This is found in the ventral visual cortical stream (Rolls 2012d). In the ventromedial prefrontal cortex, the highest degree of non-linearity, at the end of the processing stream, may be reflected in the implementation of decision-making between stimuli of different value in medial prefrontal cortex area 10 (see Section 3.12).

3.12 Value representations in the orbitofrontal cortex and neuroeconomic decision-making

3.12.1 Choosing between rewards with different value

As we have seen in this Chapter, neurons in the orbitofrontal cortex represent value (or outcome, the value of the reward or punisher received); expected value; and negative reward prediction error. The representations of value and expected value include different representations by different neurons of positive and negative value ('reward value' and 'punisher value', and of expected value ('expected reward value' and 'expected punisher value'). The representations are of reward value in that the neuronal responses to a reward such as the taste, sight or smell of food decrease when that particular food is devalued by feeding to satiety; and when the expected reward value of a visual stimulus is altered by its reversal during learning of the value of the (taste or flavor) outcome that is expected when the discriminative visual or olfactory stimulus is presented (Rolls 2014a, Rolls & Grabenhorst 2008).

Thus the brain maintains representations of the values of different stimuli (including abstract reinforcers such as money (O'Doherty, Kringelbach, Rolls, Hornak & Andrews 2001a, Rolls, McCabe & Redoute 2008e, Xie, Jia, Rolls, Liu, Banaschewski, Barker, Bodke, Bromberg, C., Quinlan, Desrivieres, Flor, Grigis, Garavan, Gowland, Heinz, Hohmann, Ittermann, Martinot, Martinot, Nees, Papadopoulos Orfanos, Paus, Poustka, Frohner, Smolka, Walter, Whelan, Schumann, Feng & IMAGEN 2019)), and these representations are in the orbitofrontal cortex (Rolls 2014a, Rolls 2018b, Rolls & Grabenhorst 2008, Grabenhorst & Rolls 2011). We have argued and produced evidence that these reward value representations are on a common scale to facilitate the decision-making process (Grabenhorst, D'Souza, Parris, Rolls & Passingham 2010a, Grabenhorst & Rolls 2011) (see Section 3.12.2).

In slightly different terminology, value represents a common unit of measure to make a comparison between these reinforcing stimuli or 'goods' (Padoa-Schioppa 2011, Padoa-Schioppa & Conen 2017). In that terminology, a 'commodity' is a unitary amount of a specified good independently of the circumstances in which it is available (e.g. quantity, cost, delay, etc.). The value of each good is computed at the time of choice on the basis of multiple 'determinants', which include the specific commodity, its quantity, the current motivational state, the cost of obtaining it, the behavioural context of choice (i.e. the other choices that are currently available), etc. The collection of these determinants thus defines the value of the 'good'.

The hypothesis is that while choosing, individuals compute the values of different options independently of one another. It is argued that the 'net reward value', i.e. the value of each good minus the cost of obtaining it, must be computed and represented on a common scale of value as the input to the decision-making process, which makes the choice (Grabenhorst & Rolls 2011). The reason that the net value must be computed is that the decision-making process itself, performed it is suggested by an attractor decision-making network (Section 3.13), cannot by itself receive as inputs separate values and costs for each choice, for these variables related to a specific choice could not be related to each other in the decision-making attractor network.

A brain region that does appear to compute the actions needed to obtain a stimulus with the particular value, and which takes into account the costs of actions (which we have termed the extrinsic costs (Grabenhorst & Rolls 2011)), is the cingulate cortex (Rushworth, Noonan, Boorman, Walton & Behrens 2011, Grabenhorst & Rolls 2011), which receives value information about the goods in its anterior cingulate part from the orbitofrontal cortex (Rolls 2005, Rolls 2009c, Grabenhorst & Rolls 2011). It is argued that the computation of net value in the orbitofrontal cortex does not depend on the sensori-motor contingencies of choice (the spatial configuration of the offers or the specific action that will implement the choice outcome), for the behavioural responses and actions are not represented in the orbitofrontal cortex, which represents the value of stimuli, and does not represent actions and responses (Thorpe, Rolls & Maddison 1983, Rolls 2005, Padoa-Schioppa 2011, Padoa-Schioppa & Conen 2017). These action contingencies may, however, affect values in the form of action costs. In particular, the actions necessary to obtain different goods often bear different costs. It is still an interesting issue about whether these 'extrinsic costs' (the costs of the actions necessary to obtain a reward (Grabenhorst & Rolls 2011)) are represented in the orbitofrontal cortex.

The extrinsic costs that influence the value of a good and the value of a choice include
1. The action costs, including the difficulty of the actions needed to obtain the good, as just described;
2. the time delay (with future rewards being discounted as a function of the length of the delay, and differently discounted by different individuals);
3. the 'risk', i.e. the probability that the reward will be obtained;
4. the amount of the good obtained if it is chosen;
5. the quality of the good, e.g. one juice may be preferred over another;
6. ambiguity (i.e. poor knowledge about the probability that a reward if chosen will be obtained).

Intrinsic or internal costs and related factors that influence the value of stimuli include (Grabenhorst & Rolls 2011, Padoa-Schioppa 2011, Padoa-Schioppa & Conen 2017)
1. motivational state;
2. patience vs impatience or impulsiveness;
3. risk attitude, that is choice when the outcome is probabilistic, for example whether one is likely to gamble;
4. ambiguity attitude;
5. whether the stimulus which may have pleasant components has in addition unpleasant components.

Further factors important in understanding choices in the field of neuroeconomics, many described in more detail below, are:
The value of each good must be computed 'online' at the time of choice, for value is influenced by for example motivational state.
While choosing, individuals normally compute the values of different goods independently of one another. Such 'menu invariance' implies transitive preferences (Padoa-Schioppa 2011, Padoa-Schioppa & Conen 2017).
Absolute value is important for long-term choice and transitive preferences. This may be represented in the orbitofrontal cortex.
Relative value is useful for short-term choice, for example on a particular trial or a block of trials, and may be separately represented in the orbitofrontal cortex.

In one neuroeconomics study that illustrates how the responses of orbitofrontal cortex neurons encode the value of a stimulus or choice, the value of the choice was manipulated by providing different numbers of drops of juice (quantity) of different quality (e.g. grape juice (A) and peppermint tea (B), which were termed commodities) to monkeys (Padoa-Schioppa & Assad 2006). The monkey preferred juice A. When offered one drop of juice A versus one drop of juice B (offer 1A:1B), the animals chose juice A. However, the animals were thirsty: they generally preferred larger amounts of juice to smaller amounts of juice. The amounts of

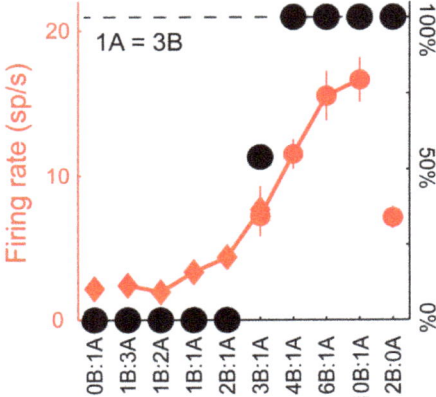

Fig. 3.55 Orbitofrontal cortex neuron encoding the offer value. On individual trials, the monkey was offered different numbers of drops of peppermint tea (juice B) versus 1 drop of grape juice (juice A). Black circles indicate the behavioural choice pattern (relative value in the upper left) and red symbols indicate the neuronal firing rate when the offer of different amounts of juice B was made vs 1 drop of juice A (1A). Red diamonds and circles refer, respectively, to trials in which the animal chose juice A and juice B. There is a sigmoid relationship between the firing rate of the neuron and the quantity of juice B offered to the monkey. (Reproduced from Padoa-Schioppa, C., Neurobiology of economic choice: a good-based model, Annual Review of Neuroscience, 34, pp. 333–359 © 2011, Annual Reviews.)

the two juices offered against each other varied from trial to trial, which induced a commodity quantity trade-off in the choice pattern. For example in one session (Fig. 3.55), offer types (indicated by the number of small squares on a screen that were available for A and for B) included 0B:1A, 1B:2A, 1B:1A, 2B:1A, 3B:1A, 4B:1A, 6B:1A, 10B:1A and 3B:0A. The monkey generally chose 1A when 1B or 2B were available as the alternative, it was roughly indifferent between the two juices when offered 3B:1A, and it chose B when 4B, 6B or 10B were available (Fig. 3.55). In other words, the monkey assigned to 1A a value roughly equal to the value it assigned to 3B. A neuron recorded in the orbitofrontal cortex responded with a low rate (several spikes/s) when the offer was 2B or less, at an intermediate rate (approximately 10 spikes/s) when the offer was 3B or 4B, and at a high rate (approximately 17 spikes/s) when the offer was 6B or higher relative to 1A (Fig. 3.55). The neuron thus encoded the value of the offer, where the value assigned by the monkey reflected a commodity × quantity tradeoff.

The offer value neurons respond when the visual stimulus indicating the taste/flavor reward that will be obtained is shown (Padoa-Schioppa & Assad 2006, Padoa-Schioppa 2011, Padoa-Schioppa & Conen 2017). They thus correspond to the orbitofrontal cortex neurons described by Rolls and colleagues that respond to a visual stimulus, for example in a visual discrimination task, that indicates the value of the reward or punisher that will be obtained (Thorpe, Rolls & Maddison 1983, Rolls, Critchley, Mason & Wakeman 1996a, Critchley & Rolls 1996c). These visual neurons reflect reward value in that they respond to a particular visual stimulus when the value is high, and gradually respond less to the visual stimulus as gradually it becomes devalued by feeding to satiety (Critchley & Rolls 1996c) (Fig. 3.25). These visual neurons also respond to a visual stimulus when it signifies a high value, and do not respond when it is devalued by visual discrimination reversal learning so that it signifies after learning a low reward value (Rolls, Critchley, Mason & Wakeman 1996a) (Fig. 3.22). In addition, these studies show that other neurons reflect the punisher value of a visual stimulus, responding for example to a visual stimulus when it signifies the punisher of a taste of saline if the visual stimulus is selected (Fig. 3.23) (Thorpe, Rolls & Maddison 1983, Rolls, Critchley, Mason & Wakeman 1996a).

Padoa-Schioppa & Assad (2006) also described neurons that in the same task responded when the juice taste reward was delivered. Their taste neurons reflected value, in that they had for example a large response when 4B or greater was delivered, an intermediate response when 3B was delivered, and no response when 2B or less was delivered (Fig. 3.55) (Padoa-Schioppa 2011). These neurons again correspond to the taste reward neurons of Rolls and colleagues analysed in the orbitofrontal cortex (Rolls, Yaxley & Sienkiewicz 1990, Rolls, Critchley, Verhagen & Kadohisa 2010a), which respond to a taste when it has a high value, and gradually respond less to that taste when it is gradually devalued by feeding to satiety (Rolls, Sienkiewicz & Yaxley (1989), e.g. Fig. 3.5).

It is of interest that the visual reward and taste reward neurons in the orbitofrontal cortex described by Rolls and colleagues maintain their firing almost unchanged to other visual or taste stimuli when one visual or taste stimulus is devalued (Rolls, Sienkiewicz & Yaxley 1989, Critchley & Rolls 1996c) (e.g. Fig. 3.5). These neurons thus reflect primarily *absolute reward value*, in that their firing rate to other rewards is little influenced when one of the visual or taste rewards on offer is devalued (see further Section 3.12.3). However, the small increase in firing rate sometimes found in sensory-specific satiety experiments to visual or taste food stimuli that have not been fed to satiety (Rolls, Sienkiewicz & Yaxley 1989, Critchley & Rolls 1996c) (e.g. Fig. 3.25) may reflect a small proportion of *relative reward value* in the representations provided by these visual and taste orbitofrontal cortex neurons.

In the experiment illustrated in Fig. 3.55, offers varied on two dimensions: juice type (commodity), and juice amount (quantity). The same method can be applied when offers vary on other dimensions, such as probability, cost, delay, etc. For example, Kable & Glimcher (2007) conducted on human subjects an experiment on *temporal discounting*. People and animals often prefer smaller rewards delivered earlier to larger rewards delivered later – an important phenomenon with broad societal implications. In the study of Kable and Glimcher, subjects chose in each trial between a small amount of money delivered immediately and a larger amount of money delivered at a later time. For given delivery time t, the amount of money was varied, and the indifference point was identified: the amount of money delivered at time t such that the subject would be indifferent between the two options. This procedure was repeated for different delivery times t. Indifference points – fitted with a hyperbolic function – provided a measure of the subjective value choosers assigned to time-discounted money. The results of the fMRI experiment showed that the activation in the ventromedial prefrontal cortex (vmPFC) reflected the time-discounted values.

An interesting procedure to measure indifference points is to perform a 'second price auction'. For example in a study by Plassmann, O'Doherty & Rangel (2007), hungry human subjects were asked to declare the highest price they would be willing to pay for a given food (i.e., their indifference point, also called 'reservation price'). Normally, people would try to save money and declare a price lower than their true reservation price. However, second price auctions discourage them from doing so by randomly generating a second price after the subjects have declared their own price. If the second price is lower than the declared price, subjects get to buy the food and pay the second price; if the second price is higher than the declared price, subjects do not get to buy the food at all. In these conditions, the optimal strategy for subjects is to declare their true reservation price. This procedure thus measures for each subject the indifference point between food and money. Using this measure, Plassmann et al. (2007) confirmed that the BOLD signal in the orbitofrontal cortex reflects the subjective value assigned to different foods.

In summary, to measure the neural representation of subjective value, it is necessary to let the subject choose between alternative offers, infer values from the indifference point, and use that measure to interpret neural signals.

The findings are of course consistent with the reward value representations described previously in the orbitofrontal cortex based on neuronal recordings that show the encoding of value (Rolls, Sienkiewicz & Yaxley 1989, Critchley & Rolls 1996c, Rolls, Critchley, Browning, Hernadi & Lenard 1999, Rolls, Critchley, Verhagen & Kadohisa 2010a), and on BOLD signal activations in the human orbitofrontal cortex that are correlated with subjective pleasantness (Kringelbach, O'Doherty, Rolls & Andrews 2003, Grabenhorst, Rolls & Bilderbeck 2008a, Grabenhorst & Rolls 2008, Grabenhorst, Rolls, Parris & D'Souza 2010b).

A neuronal representation of value can be said to be 'abstract' (i.e., in the space of goods) if two conditions are met (Padoa-Schioppa 2011, Padoa-Schioppa & Conen 2017).

First, the encoding by neurons should be *independent of the sensori-motor contingencies* of choice, so that the neurons do not just encode movements. The relation of orbitofrontal cortex neuronal activity to the reward value of sensory stimuli including taste, olfactory, oral texture, and visual stimuli, and not to movements, for example of the mouth or arm, has been made clear since our earliest reports (Thorpe, Rolls & Maddison 1983, Rolls, Yaxley & Sienkiewicz 1990, Verhagen, Rolls & Kadohisa 2003, Rolls 2005), and has been confirmed by Padoa-Schioppa & Assad (2006), who found that less than 5% of OFC neurons were significantly modulated by the spatial configuration of the offers on the monitor or by the direction of the eye movement. Similar independence of OFC representations of value from the details of actions has also been reported by others (Kennerley & Wallis 2009, Roesch & Olson 2005, Grattan & Glimcher 2014).

Second, the encoding should be *domain general*. In other words, the activity should represent the value of the good affected by all the relevant determinants (commodity, quantity, risk, cost, etc.). Current evidence for such an abstract representation is convincing for two brain areas, the orbitofrontal cortex (OFC) and the closely related ventromedial prefrontal cortex (vmPFC). Evidence that commodity and quantity affect value (subjective value, the value to the individual) and the representation in the OFC similarly has been described above (Padoa-Schioppa & Assad 2006, Padoa-Schioppa 2011, Padoa-Schioppa & Conen 2017) (see Fig. 3.55). The effects of risk, i.e. the probability of obtaining the good or reward, on subjective value have been shown to be reflected in the activations found in the human orbitofrontal cortex (Rolls, McCabe & Redoute 2008e, Peters & Buchel 2009). Under risk, the probabilities of different outcomes can be estimated, whereas under ambiguity, even these probabilities are not known. Choices of monetary offers under ambiguity vs risk (which are differently weighted in different subjects) also trade off as predicted by subjective value representations in the vmPFC (Levy, Snell, Nelson, Rustichini & Glimcher 2010). The delay of a reward decreases the value of the delayed reward and activations in the human vmPFC in a corresponding way (Kable & Glimcher 2007), and consistent results have been found at the single neuron level in monkeys (Roesch & Olson 2005). The cost in terms of the effort involved in obtaining a reward also decreases the neuronal responses in the OFC to a reward (Kennerley, Dahmubed, Lara & Wallis 2009), providing evidence that subjective value representations in the OFC do reflect the difficulty of the actions required to obtain the reward (though not the details of the actions themselves). This is an indication that what we have also termed the 'net value' of a reward, that is the value of the reward minus the cost / effort required to obtain it, needs to be represented, for this 'net value' input is what is required to the decision-making network (Grabenhorst & Rolls 2011, Rolls 2014a, Rolls 2016c). This is needed because the attractor decision-making network cannot relate separate inputs for the rewards and for the costs of several alternatives, for which cost was to be bound to each reward could not be implemented in the decision-making network.

There is thus considerable evidence that the orbitofrontal cortex (OFC) and adjoining ventromedial prefrontal cortex (vmPFC) provide an abstract representation of value. Important properties of the representation are that the subjective value, the value to the individual, is represented and not the actions required to obtain the reward or 'good'; and that the representation is domain general, that is reflects the value when it is altered in a number of ways including the magnitude of the good, risk, delay, and the cost/effort required to obtain the good. The single neuron data, including much that we have obtained, indicates that the representation at the neuronal level is specific for each different type of reward or good, with a common scale of value, but no conversion into a common currency, as described further in Section 3.12.2. The view that there is a representation of value in the orbitofrontal cortex and vmPFC, which may be the source of value effects in other brain regions, has now been accepted by Levy & Glimcher (2012). However, as the data that they review is from fMRI studies, they are not able to make the distinction as clear about no conversion into a common currency, for the fMRI activations reflect the responses of very many different single neurons, and do not provided clear evidence that different types of reward are represented by separate neurons in a sparse distributed representation (Rolls 2014a, Rolls & Treves 2011, Rolls, Critchley, Verhagen & Kadohisa 2010a).

The effect of the value representations in the orbitofrontal cortex on other brain areas is indeed a point of great interest. As described in Chapter 2 and Section 5.1, there are projections from the orbitofrontal cortex to the anterior cingulate cortex, with many rewards represented in the human pregenual cingulate cortex, and many punishers in the anterodorsal cingulate cortex (Rolls 2005, Rolls & Grabenhorst 2008, Grabenhorst & Rolls 2011) (Fig. 3.54). Indeed, we (Rolls 2005, Rolls & Grabenhorst 2008, Rolls 2009c, Grabenhorst & Rolls 2011) have argued that the function of the value representation in the anterior cingulate cortex is to provide the representation of (reward) outcome necessary for action–outcome learning implemented in the cingulate cortex, as described in Section 5.1. In this context, it is of interest that single neurons in the monkey anterior cingulate cortex encoded post-decision variables such as chosen value and chosen juice taste value, but not pre-decision variables such as offer value (e.g. the sight of the food or of a symbol that indicated what was available for choice) (Cai & Padoa-Schioppa 2012). This is in contrast to the orbitofrontal cortex, in which the offer value is also encoded. This evidence is thus consistent with the hypothesis that the OFC represents subjective value in a way that can be an input to a choice decision-making system (in for example medial prefrontal cortex area 10 / vmPFC) because the OFC represents the expected value of the outcome (e.g. the sight of food, or an offer value (Thorpe, Rolls & Maddison 1983, Rolls, Critchley, Mason & Wakeman 1996a, Rolls, McCabe & Redoute 2008e, Padoa-Schioppa & Assad 2006, Padoa-Schioppa 2011, Padoa-Schioppa & Conen 2017)), whereas the cingulate cortex is involved in learning associations between actions and outcomes such as whether a juice or monetary reward was obtained (Section 5.1).

It is of interest that insofar as a representation of value exists in rodents (Schoenbaum, Roesch, Stalnaker & Takahashi 2009), it does not appear to meet the conditions for abstraction described above (Padoa-Schioppa 2011, Padoa-Schioppa & Conen 2017). For example, neurons in the rodent OFC may be spatially selective and thus represent responses (Feierstein, Quirk, Uchida, Sosulski & Mainen 2006, Roesch, Taylor & Schoenbaum 2006). Further, experiments that manipulated two determinants of value found that different neuronal populations in the rat OFC represent reward magnitude and time delay – a striking difference with primates (Roesch & Olson 2005, Roesch, Taylor & Schoenbaum 2006). Differences in the anatomy and connections of the rat from the primate orbitofrontal cortex are apparent (e.g. with the rat having only agranular regions (Wise 2008), see Fig. 1.3 and Chapter 8), and it is possible that an abstract representation of value may have emerged later in evolution in parallel with the expansion of the frontal lobes.

3.12.2 A common scale of value for different goods in the orbitofrontal cortex, but no conversion to a common currency

3.12.2.1 Reward-specific / value-specific representations

Single neurons in the orbitofrontal cortex encode different specific rewards (Rolls 2014a, Rolls & Grabenhorst 2008, Grabenhorst & Rolls 2011). They do this by responding to different combinations of taste, olfactory, somatosensory, visual, and auditory stimuli including socially relevant stimuli such as face expression (Rolls 2005, Rolls, Critchley, Browning & Inoue 2006a, Rolls & Grabenhorst 2008, Rolls 2014a, Rolls 2018b). Part of the adaptive utility of this reward-specific representation is that it provides for sensory-specific satiety as implemented by a decrease in the responsiveness of reward-specific neurons (Rolls 2014a, Rolls & Grabenhorst 2008). This is a fundamental property of every reward system that helps to ensure that a variety of different rewards is selected over time. Representations of both reward outcome and expected value are specific for the particular reward: not only do different neurons respond to different primary reinforcers, but different neurons also encode the conditioned stimuli for different outcomes, with different neurons responding for example to the sight or odour of stimuli based on the outcome that is expected (Thorpe et al. 1983, Rolls et al. 1996a).

3.12.2.2 A common scale for different specific rewards

A classical view of economic decision theory (Bernoulli 1738) implies that decision-makers convert the value of different goods into a common scale of utility. Ecological (McFarland & Sibly 1975), psychological (Cabanac 1992), and some neuroeconomic (Montague & Berns 2002, Sescousse, Li & Dreher 2015) approaches further suggest that the values of different kinds of rewards are converted into a common currency. We have argued that different specific rewards must be represented on the same scale, but not converted into a common currency, as the specific goal selected (i.e. the particular reward selected) must be the output of the decision process so that the appropriate action for that particular goal can then be chosen (Rolls 2005, Rolls 2016c, Rolls & Grabenhorst 2008, Grabenhorst & Rolls 2011, Rolls 2014a, Rolls 2016c). The key difference between the two concepts of common currency and common scaling lies in the specificity with which rewards are represented at the level of single neurons. While a common currency view implies convergence of different types of rewards onto the same neurons (a process in which information about reward identity is lost), a common scaling view implies that different rewards are represented by different neurons (thereby retaining reward identity in information processing), with the activity of the different neurons scaled to be in the same value range.

To investigate the possibility of common scaling, we performed an fMRI study in which we were able to show that even fundamentally different primary rewards, taste in the mouth and warmth on the hand, produced activations in the human OFC that were scaled to the same range as evaluated by reports made during the neuroimaging of the subjective pleasantness of the set of stimuli (Grabenhorst, D'Souza, Parris, Rolls & Passingham 2010a) (Fig. 3.56). In this case, value was measured by human subjective ratings on the same scale of pleasantness.

A different study found that the decision value for different categories of goods (food, non-food consumables, and monetary gambles) during purchasing decisions correlated with activations in the adjacent vmPFC (Chib, Rangel, Shimojo & O'Doherty 2009). Further fMRI studies with similar indications are reviewed by Levy & Glimcher (2012).

Importantly, because of the limited spatial resolution of fMRI, these studies do not answer whether it is the same or different neurons in these areas that encode the value of different rewards. fMRI investigations thus do not address the issue of whether there is a common currency (cf. Berridge & Kringelbach (2015)), because so many neurons are reflected in fMRI signals that many neurons that might be responding specifically would be summed together.

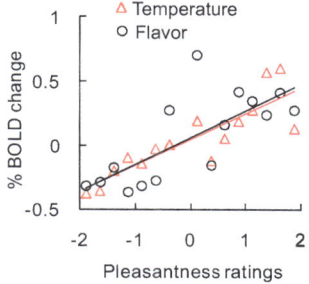

Fig. 3.56 A common scale for the subjective pleasure for different primary rewards: Neural activations in the orbitofrontal cortex correlate with the subjective pleasantness ratings for flavor stimuli in the mouth and somatosensory temperature stimuli delivered to the hand. The regression lines describing the relationship between neural activity (% BOLD signal change) and subjective pleasantness ratings were indistinguishable for both types of reward. (Reprinted from NeuroImage, 51 (3), Fabian Grabenhorst, Arun A. D'Souza, Benjamin A. Parris, Edmund T. Rolls, and Richard E. Passingham, A common neural scale for the subjective pleasantness of different primary rewards, pp. 1265–74, Copyright (2010), with permission from Elsevier.)

However, as shown most clearly by single neuron recording studies, the representations in the OFC provide evidence about the exact nature of each reward (Rolls 2014a, Rolls & Grabenhorst 2008, Grabenhorst & Rolls 2011). Moreover, in economic decision-making, neurons in the macaque OFC encode the economic value of the specific choice options on offer, for example different juice rewards (Padoa-Schioppa & Assad 2006). For many of these 'offer value' neurons, the relationship between neuronal firing rate and value was invariant with respect to the different types of juice that were available (Padoa-Schioppa & Assad 2008), suggesting that different types of juice are evaluated on a common value scale.

With our current computational understanding of how decisions are made in attractor neural networks (Section 3.13 (Deco & Rolls 2006, Wang 2008, Rolls 2016c, Rolls & Deco 2010, Deco, Rolls, Albantakis & Romo 2013, Rolls 2014a, Rolls 2016c, Rolls 2018b)), it is important that different rewards are expressed on a similar scale for decision-making networks to operate correctly but retain information about the identity of the specific reward. The computational reason is that one type of reward (e.g. food reward) should not dominate all other types of reward and always win in the competition, as this would be maladaptive. Making different rewards approximately equally rewarding makes it likely that a range of different rewards will be selected over time (and depending on factors such as motivational state), which is adaptive and essential for survival (Rolls 2014a). The exact scaling into a decision-making attractor network will be set by the number of inputs from each source, their firing rates, and the strengths of the synapses that introduce the different inputs into the decision-making network. Importantly, common scaling need not imply conversion into a new representation that is of a common currency of general reward (Rolls & Grabenhorst 2008, Grabenhorst & Rolls 2011). In the decision process itself it is important to know which reward has won, and the mechanism is likely to involve competition between different rewards represented close together in the cerebral cortex, with one of the types of reward winning the competition, rather than convergence of different rewards onto the same neuron (Rolls 2016c, Rolls 2014a, Rolls & Deco 2010). A great advantage is that whichever attractor in the decision-making network wins, has the additional property that it represents and maintains active in an attractor short-term memory the specific reward that has won, and this allows behaviour to be directed to perform actions to obtain that reward. The continuing firing of the specific reward decision attractor maintains active the goal for the action to direct the action until the action is completed. If the representation was in a common currency, the action system would have no evidence about the goal (e.g. food reward, monetary reward) that actions should be performed to acquire. Actions are typically different for different goals.

This brain organization, with specific value systems scaled on a common scale by neuronal representations in the orbitofrontal cortex but with no conversion to a common currency is an elegant aspect of brain design. One of the features of this book is that it describes this organization.

This organization may be compared with that proposed by Glimcher (2011a), where he proposes (page 407) that fairly direct inputs from sensory transduction systems to the dopamine neurons carry 'experienced subjective value', and points to evidence that the serotonergic neurons of the midbrain raphe also encode 'experienced SV' for primary rewards. This is completely different to the organization described in this book, in which representations through Tier 1 of cortical areas build invariant representations of stimuli and objects in the world that do not reflect reward value. Then in Tier 2, mainly the orbitofrontal cortex, reward value representations are built, that are specific to different types of reward (Fig. 2.2). It is these specific reward systems that I argue provide the inputs to reward-related decision-making systems (in Tier 3). Moreover, inputs to the dopamine neurons, insofar as they reflect reward prediction error, would be likely to receive their inputs from the orbitofrontal cortex, perhaps via the ventral striatum (Rolls 2014a, Rolls 2016c, Rolls 2017a). However, for Glimcher (2011a), the dopamine neurons seem to carry the reward signal to other parts of the brain. That is not what the evidence described in this book shows, for, apart from other considerations, the dopamine neurons would be poor at carrying any specific reward signal of the type that is needed as the input to a decision mechanism for choosing between different rewards, and that are represented in the orbitofrontal cortex (Rolls 2014a, Rolls 2016c, Rolls 2017a) (Section 5.2.4).

3.12.2.3 An 'ultimate' evolutionary approach to reward value scaling

My approach instead is to produce a theory in which different specific rewards are encoded by different neurons in the orbitofrontal cortex, with the different rewards represented on the same scale of value. What is the 'ultimate' explanation for how the scale is set to be appropriate for different rewards?

My hypothesis is that the scaling of each type of primary reward is defined by the fitness provided to the genes that specify in the process of evolution each type of primary reward (Rolls 2014a) (Chapter 6). If genes made one type of reward value too high, that would decrease the fitness of those genes, as an animal might for example always find eating, but not reproducing, most rewarding. So there are processes in evolution to ensure that the magnitude of each type of gene-specified reward is set to a value that, in combination with other rewards, maximizes reproductive success. The concept is that genes are in competition with each other, and must make compromises with each other, to optimize their reproductive success.

Of course, due to the variation that is part of the process of evolution by natural selection, different individuals will have a different profile of values for each gene-specified reward, leading to individual differences in behaviour and leading to a basis for understanding personality (Rolls 2014a).

In addition to this genetic specification of rewards and of the value of each on a common scale, there are many heuristics that also contribute to the successful operation of this system, which is at the heart of emotion and emotion-related decision-making. These heuristics include sensory-specific satiety, to ensure that different types of reward are sampled, which of course is adaptive; and incentive motivation, the increase in the value of a reward after its initial presentation, which helps animals to lock efficiently onto one reward for more than too brief periods of time for efficiency. Another useful adaptation relevant to this 'ultimate' account of value scaling is relearning of the value of genetically programmed rewards, for example *taste aversion learning*, in which an innately rewarding taste can be reconfigured to be treated as aversive if the taste is paired with sickness (Scott 2011). In an analogous way, *conditioned appetite and conditioned satiety* allow gene-specified flavour rewards to be recalibrated in terms of the amount of energy with which the rewarding stimulus is associated (Booth 1985).

Of course gene-specified 'primary' rewards may provide a foundation, and many other stimuli can become rewarding by virtue of associations with these primary rewards. Examples include stimuli associated with wealth, power, and status, which themselves may be genetically specified to be rewarding because of their value (to the relevant genes) for promoting reproductive success (of those genes) (Rolls 2014a) (Chapter 6).

The different gene-specified rewards can themselves be regarded as heuristics to optimize the reproductive success of the genes. For example, the steeper loss than gain subjective value function in Prospect theory (Kahneman & Tversky 1979, Tversky & Kahneman 1992) (reviewed by Glimcher (2011a) and Fox & Poldrack (2009)) can be understood as a biological adaptation to the situation in which a single loss to an individual such as an injury or loss of reputation might spell disaster in terms of reproductive success, whereas each gain in value may be of benefit to but not crucial to reproductive success, as there will remain other opportunities for gains to be made (Rolls 2014a). The gene-specified value system can be seen to be quite different to one that a rational agent might use when dealing with economic gains and losses, where rational calculations might lead to a strategy where sensitivity to losses and gains is much more equal, as this might optimize long-term economic success. This really highlights a major difference between classical economic approaches that assume a rational agent performing calculations about economic benefit, and the much more biologically realistic interpretation of much economic decision-making as frequently (unless explicit rational calculations are relied upon) involving choices influenced by the gene-specified heuristic value in evolution of different types of economic choice. In the biologically plausible case, there may be many types of value and potential costs associated with a stimulus, and these influences on value both combine and compete with each other to influence whether that stimulus, or another stimulus, is chosen. Thus in the biologically realistic economic choice situation, many factors may influence the value of a stimulus, and it may be a simplification to think of a single parameter, such as economic gain, being optimized.

This approach, with a specification of many different specific and competing rewards specified by different competing ('selfish') genes, provides a rich basis for understanding both emotion, decision-making, and the specification of value for both emotion and for decision-making including economic decision-making (Rolls 2014a).

3.12.3 Absolute value and relative value are both represented in the orbitofrontal cortex

For economic decision-making it is useful to have separate representations of absolute and relative valuation signals, as described next.

3.12.3.1 A representation of absolute reward value: menu invariance

A representation of the *absolute value* of rewards is important for stable long-term preferences and consistent economic choices (Padoa-Schioppa & Assad 2008, Padoa-Schioppa 2011, Padoa-Schioppa & Conen 2017, Glimcher, Camerer, Fehr & Poldrack 2009). Such a representation should not be influenced by the value of other available rewards. Absolute value enables comparison of the value of different goods that may be available at different times in the long timescale of days or more. There is evidence for absolute value coding in the orbitofrontal cortex. For example, in sensory-specific satiety experiments, the responses of neurons to the food eaten to satiety decrease to zero, while the responses of the neurons to other stimuli changes rather little, even though their relative value has changed (see e.g. Fig. 3.5 (Rolls, Sienkiewicz & Yaxley 1989)). Indeed, as satiety progresses, the neuronal responses to the food gradually decrease, and so does whether and how vigorously the animal

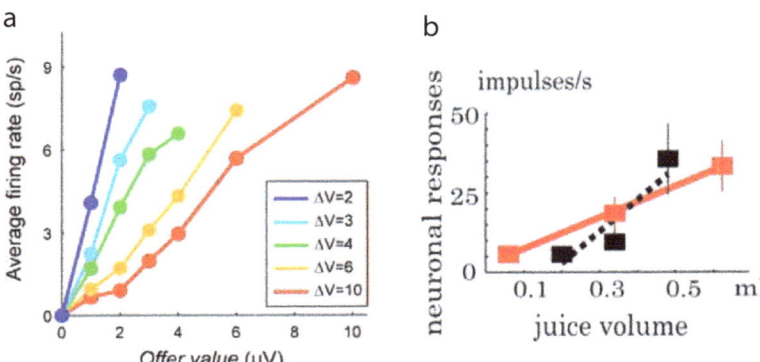

Fig. 3.57 Scaling of value: a representation of relative reward value. (a) Padoa-Schioppa (2009) found that some neurons in the orbitofrontal cortex that encode the offer value of different types of juice adapt their sensitivity to the value range of juice rewards available in a given session, while keeping their neuronal activity range constant. Each line shows the average neuronal response for a given value range. (b) Kobayashi et al. (2010) found that neurons in the orbitofrontal cortex adapt their sensitivity of value coding to the statistical distribution of reward values, in that the reward sensitivity slope adapted to the standard deviation of the probability distribution of juice volumes available in different groups of trials (solid vs dashed line). These findings indicate that the range of the value scale in the orbitofrontal cortex can be adjusted to reflect the range of rewards that are available at a given time. Reproduced with permission. ((a) Reproduced from Padoa-Schioppa, C., Range-adapting representation of economic value in the orbitofrontal cortex. Journal of Neuroscience 29 (44) pp. 14004–14014, Ⓒ 2009, The Society for Neuroscience. (b) Reproduced from Kobayashi, S., Pinto de Carvalho, O. and Schultz, W., Adaptation of reward sensitivity in orbitofrontal neurons, Journal of Neuroscience 30 (2) pp. 534–544, Ⓒ 2010, The Society for Neuroscience.)

will select that food for ingestion, so that the neuronal firing encodes exactly how rewarding the stimulus is, not its relative value relative for example to no reward (see e.g. Fig. 3.5). In another type of experiment, it was found that the responses of some orbitofrontal cortex neurons that encoded the value of a specific stimulus did not depend on what other stimuli were available at the same time (Padoa-Schioppa & Assad 2008). This has been referred to as *menu invariance*. In the experiment, juices of three types A, B, and C could be offered as a choice between any two on a given trial, viz A:B, B:C, and C:A. The firing rate to for example juice C was not affected by whether the choice was between C and A or B.

This absolute value representation in the orbitofrontal cortex may provide a neurobiological foundation for *transitivity*, a fundamental trait of economic choice (Padoa-Schioppa & Assad 2008). Transitivity of choice refers to a situation in which if A is preferred to B (A>B), and B is preferred to C, then A should be preferred to C. Further, preference transitivity is a hallmark of rational choice behaviour and one of the most fundamental assumptions of economic theory (Kreps 1990).

3.12.3.2 A representation of relative reward value

In contrast, to select the option with the highest subjective value in a specific choice situation perhaps in the same block of trials, it may be useful to represent the *relative value* of each option. For example, in the parietal cortex, neurons encode the relative value of the options associated with specific eye movements (Kable & Glimcher 2009). The apparent difference in value coding between the orbitofrontal cortex and parietal cortex has led to the suggestion that absolute value signals encoded in the orbitofrontal cortex are subsequently rescaled in the parietal cortex to encode relative value in order to maximize the difference between the choice options for action selection (Kable & Glimcher 2009). However, there is also evidence for relative encoding of value in the orbitofrontal cortex, in that neuronal responses to a food reward can depend on the value of the other reward that is available in a block of trials (Tremblay & Schultz 1999, Padoa-Schioppa 2009, Kobayashi, Pinto de Carvalho & Schultz 2010), as described next.

Some neurons in the orbitofrontal cortex show an adaptive *scaling of reward value*. These neurons adapt the sensitivity with which reward value is encoded to the range of values that is available at a given time (Padoa-Schioppa 2009, Kobayashi et al. 2010). The basic result is illustrated in Fig. 3.57a, which depicts the activity of 937 offer value neurons from the orbitofrontal cortex (Padoa-Schioppa 2009). Different neurons were recorded in different sessions and the range of values offered to the monkey varied from session to session. What was found was that the distribution of firing rate responses measured for the population across sessions did not depend on the range of values offered to the monkey within a session. In other words, orbitofrontal cortex neurons adapted their gain (i.e., the slope of the relation between the firing rate and the reward value) in such a way that a given range of firing rates described different ranges of values in different behavioural conditions. Kobayashi et al. (2010) showed that this adaptation to the range of rewards available at any one time (Fig. 3.57b) can take place within 15 trials. Thus relative reward value is represented by some neurons in the orbitofrontal cortex.

This scaling of value may be useful when values computed in different behavioural conditions can vary substantially. For example the same individual might choose sometimes between goods worth a few dollars and at other times between goods worth many thousands of dollars (e.g. when choosing between different houses for sale). However, any representation of value is ultimately limited to a finite range of neuronal firing rates, typically in the region of 0–50 spikes/s in the orbitofrontal cortex. The scaling of reward value by orbitofrontal cortex neurons may, for a given range of possible values, produce an optimal (i.e. maximally sensitive) representation of value at any one time that would fully exploit the range of possible firing rates. This is a similar hypothesis to that of the regression of emotional, that is reward-produced, states towards an average level that may occur in order to allow an individual, whatever the environment, to be maximally sensitive to a change of reward value, so that a local reward gradient can be climbed efficiently (Rolls 2014a).

This adaptive *scaling of reward value* is also evident in positive and negative contrast effects, which also make the system optimally sensitive to the local reward gradient, by dynamically altering the sensitivity of the reward system so that small changes can be detected (Rolls 2014a).

3.12.3.3 Both relative and absolute reward are represented in the orbitofrontal cortex

As a comment on the relative and absolute value representations described in Sections 3.12.3.1 and 3.12.3.2, it should be noted that the 'absolute value' representation described in Section 3.12.3.1 was found in an experiment where the different values were being offered close together in time, whereas the 'relative reward' value representation described was found after a number of trials, approximately 15 (Padoa-Schioppa 2009, Kobayashi et al. 2010), had been allowed for rescaling. The two findings are therefore not necessarily inconsistent, and might just show that the value system in the orbitofrontal cortex can rescale given a number of trials where the values available in the task are found to be within a given range.

Given that representations of both absolute value and relative value are needed for economic decision-making, Grabenhorst & Rolls (2009) tested explicitly whether both types of representation are present *simultaneously* in the human orbitofrontal cortex. In a task in which two odours were successively delivered on each trial, we found that BOLD activations to the second odour in the antero-lateral orbitofrontal cortex tracked the relative subjective pleasantness (i.e. the pleasantness of the second odour relative to the pleasantness of the first odour on that trial) (Fig. 3.58). In contrast, in the medial and mid-orbitofrontal cortex, activations tracked the absolute pleasantness of the odour, which was obtained across the whole experiment and very probably reflected the long-term pleasantness / value of the odour (Fig. 3.58). Thus, both relative and absolute subjective value signals, both of which provide important

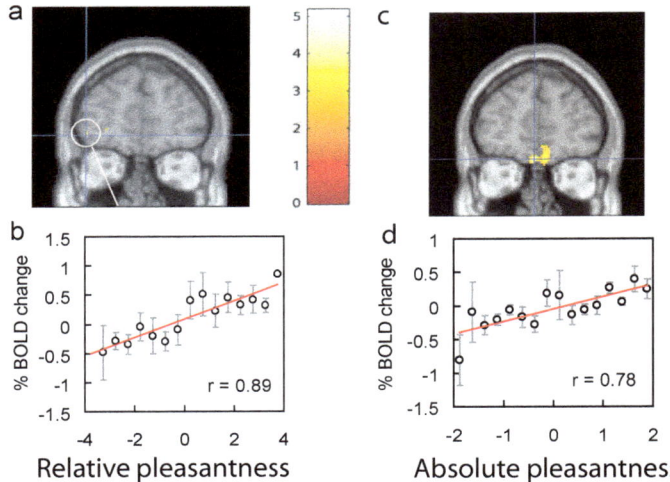

Fig. 3.58 Absolute and relative value representations in the human orbitofrontal cortex. On each trial, the subjects rated the pleasantness (value) of the second odour of a pair of 4 odours used in the experiment. a-b. Relative pleasantness: positive correlation between the BOLD signal and the difference in pleasantness of the second odor compared to the first odor. a. A significant correlation was found in the anterior lateral orbitofrontal cortex at [-44 48 -8]. b. There was a positive correlation between the BOLD signal in this brain region measured at the time of the second odor and the difference in the pleasantness of the second odor compared to the first (i.e. positive values on the abscissa are when the second odor is more pleasant) (r=0.89). c-d. Absolute pleasantness: positive correlation between the BOLD signal and the absolute value of the pleasantness ratings given to the (second) odor in (c) the medial orbitofrontal cortex [-2 50 -20]. d. The correlation between the BOLD signal in the medial orbitofrontal cortex and the pleasantness ratings (r=0.78). (Reprinted from NeuroImage, 48 (1), Fabian Grabenhorst and Edmund T. Rolls, Different representations of relative and absolute subjective value in the human brain, pp. 258–68, Copyright 2009, with permission from Elsevier.)

inputs to decision-making processes, are separately and simultaneously represented in the human orbitofrontal cortex, and both representations are of the type important in economic decision-making (Grabenhorst & Rolls 2009).

In sensory-specific satiety experiments, it is found that neuronal responses to the taste or flavour eaten to satiety decrease to zero. However, it is of interest that there is often a small increase in the firing rates of the neurons to the other stimuli not eaten to satiety (see example in Fig. 3.25). This may reflect a small degree of relative value encoding in these neurons. The same small effect is sometimes evident in human subjective pleasantness ratings during sensory-specific satiety experiments (e.g. Rolls, Rolls, Rowe & Sweeney (1981a)).

Thus separate representations are found of absolute, long-term, value, and of relative value as it depends on the behavioural context of the current choice.

My assessment, based on evidence from the thousands of neurons that I have recorded in the orbitofrontal cortex, is that absolute value is the more dominant representation. For example, the neuron illustrated in Fig. 3.5 (Rolls et al. 1989) showed almost no alteration in its firing to fruit juice (blackcurrant juice, BJ) when the other item on the 'menu', glucose solution, was devalued by feeding glucose to satiety. This is thus 'menu invariance', and reflects a representation of absolute value. Any increase in firing of such a neuron to the foods not fed to satiety (which might reflect relative value) is typically small. Similarly, when a fat stimulus (cream) was fed to satiety and an orbitofrontal cortex neuron stopped responding to the cream, the same neuron changed its response very little to the taste of glucose, which remained rewarding (Rolls, Critchley, Browning, Hernadi & Lenard 1999)). The same type of absolute value representation is found in neurons in a region that receives from the orbitofrontal cortex, the lateral hypothalamus (Rolls, Murzi, Yaxley, Thorpe & Simpson 1986)).

Correspondingly, from a computational neuroscience perspective, an absolute value representation is much more important than a relative value representation, for absolute value is needed for transitivity of choice and choices between rewards available in the long term; and a choice decision-making network can make choices based on absolute value, and has no need for a partial solution to the decision problem to be performed by a relative value representation, as described in Section 3.13.

3.12.4 The representation of expected reward value, uncertainty, and risk

Decision under uncertainty refers to choice when the probabilities and magnitudes of the expected rewards and punishers available for each choice are not made known explicitly to the subject, but must be discovered by sampling the choices. Examples of such decision tasks include the probabilistic monetary reward and loss tasks by which the representation of monetary reward value and monetary loss value in the orbitofrontal cortex was discovered (O'Doherty, Kringelbach, Rolls, Hornak & Andrews (2001a) (see Section 3.6), which was also used to investigate the sensitivity of patients with orbitofrontal cortex damage to changes in the probability of the reward and loss outcomes of particular choices (Hornak, O'Doherty, Bramham, Rolls, Morris, Bullock & Polkey 2004) (see Section 4.2), the Iowa Gambling task (Bechara, Damasio, Damasio & Anderson 1994, Bechara, Tranel, Damasio & Damasio 1996, Bechara, Damasio, Tranel & Damasio 1997, Damasio 1994, Bechara, Damasio, Tranel & Damasio 2005), probabilistic tasks used to compare brain areas sensitive to reward outcome, expected value, and errors between these (Rolls, McCabe & Redoute 2008e), and all decision tasks in non-human animals in which explicit instructions about the probabilities and possible outcomes cannot be provided. Further examples include investing in the stock market, and betting on the outcome in a sport. This is also known as decision under ambiguity.

Decision under risk refers to choice when the probability distributions and magnitudes of the expected rewards and punishers available for each choice are made known explicitly by instruction to the subject. Examples include betting on the flip of a coin, or entering a lottery with a known number of tickets.

We have seen that in microeconomics, **expected value** (and possibly **expected utility**), can be thought of as the probability of obtaining the reward multiplied by the reward value (Glimcher 2003, Glimcher 2004, Kahneman & Tversky 1984). If the probability of obtaining a reward is low, then we are less likely to choose it than when the probability is high.

Some dopamine neurons show increasing responses to conditioned stimuli predicting reward with increasing probability (Fiorillo, Tobler & Schultz 2003), and decrease their firing to predicted reward omission (Tobler, Dickinson & Schultz 2003). Their responses may thus reflect expected value. However, it also appears that at least some dopamine neurons have activity that is high when reward uncertainty is high (which occurs when reward probability is 0.5) (Fiorillo et al. 2003). As described by Rolls (2014a), this dual coding (of positive reward prediction error, and of reward uncertainty) raises problems in how receiving neurons might use this multiplexed information.

Parietal cortex neurons with activity that precedes eye movements in for example area LIP show more activity if the expected utility is high (Glimcher 2003, Glimcher 2004, Platt & Glimcher 1999, McCoy & Platt 2005a). This modulation or responsiveness by expected utility, as influenced by both probability and reward value, of neurons studied in oculomotor tasks has been found in a number of areas with oculomotor-related activity, including the cingulate cortex and the superior colliculus (McCoy & Platt 2005a, Platt & Padoa-Schioppa 2009).

For both the dopamine and the parietal cortex neurons, it seems unlikely that the actual computation of probability multiplied by reward value is performed in those areas, as reward stimuli are not known to be encoded there. It is likely, as we have seen, that expected value, reflecting reward magnitude and probability, is reflected in the activity of neurons in the orbitofrontal cortex.

The following is consistent with this hypothesis that the orbitofrontal cortex is involved in making these computations. In decision-making under risk, the outcomes are uncertain. Uncertain reward outcomes are characterised by statistical parameters that capture the numerical values of the underlying probability distributions of reward values, including the expected value, risk (variance), and probability. During decision-making in response to visual cues predicting uncertain rewards, separate subpopulations of macaque orbitofrontal cortex neurons predominantly code the prediction of one statistical parameter, with few neurons showing combined coding. These signals may then be combined to encode an integrated expected value signal (O'Neill & Schultz 2018). Further, risky decision-making is altered in humans and animals with damage to the orbitofrontal cortex (Clark, Bechara, Damasio, Aitken, Sahakian & Robbins 2008).

3.12.5 Delay of reward, emotional choice, and rational choice

Another factor that can influence decisions for rewards is the delay before the reward is obtained. If the reward will not be available for a long time, then we discount the reward value, and this is termed *temporal discounting*. Most models assume an exponential decrease in the reward value as a function of the delay until the reward is obtained, as rational choice entails treating each moment of delay equally (Frederick, Loewenstein & O'Donoghue 2002, McClure, Laibson, Loewenstein & Cohen 2004). Impulsive preference changes may reflect a disproportionate valuation of rewards available in the immediate future (Ainslie 1992, Benabou & Pycia 2002, Rachlin 2000, Montague & Berns 2002, Metcalfe & Mischel 1999). It is possible that there are two systems that influence decisions in these circumstances.

One is a rational, logic-based, system requiring syntactic manipulation of symbols that can treat each moment of delay equally, and calculate choice based on an exponential decrease of reward value with increasing delay (see Section 6.4). This rational decision system might involve language or mathematical systems in the brain, and the ability to hold several items in a working memory while the trade-offs of different long-term courses of action are compared.

A different more emotion-based system that can operate implicitly might operate according to heuristics that have become built into the system during evolution that might value disproportionately immediate rewards compared to delayed rewards. This emotion-based system might involve the orbitofrontal cortex, which as we have seen represents different types of reward and punisher (e.g. monetary gain and loss), and lesions of which in humans lead to impairments in changing behaviour when rewards are received less often for particular choices (Hornak, O'Doherty, Bramham, Rolls, Morris, Bullock & Polkey 2004, Berlin, Rolls & Kischka 2004), to impulsive choices (Berlin, Rolls & Iversen 2005), and to impairments in gambling tasks (Bechara et al. 1994, Bechara, Damasio, Tranel & Anderson 1998). This suggested dissociation of decision systems is the same concept as that encompassed by the hypothesis of dual routes to action considered in Section 6.4 and by Rolls (1999a), Rolls (2014a), and Rolls (2019b).

Consistent with the point being made about evolutionarily old emotion-based decision systems vs a recent rational system present in humans is that humans trade off immediate costs/benefits against cost/benefits that are delayed by as much as decades, whereas non-human primates have not been observed to engage in unpreprogrammed delay of gratification involving more than a few minutes (Rachlin 1989, Kagel, Battalio & Green 1995)[3].

---

[3] Seasonal food storage is not an exception, in that it appears to be stereotyped and instinctive, and hence is unlike the generalizable nature of human planning (McClure, Laibson, Loewenstein & Cohen 2004).

Moreover, individual differences in sensitivity to rewards and punishers could lead to personality differences with respect to impulsive behaviour (Rolls 2014a), and indeed patients with Borderline Personality Disorder behave similarly with respect to their impulsive behaviour to patients with orbitofrontal cortex lesions (Berlin, Rolls & Kischka 2004, Berlin & Rolls 2004, Berlin, Rolls & Iversen 2005).

Consistent with dual emotional and rational bases for decisions in humans, a 'quasi-hyperbolic' time discounting function that splices together two discounting functions – an emotional one that distinguishes sharply between present and future, and a rational one that discounts exponentially and more shallowly – provides a good fit to experimental data including retirement saving, credit-card borrowing, and procrastination (Laibson 1997, Angeletos, Laibson, Repetto, Tobacman & Weinberg 2001, O'Donoghue & Rabin 1999). This dual mechanism process can be modelled formally by

$$r(t) = \beta \gamma^t r(0) \tag{3.1}$$

where $r(t)$ is the time discounted reward value at time t, and $r(0)$ is the reward value if received immediately at time $t = 0$ (McClure, Laibson, Loewenstein & Cohen 2004). β ($0 < \beta \leq 1$) (or in fact its inverse) represents the uniform downweighting of future compared to immediate rewards, and is the parameter that encompasses the effects of emotion on decision-making in this formulation. β is 1 at time zero, and is set to a value that scales a reward at any future time relative to the value at time 0. If $\beta = 0.8$, this indicates that relative to a reward of value r at time zero, the reward at any future time would have a value of 0.8. In this sense, it models the role of emotion in decision-making as down-valuing a reward at any future time compared to immediately by a uniform discounting factor β. The γ ($\gamma \leq 1$) parameter is the discount rate in the standard exponential formula that treats a given delay equivalently independently of when it occurs (i.e. in any time interval, the value decreases by a fixed proportion of the value it has already reached), and encompasses the rational route to decision-making. In the model, it produces exponential decay of the value of a reward according to how long it is delayed. It is used in the model to capture the effects of long-term economic planning for the future.

McClure, Laibson, Loewenstein & Cohen (2004) performed an fMRI investigation in which smaller immediate rewards (today) could be chosen vs larger delayed rewards (given after delays of up to six weeks). (The monetary rewards were in the range $5–$40.) Brain areas that showed more activation for immediate vs delayed rewards (and reflected the β emotional parameter) included the medial orbitofrontal cortex, the medial prefrontal cortex/pregenual cingulate cortex, and the ventral striatum. Brain areas where activations reflected the decisions being made and the decision difficulty but which were not preferentially activated in relation to the immediate reward parameter β included the lateral prefrontal cortex (a brain region implicated in higher level cognitive functions including working memory and executive functions (Miller & Cohen 2001, Deco & Rolls 2003, Passingham & Wise 2012)), and a part of the parietal cortex implicated in numerical processing (Dehaene, Dehaene-Lambertz & Cohen 1998). (Activations in these prefrontal and parietal areas reflect the effects of the γ^t variable in Equation 3.1.) Thus emotional decisions that emphasize the importance of immediate rewards may preferentially activate reward-related areas ('β areas') such as the medial orbitofrontal cortex, pregenual cingulate cortex, and the ventral striatum, whereas difficult decisions requiring cost–benefit analysis about the value of long-term rewards preferentially activate a more cognitive system ('γ areas') that may be involved in rational thought and multistep calculation.

3.13 Decision-making mechanisms in the orbitofrontal cortex and elsewhere in the brain

3.13.1 Introduction

We have seen in earlier parts of this Chapter how the reward value of stimuli is represented on a continuous scale in the orbitofrontal cortex. For example, the firing rate of orbitofrontal cortex neurons with food-related responses decreases steadily as monkeys are fed to satiety, and similarly, activations in the medial orbitofrontal cortex to food become smaller as humans are fed to satiety, and indeed the activations are linearly related to the subjective pleasure (measured by the pleasantness rating on every trial) produced by the taste or flavour of food. Similarly, activations in the human orbitofrontal cortex are linearly related to how much money is won on a trial.

However, we almost always need to choose between different rewards that may be available, that is between different stimuli that produce different emotional states and that lead to different actions. How do we compare the reward values, and take a decision for one of the rewards on each occasion? It is very important that we make a real choice on a particular occasion, for the medieval tale told by Duns Scotus was of a donkey situated between two equidistant delicious food rewards that might never make a decision and might starve. The implication is that on each particular occasion, even if the rewards are almost equal, there has to be a mechanism in the brain to make a definite and fast choice on one trial, and then stay with that choice until the reward is obtained. Staying with a choice is adaptive, for if we took a decision and then changed our minds and kept dithering, we might never get the reward, which might disappear, or be gained by others. That also underlines that there is often adaptive value in having a decision-making mechanism that operates fast. Another desirable property of the decision-making process might be that some probabilistic component to the decision-making might be advantageous, for if we occasionally sample an option that on average has not paid off as well as another, we would be able to discover whether the rewards available for different choices had changed, which is likely to apply often in the real world [4]. Another desirable property of the decision mechanism is that it should be separate from the system that represents the reward value on a continuous scale, for at the same time that we can report on the continuous value of two rewards, we can make a decision on an individual trial to choose one or the other. This implies separate representations. Separate representations may also be useful because the inhibitory neurons need to respond differently for these two types of process. Another desirable property is that once a decision has been made about the goal that is chosen, it is likely to be useful to maintain that decision as a short-term memory, as it is then the goal for actions that need to be organized and performed over time to obtain the chosen goal. We will see that all of these are properties of the biologically plausible approach to decision-making described here.

In Section 3.13.2, a biologically plausible model of decision-making is described, and it is shown how it can be used to help understand reward-related decision-making mechanisms in parts of the orbitofrontal cortex (Section 3.13.3), and other types of decision in other brain regions. Section 3.13.3 shows how confidence in decisions is implemented in the decision-making network described, even before feedback about the decision is provided in a particular trial, and how decisions may be corrected if decision confidence is low. Other, phenomenal, models of decision-making that provide mathematical models that attempt to capture the phenomena but without a biological implementation of the mechanisms are

---

[4]To the extent that decision-making by other individuals is probabilistic, then checking options that may not have worked earlier is likely to be another part of the adaptive value of sometimes, probabilistically, choosing the less favoured option.

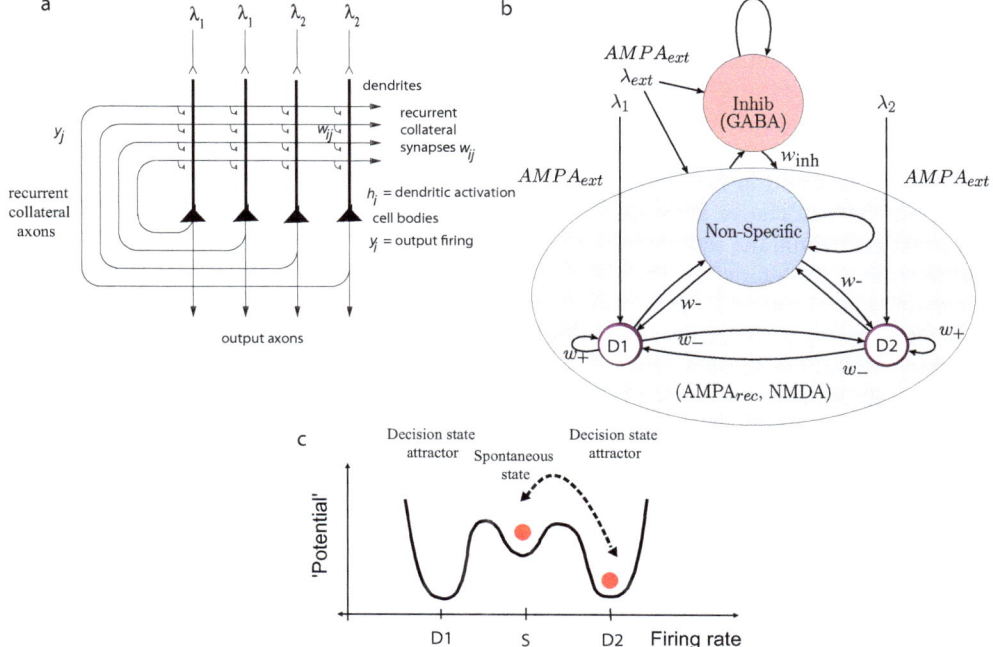

Fig. 3.59 (a) Attractor or autoassociation single network architecture for decision-making. The cell body of each neuron is shown as a triangle (like a cortical pyramidal cell), the dendrite is vertical, and receives recurrent collateral synaptic connections w_{ij} from the other neurons. The evidence for decision 1 is applied via the λ_1 inputs, and for decision 2 via the λ_2 inputs. The synaptic weights w_{ij} have been associatively modified during training in the presence of λ_1 and at a different time of λ_2. When λ_1 and λ_2 are applied, each attractor competes through the inhibitory interneurons (not shown), until one wins the competition, and the network falls into one of the high firing rate attractors that represents the decision. The noise in the network caused by the random spiking times of the neurons (for a given mean rate) means that on some trials, for given inputs, the neurons in the decision 1 (D1) attractor are more likely to win, and on other trials the neurons in the decision 2 (D2) attractor are more likely to win. This makes the decision-making probabilistic, for, as shown in (c), the noise influences when the system will jump out of the spontaneous firing stable (low energy) state S, and whether it jumps into the high firing state for decision 1 (D1) or decision 2 (D2). (b) The architecture of the integrate-and-fire network used to model decision-making (see text). The synaptic weights between the neural populations (decision pools D1 and D2, the non-specific pool, and the inhibitory pool) are 1 except where indicated. In particular, the recurrent weights, indicated by a recurrent arrow, between the neurons within an attractor decision-making pool have strong weights w_+, and between the different pools have the weak strength w_-. (c) A multistable 'effective energy landscape' for decision-making with stable states shown as low 'potential' basins. Even when the inputs are being applied to the network, the spontaneous firing rate state is stable, and noise provokes transitions from the low firing rate spontaneous state S into the high firing rate decision attractor state D1 or D2. If the noise is greater, the escaping time to a decision state, and thus the decision or reaction time, will be shorter (see Rolls and Deco 2010; Rolls 2016c).

described by Rolls (2014a) and Deco et al. (2013), as are rate models that move towards a firing rate description of decision-making. Section 9.2 provides an introduction to autoassociation or attractor networks that provide the basis of a mechanism for decision-making, and the equations for the implementation of the integrate-and fire decision-making model described here are provided in Section 9.3 (see also Wang (2002), Deco & Rolls (2006); *The Noisy Brain* (Rolls & Deco 2010), *Emotion and Decision-Making Explained* (Rolls 2014a), and *Cerebral Cortex: Principles of Operation* (Rolls 2016c) for fuller treatments of stochastic neurodynamics including those that apply to decision-making).

3.13.2 Decision-making in an attractor network

3.13.2.1 An attractor decision-making network

Consider the architecture shown in Fig. 3.59a. A set of cortical neurons has recurrent collateral excitatory synaptic connections w_{ij} from the other neurons. The evidence for decision 1 is applied via the λ_1 inputs, and for decision 2 via the λ_2 inputs. The synaptic weights w_{ij} have been associatively modified during training in the presence of λ_1 and at a different time of λ_2. The Hebbian or associative synaptic modification is such that if the presynaptic terminal and the postsynaptic neuron are simultaneously active, the synaptic connections become stronger. There are inhibitory neurons (not shown in Fig. 3.59a) that keep the total firing in the network within bounds, and in fact implement competition between the neuronal populations. As a result of the associative synaptic modification (specified in Equation 9.5), there are strong connections within the set of neurons activated by λ_1, and strong connections within the set of neurons activated by λ_2. These strengthened synapses provide positive feedback, so that if the whole or part of λ_1 is applied, that set of neurons becomes active, and maintains its activity for a long period even when the input λ_1 is removed. The neurons activated by λ_1 if firing inhibit the neurons activated by λ_2 through the inhibitory interneurons, so that just one population wins the competition and maintains its activity. This thus provides a model of memory, and its retrieval. This is called an attractor network, because a subset of the neurons within either population is sufficient to attract the system into a state in which all the neurons in that population are active, by using the strengthened recurrent collateral connections. The properties of attractor or autoassociation networks are described in Section 9.2 and elsewhere (Rolls 2016c, Hertz, Krogh & Palmer 1991, Hopfield 1982).

For decision-making, when λ_1 and λ_2 are applied simultaneously, each attractor competes through the inhibitory interneurons (not shown), until one wins the competition, and the network falls into one of the high firing rate attractors that represents the decision. When the network starts from a state of spontaneous firing, the biasing inputs encourage one of the attractors to gradually win the competition, but this process is influenced by the Poisson-like firing (spiking) of the neurons, so that which attractor wins is probabilistic. (Poisson-like indicates that the firing times are random for a given mean firing rate.) If the evidence in favour of the two decisions is equal, the network chooses each decision probabilistically on 50% of the trials. The model shows how probabilistic decision-making could be implemented in the brain. The model also shows how the evidence can be accumulated over long periods of time because of the integrating action of the attractor short-term memory network, with the recurrent collaterals feeding back information to be combined with the continuing inputs λ_1 and λ_2. The model produces shorter reaction or decision times as a function of the magnitude of the difference between the evidence for the two decisions: difficult decisions take longer, partly because the firing rates take longer to reach a decision threshold if the difference between the inputs is small.

3.13.2.2 An integrate-and-fire implementation of the attractor network for probabilistic decision-making

Because cortical neurons have almost random firing times for a given mean firing rate, i.e. the firing times follow approximately a Poisson distribution (Rolls & Treves 2011), the mean firing rates over short periods (e.g. 20–100 ms) of all the neurons in one of the decision-making populations may be higher than in the other population. These are referred to as statistical fluctuations. These fluctuations can result in the mean rate of one decision population increasing more than the other on a single trial, and influencing which decision is taken on that trial. To model these neuronal spiking time related fluctuations, we need an implementation of the decision-making network that incorporates spiking times. A simple such model is an integrate-and-fire model, which models the synapses and the membrane potentials as dynamical variables, and then produces a spike (not itself modelled to keep the implementation simple) which is then transmitted to the other neurons.

A leaky integrate-and-fire neuron along the lines just introduced can be modelled as shown schematically in Fig. 3.60. The model describes the depolarization of the membrane potential

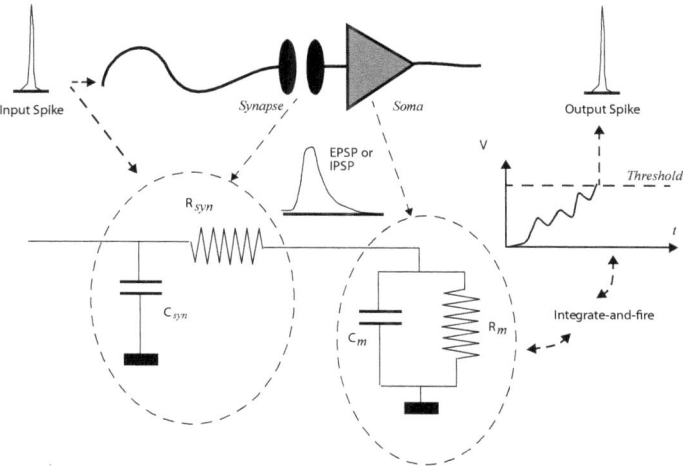

Fig. 3.60 Integrate-and-fire neuron. The basic circuit of an integrate-and-fire model consists of the neuron's membrane capacitance C_m in parallel with the membrane's resistance R_m (the reciprocal of the membrane conductance g_m) driven by a synaptic current with a conductance and time constant determined by the synaptic resistance R_{syn} (the reciprocal of the synaptic conductance g_j) and capacitance C_{syn} shown in the figure. These effects produce excitatory or inhibitory postsynaptic potentials, EPSPs or IPSPs. These potentials are integrated by the cell, and if a threshold V_{thr} is reached a δ-pulse (spike) is fired and transmitted to other neurons, and the membrane potential is reset. (Reproduced from Gustavo Deco and Edmund T. Rolls, Attention and working memory: a dynamical model of neuronal activity in the prefrontal cortex, European Journal of Neuroscience, 18 (8) pp. 2374–2390, Copyright © 2003, John Wiley and Sons.)

V (which typically is dynamically changing as a result of the synaptic effects described below between approximately −70 and −50 mV) until threshold V_{thr} (typically −50 mV) is reached when a spike is emitted and the potential is reset to V_{reset} (typically −55 mV). The membrane time constant τ_m is set by the membrane capacitance C_m and the membrane leakage conductance g_m where $\tau_m = C_m/g_m$. Changes in the membrane potential V (see right of Fig. 3.60) are produced by the input spikes operating through the dynamically modelled synapses (left of Fig. 3.60). There are very many such synapses, and the input currents produced from all these synapses result in excitatory postsynaptic potentials (EPSPs) and inhibitory postsynaptic potentials (IPSPs) that are summed by the integrate-and-fire neuron. When the threshold for firing is reached by the membrane potential V, a spike is emitted. The equations for the implementation are given in Section 9.3.

An attractor network model of decision-making using integrate-and-fire neurons was developed by Wang (2002), based on a neurodynamical model introduced by Brunel & Wang (2001). The model has been extended and successfully applied to several experimental paradigms including attention and short-term memory as well as decision-making (Rolls & Deco 2002, Deco & Rolls 2002, Deco & Rolls 2003, Deco & Rolls 2004, Deco, Rolls & Horwitz 2004, Szabo, Almeida, Deco & Stetter 2004, Deco & Rolls 2005c, Deco & Rolls 2006, Wang 2008, Rolls, Grabenhorst & Deco 2010b, Rolls, Grabenhorst & Deco 2010c, Rolls & Deco 2010, Smerieri, Rolls & Feng 2010, Deco, Rolls & Romo 2010, Rolls & Deco 2011, Rolls 2012a, Martinez-Garcia, Rolls, Deco & Romo 2011, Rolls, Dempere-Marco & Deco 2013, Deco, Rolls, Albantakis & Romo 2013, Rolls & Deco 2015b, Rolls & Deco 2015a, Rolls & Deco 2016, Rolls & Mills 2019).

In this framework, probabilistic decision-making is modelled by an attractor single network organized into a discrete set of neuronal populations or pools, as illustrated in Fig. 3.59b. The network contains N_{E} (excitatory) pyramidal cells and N_{I} inhibitory interneurons. In the simulations, we often use $N_{\mathrm{E}} = 800$ and $N_{\mathrm{I}} = 200$, consistent with the neurophysiologically observed proportion of 80% pyramidal cells versus 20% interneurons (Abeles 1991, Rolls 2016c) for a network with 1000 neurons, but effects of the number of neurons N in the network can be investigated. The neurons are fully connected (with synaptic strengths that are 1.0 unless specified otherwise). In the network illustrated in Fig. 3.59b, there are two decision-making populations, D1 and D2, each with 10% of the excitatory neurons, but the number of decision populations can be altered as needed. The recurrent synaptic connections within a decision population (indicated by the recurrent arrows in Fig. 3.59b) have a high strength of w_+ (typically 2.1), so that the population is self-sustaining in its activity, once started, and is at a biologically realistic firing rate. The remainder of the excitatory neurons are in a non-specific pool (NS), which represent other neurons in the cortex that are not involved in the particular task but fire spontaneously and contribute to the background noise (randomness) caused by the Poisson-like firing of the integrate-and-fire neurons. Their connections to the decision-making pools and the connections between the different decision-making pools are set to a value w_- which is calculated as a fraction of w_+ to make the total excitation in the network constant so that it balances the inhibition and produces a mean spontaneous firing rate for all the excitatory neurons of 3 spikes/s when no inputs λ_1 etc. have been applied (Brunel & Wang 2001, Wang 2002, Deco & Rolls 2006). A typical value for w_- is 0.86. These synaptic connection strengths are prescribed, but are generally consistent with a Hebbian associative learning process, in which synapses are strengthened when there is both presynaptic and postsynaptic activity (Equation 9.5). In this way, the synapses between neurons within a decision-making pool, which tend to be firing at the same time due to the λ inputs, are strong, and the synapses between neurons in different pools, which tend to be active at different times, are weaker.

All the excitatory synapses between the excitatory neurons use glutamate as a transmitter and have short time constant (τ_{AMPA}=10 ms) receptors that open ion channels, and long time constant (τ_{NMDA}=100 ms) receptors that open voltage-dependent ion channels, both of which inject currents into a neuron and produce depolarization in the direction of the firing threshold. (Details are provided in Section 9.3, and further background to these networks is provided by Rolls (2016c) and Rolls & Deco (2010).) The inclusion of the long time constant NMDA receptors in the model helps to maintain the persistence of the high firing rate attractor state (Wang 1999), and also prevents gamma oscillations, which arise only if the NMDA receptor contribution is insufficient (Brunel & Wang 2003, Rolls, Webb & Deco 2012, Wang 2010). [I hypothesize that in evolution the NMDA to AMPA channel conductance ratios have been set to a level that minimizes gamma oscillations consistent with the need to allow AMPA to be sufficiently strong to ensure rapid processing into attractor states (Battaglia & Treves 1998, Panzeri, Rolls, Battaglia & Lavis 2001).] The inhibitory neurons use GABA as a transmitter which hyperpolarizes the neurons, with the strength of w_{inh} typically 1.0 (Fig. 3.59b).

The evidence λ_1 for decision 1 is applied to pool D1 through 800 synapses onto each neuron, and the evidence λ_2 for decision 2 is applied to pool D2 in the same way (Fig. 3.59b). The same sets of 800 synapses on every neuron in the network also receive external inputs at a rate λ_{ext}=3 spikes/s, a typical firing rate for the spontaneous activity of cortical neurons, to reflect background activity from other cortical areas. The distribution of these inputs onto each neuron over time is what would be produced by Poisson spikes trains at 3 spikes/s on each of the 800 externally connected synapses onto each neuron, and this is one of the sources of noise in the network. Another of the sources of noise (randomness) in the network is the almost Poisson distributed spike times of the neurons in the network. As the network become larger and approaches an infinite number of neurons, the statistical fluctuations caused by this source of noise in the network become smoothed out and disappear, as described in more detail elsewhere (Rolls 2016c).

3.13.3 Analyses of reward-related decision-making mechanisms in the orbitofrontal cortex

In this Section fMRI evidence to investigate decision-making mechanisms in the orbitofrontal cortex is considered. These investigations test whether the decision-making is consistent with the mechanisms described in Section 3.13.2.

The analyses relate to the ways in which probabilistic decision-making is influenced by the easiness vs the difficulty of the decision, and how confidence in a decision emerges as a property of the neuronal attractor network decision-making process.

To address these issues, we first simulated integrate-and-fire models of attractor-based choice decision-making, and predicted from them the neuronal firing rates in the decision attractor populations and the fMRI BOLD signals on easy vs difficult trials (Rolls, Grabenhorst & Deco 2010b). We then performed two fMRI investigations of decision-making about the reward value and subjective pleasantness of thermal and olfactory stimuli, and showed that areas implicated by other analyses in decision-making (Rolls & Grabenhorst 2008, Grabenhorst, Rolls & Parris 2008b, Rolls, Grabenhorst & Parris 2010d) do show the predicted difference between activations on easy vs difficult trials in the orbitofrontal cortex (Rolls, Grabenhorst & Deco 2010b).

3.13.3.1 Neuronal responses on difficult vs easy trials, and decision confidence

Figure 3.61a and e show the mean firing rates of the two neuronal populations D1 and D2 for two trial types, easy trials (ΔI=160 Hz) and difficult trials (ΔI=0) (where ΔI is the difference in spikes/s summed across all synapses to each neuron between the two inputs, λ_1 to population D1, and λ_2 to population D2). The results are shown for correct trials, that is, trials on which the D1 population won the competition and fired with a rate of > 10 spikes/s more than the rate of D2 for the last 1000 ms of the simulation runs. Figure 3.61b shows the mean firing rates of the four populations of neurons on a difficult trial, and Fig. 3.61c shows the rastergrams for the same trial, for which the energy landscape is also shown in Fig. 3.59d. Figure 3.61d shows the firing rates on another difficult trial (ΔI=0) to illustrate the variability shown from trial to trial, with on this trial prolonged competition between the D1 and D2 attractors until the D1 attractor finally won after approximately 1100 ms. Figure 3.61f shows firing rate plots for the four neuronal populations on an example of a single easy trial (ΔI=160), Fig. 3.61g shows the synaptic currents in the four neuronal populations on the same trial, and Fig. 3.61h shows rastergrams for the same trial (Rolls, Grabenhorst & Deco 2010b).

Three important points are made by the results shown in Fig. 3.61. First, the network falls into its decision attractor faster on easy trials than on difficult trials. We would accordingly expect reaction times to be shorter on easy than on difficult trials. We might also expect the BOLD signal related to the activity of the network to be higher on easy than on difficult trials because it starts sooner on easy trials.

Second, the mean firing rate after the network has settled into the correct decision attractor is higher on easy than on difficult trials. We might therefore expect the BOLD signal related to the activity of the network to be higher on easy than on difficult trials because the maintained activity in the attractor is higher on easy trials. This shows that the exact firing rate in the attractor is a result not only of the internal recurrent collateral effect, but also of the external input to the neurons, which in Fig. 3.61a is 32 Hz to each neuron (summed across all synapses) of D1 and D2, but in Fig. 3.61e is increased by a further 80 Hz to D1, and decreased (from the 32 Hz added) by 80 Hz to D2 (i.e. the total external input to the network is the same, but ΔI=0 for Fig. 3.61a, and ΔI=160 for Fig. 3.61b).

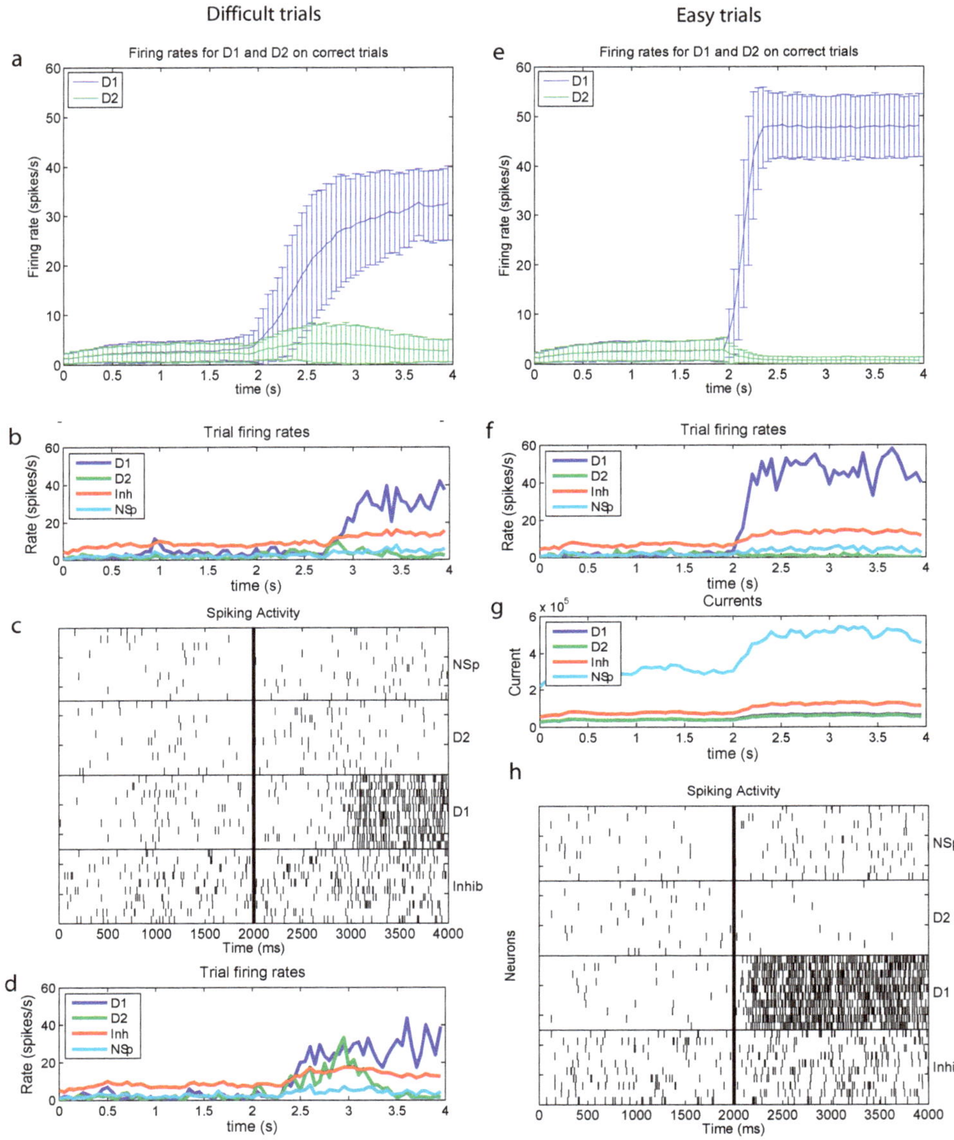

Fig. 3.61 (a) and (e) Firing rates (mean ± sd) for difficult (ΔI=0) and easy (ΔI=160) trials. The period 0–2 s is the spontaneous firing, and the decision cues were turned on at time = 2 s. D1: firing rate of the D1 population of neurons on correct trials on which the D1 population won. D2: firing rate of the D2 population of neurons on the correct trials on which the D1 population won. A correct trial was one in which in which the mean rate of the D1 attractor averaged > 10 spikes/s for the last 1000 ms of the simulation runs. (b) The mean firing rates of the four populations of neurons on a difficult trial. Inh is the inhibitory population that uses GABA as a transmitter. NSp is the non-specific population of neurons (see Fig. 3.59). (c) Rastergrams for the trial shown in b. 10 neurons from each of the four pools of neurons are shown. (d) The firing rates on another difficult trial (ΔI=0) showing prolonged competition between the D1 and D2 attractors until the D1 attractor finally wins after approximately 1100 ms. (f) Firing rate plots for the 4 neuronal populations on a single easy trial (ΔI=160). (g) The synaptic currents in the four neuronal populations on the trial shown in f. (h) Rastergrams for the easy trial shown in f and g. 10 neurons from each of the four pools of neurons are shown. (Reprinted from NeuroImage, 33 (2), Edmund T. Rolls, Fabian Grabenhorst, and Gustavo Deco, Choice, difficulty, and confidence in the brain, pp. 694–706, Copyright 2010, with permission from Elsevier.)

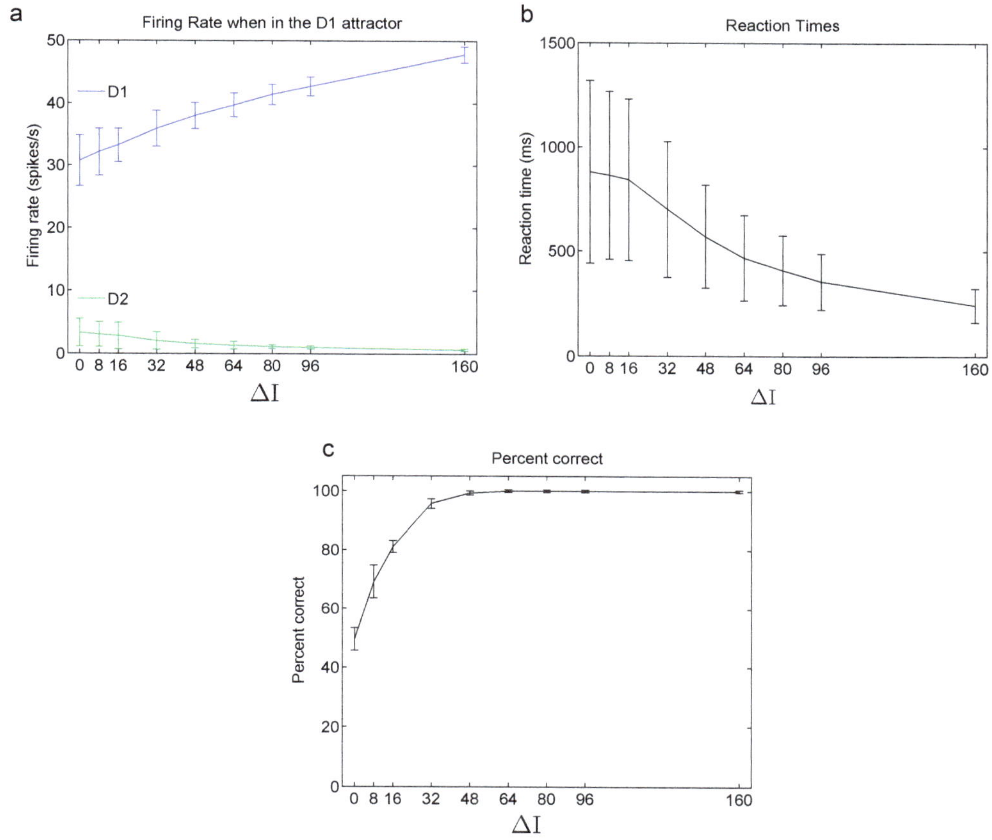

Fig. 3.62 (a) Firing rates (mean ± sd) on correct trials when in the D1 attractor as a function of ΔI. ΔI=0 corresponds to difficult, and ΔI=160 spikes/s corresponds to easy. The firing rates for both the winning population D1 and for the losing population D2 are shown for correct trials by thick lines. All the results are for 1000 simulation trials for each parameter value, and all the results shown are statistically highly significant. (b) Reaction times (mean ± sd) for the D1 population to win on correct trials as a function of the difference in inputs ΔI to D1 and D2. (c) Per cent correct performance, i.e. the percentage of trials on which the D1 population won, as a function of the difference in inputs ΔI to D1 and D2. The mean was calculated over 1000 trials, and the standard deviation was estimated by the variation in 10 groups each of 100 trials. (Reprinted from NeuroImage, 33 (2), Edmund T. Rolls, Fabian Grabenhorst, and Gustavo Deco, Choice, difficulty, and confidence in the brain, pp. 694–706, Copyright 2010, with permission from Elsevier.)

Third, the variability of the firing rate is high, with the standard deviations of the mean firing rate calculated in 50 ms epochs indicated in order to quantify the variability. The large standard deviations on difficult trials for the first second after the decision cues are applied at t=2 s reflects the fact that on some trials the network has entered an attractor state after 1000 ms, but on other trials it has not yet reached the attractor, although it does so later. This trial by trial variability is indicated by the firing rates on individual trials and the rastergrams in the lower part of Fig. 3.61. The effects evident in Fig. 3.61 are quantified, and elucidated over a range of values for ΔI, next.

Figure 3.62a shows the firing rates (mean ± sd) on correct trials when in the D1 attractor as a function of ΔI. ΔI=0 corresponds to the most difficult decision, and ΔI=160 corresponds to easy. The firing rates for both the winning population D1 and for the losing population D2 are shown. The firing rates were measured in the last 1 s of firing, i.e. between t=3 and t=4 s. It is clear that the mean firing rate of the winning population increases monotonically as ΔI increases, and interestingly, the increase is approximately linear (Pearson $r = 0.995$, p<10^{-6}). The higher mean firing rates as ΔI increases are due not only to higher peak firing, but also to the fact that the variability becomes less as ΔI increases ($r = -0.95$, p<10^{-4}), reflecting the fact that the system is more noisy and unstable with low ΔI, whereas the firing rate in the attractor is maintained more stably with smaller statistical fluctuations against the Poisson effects of the random spike timings at high ΔI. (The measure of variation indicated in the figure is the standard deviation, and this is shown here unless otherwise stated to quantify the degree of variation, which is a fundamental aspect of the operation of these neuronal decision-making networks.)

As shown in Fig. 3.62a, the firing rates of the losing population decrease as ΔI increases. The decrease of firing rate of the losing population is due in part to feedback inhibition through the inhibitory neurons by the winning population. Thus the difference of firing rates between the winning and losing populations, as well as the firing rate of the winning population D1, both clearly reflect ΔI, and in a sense the confidence in the decision.

The increase of the firing rate when in the D1 attractor (upper thick line) as ΔI increases thus can be related to the confidence in the decision, and, as will be shown next in Fig. 3.62b, the performance as shown by the percentage of correct choices. The firing rate of the losing attractor (D2, lower thick line) decreases as ΔI increases, due to feedback inhibition from the winning D1 attractor, and thus the difference in the firing rates of the two attractors also reflects well the decision confidence.

I emphasize from these findings (Rolls, Grabenhorst & Deco 2010b) that the firing rate of the winning attractor reflects ΔI, and thus the confidence in the decision which is closely related to ΔI.

3.13.3.2 Decision times of the neuronal responses

The time for the network to reach the correct D1 attractor, i.e. the reaction or decision time of the network, is shown as a function of ΔI in Fig. 3.62b (mean $\pm$ sd). Interestingly, the reaction time continues to decrease ($r = -0.95$, p<10^{-4}) over a wide range of ΔI, even when as shown in Fig. 3.62c the network is starting to perform at 100% correct. The decreasing reaction time as ΔI increases is attributable to the altered 'effective energy landscape' (Rolls 2016c): a larger input to D1 tends to produce occasionally higher firing rates, and these statistically are more likely to induce a significant depression in the landscape towards which the network flows sooner than with low ΔI. Correspondingly, the variability (quantified by the standard deviation) of the reaction times is greatest at low ΔI, and decreases as ΔI increases ($r = -0.95$, p<10^{-4}). This variability would not be found with a deterministic system (i.e. the standard deviations would be 0 throughout, and such systems include those investigated with mean-field analyses), and is entirely due to the random statistical fluctuations caused by the random spiking of the neurons in the integrate-and-fire network.

3.13.3.3 Percentage correct

At $\Delta I=0$, there is no influence on the network to fall more into attractor D1 representing decision 1 than attractor D2 representing decision 2, and its decisions are at chance, with approximately 50% of decisions being for D1. As ΔI increases, the proportion of trials on which D1 is reached increases. The relation between ΔI and percentage correct is shown in Fig. 3.62c. Interestingly, the performance becomes 100% correct with $\Delta I=64$, whereas as shown in Figs. 3.62a and b the firing rates while in the D1 attractor (and therefore potentially the BOLD signal), continue to increase as ΔI increases further, and the reaction times continue to decrease as ΔI increases further. It is a clear prediction for neurophysiological and behavioural measures that the firing rates with decisions made by this attractor process continue to increase as ΔI is increased beyond the level for very good performance as indicated by the percentage of correct decisions, and the neuronal and behavioural reaction times continue to decrease as ΔI is increased beyond the level for very good performance.

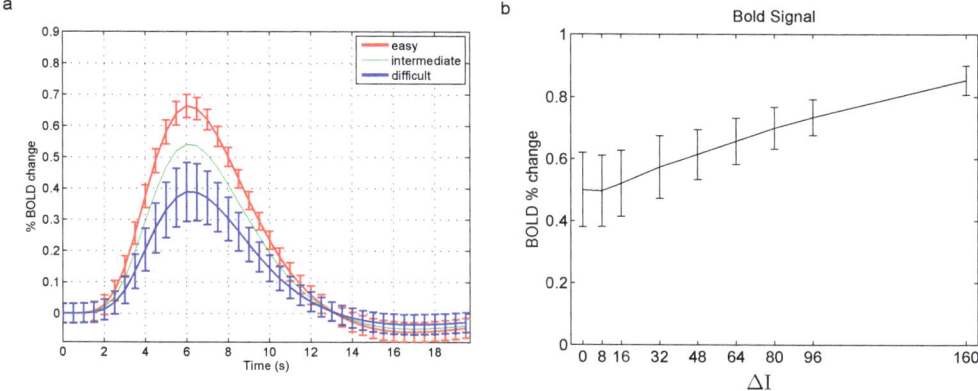

Fig. 3.63 (a) The percentage change in the simulated BOLD signal on easy trials (ΔI=160 spikes/s), on intermediate trials (ΔI=80), and on difficult trials (ΔI=0). The mean $\pm$ sd are shown for the easy and difficult trials. The percentage change in the BOLD signal was calculated from the firing rates of the D1 and D2 populations, and analogous effects were found with calculation from the synaptic currents averaged for example across all 4 populations of neurons. (b) The percentage change in the BOLD signal (peak mean $\pm$ sd) averaged across correct and incorrect trials as a function of ΔI. ΔI=0 corresponds to difficult, and ΔI=160 corresponds to easy. The percent change was measured as the change from the level of activity in a period of 1 s immediately before the decision cues were applied at t=0 s, and was calculated from the firing rates of the neurons in the D1 and D2 populations. The BOLD per cent change scaling is arbitrary, and is set so that the lowest value for the peak of a BOLD response is 0.5%. (Reprinted from NeuroImage, 33 (2), Edmund T. Rolls, Fabian Grabenhorst, and Gustavo Deco, Choice, difficulty, and confidence in the brain, pp. 694–706, Copyright 2010, with permission from Elsevier.)

Figure 3.62c also shows that the variability in the percentage correct (in this case measured over blocks of 100 trials) is large with ΔI=0, and decreases as ΔI increases. This is consistent with unbiased effects of the noise producing very variable effects in the energy landscape at ΔI=0, but in the external inputs biasing the energy landscape more and more as ΔI increases, so that the flow is much more likely to be towards the D1 attractor.

3.13.3.4 Prediction of the BOLD signals on difficult vs easy decision-making trials

It is now shown how this model makes predictions for the fMRI BOLD signals that would occur in brain areas in which decision-making processing of the type described is taking place. The BOLD signals were predicted from the firing rates of the neurons in the network (or from the synaptic currents flowing in the neurons as described later) by convolving the neuronal activity with the haemodynamic response function.

As shown in Fig. 3.63a, the predicted fMRI response is larger for easy ($\Delta I = 160$ spikes/s) than for difficult trials (ΔI=0), with intermediate trials (ΔI=80) producing an intermediate fMRI response. The difference in the peak response for ΔI=0 and ΔI=160 is highly significant ($p \ll 0.001$). Importantly, the BOLD response is inherently variable from brain regions associated with this type of decision-making process, and this is nothing to do with the noise arising in the measurement of the BOLD response with a scanner. If the system were deterministic, the standard deviations, shown as a measure of the variability in Fig. 3.63a, would be 0. It is the statistical fluctuations caused by the noisy (random) spike timings of the neurons that account for the variability in the BOLD signals in Fig. 3.63a. Interestingly, the variability is larger on the difficult trials (ΔI=0) than on the easy trials (ΔI=160), as shown in Fig. 3.63a, and indeed this also can be taken as an indicator that attractor decision-making processes of the type described here are taking place in a brain region.

Figure 3.63b shows that the percentage change in the BOLD signal (peak mean $\pm$ sd) averaged across correct and incorrect trials increases monotonically as a function of ΔI. This again can be taken as an indicator (provided that fMRI signal saturation effects are minimized)

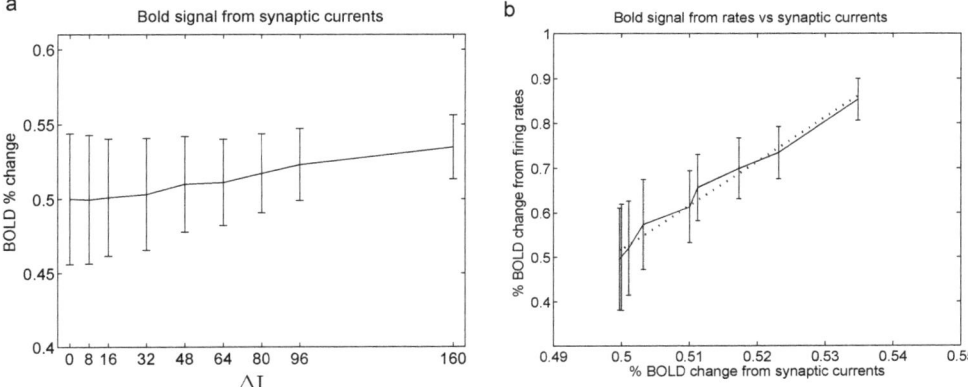

Fig. 3.64 (a) The percentage change of the BOLD signal (mean ± sd) calculated from the synaptic currents in all populations of neurons in the network (D1, D2, GABA, and non-specific, see Fig. 3.59). (Analogous results were found when the currents were calculated from the D1 and D2 populations; or from the D1, D2 and GABA populations.) (b) The relation between the BOLD current predicted from the firing rates and from the synaptic currents (r=0.99, p<10^{-6}) for values of ΔI between 0 and 160. The fitted linear regression line is shown. The BOLD per cent change scaling is arbitrary, and is set so that the lowest value is 0.5%. (Reprinted from NeuroImage, 33 (2), Edmund T. Rolls, Fabian Grabenhorst, and Gustavo Deco, Choice, difficulty, and confidence in the brain, pp. 694–706, Copyright 2010, with permission from Elsevier.)

that attractor decision-making processes of the type described here are taking place in a brain region. The percentage change in Fig. 3.63b was calculated by convolution of the firing rates of the neurons in the D1 and D2 populations with the haemodynamic response function. Interestingly, the percentage change in the BOLD signal is approximately linearly related throughout this range to ΔI (r=0.995, p<10^{-7}). The effects shown in Figs. 3.63a and b can be related to the earlier onset of a high firing rate attractor state when ΔI is larger (see Figs. 3.61 and 3.62b), and to a higher firing rate when in the attractor state (as shown in Figs. 3.61 and 3.62a). As expected from the decrease in the variability of the neuronal activity as ΔI increases (Fig. 3.62a), the variability (standard deviation) in the predicted BOLD signal also decreases as ΔI increases, as shown in Fig. 3.63b (r=0.955, p<10^{-4}).

3.13.4 Neuroimaging investigations of decision-making in the orbitofrontal cortex

Two functional neuroimaging investigations were performed to test the predictions of the model just described. Task difficulty was altered parametrically to determine whether there was a close relation between the BOLD signal and task difficulty (Rolls, Grabenhorst & Deco 2010b), and whether this was present especially in brain areas implicated in choice decision-making by other criteria (Grabenhorst, Rolls & Parris 2008b, Rolls, Grabenhorst & Parris 2010d). The decisions were about the pleasantness of olfactory (Rolls, Grabenhorst & Parris 2010d) or thermal (Grabenhorst, Rolls & Parris 2008b) stimuli.

3.13.4.1 Olfactory pleasantness decision task

The olfactory decision-making task illustrated in Fig. 3.65 was used (Rolls, Grabenhorst & Parris 2010d). ΔI, the difference in pleasantness of the two stimuli between which a decision was being made, was obtained for each trial by the absolute value of the difference in the (average) rated pleasantness of that pair of stimuli for each subject. Thus, two odours of similar pleasantness would have a small ΔI, and two odours of different pleasantness would have a large ΔI. This measure thus reflects the difficulty of the decision, and is independent of whether the second odour happened to be pleasant or unpleasant. This value for ΔI on

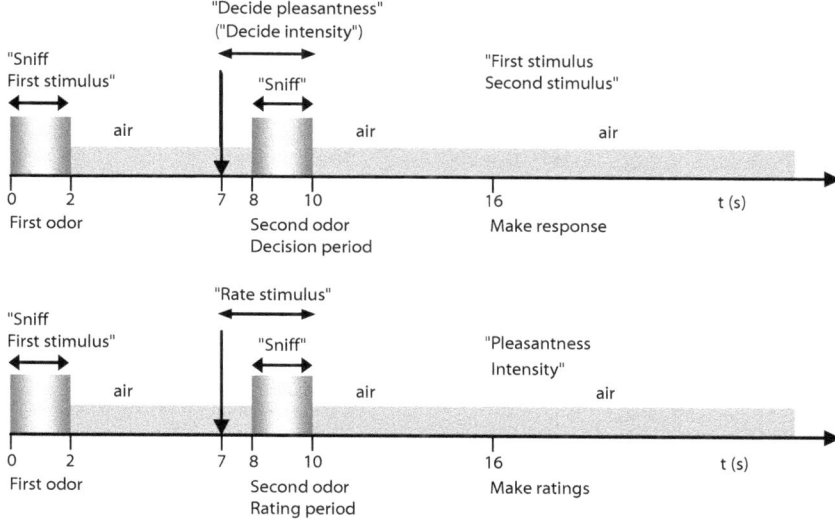

Fig. 3.65 Task design for trials of the olfactory task. On decision trials (upper), the task required a binary choice decision starting during the second odour about which of the two odours was more pleasant, or (on different trials, as indicated by the instruction at $t=7$ s) more intense. On rating trials (lower), identical stimuli were used, but no decision was required, and instead participants rated the second odour for pleasantness and intensity on continuous analog visual rating scales. The trial types were identical until $t=7$ s, when the instruction indicated whether the trial type was decide or rate. The second odour was delivered at $t=8$ s, the subjects were deciding or rating at that time, and the imaging was with respect to this period starting at $t=8$ s. No responses to indicate the decision made or the rating value could be made until t=16 s. (Reproduced from Edmund T. Rolls, Fabian Grabenhorst, Benjamin A. Parris, 'Neural Systems Underlying Decisions about Affective Odors', Journal of Cognitive Neuroscience, 22:5 (May, 2010), pp. 1069-1082. © 2010 by the Massachusetts Institute of Technology, published by the MIT Press.)

every trial was used to investigate whether at brain sites where there was more activation on easy vs difficult trials (as shown by a contrast analysis), the BOLD signal was related to ΔI. Because the stimuli were randomized, the analysis did not reflect the pleasantness or unpleasantness of the second odour, but only how different it was in pleasantness from the first odour, independently of the sign of the difference. The regressor was thus decision difficulty.

3.13.4.2 Temperature pleasantness decision task

Warm and cool thermal stimuli, and mixtures of them, were applied to the hand. In a previous investigation of the same dataset, we compared brain responses when participants were taking decisions about whether they would select a thermal stimulus (yes vs no), with activations to the same stimuli on different trials when only affective ratings were required and there was no decision about whether the participants would say yes or no to the stimuli if they were available in the future (Grabenhorst, Rolls & Parris 2008b). In the investigation on task difficulty, we analysed data only on decision trials, and the analyses were about how activations with the stimuli were related to the difficulty of the decision (Rolls, Grabenhorst & Deco 2010b), which was not investigated previously. Both the decision and rating trials were identical from the start of each trial at t=0 s until t=5 s when a visual stimulus was shown for 1 s stating 'decide' or 'rate' the thermal stimulus being applied, and at t=6 s a green cross appeared until t=10 s. On decide trials from t=6 until t=10 s the participants had to decide whether yes or no was the decision on that trial. At t=10 s a visual stimulus with yes above no or vice versa in random order was shown for 2 s, and the participant had to press the upper or lower button on the button box as appropriate to indicate the response. On rating trials from t=6 until t=10 s the participants had to encode the pleasantness and intensity of the thermal stimulus being applied, so that the ratings could be made later. On rating trials at t=10 s the pleasantness rating could be made using the same button box, and then the intensity rating was made. The thermal stimuli were a warm pleasant stimulus (41C) applied to the hand ('warm2'), a cool unpleasant stimulus (12C) applied to the hand ('cold'), a combined warm and cold stimulus ('warm2+cold'), and a second combination designed to be less pleasant (39C + 12C) ('warm1+cold'), delivered with Peltier devices as described previously (Grabenhorst, Rolls & Parris 2008b).

ΔI for the thermal stimuli was the absolute value of the pleasantness rating, based on the concept that it is more difficult to choose whether a stimulus should be repeated in future if it is close to neutral (0) in rated pleasantness, versus is rated as being pleasant (with the maximum pleasantness being +2), or as being unpleasant (with the most unpleasant being −2).

3.13.4.3 fMRI analyses

The criteria used to identify regions involved in choice decision-making in earlier investigations with the same data set were that a brain region should show more brain activity with identical stimuli on trials on which a choice decision was being made than when the continuous affective value of the stimuli were being rated, but no choice was being made between stimuli, or about whether the stimulus would be chosen again (Grabenhorst, Rolls & Parris 2008b, Rolls, Grabenhorst & Parris 2010d, Rolls & Grabenhorst 2008). For the olfactory task, a contrast of decision vs rating trials showed activations in the medial prefrontal cortex medial area 10 at [2 50 −12] z=3.78 p<0.001 (Rolls, Grabenhorst & Parris 2010d). For the thermal task, a contrast of decision vs rating trials showed activations in the medial prefrontal cortex medial area 10, at [6 54 −8] z=3.24 p=0.022 (Grabenhorst, Rolls & Parris 2008b).

3.13.4.4 Brain areas with activations related to easiness and confidence

Figure 3.66 shows experimental data with the fMRI BOLD signal measured on easy and difficult trials of the olfactory affective decision task (left) and the thermal affective decision task (right) (Rolls, Grabenhorst & Deco 2010b). The upper records are for prefrontal cortex medial area 10 in a region identified by the following criterion as being involved in choice decision-making. The criterion was that a brain region for identical stimuli should show more activity when a choice decision was being made than when a rating on a continuous scale of affective value was being made. Figure 3.66 shows for medial prefrontal cortex area 10 that there is a larger BOLD signal on easy than on difficult trials. The top diagram shows the medial prefrontal area activated in this contrast for decisions about which olfactory stimulus was more pleasant (yellow), and for decisions about whether the thermal stimulus would be chosen in future based on whether it was pleasant or unpleasant (red).

In more detail, for the thermal stimuli, the contrast was the warm2 and the cold trials (which were both easy in that the percentage of the choices were far from the chance value of 50%, and in particular were 96±1% (mean±sem) for the warm, and 18±6% for the cold), versus the mixed stimulus of warm2+cold (which was difficult in that the percentage of choices of 'Yes, it would be chosen in future' was 64±9%). For the temperature easy vs difficult decisions about pleasantness, the activation in medial area 10 had peaks at [4 42 −4] z=3.59 p=0.020 and [6 52 −4] z=3.09 p=0.045.

For the olfactory decision task, the activations in medial area 10 for easy vs difficult choices were at [−4 62 −2] z=2.84 p=0.046, confirmed in a finite impulse response (FIR) analysis with a peak at 6–8 s after the decision time at [−4 54 −6] z=3.50 p=0.002. (In the olfactory task, the easy trials were those in which one of the pair of odours was from the pleasant set, and the other from the unpleasant set. The mean difference in pleasantness, corresponding to ΔI, was 1.76±0.25 (mean±sem). The difficult trials were those in which both odours on a trial were from the pleasant set, or from the unpleasant set. The mean difference in pleasantness, corresponding to ΔI, was 0.72±0.16. For easy trials, the percentage correct was 90±2, and

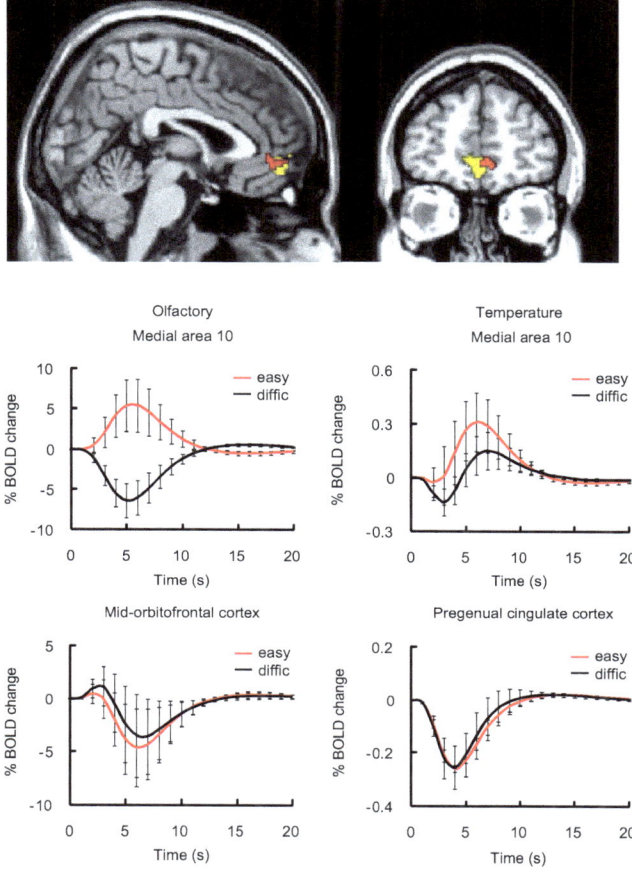

Fig. 3.66 Top: Medial prefrontal cortex area 10 / VMPFC area activated on easy vs difficult trials in the olfactory pleasantness decision task (yellow) and the thermal pleasantness decision task (red). Middle: experimental data showing the BOLD signal in medial area 10 on easy and difficult trials of the olfactory affective decision task (left) and the thermal affective decision task (right). This medial area 10 was a region identified by other criteria (see text) as being involved in choice decision-making. Bottom: The BOLD signal for the same easy and difficult trials, but in parts of the pregenual cingulate and mid-orbitofrontal cortex implicated by other criteria (see text) in representing the subjective reward value of the stimuli on a continuous scale, but not in making choice decisions between the stimuli, or about whether to choose the stimulus in future. (Reprinted from NeuroImage, 53 (2), Edmund T. Rolls, Fabian Grabenhorst, and Gustavo Deco, Choice, difficulty, and confidence in the brain, pp. 694–706, Copyright 2010, with permission from Elsevier.)

for difficult trials was 59±8.) No other significant effects in the a priori regions of interest (Grabenhorst, Rolls & Parris 2008b, Rolls, Grabenhorst & Parris 2010d) were found for the easy vs difficult trial contrast in either the thermal or olfactory reward decision task (Rolls, Grabenhorst & Deco 2010b).

The lower records in Fig. 3.66 are for the same easy and difficult trials, but in parts of the pregenual cingulate and mid-orbitofrontal cortex implicated by the same criteria in representing the subjective reward value of the stimuli, but not in making choice decisions between the stimuli. [For the pregenual cingulate cortex, there was a correlation of the activations with the subjective ratings of pleasantness of the thermal stimuli at [4 38 −2] z=4.24 p=0.001. For the mid-orbitofrontal cortex, there was a correlation of the activations with the subjective ratings of pleasantness of the thermal stimuli at [40 36 −12] z=3.13 p=0.024.] The BOLD signal was similar in these brain regions for easy and difficult trials, as shown in Fig. 3.66, and there was no effect in the contrast between easy and difficult trials.

Figure 3.67 shows the experimental fMRI data with the change in the BOLD signal for

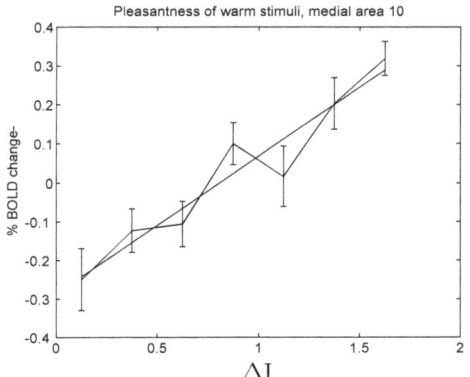 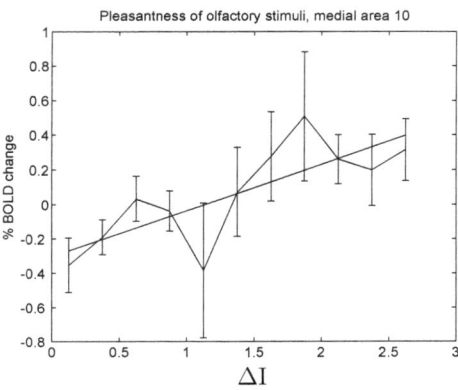

Fig. 3.67 Experimental fMRI data showing the change in the BOLD signal (mean±sem, with the fitted linear regression line shown) as a function of ΔI, the difference in pleasantness of warm stimuli or olfactory stimuli about which decision was being made, for medial prefrontal cortex area 10 / VMPFC. (Reprinted from NeuroImage, 53 (2), Edmund T. Rolls, Fabian Grabenhorst, and Gustavo Deco, Choice, difficulty, and confidence in the brain, pp. 694–706, Copyright 2010, with permission from Elsevier.)

medial prefrontal cortex area 10 indicated as a function of ΔI, the difference in pleasantness of warm stimuli or olfactory stimuli about which decision was being made, and thus the easiness of the decision. For the olfactory decision task, ΔI was the difference in pleasantness (for a given subject) between the mean pleasantness of the first odour and the mean pleasantness of the second odour between which decision was being taken, about which was more pleasant (Rolls et al. 2010b). It is shown in Fig. 3.67 (right) that there was a clear and approximately linear relation between the BOLD signal and ΔI for the olfactory pleasantness decision-making task ($r = 0.77, p = 0.005$). The coordinates for these data were as given for Fig. 3.66.

For the warm decision task, ΔI was the difference in mean pleasantness for a given subject from 0 for a given thermal stimulus about which a decision was being made about whether it should or should not be repeated in future (Grabenhorst et al. 2008b). It is shown in Fig. 3.67 (left) that there was a clear and approximately linear relation between the BOLD signal and ΔI for the thermal pleasantness decision-making task ($r = 0.96, p < 0.001$). The coordinates for these data were as given for Fig. 3.66.

If one makes a correct decision, consistent with the evidence, then one's confidence is higher than when one makes an incorrect decision (as shown by confidence ratings) (Vickers 1979, Vickers & Packer 1982). Consistent with this, the probability that a rat will abort a trial to try again is higher if a decision just made is incorrect (Kepecs, Uchida, Zariwala & Mainen 2008). This occurs before the outcome of the choice is made known to the subject.

Why does this occur, and in which brain regions is the underlying processing implemented? It has been shown that the integrate-and-fire attractor decision-making network described here predicts higher and shorter latency neuronal responses, and higher BOLD signals, in brain areas involved in making choices, on correct than on error trials, and how these changes vary with ΔI and thus compute decision confidence. The reason for this behaviour of the choice attractor network is that on correct trials, when the network influenced by the spiking noise has reached an attractor state supported by the recurrent connections between the neurons, the external inputs to the network that provide the evidence for the decision will have firing rates that are consistent with the decision, so the firing rate of the winning attractor will be higher when the correct attractor (given the evidence) wins the competition than when the incorrect attractor wins the competition (Rolls, Grabenhorst & Deco 2010c). For this effect to remain present after the choice, the decision stimuli, or a short-term memory of them, need of course to be present, providing an on-going bias to the decision-making network that is consistent (on correct trials) or inconsistent (on error trials) with the decision just taken.

It has been shown in an experimental fMRI investigation that this BOLD signature of correct vs incorrect decisions, which reflects confidence in whether a decision just taken is correct, is found in the medial prefrontal cortex area 10, the posterior and subgenual cingulate cortex, and the dorsolateral prefrontal cortex, but not in the mid-orbitofrontal cortex, where activations instead reflect the pleasantness or subjective affective value of the stimuli used as inputs to the choice decision-making process (Rolls, Grabenhorst & Deco 2010c). This approach to decision-making, in contrast to phenomenal mathematical models of decision-making as an accumulation or diffusion process (Vickers 1979, Vickers & Packer 1982, Ratcliff & Rouder 1998, Ratcliff, Zandt & McKoon 1999, Usher & McClelland 2001), thus makes testable predictions about how correct vs error performance is implemented in the brain, and these predictions are supported by experimental results showing that areas involved in choice decision-making (or that receive from them) have activity consistent with these predictions, and that other areas not involved in the choice-making part of the process do not.

In conclusion, these analyses show that the signature of an attractor decision-making network, increasing BOLD signals as a function of ΔI on correct trials, and decreasing on error trials, is found in the medial prefrontal cortex area 10 / ventromedial prefrontal cortex, VMPFC (Rolls, Grabenhorst & Deco 2010b, Rolls, Grabenhorst & Deco 2010c). This is an area implicated by other evidence in decision-making between stimuli of different value (Grabenhorst et al. 2008b, Rolls 2014a). The same signature was not found in other parts of the orbitofrontal cortex that are implicated in representing reward value on a continuous scale. In addition, the fMRI investigations provide support for this attractor model of decision-making, for the model makes predictions consistent with the empirical data. Consistent with these investigations, in macaques single neurons in the ventromedial prefrontal cortex (corresponding to the medial area 10 region described) rapidly come to signal the value of the chosen offer, suggesting that a circuit in the VMPFC serves to produce a choice (Strait, Blanchard & Hayden 2014), and consistent with the attractor model of decision-making (Rolls 2016c, Rolls 2014a, Deco, Rolls, Albantakis & Romo 2013). Neurons that respond to chosen value in a decision task with a delay between the two reward options have also been described in area 13, and these neurons may respond to the difference in reward value when the second option is shown (Setogawa, Mizuhiki, Matsumoto, Akizawa, Kuboki, Richmond & Shidara 2019).

Further comparison of this model of decision-making with other approaches to decision-making is provided elsewhere (Rolls 2016c, Rolls 2014a, Deco, Rolls, Albantakis & Romo 2013).

3.14 A representation of novel visual stimuli, and memory-related effects, in the orbitofrontal cortex

A population of neurons has been discovered in the primate orbitofrontal cortex that responds to novel but not familiar visual stimuli, and takes typically a few trials to habituate (Rolls, Browning, Inoue & Hernadi 2005a). The memories of these neurons last for at least 24 h. Exactly what role these neurons have in memory is not yet known, but there are connections from the area in which these neurons are recorded to the temporal lobe, and activations in a corresponding orbitofrontal cortex area in humans are found when new visual stimuli must be encoded in memory (Frey & Petrides 2002b, Frey & Petrides 2003, Petrides 2007).

The human ventromedial prefrontal cortex (which includes area 14 (Mackey & Petrides 2014)) is implicated in some aspects of memory including autobiographical memory, in that

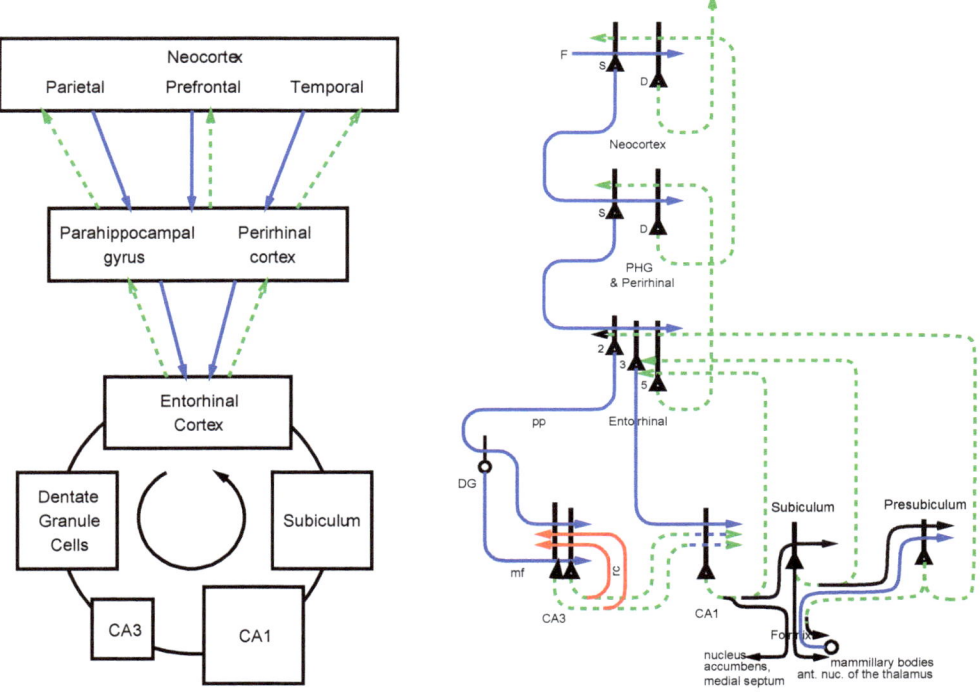

Fig. 3.68 Forward connections (blue solid lines) from areas of cerebral association neocortex via the parahippocampal gyrus and perirhinal cortex, and entorhinal cortex, to the hippocampus; and backprojections (green dashed lines) via the hippocampal CA1 pyramidal cells, subiculum, and parahippocampal gyrus to the neocortex. There is great convergence in the forward connections down to the single network implemented in the CA3 pyramidal cells; and great divergence again in the backprojections. Left: block diagram. Right: more detailed representation of some of the principal excitatory neurons in the pathways. Abbreviations: D, deep pyramidal cells; DG, dentate granule cells; F, forward inputs to areas of the association cortex from preceding cortical areas in the hierarchy. mf: mossy fibres; PHG, parahippocampal gyrus and perirhinal cortex; pp, perforant path; rc, recurrent collaterals of the CA3 hippocampal pyramidal cells shown in red; S, superficial pyramidal cells; 2, pyramidal cells in layer 2 of the entorhinal cortex; 3, pyramidal cells in layer 3 of the entorhinal cortex; 5, 6, pyramidal cells in the deep layers of the entorhinal cortex. The thick lines above the cell bodies represent the dendrites.

activations are found during memory retrieval (Barry, Chadwick & Maguire 2018, Bonnici & Maguire 2018), and in that damage in this region may impair memory, in addition to its effects on emotion (McCormick, Ciaramelli, De Luca & Maguire 2018). In a study on navigation, it was found that humans with damage to the ventromedial prefrontal cortex were impaired, and what was of interest was that the errors were frequently related to navigating to the incorrect goal (Ciaramelli 2008). I suggest that this may provide a framework for understanding how memory, and navigation tasks (which require memory of the goal) may relate to the functions of the orbitofrontal / ventromedial prefrontal cortex. It may be because the goals, the rewards, of the navigation or memory task are represented in the orbitofrontal / ventromedial prefrontal cortex, and if the value or goal representations are disrupted, this may be the reason why some memory or navigation tasks are impaired.

This concept also provides an account for why the orbitofrontal cortex / ventromedial prefrontal cortex may be activated in memory tasks. The theory of the hippocampus and memory is that inputs from the dorsal stream about space and action, from the ventral stream about objects and people, and from the orbitofrontal cortex about rewards, reach the hippocampal system via the routes shown in Fig. 5.3 (Rolls 1989a, Rolls 1989b, Rolls 1990b, Treves & Rolls 1994, Rolls 1996a, Kesner & Rolls 2015, Rolls 2016c, Rolls 2018a, Rolls & Wirth 2018). In the hippocampus, these different inputs that are present in an event can be associated together in the CA3 recurrent collateral autoassociation / attractor network (Fig.

3.68). During recall, an input from any one of these systems, for example about a person, may trigger the recall of the other components, e.g. about where, and about the reward / emotional states, in the process known as completion to produce the whole episodic memory event. The backprojections to each of the cortical systems that provide inputs to the hippocampus then provide a mechanism for the neuronal firing states to be recalled in the neocortical areas that provide inputs to the hippocampus. These neocortical areas include the orbitofrontal / ventromedial prefrontal cortex, where the reward / affective state component will be retrieved during memory recall. It is suggested that this provides an account for why the orbitofrontal cortex / ventromedial prefrontal cortex may be activated during memory recall. The memory recall includes autobiographical memory, and that type of memory recall might be expected to produce strong activations in the orbitofrontal cortex during memory recall, because of their affective components.

3.15 Deep brain stimulation of the orbitofrontal cortex

Olds & Milner (1954) discovered that rats would learn to stimulate electrically some regions of the brain, including the lateral hypothalamus. James Olds noticed that rats would return to a corner of an open field apparatus where stimulation had just been given. He stimulated the rat whenever it went to the corner and found that the animals rapidly learned to go there to obtain the stimulation, by making delivery of it contingent on other types of behaviour, such as pressing a lever in a Skinner box or crossing a shock grid (Olds 1977).

We extended that discovery to primates, to macaques (Rolls et al. 1980, Rolls 2005). The stimulation protocol is that 0.5 s trains of 0.5 ms pulses are applied at 100 Hz. The macaque (or squirrel monkey) quickly learns to press a lever, or perform any other instrumental response, to obtain a train of stimulation of this type for every response. The macaques will continue to do this for hours at a time, pressing typically quite rapidly, with a press every few seconds.

One group of brain-stimulation reward sites is located along the general course of the medial forebrain bundle, passing lateral to the midline from the ventral tegmental area of the midbrain posteriorly (near the dopamine neurons), through the lateral hypothalamus, preoptic area and nucleus accumbens, toward the prefrontal cortex (orbitofrontal cortex in the monkey) anteriorly (Fig. 3.69) (Olds & Olds 1965, Rolls 1971, Rolls 1974, Rolls 1975, Rolls 1976, Rolls & Cooper 1974, Mora, Avrith & Rolls 1980, Rolls, Burton & Mora 1980). The dopamine neurons are unlikely to be the key neurons directly activated by this stimulation, because it is likely that dopamine neurons cannot follow rates as high as 100 Hz, and the stimulation becomes more rewarding as the stimulation frequency is increased from 25 Hz to 200 Hz. However, it is likely that the dopamine neurons are indirectly activated by the stimulation at these rewarding brain sites. (Much more detailed evidence on brain-stimulation reward is available in Chapter 7 of my book *Emotion Explained* (Rolls 2005), which I have made available at my website www.oxcns.org.)

A second group of self-stimulation sites is in limbic and related areas such as the amygdala, nucleus accumbens, and prefrontal cortex (orbitofrontal cortex in the monkey) (Rolls 1974, Rolls 1975, Rolls 1976, Rolls, Burton & Mora 1980, Mora, Avrith & Rolls 1980). This group of sites is highly interconnected neurophysiologically with the first group lying along the general course of the medial forebrain bundle, in that stimulation in any one of these reward sites activates neurons in the others in primates (Rolls, Burton & Mora 1980) (see below).

By recording from single neurons while stimulation is delivered at the threshold current

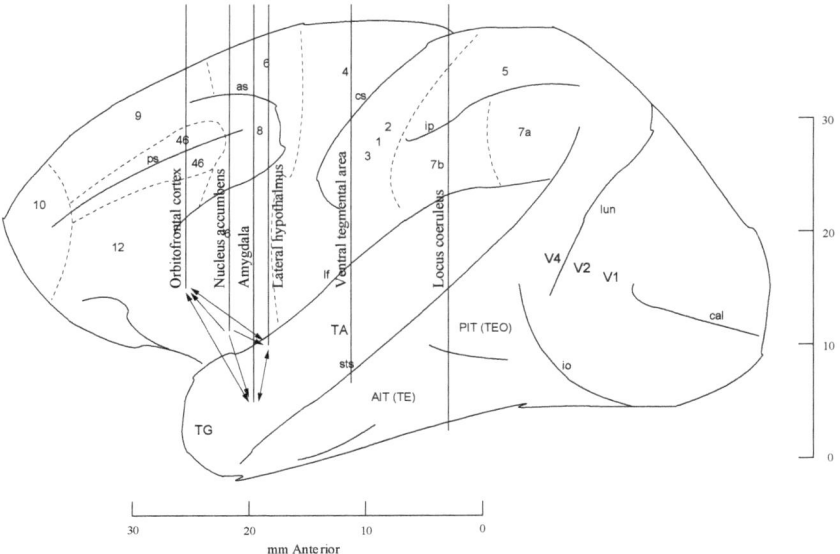

Fig. 3.69 Some brain sites in primates at which electrical stimulation of the brain can produce reward. The arrows indicate that stimulation at any one of these sites activates neurons in all of the other sites connected by arrows, as shown by Rolls, Burton and Mora (1980). The scales show the stereotaxic base planes. Abbreviations as in Fig. 2.1.

to self-stimulation electrodes[5], it is possible to determine which neural systems are actually activated by brain-stimulation reward. In the rat it is clear that during hypothalamic self-stimulation, neurons in the prefrontal cortex, amygdala and some areas of the brainstem, as well as in the hypothalamus itself, are activated (Rolls 1974, Rolls 1975, Rolls 1976, Ito 1976). In the monkey it has been found that neurons in the lateral hypothalamus, orbitofrontal cortex, amygdala, nucleus accumbens, and ventral tegmental area are activated during self-stimulation of any one of these sites or of the nucleus accumbens (see Fig. 3.69) (Rolls 1974, Rolls 1975, Rolls 1976, Rolls, Burton & Mora 1980, Rolls 2005). Thus in the monkey, there is a highly interconnected set of structures, stimulation in any one of which will support self-stimulation and will activate neurons in the other structures.

The orbitofrontal cortex is one of the brain regions in which excellent self-stimulation is produced in primates (Mora, Avrith, Phillips & Rolls 1979, Phillips, Mora & Rolls 1979, Phillips, Mora & Rolls 1981, Rolls, Burton & Mora 1980, Mora, Avrith & Rolls 1980). The self-stimulation is like lateral hypothalamic self-stimulation in that it is learned rapidly, and occurs at a high rate. It has been shown that the self-stimulation of the orbitofrontal cortex is hunger-dependent, in that feeding a monkey to satiety produces great attenuation of orbitofrontal cortex self-stimulation (Mora, Avrith, Phillips & Rolls 1979). Of all the brain-stimulation reward sites studied in the monkey, it is the one at which feeding to satiety has the most profound effect in reducing self-stimulation (Rolls, Burton and Mora 1980). The orbitofrontal self-stimulation pulses have also been shown to drive neurons strongly in the lateral hypothalamus with latencies of only a few ms (Rolls 1975, Rolls 1976, Rolls, Burton & Mora 1980). Conversely, single neurons in the primate orbitofrontal cortex are activated from brain-stimulation reward sites in the lateral hypothalamus. These neuronal activations were typically trans-synaptic with latencies of 2–10 ms. On the basis of these findings, it was suggested that orbitofrontal cortex stimulation in primates is rewarding because it taps into food-reward mechanisms.

---

[5]The threshold current for self-stimulation is the minimum amount of current for a given stimulation pulse-width required to produce self-stimulation at a given self-stimulation site.

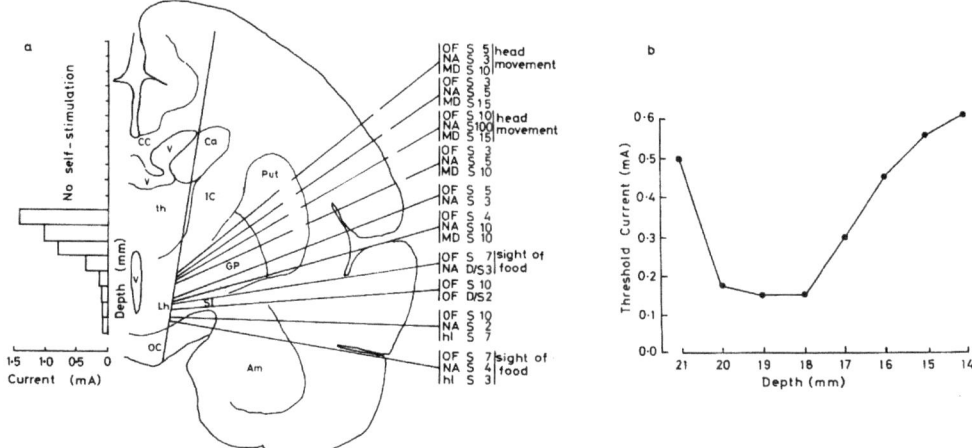

Fig. 3.70 a. Neurons activated by both brain-stimulation reward and the sight of food were found at the lower end of this microelectrode track in the macaque lateral hypothalamus. Neurons higher up the track in the globus pallidus were activated by brain-stimulation reward and also by head movements. The neurons were trans-synaptically (S) or possibly in some cases directly (D/S) activated with the latencies shown in ms from self-stimulation sites in the orbitofrontal cortex (OF), nucleus accumbens (NA), mediodorsal nucleus of the thalamus (MD), or lateral hypothalamus (hl). b. Self-stimulation through the recording microelectrode occurred with low currents if the microelectrode was in the hypothalamus close to the neurons activated by the sight of food. Am - amygdala; Ca - caudate; CC - corpus callosum; Gp - globus pallidus; Lh - lateral hypothalamus; OC - optic chiasm; Put - putamen; V - ventricle. (Modified from Rolls 1975; Reprinted from Brain Research, 194 (2), E.T. Rolls, M.J. Burton, and F. Mora, Neurophysiological analysis of brain-stimulation reward in the monkey, pp. 339–357, Copyright © 1980 Published by Elsevier B.V.)

We wished to test this hypothesis, and therefore recorded from these neurons activated from brain-stimulation reward sites when the macaques were awake, and we could offer the macaques natural rewards such as food. This very rapidly led to the discovery that the taste, and even the sight, of food, often activated these neurons that were activated from brain-stimulation reward sites (Rolls et al. 1980). This discovery was originally made by recordings in the lateral hypothalamus, where we discovered food reward related neurons, but that was quickly extended to the orbitofrontal cortex, in which we also discovered food reward related neurons (Rolls, Burton & Mora 1980, Thorpe, Rolls & Maddison 1983), and that discovery led to all the other discoveries about taste, olfactory and visual reward systems in macaques and humans described in the earlier parts of this Chapter.

Rewarding electrical stimulation of the macaque orbitofrontal cortex can activate lateral hypothalamic feeding-related neurons, which respond for example to the sight or taste of food (Rolls et al. 1980). An example of an experiment of this type is illustrated in Fig. 3.70. As the recording electrode was lowered into the lateral hypothalamus, a brain region essential for feeding (Rolls 2014a, Rolls 2005), single neurons were found to be activated with the latencies shown in ms from reward sites in the orbitofrontal cortex (OFC) and nucleus accumbens (NA) (Rolls et al. 1980). Two of the neurons in the lateral hypothalamus responded to the sight of food. Thus brain-stimulation reward of the orbitofrontal cortex activated lateral hypothalamic food-related reward neurons. (They were shown to be reward-related by the finding that these neurons only respond to the sight of food when the monkey is hungry (Rolls et al. 1986).) Moreover, electrical stimulation through the recording microelectrode could support brain-stimulation reward at low currents when the microelectrode was close to the food reward-related neurons in the lateral hypothalamus, as shown in Fig. 3.70. The hypothesis that all these discoveries support is that the food reward is decoded in the orbitofrontal cortex, as described earlier in this Chapter, and that orbitofrontal cortex neurons send that information to the lateral hypothalamus, which is a key part of the feeding system where external signals about the sight and taste of food are integrated with internal signals about plasma glucose, leptin, ghrelin, and other hormones (Rolls 2014a, Rolls 2016f). However, an important part of the concept here is that some of the satiety and hunger signals must reach the orbitofrontal cortex etc, via for example the hypothalamus and visceral insula, to account for the fact that orbitofrontal cortex taste, olfactory, and sight of food-related neurons do encode food reward, in that their responses are decreased to zero by feeding to satiety (Rolls, Sienkiewicz & Yaxley 1989, Critchley & Rolls 1996c).

It has been shown that electrical stimulation of the human orbitofrontal cortex can also produce reward and raise mood (Rao et al. 2018). Although the title of that study emphasised the lateral orbitofrontal cortex, many of the sites were in the middle part of the orbitofrontal cortex, areas 13 and 11, which we categorise as medial orbitofrontal cortex, and is the area activated by many rewards. It is likely that these medial orbitofrontal cortex sites will produce better reward in humans than stimulation in the lateral orbitofrontal cortex BA12/47, for these lateral sites are activated by unpleasant stimuli and by not obtaining expected rewards, as described above. The medial (/ middle) orbitofrontal cortex may for all the reasons described in this Chapter be a key area of interest for deep brain stimulation to help relieve depression, as described in Chapter 7. In addition, consistent with our neurophysiological and neuroimaging investigations, electrical stimulation of the human orbitofrontal cortex may produce gustatory and olfactory sensations (Yih, Beam, Fox & Parvizi 2019).

3.16 The orbitofrontal cortex and addiction

Orbitofrontal cortex reward mechanisms may be important in several types of addiction.

Dopamine projections reach the orbitofrontal cortex. One way in which dopaminergic activation produced by the psychomotor stimulants such as amphetamine and cocaine produces reward is by activating the reward mechanisms just discussed in the orbitofrontal cortex (Phillips, Mora & Rolls 1981, Voellm, De Araujo, Cowen, Rolls, Kringelbach, Smith, Jezzard, Heal & Matthews 2004), and regions to which it projects such as the nucleus accumbens which is part of the ventral striatum (Phillips, Blaha & Fibiger 1989, Phillips & Fibiger 1990) (see further Section 5.3, Koob & Volkow (2016), and Nutt, Lingford-Hughes, Erritzoe & Stokes (2015)). In more detail, macaques will self-administer amphetamine to the orbitofrontal cortex (Phillips et al. 1981), and intravenous administration of amphetamine to drug-naive humans activates the orbitofrontal cortex (Voellm et al. 2004) (see further Section 5.2.2).

Another example is smoking, in which there is low functional connectivity of the lateral orbitofrontal cortex, which may promote impulsiveness and the administration of nicotine which may act to increase activity generally in the brain, in that those who tend to smoke have low overall functional connectivity (Cheng et al. 2019).

Another example is drinking alcohol, in which there is high functional connectivity of the medial orbitofrontal cortex (Cheng et al. 2019), which may promote sensation-seeking (Wan et al. 2019). These results were obtained in a study with more than 2000 participants.

Increased impulsivity was found in smokers, associated with decreased functional connectivity of the non-reward-related lateral orbitofrontal cortex; and increased impulsivity was found in high amount drinkers, associated with increased functional connectivity of the reward-related medial orbitofrontal cortex (Wan et al. 2019).

Further, the functional connectivities in 14-year-old non-smokers (and also in 14-year-old female low-drinkers) were related to who would smoke or drink at age 19. An implication is that these differences in brain functional connectivities play a role in smoking and drinking, together with other factors (Cheng et al. 2019).

These investigations emphasize that there are different brain systems that are involved in different types of addiction, and that several involve the orbitofrontal cortex.

Given the research described in this Chapter on the functions of the primate including human orbitofrontal cortex, a synthesis is provided in Chapter 10, and some points for possible future research are also considered in Chapter 10.

4 Orbitofrontal cortex damage effects in humans and other primates

4.1 Non-human primates

4.1.1 Emotion and reward-related learning impairments

Damage to the caudal orbitofrontal cortex in the monkey produces emotional changes. These include reduced aggression to humans and to stimuli such as a snake and a doll, a reduced tendency to reject foods such as meat (Butter et al. 1970, Butter & Snyder 1972, Butter et al. 1969), and a failure to display the normal preference ranking for different foods (Baylis & Gaffan 1991). Emotional responses to an artificial snake are impaired by both orbitofrontal cortex and amygdala lesions (Murray & Izquierdo 2007).

These changes that follow frontal lobe damage may be related to a failure to react normally to and learn from non-reward in a number of different situations. This failure is evident as a tendency to respond when responses are inappropriate, e.g. no longer rewarded. In particular, macaques with lesions of the orbitofrontal cortex are impaired at tasks that involve learning about which stimuli are rewarding and which are not, and especially in altering behaviour when reinforcement contingencies change. The monkeys may respond when responses are inappropriate, e.g. no longer rewarded, or may respond to a non-rewarded stimulus. For example, monkeys with orbitofrontal cortex damage are impaired on Go/NoGo task performance, in that they Go on the NoGo trials (Iversen & Mishkin 1970)[6], and in an object-reversal task in that they respond to the object that was formerly rewarded with food, and in extinction in that they continue to respond to an object that is no longer rewarded (Butter 1969, Jones & Mishkin 1972, Meunier, Bachevalier & Mishkin 1997)[7].

---

[6]In a Go/NoGo task, on a Go trial one visual stimulus is shown, and a response such as licking a tube can be made to obtain a food reward; and on a NoGo trial, a different visual stimulus is shown, and no response must be made otherwise a punishment, of for example a taste of aversive saline, is obtained (Thorpe, Rolls & Maddison 1983, Rolls, Critchley, Mason & Wakeman 1996a). The task tests for stimulus–reward associations, in that one visual stimulus is associated with food reward, and the other with saline punishment if a response is made. There is a different version of a Go/NoGo task on which on NoGo trials no response must be made in order to obtain reward, and this version of the task with symmetrical reinforcement tests for whether one visual stimulus can be mapped to one behaviour, a response, and another visual stimulus to another behaviour, not responding, in order to obtain reward. Unless otherwise specified, it is the first version of the task that uses asymmetrical reinforcement and that tests for stimulus–reinforcer associations that is referred to in this book.

[7]In a visual discrimination reversal task as run in neurophysiological experiments (Thorpe, Rolls & Maddison 1983, Rolls, Critchley, Mason & Wakeman 1996a), on a trial on which one visual stimulus is shown, the S+ or positive discriminative stimulus S^D, a response such as licking a tube can be made to obtain a food reward; and on a trial on which the other visual stimulus is shown, the S– or negative discriminative stimulus S^Δ, no response must be made otherwise a punisher, of for example a taste of aversive saline, is obtained (Thorpe et al. 1983, Rolls et al. 1996a). After good performance is obtained, the reward association is reversed, so that the visual stimulus that was formerly an S+ becomes an S–, and vice versa. Behaviour typically reverses over a number of trials, so that the new S+ become the stimulus that is worked for. The task tests for the ability to reverse stimulus–reward associations based on a changed of expected value, and if reversal occurs, shows for example that the neuron being recorded encodes the reinforcement association of the visual stimuli, and not the physical identity of visual stimuli. The improvement in reversal learning performance so that after a number of reversal a reversal can take place in as little as one trial (Thorpe, Rolls & Maddison 1983) is referred to as reversal learning set (Deco & Rolls 2005a).

There is some evidence for dissociation of function within the orbitofrontal cortex, in that lesions to the inferior convexity produced Go/NoGo and object reversal deficits, whereas damage to the caudal orbitofrontal cortex, area 13, produced the extinction deficit (Rosenkilde 1979). The visual discrimination reversal learning deficit shown by monkeys with orbitofrontal cortex damage (Jones & Mishkin 1972, Baylis & Gaffan 1991, Murray & Izquierdo 2007) may be due at least in part to the tendency of these monkeys not to withhold responses to non-rewarded stimuli (Jones & Mishkin 1972) including objects that were previously rewarded during reversal (Rudebeck & Murray 2011), and including foods that are not normally accepted (Butter et al. 1969, Baylis & Gaffan 1991). Consistently, orbitofrontal cortex (but not amygdala lesions) impaired instrumental extinction (Murray & Izquierdo 2007).

4.1.2 Impairment of reward value as altered by selective satiation, reward size, and delay of reward

As described in Chapter 3, selective satiation, which produces sensory-specific satiety, is a way of measuring reward value. Reducing the value of a food stimulus by feeding to satiety decreases the responses of orbitofrontal cortex neurons (and activations in humans) selectively to the food with which satiety was produced, providing direct evidence for value representations in the orbitofrontal cortex (Rolls, Sienkiewicz & Yaxley 1989, Critchley & Rolls 1996a, Kringelbach, O'Doherty, Rolls & Andrews 2003, Rolls & Grabenhorst 2008, Grabenhorst & Rolls 2011).

Consistent with this, lesions of areas 11/13 (but not area 14), disrupted the rapid updating of object value during selective satiation (Rudebeck & Murray 2011, Rudebeck et al. 2017, Murray & Rudebeck 2018). A further finding is that area 13 inactivation impairs the updating of value representations during satiation, and that inactivation of area 11 impairs the selection of goals in the choice process (Murray, Moylan, Saleem, Basile & Turchi 2015).

Further, and in relation to neuroeconomics, the estimation of predicted reward value as influenced by reward size, and delay to reward, or both, is impaired by orbitofrontal cortex lesions in macaques (Simmons, Minamimoto, Murray & Richmond 2010).

These effects of damage to the orbitofrontal cortex are thus consistent with the neurophysiology and neuroimaging described in Chapter 3.

4.1.3 Credit assignment vs the comparison of choices

In further analyses, an impairment in the stimulus-reinforcer associations learned on individual trials has been described following lesions to the mid and lateral parts of the orbitofrontal cortex (Noonan, Walton, Behrens, Sallet, Buckley & Rushworth 2010, Walton, Behrens, Buckley, Rudebeck & Rushworth 2010, Noonan, Kolling, Walton & Rushworth 2012). (Care is needed in the description of the lesions in this study. These authors follow an anatomical hypothesis (Carmichael & Price 1996) that separates a medial but in fact primarily cingulate cortex network, from a lateral primarily orbitofrontal cortex network. The 'lateral' network does not mean lateral orbitofrontal cortex. The so-called 'lateral' network referred to in this study (Noonan et al. 2010, Walton et al. 2010, Noonan et al. 2012) in fact included much of areas 11 and 13, as well as parts of area 12.) The deficit produced by these lesions of the middle and lateral orbitofrontal cortex impaired what was described as credit assignment: the ability to assign reward outcomes to particular stimulus choices. Normal monkeys attribute expected value to a stimulus as a function of the precise history of reward received in association with the choice of that particular stimulus, in accordance with Thorndike's 'Law of Effect'. In contrast, animals with these orbitofrontal cortex lesions were no longer able to associate a reward outcome with the corresponding stimulus on which it was contingent. Instead, animals valued a particular stimulus as a proximity-weighted function of the history of all rewards received approximately at the time of choice, even when the rewards were actually caused by choices of the alternative stimuli on preceding and subsequent trials, a phenomenon that Thorndike termed 'Spread of Effect'.

This is thus consistent with the hypothesis that the orbitofrontal cortex is involved in associating correctly stimuli and reward to produce the correct expected value, one of the key concepts developed from the neurophysiological investigations described in Chapter 3.

In contrast, in the same study, 'medial' lesions (in fact mainly of the gyrus rectus area 14 which is included in the cingulate network, and in an area sometimes termed ventromedial prefrontal cortex) appeared to impair reward-guided decision-making because they disrupt the comparison of choice values (Noonan et al. 2010, Walton et al. 2010, Noonan et al. 2012). Rather than choosing the highest value option, macaques with these 'ventromedial prefrontal cortex' lesions were more likely than controls to choose the second best option (out of three options).

This is consistent with the identification of an area in the human ventral medial prefrontal cortex area 10 or 'ventromedial prefrontal cortex' (VMPFC) that is implicated in neuroimaging studies in the mechanisms of choice decision-making between rewards (Rolls et al. 2010b, Rolls et al. 2010c), described in Section 3.13.

4.1.4 Rapid reversal learning

The neurophysiological and neuroimaging investigations described in Chapter 3 and elsewhere (Rolls 2017c, Rolls 2014a, Rolls 2018b) provide evidence for a mechanism for one-trial reversal learning in the primate including human orbitofrontal cortex. This type of process may be important for rapidly updating reward value representations that are very important in primate including human social behaviour. This rapid reversal learning can be studied using reversal learning set, the process by which during repeated reversal learning, performance gradually improves until reversal can occur in one trial. It is important that after reversal learning set has been acquired, when the contingency is reversed, the individual (human or non-human primate) makes a response to the current S+ expecting to get reward, but instead obtains the punisher. On the very first subsequent trial on which the pre-reversal S– is shown, the individual will perform a response to it expecting now to get reward, *even though the post-reversal S+ has not since the reversal been associated with reward to produce associative learning (using for example long-term potentiation) for the post-reversal S+.* (This is in fact illustrated in Fig. 3.46 on page 76.) To implement this very rapid stimulus–reinforcer association reversal, a rule-based process requires the current rule to be held in mind, in short-term memory. This, and non-reward neurons that maintain their firing for many seconds as illustrated in Fig. 3.46, may be developments provided for by the evolution of granular orbitofrontal cortex areas in primates (see Section 1.2 and Chapter 9).

It is this rule-based, one-trial, visual reversal learning that is the type of emotion-related learning to which the primate including human orbitofrontal cortex makes an important contribution. (Claims that the orbitofrontal cortex is not involved in reversal learning in rodents (Stalnaker, Cooch & Schoenbaum 2015) have not adequately dealt with this point, as it is not clear that this type of learning occurs in rodents, as described in Chapter 8.) Moreover, when assessing the effects of lesions of the orbitofrontal cortex on this type of learning in primates, it appears to be important that the lateral orbitofrontal cortex area 12 is included in the lesion (which it not always is (Murray & Izquierdo 2007, Rudebeck & Murray 2014)), because that is where a focus appears to be of the non-reward reversal-related effects in primates including humans in tasks that often involve probabilistic situations (Kringelbach & Rolls 2003, O'Doherty, Kringelbach, Rolls, Hornak & Andrews 2001a, Chau,

Sallet, Papageorgiou, Noonan, Bell, Walton & Rushworth 2015). Indeed, earlier research in which the lesions included the lateral orbitofrontal cortex did demonstrate deficits in reversal learning and extinction (Iversen & Mishkin 1970, Butter 1969).

More recent research is showing that in macaques lateral orbitofrontal cortex lesions (sometimes termed ventrolateral prefrontal cortex, VLPFC) do impair choices based on probabilities of reward (Rudebeck, Saunders, Lundgren & Murray 2017, Murray & Rudebeck 2018), which benefits from sensitivity to non-reward and the ability to remember previous rewards and non-rewards received for a choice. The task was a three-armed bandit task in which the probability of obtaining reward for each of the three options changed during the task. In that the macaques with these lateral orbitofrontal cortex lesions failed to respond to the change in the probability of less reward for some options and more reward for others, the macaques were not responding appropriately to the decreases and increases in the reward available for the different options. This is consistent with the concept that the orbitofrontal cortex is involved in responding to non-reward as well as expected reward that is based on the neurophysiological and neuroimaging studies described in Chapter 3 and elsewhere (Rolls 2017c, Rolls 2016e, Rolls 2014a, Thorpe et al. 1983, Rolls 2018b). Further, this is in line with the importance of the cortex for holding items in short-term memory in attractor networks (Rolls 2016c), which is what I propose contributes to the rule based non-reward-related functionality of the lateral orbitofrontal cortex, with these short-term memories also useful for probabilistic reward-related learning, and remembering the rewards delivered on the previous trials.

However, the task used in the lesion study (Rudebeck et al. 2017, Murray & Rudebeck 2018) was a probabilistic reward choice task, and the switching between the options took many trials. The hypothesis that I have developed is that the orbitofrontal cortex, and especially its lateral part, is especially important in very rapid reversal, in as little as one trial, which has many advantages in enabling primates including humans to rapidly update their behaviour in for example social situations. It would accordingly be a useful investigation in a future macaque study to analyze which parts of the orbitofrontal cortex if damaged affect this type of very rapid reversal of reward expectations and behaviour.

The lesions in the experiment (Rudebeck et al. 2017, Murray & Rudebeck 2018) on the adjustment of choices to reflect reward probability in the three-armed bandit task (Rudebeck et al. 2017) were termed ventrolateral frontal cortex lesions (VLFC), and included at least parts of area 12 the lateral orbitofrontal cortex (Fig. 1.2) which is implicated in reversal learning (Kringelbach & Rolls 2003, O'Doherty et al. 2001a, Chau et al. 2015, Rolls 2017c, Rolls 2016e, Thorpe et al. 1983), but also appeared to extend considerably round the convexity of the orbitofrontal cortex to include parts of the ventrolateral prefrontal cortex, which in humans would probably include parts of the inferior frontal gyrus.

This highlights an issue with lesion studies: sometimes the choice of the part of the brain to lesion may lead to what appear to be confusing results. For example, at one time it was held that orbitofrontal cortex lesions do not affect reward-related learning and its reversal (Murray & Izquierdo 2007, Rudebeck & Murray 2014), but in some of those studies the lesions were only of the medial orbitofrontal cortex areas such as 13 and 11, and did not include the lateral orbitofrontal cortex area 12. It may be useful in future to guide lesion studies in non-human primates by knowledge of where different types of activated neuron are, and by fMRI, rather than by predetermined ideas of suitable definitions of for example 'the orbitofrontal cortex', when this may not include the lateral orbitofrontal cortex area 12.

For clarification, the areas of the orbitofrontal cortex are shown in Fig. 1.2, and include what is termed medial orbitofrontal cortex in this book, areas 13 and 11; and what is termed lateral orbitofrontal cortex in this book, area 12 (with the latter termed area 12/47 in humans)[8]. This division of the orbitofrontal cortex is supported not only by the architecture and connections of the medial and lateral orbitofrontal cortex described in Chapters 1 and 2, but also by the finding that the automated anatomical atlas (AAL2 (Rolls et al. 2015a)) regions in areas 11 and 13 have high functional connectivity with each other and not with the lateral orbitofrontal area 12, and by the finding that the regions within area 12 have high functional connectivity with each other but not with those in areas 13 and 11 (Rolls, Cheng, Gilson, Qiu, Hu, Ruan, Li, Huang, Yang, Tsai, Zhang, Zhuang, Lin, Deco, Xie & Feng 2018b).

Lesions more laterally, in for example the inferior convexity prefrontal cortex which receives from the inferior temporal visual cortex (Saleem, Miller & Price 2014a), can influence tasks in which objects must be remembered for short periods, e.g. delayed matching to sample and delayed matching to non-sample tasks (Passingham 1975, Mishkin & Manning 1978, Kowalska, Bachevalier & Mishkin 1991), and neurons in this region may help to implement this visual object short-term memory by holding the representation active during the delay period (Rosenkilde et al. 1981, Wilson, O'Sclaidhe & Goldman-Rakic 1993). Whether this inferior convexity area is specifically involved in a short-term object memory is not yet clear (Passingham & Wise 2012). It should be noted that this short-term memory system for objects (which receives inputs from the temporal lobe visual cortical areas in which objects are represented) is different from the short-term memory system in the dorsolateral part of the prefrontal cortex, which is concerned with spatial short-term memories, consistent with its inputs from the parietal cortex (Williams, Rolls, Leonard & Stern 1993, Saleem, Miller & Price 2014b, Deco & Rolls 2003, Deco, Rolls & Horwitz 2004, Deco, Rolls & Romo 2010, Miller 2013, Lundqvist, Herman & Miller 2018). In any case, it is worth noting that the lateral inferior convexity part of the prefrontal cortex could be involved in a function related to the short-term memory for objects. This does not exclude this part of the prefrontal cortex from, in addition, being part of the more orbitofrontal system involved in visual to reinforcer association learning and reversal.

4.2 Humans

4.2.1 Introduction

In Chapter 3 we have considered evidence from neuroimaging on the functions of the human orbitofrontal cortex in emotion and motivation. In this Section we consider complementary evidence from the effects of damage to the human orbitofrontal cortex. In humans, euphoria, irresponsibility, lack of affect, and impulsiveness can follow frontal lobe damage (Kolb & Whishaw 2015, Damasio 1994, Eslinger & Damasio 1985), particularly orbitofrontal cortex damage (Rolls, Hornak, Wade & McGrath 1994a, Hornak, Bramham, Rolls, Morris, O'Doherty, Bullock & Polkey 2003, Berlin, Rolls & Kischka 2004, Berlin, Rolls & Iversen 2005).

It is of interest that a number of the symptoms of frontal lobe damage in humans appear to be related to the functions described in Chapter 3 of representing primary reinforcers,

---

[8]Confusingly, Murray & Rudebeck (2018) refer to the gyrus rectus area 14 (which is closely related to the anterior cingulate cortex (Carmichael & Price 1996)) as 'medial orbitofrontal cortex'; to areas 11 and 13 as 'lateral orbitofrontal cortex'; and area 12 as part of the 'ventrolateral prefrontal cortex'. In another paper (Rudebeck & Murray 2014) they refer to the medial one third of the orbital surface as 'Medial OFC'; to the middle one third as 'Lateral OFC' even though most of it is areas 13 and 11; and leave blank and do not discuss area 12, which is the lateral OFC. Carmichael & Price (1996) did distinguish a medial prefrontal cortex network, which was largely cingulate, from a lateral prefrontal cortex network which was largely orbitofrontal cortex, but that is a different issue to what is medial and what is lateral orbitofrontal cortex. The definitions of medial and lateral orbitofrontal cortex are provided in Section 1.1.2 and Fig. 1.2.

and of altering behaviour when stimulus–reinforcement associations alter, as described next. Thus, humans with frontal lobe damage can show impairments in a number of tasks in which an alteration of behavioural strategy is required in response to a change in environmental reinforcement contingencies (Goodglass & Kaplan 1979, Jouandet & Gazzaniga 1979, Kolb & Whishaw 2015, Zald & Rauch 2006). For example, Milner (1963) showed that in the Wisconsin card sorting task (in which cards are to be sorted according to the colour, shape, or number of items on each card depending on whether the examiner says 'right' or 'wrong' to each placement), frontal patients either had difficulty in determining the first sorting principle, or in shifting to a second principle when required to. Also, in stylus mazes frontal patients have difficulty in changing direction when a sound indicates that the correct path has been left (Milner 1982). It is of interest that, in both types of test, frontal patients may be able to verbalize the correct rules yet may be unable to correct their behavioural sets or strategies appropriately.

Some of the personality changes that can follow frontal lobe damage may be related to a similar type of dysfunction. For example, the euphoria, irresponsibility, lack of affect, and lack of concern for the present or future that can follow frontal lobe damage (see Zald & Rauch (2006) and Section 1.1.1 may also be related to a dysfunction in altering behaviour appropriately in response to a change in reinforcement contingencies. Indeed, in so far as the orbitofrontal cortex is involved in the disconnection of stimulus–reinforcer associations, and such associations are important in learned emotional responses (see above), then it follows that the orbitofrontal cortex is involved in emotional responses by correcting stimulus–reinforcer associations when they become inappropriate (see below). A failure of this process might be reflected in effects such as impulsive behaviour, and a failure to respond appropriately to corrective feedback received from the environment.

4.2.2   Reward valuation, and reversal learning

The hypotheses about the role of the orbitofrontal cortex in the rapid alteration of stimulus–reinforcer associations, and the functions more generally of the orbitofrontal cortex in human behaviour, have been investigated in studies in humans with damage to the ventral parts of the frontal lobe. (The description ventral is given to indicate that there was pathology in the orbitofrontal or related parts of the frontal lobe, and not in the more dorso-lateral parts of the frontal lobe.) A task that was directed at assessing the rapid alteration of stimulus–reinforcer associations was used, because the findings above indicate that the orbitofrontal cortex is involved in this type of learning. This was used instead of the Wisconsin card sorting task, which requires patients to shift from category (or dimension) to category, e.g. from colour to shape. The task used was visual discrimination reversal, in which patients could learn to obtain points by touching one stimulus when it appeared on a video monitor, but had to withhold a response when a different visual stimulus appeared, otherwise a point was lost. After the subjects had acquired the visual discrimination, the reinforcement contingencies unexpectedly reversed. The patients with ventral frontal lesions made more errors in the reversal (or in a similar extinction) task, and completed fewer reversals, than control patients with damage elsewhere in the frontal lobes or in other brain regions (Rolls, Hornak, Wade & McGrath 1994a) (see Fig. 4.1). A reversal deficit in a similar task in patients with ventromedial frontal cortex damage was also reported by Fellows & Farah (2003).

An important aspect of the findings of Rolls, Hornak, Wade & McGrath (1994a) was that the reversal learning impairment correlated highly with the socially inappropriate or disinhibited behaviour of the patients, and also with their subjective evaluation of the changes in their emotional state since the brain damage. The patients were not impaired at other types of memory task, such as paired associate learning. It is of interest that the patients can often

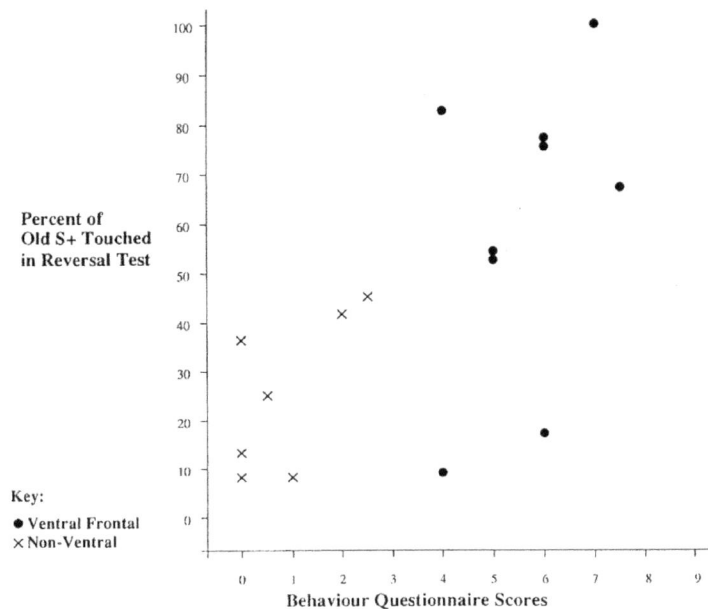

Fig. 4.1 Visual discrimination reversal performance in humans with damage to the ventral part of the frontal lobe. The task was to touch the screen when one image, the S+, was shown in order to obtain a point; and to refrain from touching the screen when a different visual stimulus, the S−, was shown in order to obtain a point. The scattergraph shows that during the reversal the group with ventral damage were more likely to touch the previously rewarded stimulus (Old S+), and that this was related to the score on a Behaviour Questionnaire. Each point represents one patient in the ventral frontal group or in a control group. The Behaviour Questionnaire rating reflected high ratings on at least some of the following: disinhibited or socially inappropriate behaviour; misinterpretation of other people's moods; impulsiveness; unconcern about or underestimation of the seriousness of his condition; and lack of initiative. (Reproduced from Journal of Neurology, Neurosurgery and Psychiatry, 57 (2), pp. 1518–25, Emotion-related learning in patients with social and emotional changes associated with frontal lobe damage, E. T. Rolls, J. Hornak, D. Wade, J. McGrath, ©1994, BMJ Publishing Group Ltd. with permission.)

verbalize the correct response, yet commit the incorrect action. This is consistent with the hypothesis that the orbitofrontal cortex is normally involved in executing behaviour when the behaviour is performed by evaluating the reinforcement associations of environmental stimuli (see below). The orbitofrontal cortex seems to be involved in this in both humans and non-human primates, when the learning must be performed rapidly, in, for example, acquisition, and during reversal.

To seek positive confirmation that effects on stimulus–reinforcer association learning and reversal were related to orbitofrontal cortex damage rather than to any other associated pathology, a new reversal-learning task was used with a group of patients with discrete, surgically produced, lesions of the orbitofrontal cortex. In the new visual discrimination task (the same as that used in our monetary reward functional neuroimaging task, O'Doherty, Kringelbach, Rolls, Hornak & Andrews (2001a)), two stimuli are always present on the video monitor and the patient obtains 'monetary' reward by touching the correct stimulus, and loses 'money' by touching the incorrect stimulus. This design controls for an effect of the lesion in simply increasing the probability that any response will be made (cf. Aron, Fletcher, Bullmore, Sahakian & Robbins (2003) and Clark, Cools & Robbins (2004)). The task also used probabilistic amounts of reward and punishment on each trial, to make it harder to use a verbal strategy with an explicit rule. The task also had the advantage that it was the same as that used in our human functional neuroimaging study that had showed activation of the orbitofrontal cortex by monetary gain or loss (O'Doherty et al. 2001a). It was found that a group of patients with bilateral orbitofrontal cortex lesions were severely impaired at the

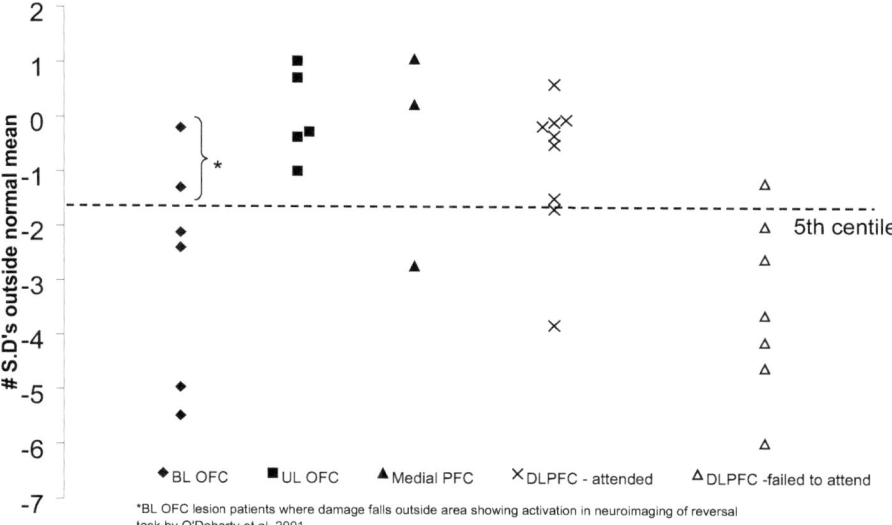

Fig. 4.2 Visual discrimination reversal performance on the probabilistic reversal task in humans with damage to different parts of the ventral part of the frontal lobe. Lesion groups: BL OFC: Bilateral Orbitofrontal cortex; UL OFC: Unilateral Orbitofrontal cortex; Medial PFC: Medial prefrontal cortex; DLPFC: Dorsolateral prefrontal cortex. The patients with bilateral damage to the orbitofrontal cortex performed poorly at the task. Patients with lesions of the dorsolateral prefrontal cortex performed poorly only if they had an attention deficit and failed to pay attention to the part of the display that informed them whether they had won on the current trial of the task. (Attended/Failed to attend: The patient attended/failed to attend to the crucial feedback during the reversal test, namely the amount won or lost on each trial.) (Reproduced from Edmund T. Rolls, J. Hornak, J. O'Doherty, J. Bramham, R. G. Morris, P. R. Bullock, and C. E. Polkey, 'Reward-related Reversal Learning after Surgical Excisions in Orbital-frontal or Dorsolateral Prefrontal Cortex in Humans', Journal of Cognitive Neuroscience, 16:3 (April, 2004), pp. 463–478. © 2004 by the Massachusetts Institute of Technology, published by the MIT Press.)

reversal task, in that they accumulated less money (Hornak, O'Doherty, Bramham, Rolls, Morris, Bullock & Polkey 2004) (see Fig. 4.2). These patients often failed to switch their choice of stimulus after a large loss; and often did switch their choice even though they had just received a reward, and this has been quantified in a more recent study (Berlin, Rolls & Kischka 2004). The investigation showed that the impairment was only obtained with bilateral orbitofrontal cortex damage, in that patients with unilateral orbitofrontal cortex (or medial prefrontal cortex) lesions were not impaired in the reversal task (see Fig. 4.2). The importance of the failure to rapidly learn about the value of stimuli from negative feedback has also been described as a critical difficulty for patients with orbitofrontal cortex lesions (Fellows 2007, Wheeler & Fellows 2008, Fellows 2011), and has been contrasted with the effects of lesions to the anterior cingulate cortex which impair the use of feedback to learn about actions (Fellows 2011, Camille, Tsuchida & Fellows 2011) (see Section 5.1).

As described in Chapter 3, these results are complemented by neuroimaging results with fMRI in normal subjects, which showed that in the same task, activation of the medial orbitofrontal cortex was correlated with how much money was won on single trials, and activation of the lateral orbitofrontal cortex was correlated with how much money was lost on single trials (O'Doherty, Kringelbach, Rolls, Hornak & Andrews 2001a) (Figs. 3.43 and 3.44). Together, these results on the effects of brain damage to the orbitofrontal cortex, and these and other complementary neuroimaging results, provide evidence that at least part of the function of the orbitofrontal cortex in emotion, social behaviour, and decision-making is related to representing reinforcers, detecting changes in the reinforcers being received, using these changes to rapidly reset stimulus–reinforcer associations, and rapidly changing behaviour as a result.

Bechara and colleagues also have findings that are consistent with those described above in patients with frontal lobe damage when they perform a gambling task (Bechara et al. 1994, Bechara et al. 1996, Bechara et al. 1997, Damasio 1994, Bechara et al. 2005, Glascher, Adolphs, Damasio, Bechara, Rudrauf, Calamia, Paul & Tranel 2012). In the Iowa gambling task subjects were asked to select cards from four decks of cards and maximize their winnings. During the task electrodermal activity (Skin Conductance Responses, SCR) of the subject was measured as an index of somatic activation. After each selection of a card, facsimile money is lost or won. Two of the four decks produce large payouts with larger penalties (and can thus be considered high-risk), while the other two decks produce small payouts but smaller penalties (low-risk). The most profitable strategy is therefore to consistently select cards from the two low-risk decks, which is the strategy adopted by normal control subjects. Patients with damage to the ventromedial part of the orbitofrontal cortex, but not the dorsolateral prefrontal cortex, would persistently draw cards from the high-risk packs, and lack anticipatory SCRs while they pondered risky choices. The task was designed to mimic aspects of real-life decision-making that patients with orbitofrontal cortex lesions find difficult. Such decisions typically involve choices between actions associated with differing magnitudes of reward and punishment where the underlying contingencies relating actions to relevant outcomes remain hidden.

Bechara et al. (1998) have reported a dissociation between subjects with different frontal lobe lesions. All subjects with orbitofrontal cortex lesions were impaired on the gambling task, while only those with the most anteriorly placed lesions were normal on working memory tasks. Other subjects with right dorsolateral/high mesial lesions were impaired on working memory tasks but not on the gambling task. Bechara, Damasio, Damasio & Lee (1999) went on to compare subjects with bilateral amygdala but not orbitofrontal cortex lesions, and subjects with orbitofrontal cortex but not amygdala lesions, and found that all subjects were impaired in the gambling task and all failed to develop anticipatory SCRs. However, while subjects with orbitofrontal cortex lesions still, in general, produced SCRs when receiving a monetary reward or punishment, the subjects with bilateral amygdala lesions failed to do so. Fellows & Farah (2005) found that patients with ventromedial prefrontal or with dorsolateral frontal lobe damage were impaired on the Iowa gambling task, yet only the ventromedial frontal damage group had a reversal deficit. (This reversal deficit can be produced in patients with small bilateral lesions of the orbitofrontal cortex, as shown by Hornak, O'Doherty, Bramham, Rolls, Morris, Bullock & Polkey (2004).) Moreover the deficit on the gambling task of the ventromedial prefrontal patients was related to the fact that in the Iowa gambling task the first few choices of a high-risk deck are rewarded, and that later, when a large loss is received from a high-risk deck, an implicit reversal is required. Thus the deficit of patients with orbitofrontal cortex / ventromedial prefrontal cortex damage in the task may be related at least in part to their failure to perform stimulus–reinforcer association reversal learning, rather than for other reasons.

In relation to real-world gambling, impulsive choice measured with a delay-discounting task (and reflecting aversion for a delayed reward) was found in problem gamblers, but impulsive action (measured with the stop-signal task, which requires withholding of a motor response), was especially impaired in pathological gambling (Brevers, Cleeremans, Verbruggen, Bechara, Kornreich, Verbanck & Noel 2012).

Credit assignment, as indexed by the normal influence of contingent relationships between choice and reward, is reduced in patients with lateral orbitofrontal cortex damage (Noonan, Chau, Rushworth & Fellows 2017). The impairment may reflect insufficient sensitivity to non-reward, consistent with the functions of the lateral orbitofrontal cortex in non-reward described in Chapter 3.

By contrast, patients with ventromedial prefrontal cortex damage made more stochastic choices than Controls when the decision was framed by valuable distracting alternatives, suggesting that choices were no longer independent of irrelevant options (Noonan et al. 2017). This is consistent with the identification of an area in the human ventral medial prefrontal cortex area 10 or 'ventromedial prefrontal cortex' (VMPFC) that is implicated in neuroimaging studies in the mechanisms of choice decision-making between rewards (Rolls et al. 2010b, Rolls et al. 2010c), described in Section 3.13. Also consistent with the neurophysiology and neuroimaging described in Chapter 3, patients with focal damage to the ventromedial prefrontal cortex showed deficits in goal-directed choice by persistently selecting actions for a food outcome that had been devalued through selective satiation (Reber, Feinstein, O'Doherty, Liljeholm, Adolphs & Tranel 2017).

Overall, a picture is beginning to emerge of how the neurophysiology and functional neuroimaging described in Chapter 3 about reward value and reward-related learning and choice are complemented by findings of the effects of lesions to the ventromedial prefrontal cortex which affect choice, vs lateral orbitofrontal cortex damage that affects behaviour to non-rewarded stimuli in humans, as well as in macaques (Section 4.1). The framework remains that the main part of the orbitofrontal cortex, areas 13 and 11, represent the reward value of stimuli; that the lateral orbitofrontal cortex, area BA 12, is involved in the effects of non-reward and punishment; and that the ventromedial prefrontal cortex, (VMPFC / the ventral part of medial area 10) is involved in choice decision-making between stimuli with different reward value. Next, evidence is described about the importance of the human orbitofrontal cortex in the subjective experiences related to emotion, and more generally in emotion.

4.2.3 Social behaviour, subjective emotional change, and personality

It is of interest that the patients with bilateral orbitofrontal cortex damage who were impaired at the visual discrimination reversal task had high scores on parts of a Social Behaviour Questionnaire in which the patients were rated on behaviours such as emotion recognition in others (e.g. their sad, angry, or disgusted mood); in interpersonal relationships (such as not caring what others think, and not being close to the family); emotional empathy (e.g. when others are happy, is not happy for them); interpersonal relationships (e.g. does not care what others think, and is not close to his family); public behaviour (is uncooperative); antisocial behaviour (is critical of and impatient with others); impulsivity (does things without thinking); and sociability (is not sociable, and has difficulty making or maintaining close relationships) (Hornak, Bramham, Rolls, Morris, O'Doherty, Bullock & Polkey 2003), all of which could reflect less behavioural sensitivity to different types of punishment and reward. Further, in a Subjective Emotional Change Questionnaire in which the patients reported on any changes in the intensity and/or frequency of their own experience of emotions, the bilateral orbitofrontal cortex surgical lesion patients with deficits in the visual discrimination reversal task reported a number of changes, including changes in sadness, anger, fear and happiness (Hornak et al. 2003).

There are likely to be individual differences in all the emotion systems in the brain, and these are likely to be important in personality (Rolls 2014a). For example, and in the context that the lateral orbitofrontal cortex is activated by many non-rewarding and punishing stimuli (Fig. 3.54), the lateral orbitofrontal cortex is recruited more in individuals with problems with 'stop inhibition', that is, in tasks in which a NoGo response must be made occasionally (Somerville, Hare & Casey 2011). Impulsiveness may be related to a relative insensitivity of this system, and not only is the orbitofrontal cortex implicated in this, but one of its output regions, the ventral striatum, is activated more strongly by incentive stimuli (of which examples might be the sight of cookies or of drugs) in people with impulsive/antisocial personalities (Buckholtz, Treadway, Cowan, Woodward, Benning, Li, Ansari, Baldwin, Schwartzman,

Shelby, Smith, Cole, Kessler & Zald 2010). Of great interest, in people who are not impulsive and who control their behaviour with the rational system, activations related to signals from the dorsolateral prefrontal cortex, involved in planning, are stronger in the head of the caudate (Buckholtz et al. 2010). An implication is that within the basal ganglia, competition between the emotional system (activating the ventral striatum) and the rational system (activating the head of the caudate) may be one way in which selection of behavioural output between the rational vs the emotional system may be made (see Sections 6.4 and 5.3). There are also interesting age-related differences in the sensitivity of these reward and punishment systems. For example, adolescents show increased responsiveness to social cues and monetary rewards than younger people or adults (Somerville et al. 2011).

An idea of how such stimulus–reinforcer learning may play an important role in normal human behaviour, and may be related to the behavioural changes seen clinically in the patients of Rolls, Hornak, Wade & McGrath (1994a) with ventral frontal lobe damage, can be provided by summarizing the behavioural ratings given by the carers of these patients (Rolls et al. 1994a). The patients were rated high on at least some of the following: disinhibition or socially inappropriate behaviour; violence, verbal abusiveness; lack of initiative; misinterpretation of other people's behaviour; anger or irritability; and lack of concern for their own condition. Such behavioural changes correlated with the stimulus–reinforcer reversal and extinction learning impairment (Rolls et al. 1994a). The suggestion thus is that the insensitivity to reinforcement changes in the learning task may be at least part of what produces the changes in behaviour found in these patients with ventral frontal lobe damage.

The more general impact on the behaviour of these patients is that their irresponsibility tended to affect their everyday lives. For example, if such patients had received their brain damage in a road traffic accident, and compensation had been awarded, the patients often tended to spend their money without appropriate concern for the future, sometimes, for example, buying a very expensive car (Rolls et al. 1994a). Such patients often find it difficult to invest in relationships too, and are sometimes described by their family as having changed personalities, in that they care less about a wide range of factors than before the brain damage. The suggestion that follows from this is that the orbitofrontal cortex may normally be involved in much social behaviour, and the ability to respond rapidly and appropriately to social reinforcers is, of course, an important aspect of primate social behaviour. When Goleman (1995) writes about emotional intelligence, the functions being performed may be those that we are now discussing, and also those concerned with face-expression decoding that are described in Section 4.2.4.

Most known cases of human orbitofrontal damage have occurred in adulthood, but two cases of damage acquired in early life were reported by Anderson, Bechara, Damasio, Tranel & Damasio (1999). The two patients showed lifelong behavioural problems, which were resistant to corrective influences. But more importantly, the patients appeared completely to lack knowledge about moral and societal conventions. Interestingly, other patients with late acquired orbitofrontal lesions have retained knowledge of such matters, even if they do not always act in accordance with this explicit knowledge. The lack of this moral knowledge and subsequent reckless behaviour in the two patients with early life damage to the orbitofrontal cortex is consistent with the hypothesis that the orbitofrontal cortex is crucial for stimulus–reinforcer association learning (Rolls 1990a, Rolls 2014a, Rolls 2012b). An implication is that, at least in part because of its importance in utilizing feedback to correct value representations, the orbitofrontal cortex becomes important in moral behaviour (Mendez 2009).

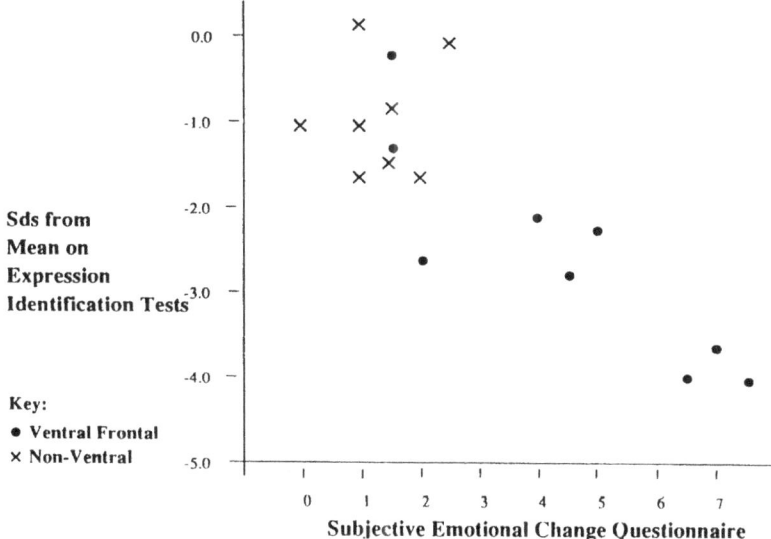

Fig. 4.3 Face expression identification deficit in humans with damage to the ventral part of the frontal lobe, and its relation to the patient's own rating of Subjective Emotional Change since the brain damage, based on sadness (or regret), anger (or frustration), fear (or anxiety), disgust, and excitement or enjoyment. (Reprinted from Neuropsychologia, 34 (4), J. Hornak, E.T. Rolls, and D. Wade, Face and voice expression identification in patients with emotional and behavioural changes following ventral frontal lobe damage, pp. 247–61, Copyright, 1996, with permission from Elsevier.)

4.2.4 Face and voice expression identification

To investigate the possible significance of face-related inputs to orbitofrontal visual neurons described in Chapter 3, we also tested the responses of these patients to faces. We included tests of face (and also voice) expression decoding, because these are ways in which the reinforcing quality of individuals is often indicated. Impairments in the identification of facial and vocal emotional expression were demonstrated in a group of patients with ventral frontal lobe damage who had socially inappropriate behaviour (Hornak, Rolls & Wade 1996, Rolls 1999b) (see Fig. 4.3). The expression identification impairments could occur independently of perceptual impairments in facial recognition, voice discrimination, or environmental sound recognition. The face and voice expression problems did not necessarily occur together in the same patients, providing an indication of separate processing. Poor performance on both expression tests was correlated with the degree of alteration of emotional experience reported by the patients. There was also a strong positive correlation between the degree of altered emotional experience and the severity of the behavioural problems (e.g. disinhibition) found in these patients. A comparison group of patients with brain damage outside the ventral frontal lobe region, without these behavioural problems, was unimpaired on the face expression identification test, was significantly less impaired at vocal expression identification, and reported little subjective emotional change (Hornak et al. 1996, Rolls 1999b). Consistent with these findings, face emotion recognition was impaired following ventromedial, but not dorsal or lateral, prefrontal cortex damage (Heberlein, Padon, Gillihan, Farah & Fellows 2008).

These findings have been extended, and it has been found that patients with face expression decoding problems do not necessarily have impairments at visual discrimination reversal, and vice versa (Hornak, Bramham, Rolls, Morris, O'Doherty, Bullock & Polkey 2003, Hornak, O'Doherty, Bramham, Rolls, Morris, Bullock & Polkey 2004). This is consistent with some topography in the orbitofrontal cortex (see Section 3.11).

To obtain clear evidence that the changes in face and voice expression identification, emotional behaviour, and subjective emotional state were related to orbitofrontal cortex damage itself, and not to damage to surrounding areas which is present in many closed head injury patients, we performed these assessments in patients with circumscribed lesions made surgically in the course of treatment (Hornak, Bramham, Rolls, Morris, O'Doherty, Bullock & Polkey 2003). This study also enabled us to determine whether there was functional specialization within the orbitofrontal cortex, and whether damage to nearby and connected areas (such as the anterior cingulate cortex) in which some of the patients had lesions could produce similar effects. We found that some patients with bilateral lesions of the orbitofrontal cortex had deficits in voice and face expression identification, and the group had impairments in social behaviour, and significant changes in their subjective emotional state (Hornak et al. 2003). The same group of patients had deficits on the probabilistic monetary reward task (Hornak et al. 2004). Some patients with unilateral damage restricted to the orbitofrontal cortex also had deficits in voice expression identification, and the group did not have significant changes in social behaviour, or in their subjective emotional state. Patients with unilateral lesions of the antero-ventral part of the anterior cingulate cortex and/or medial prefrontal cortex area BA9 were in some cases impaired on voice and face expression identification, had some change in social behaviour, and had significant changes in their subjective emotional state. Patients with dorsolateral prefrontal cortex lesions or with medial lesions outside the anterior cingulate cortex and medial prefrontal BA9 areas were unimpaired on any of these measures of emotion. In all cases in which voice expression identification was impaired, there were no deficits in control tests of the discrimination of unfamiliar voices and the recognition of environmental sounds.

These results (Hornak, Bramham, Rolls, Morris, O'Doherty, Bullock & Polkey 2003) thus confirm that damage restricted to the orbitofrontal cortex can produce impairments in face and voice expression identification, which may be primary reinforcers. The system is sensitive, in that even patients with unilateral orbitofrontal cortex lesions may be impaired. The impairment is not a generic impairment of the ability to recognize any emotions in others, in that frequently voice but not face expression identification was impaired, and vice versa. This implies some functional specialization for visual vs auditory emotion-related processing in the human orbitofrontal cortex. The results also show that the changes in social behaviour can be produced by damage restricted to the orbitofrontal cortex, in that the effects were related to the sites of the surgically produced lesions. The patients were particularly likely to be impaired on emotion recognition (they were less likely to notice when others were sad, or happy, or disgusted); on emotional empathy (they were less likely to comfort those who are sad, or afraid, or to feel happy for others who are happy); on interpersonal relationships (not caring what others think, and not being close to his/her family); and were less likely to cooperate with others; were impatient and impulsive; and had difficulty in making and keeping close relationships. The results also show that changes in subjective emotional state (including frequently sadness, anger and happiness) can be produced by damage restricted to the orbitofrontal cortex (Hornak et al. 2003). In addition, the patients with bilateral orbitofrontal cortex lesions were impaired on the probabilistic reversal learning task (Hornak et al. 2004). The findings overall thus make clear the types of deficit found in humans with orbitofrontal cortex damage, and can be easily related to underlying fundamental processes in which the orbitofrontal cortex is involved, including decoding and representing primary reinforcers, being sensitive to changes in reinforcers, and rapidly readjusting behaviour to stimuli when the reinforcers available change.

The results (Hornak et al. 2003) also extend these investigations to the anterior cingulate cortex (including some of medial prefrontal cortex area BA9) by showing that lesions in these regions can produce voice and/or face expression identification deficits, and marked changes in subjective emotional state (see Chapter 5.1).

Deficits in face expression identification following orbitofrontal cortex lesions have been confirmed (Tsuchida & Fellows 2012), with ventromedial prefrontal cortex lesions associated with an impairment in distinguishing emotional from neutral face expressions, and left ventrolateral prefrontal cortex lesions associated with an impairment in discriminating between different face expressions.

4.2.5 Orbitofrontal cortex lesions and impulsiveness: some similarities with Borderline Personality Disorder

It has also been possible to relate the functions of the orbitofrontal cortex to some psychiatric symptoms. Berlin, Rolls & Kischka (2004), Berlin & Rolls (2004) and Berlin, Rolls & Iversen (2005) compared the symptoms of patients with a personality disorder syndrome, Borderline Personality Disorder (BPD), with those of patients with lesions of the orbitofrontal cortex. The symptoms of the self-harming Borderline Personality Disorder patients include high impulsivity, affective instability, and emotionality; and low extraversion. It was found that orbitofrontal cortex and Borderline Personality Disorder patients performed similarly in that they were more impulsive, reported more inappropriate behaviours in the Frontal Behaviour Questionnaire, and had more Borderline Personality Disorder characteristics, and anger, and less happiness, than control groups (either normals, or patients with lesions outside the orbitofrontal cortex).

One of the measures of impulsiveness was the Matching Familiar Figures Test. In this standard cognitive behavioural measure of impulsivity, created by Kagan (1966), a participant selects (points to), from a set of highly similar pictures, the one that is exactly the same as the standard reference picture. High impulsiveness is reflected in short latencies to make a choice (which are typically 55 s in control subjects), and errors in the choices made. The other measure of impulsiveness was the Barratt Impulsiveness Scale (Patton, Stanford & Barratt 1995) which is a 30-item questionnaire that assesses non-planning impulsivity (attention to details), motor impulsivity (acting without thinking), and cognitive impulsivity (future oriented thinking and coping stability). Both the orbitofrontal and BPD groups were impaired at both measures of impulsiveness.

Both the orbitofrontal and BPD groups also had a faster perception of time (i.e. they underproduced time) than normal controls. This may be one factor underlying their increased impulsiveness, in that they feel that sufficient time has elapsed to initiate action.

It was of considerable interest that the BPD group, as well as the orbitofrontal group, scored highly on the Frontal Behaviour Questionnaire which assessed inappropriate behaviours typical of orbitofrontal cortex patients including disinhibition, social inappropriateness, perseveration, and uncooperativeness. Both groups were also less open to experience (i.e. less open-minded), a personality characteristic.

The orbitofrontal and BPD patients performed differently on other tasks: BPD patients were less extraverted and conscientious, and more neurotic and emotional, than all other groups. Patients with orbitofrontal cortex lesions had more severe deficits in reversing stimulus–reinforcer associations compared to all other groups and had a faster perception of time (overestimated time) than normal controls. These deficits were not related to spatial working memory functions which are impaired by dorsolateral prefrontal cortex damage.

Thus some but not other symptoms of self-harming Borderline Personality Disorder patients are similar to those of patients with orbitofrontal cortex damage. The symptoms the groups have in common include impulsiveness and the inappropriate behaviours typical of 'frontal' patients. This could imply that in BPD patients some aspects of the operation of the orbitofrontal cortex are occurring differently to the way they operate in normal control subjects. Part of the interest of this is that it may help to point towards new concepts that may be useful in the treatment of some of the symptoms of patients with Borderline Personality Disorder. On the other hand, other aspects of Borderline Personality Disorder do not appear to be related to orbitofrontal cortex functions, including the more neurotic and more emotional personality characteristics of the BPD group together with their lower extraversion and conscientious (Berlin, Rolls & Kischka 2004, Berlin & Rolls 2004, Berlin, Rolls & Iversen 2005).

There are many types of impulsiveness (Dalley & Robbins 2017), and some such as performance in the stop-signal task, which measures a type of motor impulsiveness, are associated with damage to the right inferior frontal gyrus (Aron, Robbins & Poldrack 2014). In the stop-signal task, the lateral orbitofrontal cortex and the adjoining inferior frontal gyrus are both activated (Deng, Rolls, Ji, Robbins, Banaschewski, Bokde, Bromberg, Buechel, Desrivieres, Conrod, Flor, Frouin, Gallinat, Garavan, Gowland, Heinz, Ittermann, Martinot, Lemaitre, Nees, Papadopoulos Orfanos, Poustka, Smolka, Walter, Whelan, Schumann, Feng & the Imagen consortium 2017). More generally, we have argued that one mechanism promoting impulsiveness may be under-connectedness of the lateral orbitofrontal cortex non-reward system, and another is over-connectedness of the medial orbitofrontal cortex reward system (Cheng, Rolls, Robbins, Gong, Liu, Lv, Du, Wen, Ma, Quinlan, Garavan, Artiges, Papadopoulos Orfanos, Smolka, Schumann, Kendrick & Feng 2019).

4.2.6 Frontotemporal dementia

Another case in which it is possible to relate psychiatric types of symptom to orbitofrontal cortex function is frontotemporal dementia, which is a progressive neurodegenerative disorder attacking the frontal lobes and producing major and pervasive behavioural changes in personality and social conduct resembling those produced by orbitofrontal lesions (Rahman, Sahakian, Hodges, Rogers & Robbins 1999, Hodges & Piguet 2018). Patients appear either socially disinhibited with facetiousness and inappropriate jocularity, or apathetic and withdrawn. Many patients show mental rigidity and inability to appreciate irony or other subtle aspects of language. They tend to engage in ritualistic and stereotypical behaviour, and their planning skills are invariably impaired. The dementia is accompanied by gradual withdrawal from all social interactions. Memory is usually intact but patients have difficulties with working memory and concentration. Interestingly, given the anatomy and physiology of the orbitofrontal cortex, frontotemporal dementia causes profound changes in eating habits, with escalating desire for sweet food coupled with reduced satiety, which is often followed by enormous weight gain (Piguet 2011, Hodges & Piguet 2018).

5 Orbitofrontal cortex output pathways: cingulate cortex, basal ganglia, and dopamine

The orbitofrontal cortex is involved in representing the value of stimuli. It is in a sense an output region for all the sensory systems, including taste, olfaction, visual, auditory, and somatosensory, that represent 'what' a stimulus is, and uses that information to build representations that are frequently multimodal but are in value space rather than 'what' or stimulus identity space. Orbitofrontal cortex neurons focus on value representations for stimuli, and know little about actions or behavioural responses. In this Chapter I consider the outputs of the orbitofrontal cortex to two important systems, the cingulate cortex, and basal ganglia (Section 5.3). The dopamine systems in the brain, which project strongly to the basal ganglia as well as to some cortical areas, are also considered in this Chapter, because they can be considered as output systems of the orbitofrontal cortex, as will be described in Section 5.2 (see Fig. 2.5). Other output systems for the orbitofrontal cortex include the anterior insula for autonomic responses (Critchley & Harrison 2013, Al Omran & Aziz 2014, Rolls 2016b, Quadt et al. 2018), and the inferior frontal gyrus (Rolls, Cheng, Du, Wei, Qiu, Dai, Zhou, Xie & Feng 2019a) (Section 7.4.2).

5.1 The cingulate cortex

5.1.1 Introduction to and overview of the cingulate cortex

The anterior cingulate cortex receives inputs from the orbitofrontal cortex about the value of stimuli, that is about goals including the value of outcomes (the reward received) and the expected value. The anterior cingulate cortex in combination with the mid-cingulate motor area, which contains representations of actions, interfaces actions to outcomes (rewards or punishers received) using action–outcome learning, and also takes into account the cost of actions to obtain the goal when selecting actions. The anterior and mid-cingulate cortical areas are thus relevant to emotion, for they implement the instrumental goal-directed actions that the instrumental reinforcers involved in emotion produce (Rolls 2014a, Rolls 2019d, Rolls 2019a). In the context of its representations of value, damage to the anterior cingulate areas does influence emotion.

The anterior cingulate cortex operates as a system that is aiming to obtain goals, and is taking into account the outcomes received after actions, in that it is sensitive to devaluation of the goal, and will not select an action if the goal has been devalued. This is in contrast to the basal ganglia, which implement a stimulus–motor response mapping which becomes automated as a habit after much learning, and is not sensitive to devaluation of the goal (Rolls 2014a, Rolls 2016c, Rolls 2018b).

The posterior cingulate cortex has different functions, for it is not activated in the same way as the anterior cingulate cortex by rewards and punishers, and is involved in spatio-topographical and related memory functions with its connections to parietal structures such

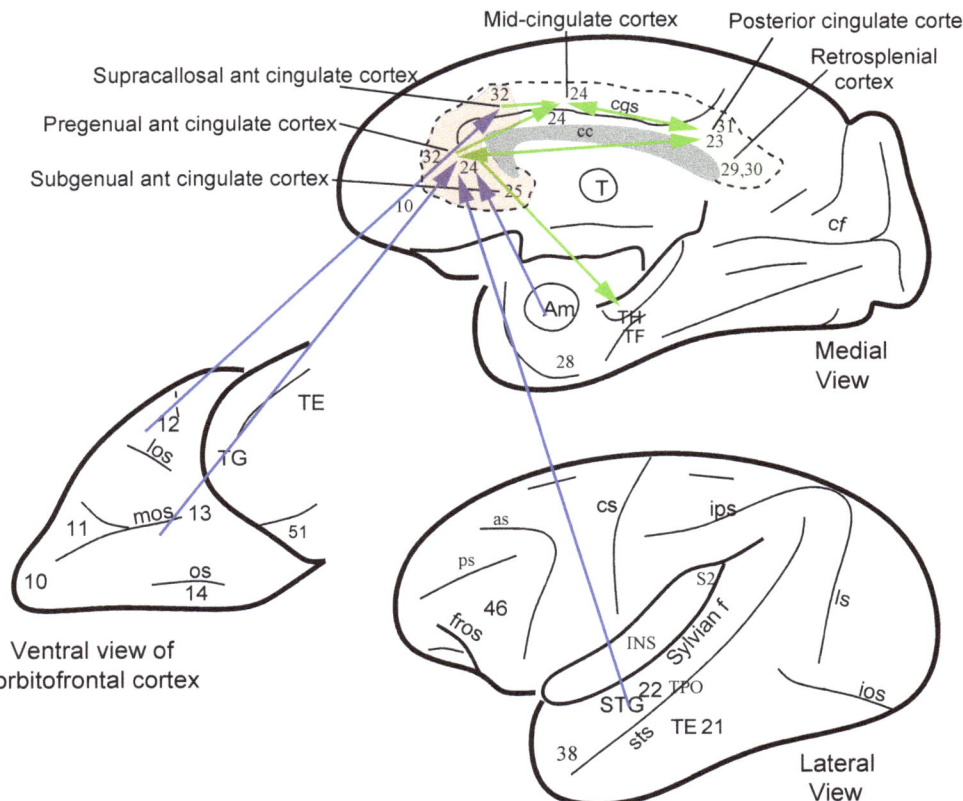

Fig. 5.1 Connections of the anterior cingulate cortex shown on views of the primate brain (see text). The anterior cingulate cortex (including the subgenual cingulate cortex area 25) is shaded in red, the posterior cingulate cortex (areas 23 and 31) and retrosplenial cortex (areas 29 and 30) in green, and the corpus callosum (cc) in grey. The arrows show the main direction of connectivity, but there are connections in both directions. Connections reach the pregenual cingulate cortex especially from the medial/mid-orbitofrontal cortex; and reach the supracallosal anterior cingulate cortex especially from the lateral orbitofrontal cortex and inferior frontal gyrus. Connections to the anterior cingulate cortex from the temporal lobe are from the (auditory) superior temporal gyrus (STG), from the visual and auditory cortex in the superior temporal sulcus; and from the amygdala. Abbreviations: as, arcuate sulcus; cf, calcarine fissure; cgs, cingulate sulcus; cs, central sulcus; ls, lunate sulcus; ios, inferior occipital sulcus; mos, medial orbital sulcus; os, orbital sulcus; ps, principal sulcus; sts, superior temporal sulcus; Sf, Sylvian (or lateral) fissure (which has been opened to reveal the insula); Am, amygdala; INS, insula; TE (21), inferior temporal visual cortex; STG (22), superior temporal gyrus auditory association cortex; TF and TH, parahippocampal cortex; TPO, multimodal cortical area in the superior temporal sulcus; 28, entorhinal cortex; 38, TG, temporal pole cortex; 13, 11, medial orbitofrontal cortex; 12, lateral orbitofrontal cortex; 10, ventral prefrontal cortex; 14, gyrus rectus; 51, olfactory (prepyriform and periamygdaloid) cortex.

as the precuneus and with the hippocampus that are involved in these functions (Vogt 2009, Cavanna & Trimble 2006, Rolls 2015d, Rolls 2018a, Rolls & Wirth 2018, Rolls 2019d, Rolls 2019a). However, the posterior cingulate cortex does have connectivity with the orbitofrontal cortex. Moreover, the functional connectivity between the lateral orbitofrontal cortex and the posterior cingulate cortex is increased in depression, and this may contribute to the increased negative rumination in depression (Cheng, Rolls, Qiu, Xie, Wei, Huang, Yang, Tsai, Li, Meng, Lin, Xie & Feng 2018b) (see Section 7.4.4). The relation of the posterior cingulate cortex to the orbitofrontal cortex is considered in Section 5.1.10.

5.1.2 Anterior cingulate cortex anatomy and connections

The anterior cingulate areas occupy approximately the anterior one third of the cingulate cortex (see Fig. 5.1) and are involved in emotion. They may be distinguished from a mid-cingulate area (i.e. further back than the anterior cingulate region and occupying approximately the middle third of the cingulate cortex) which has been termed the cingulate motor area (Vogt, Derbyshire & Jones 1996, Vogt 2009, Vogt 2016, Vogt 2019) and may be involved in action selection (Rushworth, Walton, Kennerley & Bannerman 2004, Rushworth et al. 2011). The anterior cingulate cortex includes parts of area 32 and 24, and comprises the pregenual cingulate cortex, the supracallosal anterior cingulate cortex, and area 25 the subgenual cingulate cortex (Figs. 5.1, 1.2 and 1.3) (Price 2006, Ongur, Ferry & Price 2003, Ongur & Price 2000, Carmichael & Price 1996, Vogt 2009, Vogt 2019). (The midcingulate cortex has been described as having an anterior and a posterior part, with the criteria including cytoarchitecture (Vogt 2016, Vogt 2019).)

As shown in Figs. 5.1 and 5.3, the anterior cingulate cortex receives strong inputs from the orbitofrontal cortex, and is also characterised by connections with the amygdala (Carmichael & Price 1995a, Morecraft & Tanji 2009, Vogt 2009). The anterior cingulate cortex also has connections with some temporal cortical areas involved in memory including the parahippocampal gyrus (which provides via the entorhinal cortex a bridge to the hippocampus); and with the rostral superior temporal gyrus, the auditory superior temporal gyrus, and the dorsal bank of the superior temporal sulcus (Saleem et al. 2008, Vogt 2009) (see Fig. 5.1). (The cortex in the superior temporal sulcus contains visual neurons that respond to face expression, gesture, and head movement (Hasselmo, Rolls & Baylis 1989a, Hasselmo, Rolls, Baylis & Nalwa 1989b).

In more detail, a 'medial prefrontal network' (mainly anterior cingulate cortex) selectively involves medial areas 14r, 14c, 24, 25, 32, and 10m, rostral orbital areas 10o and 11m, and agranular insular area Iai in the posterior orbital cortex in macaques (Carmichael & Price 1996). An 'orbital' prefrontal network links most of the areas within the orbital cortex, including areas Iam, Iapm, Ial, 12l, 12m, and 12r in the caudal and lateral parts of the orbital cortex, with areas 13l, 13m, and 13b in the central orbital cortex, which have further onward connections to the rostral orbital area 11l (Carmichael & Price 1996, Ongur & Price 2000, Price 2006). Several orbital areas (including 13a, 12o and 11m) have connections with both the medial and orbital networks. Many of these areas are shown in Figs. 5.1 and 1.2. It is very interesting that this medial prefrontal network (anterior cingulate cortex) has connections with the posterior cingulate / retrosplenial cortex, and parahippocampal cortex (Saleem et al. 2008), and has access to the hippocampus in this way; whereas the orbitofrontal cortex has projections to the perirhinal cortex (Saleem et al. 2008), and thus has access to the hippocampus via a more ventral route (Fig. 5.3).

A very interesting finding in relation to what follows is that the medial orbitofrontal cortex has strong functional connectivity with the pregenual cingulate cortex, in both of which rewards are represented; and that the lateral orbitofrontal cortex (and inferior frontal gyrus) has strong functional connectivity with the supracallosal, more dorsal, anterior cingulate cortex area, both of which are activated by unpleasant aversive stimuli (Rolls, Cheng, Gong, Qiu, Zhou, Zhang, Lv, Ruan, Wei, Cheng, Meng, Xie & Feng 2018c). This was shown in a resting state fMRI investigation with 254 healthy participants (Rolls et al. 2018c). Parcellation was performed based on the functional connectivity of individual anterior cingulate cortex voxels in the controls (Fig. 5.2). A pregenual and subcallosal subdivision (1, green) has strong functional connectivity with the medial orbitofrontal cortex and connected areas (Fig. 5.2), which are implicated in reward (Fig. 3.54 on page 88). The supracallosal subdivision (2, red), which is activated by unpleasant stimuli and non-reward, has strong functional connectivity with the lateral orbitofrontal cortex and adjacent inferior frontal gyrus areas (Fig. 5.2), also activated by unpleasant stimuli (Fig. 3.54) (Rolls et al. 2018c). These functional connectivities provide support for the hypothesis that the reward-related medial orbitofrontal cortex provides inputs to the pregenual cingulate cortex, also activated by rewards; and that the lateral orbitofrontal cortex, implicated in effects of non-reward and punishers, provides inputs to the supracallosal

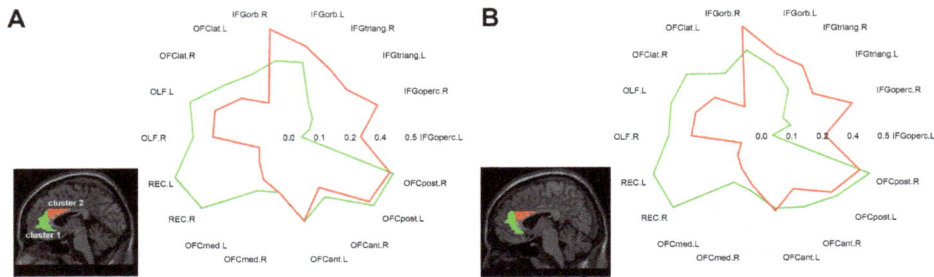

Fig. 5.2 Voxel-level parcellation of the Anterior Cingulate Cortex (ACC) based on its functional connectivity in healthy controls with other brain areas. Cluster 1 (green) is pregenual and subcallosal. Cluster 2 (red) is supracallosal. The circular plot shows the correlations of the voxels in each subdivision of the ACC with the significantly different voxels in orbitofrontal cortex automated anatomical atlas (AAL2, Rolls et al 2015)) areas. The correlations are indicated as the distance from the centre of the circular plot, with the r value for the correlation as shown. The pregenual and subcallosal subdivision (1, green) has strong functional connectivity with the medial orbitofrontal cortex and connected areas (AAL2 areas from OLF to OFCpost). The supracallosal subdivision (2, red) has strong functional connectivity with the lateral orbitofrontal cortex area IFGorb and with adjacent inferior frontal gyrus areas (IFGtriang to IFGoperc). A is left and B is right. (Adapted from Cerebral Cortex, Functional Connectivity of the Anterior Cingulate Cortex in Depression and in Health, Edmund T Rolls, Wei Cheng, Weikang Gong, Jiang Qiu, Chanjuan Zhou, Jie Zhang, Wujun Lv, Hongtao Ruan, Dongtao Wei, Ke Cheng, Jie Meng, Peng Xie, and Jianfeng Feng, pp. 652–663, Figure 5a and b, doi.org/10.1093/cercor/bhy236, Copyright © The Authors 2018.)

part of the anterior cingulate cortex, also activated by unpleasant stimuli (Rolls et al. 2018c).

The outputs of the anterior cingulate cortex reach further back in the cingulate cortex towards the mid-cingulate cortex, which includes the cingulate motor area (Vogt et al. 1996, Morecraft & Tanji 2009, Vogt 2009, Vogt 2016). The anterior cingulate cortex also projects forwards to medial prefrontal cortex area 10 (Price 2006, Ongur & Price 2000), and to temporal lobe areas including the parahippocampal gyrus, perirhinal cortex, and entorhinal cortex (Vogt 2009).

Another route for output is via the projections to the striatum / basal ganglia system.

The anterior cingulate cortex, including the subgenual cingulate cortex area 25, also has outputs that can influence autonomic/visceral function via the hypothalamus, midbrain periaqueductal gray, and insula, as does the orbitofrontal cortex (Rempel-Clower & Barbas 1998, Price 2006, Ongur & Price 2000, Critchley & Harrison 2013).

5.1.3 Anterior cingulate cortex functional neuroimaging and neuronal activity

5.1.4 A framework

The pregenual and the adjoining dorsal anterior cingulate areas can be conceptualized as a relay that allows information about expected rewards and outcomes, received from the orbitofrontal cortex, to be linked, via longitudinal connections running in the cingulum fibre bundle, to information about actions represented in the mid-cingulate cortex. The mid-cingulate cortex receives inputs about actions from the posterior cingulate cortex, which receives this information from the parietal cortex (Rolls 2019d, Rolls 2019a). The learning of action-outcome associations in the cingulate cortex enables the correct actions to be selected in future. The connections that provide for this are shown in Fig. 5.3.

Bringing together information about specific rewards with information about actions, and the costs associated with actions, is important for associating actions with the value of their outcomes and for selecting the correct action that will lead to a desired reward (Walton, Bannerman, Alterescu & Rushworth 2003, Rushworth, Buckley, Behrens, Walton & Bannerman 2007, Rolls 2009c, Rushworth, Noonan, Boorman, Walton & Behrens 2011, Grabenhorst & Rolls 2011, Rolls 2014a, Kolling, Wittmann, Behrens, Boorman, Mars &

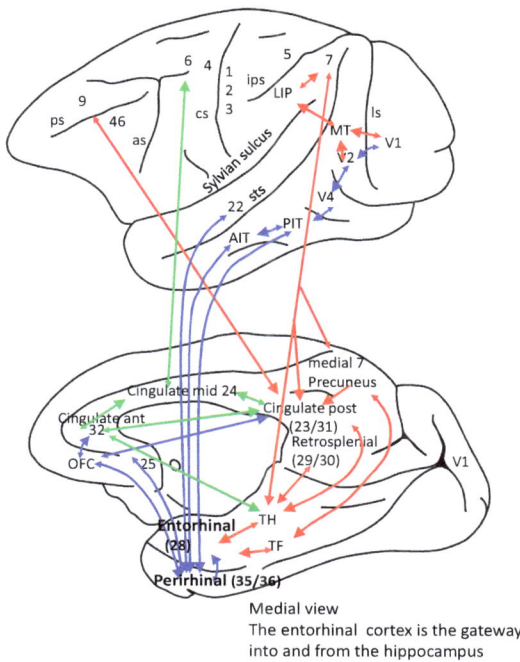

Medial view
The entorhinal cortex is the gateway
into and from the hippocampus

Fig. 5.3 The connections of the anterior and posterior cingulate cortex with their input areas, and their outputs to the hippocampal memory system. A medial view of the macaque brain is shown below, and a lateral view is above. The green arrows show the convergence of reward or outcome information from the anterior cingulate cortex (ACC) and of information about actions from the posterior cingulate cortex to the mid-cingulate motor area, which then projects to premotor areas including the premotor cortex area 6 and the supplementary motor area. This provides connectivity for action-outcome learning. The ACC receives reward outcome information from the orbitofrontal cortex (OFC). The posterior cingulate cortex receives information about actions from the parietal cortex. This cingulate connectivity is compared with that of the hippocampus, which receives information from the ventral 'what' processing stream (blue) and the dorsal 'where' or 'action' processing stream (red). The hippocampus receives its inputs via the parahippocampal gyrus (areas TF and TH), and the perirhinal cortex (areas 35 and 36), both of which in turn project to the entorhinal cortex (area 28), send inputs to the hippocampus and receive backprojections from the hippocampus. The forward inputs towards the entorhinal cortex and hippocampus are shown with large arrowheads, and the weaker return backprojections with small arrowheads. The hippocampus receives via the perirhinal cortex areas 35 and 36 which project to the lateral entorhinal cortex areas 28 from the ends of the hierarchically organised ventral visual system pathways (V1, V2, V4, PIT, AIT) that represent 'what' object is present (including also faces, and even scenes), from the anterior inferior temporal visual cortex (AIT, BA21, TE) where objects and faces are represented which receives from the posterior inferior temporal cortex (PIT, BA20, TEO); from the reward system in the orbitofrontal cortex (OFC) and amygdala, and from an area to which the OFC projects, the anterior cingulate cortex BA32 and subgenual cingulate cortex (BA25); from the high order auditory cortex (BA22); and from olfactory, taste, and somatosensory 'what' areas (not shown). These ventral 'what' pathways are shown in blue. The hippocampus also receives via the parahippocampal cortex areas TF and TH inputs (shown in red) from the dorsal visual 'where' or 'action' pathways, which reach parietal cortex area 7 via the dorsal visual stream hierarchy, including V1, V2, MT, MST, LIP, and VIP, and from areas to which they are connected, including the dorsolateral prefrontal cortex BA46 and the posterior cingulate (Cingulate post) and retrosplenial cortex. The hippocampus provides a system for all the high-order cortical regions to converge into a single network in the hippocampal CA3 region (Rolls, 2018a). Other abbreviations: as - arcuate sulcus; cs - central sulcus; ips - intraparietal sulcus; ios - inferior occipital sulcus; ls - lunate sulcus; sts - superior temporal sulcus. (Modified from Rolls 2019a.)

Rushworth 2016). Indeed, consistent with its strong connections to motor areas (Morecraft & Tanji 2009), lesions of the anterior cingulate cortex impair reward-guided action selection (Kennerley, Walton, Behrens, Buckley & Rushworth 2006, Rudebeck, Behrens, Kennerley, Baxter, Buckley, Walton & Rushworth 2008), neuroimaging studies have shown that the anterior cingulate cortex is active when outcome information guides choices (Walton, Devlin & Rushworth 2004), and single neurons in the anterior cingulate cortex encode information about both actions and outcomes including reward prediction errors for actions (Matsumoto, Matsumoto, Abe & Tanaka 2007, Luk & Wallis 2009, Kolling et al. 2016). For example, Luk & Wallis (2009) found that in a task where information about three potential outcomes (three types of juice) had to be associated on a trial-by-trial basis with two different responses (two lever movements), many neurons in the anterior cingulate cortex encoded information about both specific outcomes and specific actions.

5.1.5 Pregenual representations of reward value, and supracallosal representations of punishers and non-reward

Functional magnetic resonance neuroimaging (fMRI) studies show that there are rather separate representations of positively affective, pleasant, stimuli in the pregenual cingulate cortex (yellow in Fig. 3.54); and of negative, unpleasant, stimuli just posterior to this above the corpus callosum in the anterior cingulate cortex (white in Fig. 3.54) (Rolls 2009c, Grabenhorst & Rolls 2011). The area activated by pain is typically 10–30 mm behind and above the most anterior (i.e. pregenual) part of the anterior cingulate cortex (see e.g. Rolls, O'Doherty, Kringelbach, Francis, Bowtell & McGlone (2003d), Fig. 3.54, and Vogt & Sikes (2000) and Vogt et al. (1996)). Pleasant touch was found to activate the most anterior part of the anterior cingulate cortex, just in front of the genu (or knee) of the corpus callosum (i.e. pregenual cingulate cortex) (Rolls, O'Doherty, Kringelbach, Francis, Bowtell & McGlone 2003d, McCabe, Rolls, Bilderbeck & McGlone 2008) (Fig. 3.54). Pleasant temperature applied to the hand also produces a linear activation related to the degree of subjective pleasantness in the pregenual cingulate cortex (Grabenhorst, Rolls & Parris 2008b). Oral somatosensory stimuli such as viscosity and the pleasantness of fat texture also activate this pregenual part of the anterior cingulate cortex (De Araujo & Rolls 2004, Grabenhorst, Rolls, Parris & D'Souza 2010b). More than just somatosensory stimuli are represented, however, in that (pleasant) sweet taste also activates the pregenual anterior cingulate cortex (De Araujo & Rolls 2004, De Araujo, Kringelbach, Rolls & Hobden 2003a) where attention to pleasantness (Grabenhorst & Rolls 2008) and cognition (Grabenhorst, Rolls & Bilderbeck 2008a) also enhances activations, as do pleasant odours (Rolls, Kringelbach & De Araujo 2003c) (Fig. 3.16, and cognitive inputs that influence the pleasantness of odours (De Araujo et al. 2005) (Fig. 3.50, and also top-down inputs that produce selective attention to odour pleasantness (Rolls, Grabenhorst, Margot, da Silva & Velazco 2008a). Unpleasant odours activate further back in the anterior cingulate cortex (Rolls, Kringelbach & De Araujo 2003c) (Fig. 3.16). Activations in the pregenual cingulate cortex are also produced by the taste of water when it is rewarding because of thirst (De Araujo, Kringelbach, Rolls & McGlone 2003b), by the flavour of food (Kringelbach, O'Doherty, Rolls & Andrews 2003), and by monetary reward (O'Doherty, Kringelbach, Rolls, Hornak & Andrews 2001a) (Fig. 3.44). Moreover, the outcome value and the expected value of monetary reward activate the pregenual cingulate cortex (Rolls, McCabe & Redoute 2008e). The locations of some of these activations are shown in Fig. 3.54.

In these studies, the anterior cingulate activations were linearly related to the subjective pleasantness or unpleasantness of the stimuli, providing evidence that the anterior cingulate cortex provides a representation of value on a continuous scale (Fig. 3.54). Moreover, evidence was found that there is a common scale of value in the pregenual cingulate cortex, with the affective pleasantness of taste stimuli and of thermal stimuli applied to the hand producing identically scaled BOLD activations (Grabenhorst, D'Souza, Parris, Rolls & Passingham 2010a). The implication is that the anterior cingulate cortex contains a value representation used in decision-making, but that the decision itself may be made elsewhere. Decisions about actions that reflect the outcomes represented in the anterior cingulate cortex may be made further posterior towards the mid-cingulate cortex. Decisions about the value of stimuli may be made in the medial prefrontal cortex area 10 (or ventromedial prefrontal cortex, VMPFC) (Rolls et al. 2010b, Rolls et al. 2010c), which receives inputs from the orbitofrontal cortex and also from the anterior cingulate cortex.

Value representations in the pregenual cingulate cortex are confirmed by recording studies in monkeys (Rolls 2008d, Rolls 2009c, Kolling et al. 2016). For example, Gabbott, Verhagen, Kadohisa and Rolls found neurons in the pregenual cingulate cortex that respond to taste and it was demonstrated that the representation is of reward value, for devaluation by feeding to satiety selectively decreased neuronal responses to the food with which the animal was satiated (Rolls 2008d).

The framework then is that the value representations computed in the orbitofrontal cortex where there is little representation of action are transferred to the anterior cingulate cortex, where they can be used as the representation of reward vs non-reward or punishment outcome to be associated with representations of actions as part of goal-dependent action-outcome learning.

5.1.6 Anterior cingulate cortex and action-outcome representations

Some single neuron studies indicating encoding of actions and outcomes have often involved rather dorsal recordings above the pregenual cingulate cortex in the dorsal anterior cingulate cortex (dorsal bank of the cingulate sulcus) (Matsumoto et al. 2007, Luk & Wallis 2009, Kolling et al. 2016). In a similar area, action–outcome associations appear to be represented, in that in tasks in which there were different relations between actions and rewards, it was found that even before a response was made, while the monkey was looking at a visual cue, the activity of anterior cingulate cortex neurons depended on the expectation of reward or non-reward (25%), the intention to move or not (25%), or a combination of movement intention and reward expectation (11%) (Matsumoto, Suzuki & Tanaka 2003). Luk & Wallis (2013) described recordings in the same dorsal anterior cingulate cortex area that reflected the outcomes when monkeys made a choice of a left or right lever response to obtain a reward outcome, and also described a weak dissociation for more stimulus-outcome neurons in the orbitofrontal cortex, that is when monkeys had to choose the reward outcome based on which visual stimulus was shown. In the same dorsal anterior cingulate area neurons were more likely to take into account the costs of the actions required to obtain rewards, as well as the probability of obtaining the reward, than were neurons in the orbitofrontal cortex (Kennerley & Wallis 2009, Kennerley, Behrens & Wallis 2011, Kolling et al. 2016). In the dorsal anterior cingulate cortex, neurons may reflect evidence about the several most recent rewards, and use this to help guide choices (Kolling et al. 2016). More ventrally in the anterior cingulate cortex, neurons are more likely to reflect reward outcome rather than primarily actions, and the outcome representation trailed that in the orbitofrontal cortex (Cai & Padoa-Schioppa 2012). These findings are consistent with the hypothesis developed here and elsewhere (Rolls 2019d, Rolls 2019a) that the orbitofrontal cortex represents value but not actions, and takes decisions based on reward value, and that value information is transmitted from the orbitofrontal cortex to the anterior cingulate cortex, where there are action-related neurons, and where action-outcome learning takes place.

Foraging studies also implicate the anterior cingulate cortex in representing value, and in taking into account costs. For example, some neurons responded at higher rates when the monkeys were about to move to another foraging patch, and the threshold amount of this firing before the monkey switched to a new patch depended on the cost of switching (the delay before foraging in the new patch could resume) (Hayden, Pearson & Platt 2011). Consistent with this, the costs of actions can influence reward value representations in the macaque orbitofrontal cortex, even though the actions themselves are not represented in the orbitofrontal cortex (Cai & Padoa-Schioppa 2019).

In a neuroimaging study that provides evidence that the anterior cingulate cortex is active when outcome information guides choices made by the individual (Walton et al. 2004), the activations were relatively far back in the anterior cingulate cortex (y=22) towards the mid-cingulate cortex. This is consistent with the hypothesis that the reward value information in the pregenual cingulate cortex and the negative value representations just behind and dorsal to this in the anterior cingulate cortex are projected posteriorly towards the mid-cingulate area for interfacing to action.

5.1.7 Anterior cingulate cortex lesion effects

Lesion studies in monkeys (Rudebeck et al. 2008) and humans (Camille, Tsuchida & Fellows 2011), have demonstrated a dissociation in the role of the anterior cingulate cortex in action–outcome associations to guide behaviour; and of the orbitofrontal cortex in stimulus–outcome associations to update expected value (Rushworth, Kolling, Sallet & Mars 2012). Lesions of the anterior cingulate cortex in rats impair the ability to take into account the costs of actions, and this is supported by a neuroimaging study in humans (Croxson, Walton, O'Reilly, Behrens & Rushworth 2009).

An investigation more closely related to the understanding of emotion showed that patients with selective surgical lesions of the antero-ventral part of the anterior cingulate cortex (ACC) and/or medial BA9 were in some cases impaired on voice and face expression identification, had some change in social behaviour, such as inappropriateness, and had significant changes in their subjective emotional state (Hornak, Bramham, Rolls, Morris, O'Doherty, Bullock & Polkey 2003).

There is also neuroimaging evidence that complements the effects of lesions (Hornak et al. 2003) in suggesting a role for certain medial regions in the subjective experience of emotion. In neuroimaging studies with normal human subjects bilateral activations in medial BA9 were found as subjects viewed emotion-laden stimuli, and in both medial BA9 as well as in ventral ACC during self-generated emotional experience (i.e. in the absence of a stimulus) as subjects recalled emotions of sadness or happiness (Lane, Reiman, Ahern, Schwartz & Davidson 1997a, Lane, Reiman, Bradley, Lang, Ahern, Davidson & Schwartz 1997b, Lane, Reiman, Axelrod, Yun, Holmes & Schwartz 1998, Phillips, Drevets, Rauch & Lane 2003). On the basis of a review of imaging studies which consistently emphasize the importance of anterior and ventral regions of the anterior cingulate cortex for emotion, Bush, Luu & Posner (2000) argue that the anterior cingulate cortex can be divided into a ventral 'affective' division (which includes the subcallosal region and the part anterior to the corpus callosum), and a dorsal 'cognitive' division, a view strengthened by the demonstration of reciprocally inhibitory interactions between these two regions.

A current working hypothesis is that the affective part of the anterior cingulate cortex receives inputs about expected rewards and punishers, and about the rewards and punishers received, from the orbitofrontal cortex and amygdala. There is some segregation of the areas that receive these inputs. The anterior cingulate cortex may compare these signals, take into account the cost of actions, and utilize the value representations in action–outcome learning.

5.1.8 Subgenual cingulate cortex

The subgenual part (area 25) of the anterior cingulate cortex is, via its outputs to the hypothalamus and brainstem autonomic regions, involved in the autonomic component of emotion (Koski & Paus 2000, Barbas & Pandya 1989, Ongur & Price 2000, Gabbott, Warner, Jays & Bacon 2003, Vogt 2009). The anterior cingulate cortex is also activated in relation to autonomic events, and Nagai, Critchley, Featherstone, Trimble & Dolan (2004) have shown that there is a correlation with skin conductance, a measure of autonomic activity related to sympathetic activation, in the anterior cingulate cortex and related areas. The dorsal anterior and mid-cingulate cortical areas may be especially related to blood pressure, pupil size, heart rate, and electrodermal activity, whereas the subgenual cingulate cortex, with ventromedial prefrontal cortex, appears antisympathetic (and parasympathetic) (Critchley & Harrison 2013). The subgenual cingulate cortex is connected with the ventromedial prefrontal cortical areas (Johansen-Berg, Gutman, Behrens, Matthews, Rushworth, Katz, Lozano & Mayberg 2008).

Evidence implicating the subgenual and more generally the subcallosal cingulate cortex in depression is described in Section 7.4.3. Interestingly, neurons in the human subcallosal cingulate cortex responded to emotion categories present in visual stimuli, with more neurons responding to negatively valenced than positively valenced emotion categories (Laxton, Neimat, Davis, Womelsdorf, Hutchison, Dostrovsky, Hamani, Mayberg & Lozano 2013b).

5.1.9 Mid-cingulate cortex, the cingulate motor area, and action–outcome learning

The anterior cingulate area may be distinguished from a mid-cingulate area (i.e. further back than the perigenual cingulate region and occupying approximately the middle third of the cingulate cortex), which has been termed the cingulate motor area (Vogt et al. 1996, Vogt, Berger & Derbyshire 2003, Vogt 2009, Vogt 2016, Vogt 2019). The mid-cingulate area may be divided into an anterior or rostral cingulate motor area (24c') concerned with skeletomotor control which may be required in avoidance and fear tasks, and a posterior or caudal cingulate motor area (24d) which may be more involved in skeletomotor orientation (Vogt et al. 2003, Vogt 2016). (As has been noted above, what has been termed the anterior mid-cingulate cortex (Vogt 2016) may overlap with or be similar to what is described as the supracallosal part of the anterior cingulate cortex in this Chapter.)

This midcingulate cortex is activated by pain but, because this area is also activated in response selection tasks such as divided attention and Stroop tasks (which involve cues that cause conflict such as the word red written in green when the task is to make a response to the green colour), it is suggested that activation of this mid-cingulate area by painful stimuli was related to the response selection processes initiated by painful stimuli (Vogt et al. 1996, Derbyshire, Vogt & Jones 1998). Both the anterior cingulate and the mid-cingulate areas may be activated in functional neuroimaging studies not only by physical pain, but also by social pain, for example being excluded from a social group (Eisenberger & Lieberman 2004).

In human imaging studies it has been found that the anterior/mid-cingulate cortex is activated when there is a change in response set or when there is conflict between possible responses, but it is not activated when only stimulus selection is at issue (van Veen, Cohen, Botvinick, Stenger & Carter 2001, Rushworth, Hadland, Paus & Sipila 2002).

Some anterior/mid-cingulate neurons respond when errors are made (Niki & Watanabe 1979, Kolling et al. 2016, Procyk, Wilson, Stoll, Faraut, Petrides & Amiez 2016), or when rewards are reduced (Shima & Tanji 1998) (and activations are found in corresponding imaging studies (Bush, Vogt, Holmes, Dales, Greve, Jenike & Rosen 2002, Procyk et al. 2016)). In humans, an event-related potential (ERP), called the error related negativity (ERN), may originate in the area 24c' (Ullsperger & von Cramon 2001), and many studies provide evidence that errors made in many tasks activate the anterior/mid-cingulate cortex, whereas tasks with response conflict activate the superior frontal gyrus (Rushworth et al. 2004, Kolling et al. 2016, Procyk et al. 2016).

Correspondingly, in rodents a part of the medial prefrontal / anterior cingulate cortex termed the prelimbic cortex is involved in learning relations between behavioural responses and reinforcers, that is between actions and outcomes (Balleine & Dickinson 1998, Cardinal,

Parkinson, Hall & Everitt 2002, Killcross & Coutureau 2003a). Balleine & Dickinson (1998) showed that the sensitivity of instrumental behaviour to whether a particular action was followed by a reward was impaired by prelimbic cortex lesions. When making decisions about actions, it is important to take into account the costs as well as the benefits. There is some evidence implicating the rodent anterior cingulate cortex (prelimbic cortex) in this, in that rats with prelimbic cortex lesions were impaired in a task that required decisions about an action with a large reward but a high barrier to climb, vs an action with a lower reward but no barrier (Walton, Bannerman & Rushworth 2002, Walton et al. 2003).

5.1.10 The posterior cingulate cortex

The posterior cingulate cortex receives major inputs from parietal cortical areas that receive from the dorsal visual stream and somatosensory areas, and is involved in spatial processing and action in space (Vogt 2009, Vogt & Pandya 1987, Vogt & Laureys 2009, Rolls 2018a, Rolls & Wirth 2018, Rolls 2019d, Rolls 2019a). Interestingly, the posterior cingulate cortex also has connections with the orbitofrontal cortex (Vogt & Pandya 1987, Vogt & Laureys 2009) (Fig. 5.3). The posterior cingulate cortex is a region with strong connections in primates to the parahippocampal gyrus (areas TF and TH) and the entorhinal cortex, and thus with the hippocampal memory system (Bubb, Kinnavane & Aggleton 2017, Vogt 2009, Rolls 2018a, Rolls & Wirth 2018) (Fig. 5.3). Backprojections from the hippocampal system to posterior cingulate and parietal areas are likely to be involved in memory recall (Rolls 2016c, Rolls 2018a, Kesner & Rolls 2015).

One key and interesting concept that emerges is that orbitofrontal cortex value-related information has access to the posterior cingulate cortex and by this dorsal route into the hippocampal memory system, as well as by the ventral route via the perirhinal and (lateral) entorhinal cortex via which object-related information reaches the hippocampal memory system (Fig. 5.3) (Rolls 2018a, Rolls & Wirth 2018, Rolls 2019d, Rolls 2019a). The hippocampal memory system can then associate these three types of information, about where the object or face is present in space 'out there' using spatial view cells, combining if present information about the reward value of the object or position in space (Rolls 2016c, Kesner & Rolls 2015, Rolls 2018a, Rolls & Wirth 2018, Rolls 2019d, Rolls & Xiang 2006, Rolls, Xiang & Franco 2005b, Rolls & Xiang 2005, Rolls, Robertson & Georges-François 1997a, Rolls, Treves, Robertson, Georges-François & Panzeri 1998b, Robertson, Rolls & Georges-François 1998, Georges-François, Rolls & Robertson 1999).

Consistent with its anatomy, the posterior cingulate region (BA 23/31) (with the retrosplenial cortex BA 29/30) is consistently engaged by a range of tasks that examine episodic memory including autobiographical memory, and imagining the future; and also spatial navigation and scene processing (Leech & Sharp 2014, Auger & Maguire 2013). Self-reflection and self-imagery activate the ventral part of the posterior cingulate cortex (vPCC, the part with which we are mainly concerned here) (Kircher, Brammer, Bullmore, Simmons, Bartels & David 2002, Kircher, Senior, Phillips, Benson, Bullmore, Brammer, Simmons, Williams, Bartels & David 2000, Johnson, Baxter, Wilder, Pipe, Heiserman & Prigatano 2002, Sugiura, Watanabe, Maeda, Matsue, Fukuda & Kawashima 2005).

A second key and interesting concept is that the posterior cingulate cortex, and the retrosplenial cortex, which both are highly connected with both lateral and medial parietal cortex areas (Vogt 2009, Rolls 2018a, Rolls & Wirth 2018), provides a route for information about actions in space, represented in the parietal cortex by both visual spatial and somatosensory representations (Bisley & Goldberg 2010, Whitlock 2017), to gain access to the cingulate cortex action-outcome learning system. The resulting concept is that the cingulate cortex receives action information via the parietal to posterior cingulate cortex route, and reward information via the orbitofrontal cortex to anterior cingulate cortex route, and from this information associates actions with outcomes, can then select optimal actions given the rewards and costs, and can produce goal-directed actions via the cingulate motor area with its outputs to premotor cortical areas, as illustrated in Fig. 5.3 (Rolls 2019d, Rolls 2019a).

The posterior cingulate cortex is implicated in decision-making in that some neurons there respond when risky, uncertain choices are made (McCoy & Platt 2005b); and some neurons respond more when an expected large reward is not obtained, maintaining that firing until the next trial (Hayden, Nair, McCoy & Platt 2008) (probably reflecting input from orbitofrontal cortex error neurons that have attractor state-like persistent firing that encodes and maintains a negative reward prediction error signal (Thorpe, Rolls & Maddison 1983, Rolls & Grabenhorst 2008, Rolls 2009a, Rolls 2019d, Rolls 2019a)).

5.1.11 The cingulate cortex: synthesis

One important function of the cingulate cortex is, via the mid-cingulate motor area with its connections to neocortical motor areas, to associate actions with outcomes, as indicated by the connections shown in green in Fig. 5.3. My proposal is that convergence of reward or outcome information from the anterior cingulate cortex, and of information about actions from the posterior cingulate cortex, occurs in the cingulate cortex leading to outputs via the mid-cingulate motor area, which projects to premotor areas including the premotor cortex area 6 and the supplementary motor area (see green arrows in Fig. 5.3). This provides connectivity for action-outcome learning (Rolls 2019d, Rolls 2019a). The anterior cingulate cortex receives reward and punishment outcome information from the orbitofrontal cortex (OFC). The posterior cingulate cortex receives information about actions from the parietal cortex. Then these two types of information are brought together towards the mid-part of the cingulate cortex, the cingulate motor area, which with its connections to premotor areas can select the action that is most likely, given the action-outcome learning performed within this cingulate system, to obtain the goal, the desired outcome (Rolls 2019d). In addition, the parietal areas have projections to medial frontal areas connected with the dorsal parts of the anterior cingulate cortex (Vogt 2009), and these projections may also provide a route for action-related information to reach the cingulate action-outcome learning system (Rolls 2019d).

A second important function of the cingulate cortex is related to the hippocampal memory system (Rolls 2018a), as shown in Fig. 5.3. The anatomical connectivity shown in Fig. 5.3 provides two routes for reward-related information to reach the hippocampal memory system. The first, more direct, route is from the orbitofrontal cortex and amygdala to the perirhinal cortex with information derived from the ventral visual and auditory 'what' processing streams (blue in Fig. 5.3). The second route for reward-related information is via the anterior cingulate cortex (which receives its reward-related information from the orbitofrontal cortex) which projects to the posterior cingulate cortex and also to the parahippocampal gyrus, providing access to the hippocampal memory system via the dorsal route. There are also direct projections from the orbitofrontal cortex to the posterior cingulate cortex (green in Fig. 5.3). These concepts are further elaborated by Rolls (2019d) and Rolls (2019a).

5.2 Dopamine systems in the brain and reward prediction errors

Evidence is described in Chapter 3 that the main reward system in the primate brain is the orbitofrontal cortex (and to a lesser extent in primates the amygdala, as described in Section 6.5), in that the cortical areas in Tier 1 that represent what stimulus is present independently of reward project into the orbitofrontal cortex in Tier 2, where the stimuli are represented in terms of their reward value (Fig. 2.2). The orbitofrontal cortex represents the value of very many stimuli in a high dimensional space of stimuli, with different neurons tuned to respond to different specific rewards (such as a sweet taste, the mouth feel of a rich fatty food, or the emotional expression on a face). Moreover, the orbitofrontal cortex performs the learning of associations of stimuli with primary reinforcers, implements rapid reversal of this learning, and computes negative reward prediction error. The evidence for all of this is described in Chapter 3.

The orbitofrontal cortex then has a number of outputs, and one is indirectly to the dopamine neurons in the brainstem (Rolls 2017a), as shown in Fig. 2.5 on page 15. The dopamine neurons appear to have a quite different representation to the reward value neurons in the orbitofrontal cortex, in that they represent positive reward prediction error which may be used as a training signal for some brain systems such as the basal ganglia. The dopamine neurons do not represent the reward value of a stimulus, which is characteristic of orbitofrontal cortex neurons, but more a learning signal that operates if the reward obtained is better than expected. Also, the dopamine neurons do not appear to have firing that describes the exact nature of the reinforcer (such as a sweet taste), so are not apparently suitable for providing the goal for actions in the way that the orbitofrontal cortex to cingulate cortex system does. However, there are dopamine receptors in a number of cortical areas, including the orbitofrontal cortex, and it is quite clear that dopamine systems can be very reinforcing, and indeed are important in addiction to the psychomotor stimulants such as amphetamine and cocaine. In this context, evidence on the orbitofrontal cortex / dopamine system is considered in this section (5.2), and on orbitofrontal cortex projections to the striatum in Section 5.3.

5.2.1 Dopamine pathways

Dopamine is involved in reward systems in the brain, in that the dopamine neurons in the midbrain receive inputs from the orbitofrontal cortex via the ventral striatum to ventral pallidum, and via the ventral striatum to ventral pallidum to lateral habenula to rostromedial tegmental nucleus (Fig. 2.5) (Haber 2014, Rolls 2017a), and have then a major influence on stimulus-response habit learning in the basal ganglia (Section 5.3), and also projections to a number of cortical areas in primates, including the dorsolateral prefrontal cortex involved in working memory and executive function, and the orbitofrontal and temporal lobe cortices (Haber & Knutson 2010, Haber 2016, Haber 2014, Diamond 2007, Arnsten, Wang & Paspalas 2015, Rolls 2016c).

The dopaminergic neurons' pathways have been traced using histofluorescence and other techniques (Ungerstedt 1971, Bjorklund & Lindvall 1986, Cooper, Bloom & Roth 2003, Haber 2014, Haber 2016, Heilbronner, Rodriguez-Romaguera, Quirk, Groenewegen & Haber 2016). The mesostriatal dopamine projection (see Fig. 5.4) originates mainly (but not exclusively) from the A9 dopamine cell group in the substantia nigra, pars compacta, and projects to the (dorsal or neo-) striatum, in particular the caudate nucleus and putamen. The mesolimbic dopamine system originates mainly from the A10 cell group, and projects to the nucleus accumbens and olfactory tubercle, which together constitute the ventral striatum (see Fig. 5.4). In addition there is a mesocortical dopamine system projecting mainly from the A10 neurons to the frontal cortex, but especially in primates also to other cortical areas, including parts of the temporal cortex (Haber 2014).

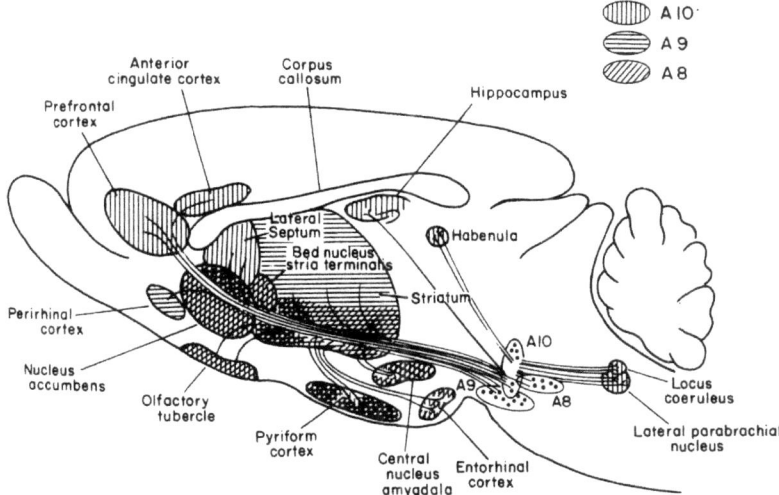

Fig. 5.4 Schematic diagram illustrating the distribution of the main central neuronal pathways containing dopamine in the rat. The stippled regions indicate the major nerve-terminal areas and their cell groups of origin. The cell groups in this figure are named according to the nomenclature of Dahlstrom and Fuxe (1965). The A9 cell group in the substantia nigra pars compacta is one of the main DA-containing cell groups, and gives rise mainly to the nigro-striatal dopamine pathway terminating in the striatum. The A10 cell group in the ventral tegmental area is the other main DA-containing cell groups, and gives rise mainly to the meso-limbic DA pathway which terminates in the nucleus accumbens and the olfactory tubercle (together known as the ventral striatum), and the meso-cortical DA pathway which terminates in prefrontal, anterior cingulate, and some other cortical areas. Reproduced from The Biochemical Basis of Neuropharmacology, 8th edition, by Jack R. Cooper, Floyd E. Bloom, and Robert H. Roth, p. 227, Figure 9.1a © Oxford University Press, 2004. Reproduced by permission of Oxford University Press.

5.2.2 Self-administration of dopaminergic substances, and addiction

In this section evidence is summarized that a major class of drug, the psychomotor stimulants such as amphetamine and cocaine and both of which stimulate the release of dopamine, can produce their reward by acting on a dopaminergic mechanism in the nucleus accumbens (part of the ventral striatum) (Everitt & Robbins 2013, Koob & Volkow 2016, Rolls 2014a), which receives a dopaminergic input from the A10 cell group in the ventral tegmental area. These drugs are addictive, and understanding their mode of action in the brain helps to clarify how these drugs produce their effects. Some of the evidence is as follows:

1. Amphetamine (which increases the release of dopamine and noradrenaline) is self administered intravenously by humans, monkeys, rats, etc.
2. Amphetamine self-injection intravenously is blocked by dopamine receptor blockers such as pimozide and spiroperidol. The implication is that the psychomotor stimulants produce their reward by causing the release of dopamine which acts on dopamine receptors. The receptor blocker at first increases the rate at which the animal will work for the intravenous injection. The reason for this is that with each lever press for amphetamine, less reward is produced than without the receptor blockade, so the animal works more to obtain the same net amount of reward. This is typical of what happens with low rate operant response behaviour when the magnitude of the reward is reduced. The rate increase is a good control which shows that the dopamine receptor blockade at the doses used does not produce its reward-reducing effect by interfering with motor responses.
3. Apomorphine (which activates D2 dopamine receptors) is self-administered intravenously.
4. Intravenous self-administration of indirect DA agonists such as D-amphetamine and cocaine is much decreased by 6-OHDA lesions of the nucleus accumbens.
5. Rats will learn to self-administer very small quantities of amphetamine to the nucleus accumbens. This effect is abolished by 6-OHDA lesions of the meso-limbic dopamine pathway.

6. Mice will learn instrumental responses to optogenetically activate dopamine neurons (Rossi, Sukharnikova, Hayrapetyan, Yang & Yin 2013).
7. Monkeys will learn to self-administer very small quantities of amphetamine to the orbitofrontal cortex (Phillips, Mora & Rolls 1981).

In rodents early on in cocaine self-administration the behaviour is under control of an action–outcome system in the nucleus accumbens core and dorsomedial striatum, whereas a dorsolateral striatum-dependent stimulus-response, habit, process controls the behaviour after repeated self-administration over several weeks (Everitt, Belin, Economidou, Pelloux, Dalley & Robbins 2008, Everitt & Robbins 2013). This evidence is supported by neuroimaging findings in humans, though these also point to the importance of the orbitofrontal cortex in addiction in humans (Everitt, Giuliano & Belin 2018).

When humans receive amphetamine, some of the main brain areas that are activated are the medial orbitofrontal cortex, and the rostral part of the anterior cingulate cortex, as well as the ventral striatum (Voellm, De Araujo, Cowen, Rolls, Kringelbach, Smith, Jezzard, Heal & Matthews 2004). This indicates that at least part of the reward and pleasure produced by the psychomotor stimulants may be being produced by activation of the medial orbitofrontal and anterior cingulate cortex, both of which receive dopamine inputs, and in both of which there are neurons and activations produced by natural rewards. Consistently, the orbitofrontal cortex as well as the areas to which it projects such as the ventral striatum are activated in cocaine (another psychomotor stimulant) addicts by exposure to drug-related conditioned stimuli associated with the cocaine (Volkow, Wang, Tomasi & Baler 2013). Also consistent with the role of the orbitofrontal cortex in the reward value of psychomotor stimulants, amphetamine is self-administered to the orbitofrontal cortex by monkeys (Phillips, Mora & Rolls 1981).

The (Pavlovian) conditioned cues that support addiction and may lead to relapse to addiction by Pavlovian-instrumental transfer (Cardinal et al. 2002) may operate in part via the orbitofrontal cortex, for Childress et al. (1999) have shown that cocaine-related cues shown visually in a video to addicts activate the orbitofrontal cortex, and also parts of the anterior cingulate and medial prefrontal cortex. These Pavlovian conditioned effects to drug cues are very important in addiction (Everitt et al. 2018), and the orbitofrontal cortex may be involved in this in humans and other primates.

Dopamine does not appear to implement the rewarding effects of some other drugs, including opiates, nicotine, and cannabis, and the evidence that dopamine implements the addictive effects even of stimulant drugs in humans needs re-evaluation (Nutt et al. 2015).

5.2.3 Behaviours associated with the release of dopamine

The functional role of dopamine can be investigated by determining what factors influence its release. It has been found that the preparatory behaviours for feeding, including foraging for food, food hoarding, and performing instrumental responses to obtain food and other reinforcers, are more associated with dopamine release than is the consummatory behaviour of feeding itself (Phillips, Vacca & Ahn 2008, Phillips, Pfaus & Blaha 1991). Dopamine may also be released in relation to movement and incentive motivation (Phillips et al. 2008).

Although the majority of the studies have focused on rewarded behaviour, there is also extensive evidence that dopamine can be released by stimuli that are aversive or stressful (Bromberg-Martin, Matsumoto & Hikosaka 2010). For example, Rada, Mark & Hoebel (1998) showed that dopamine was released in the nucleus accumbens when rats worked to escape from aversive hypothalamic stimulation.

5.2.4 Dopamine neurons and reward prediction error

There is extensive evidence that dopamine neurons may signal positive reward prediction error, that is, can respond when a reward is unexpectedly obtained, or when the reward obtained is greater than predicted, or when a stimulus predicting reward is given (Schultz 2013, Glimcher 2011b, Schultz 2016b, Schultz 2016a). The phasic response of the dopamine neurons has an initial non-selective component, and is followed with a latency that may be as long as 200 ms by a second component that is increased firing if the reward is greater than expected, and a decrease of the very low spontaneous rate if the reward is less than expected. However, the evidence for this interpretation is not fully consistent, in that some dopamine neurons respond to aversive stimuli, some to rewarding and aversive stimuli, and others to stimuli that may be salient in other ways, for example novel stimuli (Matsumoto & Hikosaka 2009a, Bromberg-Martin et al. 2010). Further, some of the positive reward prediction error neurons also increase their firing to a bitter taste in low concentrations (Schultz 2016b), even though a bitter taste can not signal a positive reward prediction error. A further complication is that the tonic, sustained, firing of the dopamine neurons has been related to reward uncertainty (Fiorillo, Tobler & Schultz 2003). Another complication is that some dopamine neurons are related to habit-based rewards, and do not signal normal positive reward prediction error (Kim, Ghazizadeh & Hikosaka 2015).

These dopamine neurons are thus very different from the reward encoding neurons in the orbitofrontal cortex that respond to the value of the outcomes, and of activations in the orbitofrontal cortex, which are linearly related to the subjective affective value of tastes, flavours etc, and are thus closely related to emotional value, as described in Chapter 3. The difference is that the dopamine neurons respond to a better than expected outcome, not to the value of the outcome. Further, the dopamine neurons may stop responding to the primary (unlearned) reinforcer or outcome quite rapidly as the task is learned, and instead respond only to the earliest indication that a trial of the task is about to begin (Schultz, Romo, Ljunberg, Mirenowicz, Hollerman & Dickinson 1995). A key difference is that orbitofrontal cortex outcome value neurons always respond to the outcome (e.g. a taste of fruit juice) even when it is expected; whereas dopamine positive error prediction neurons do not respond to the outcome if it is as expected. *Thus dopamine neurons could not convey information about a primary reward (such as a fruit juice reward outcome) and its subjective affective value if the trial is successful and the outcome was as expected. They are thus unlike, and could not perform the functions of, the reward outcome value neurons in the orbitofrontal cortex described in Chapter 3.*

These dopamine neurons are also very different from the orbitofrontal cortex negative reward prediction error neurons, which have strong increased firing when the reward outcome is *lower* than expected (as illustrated in Fig. 3.46, Thorpe, Rolls & Maddison (1983)).

Another difficulty is the issue of where dopamine neurons receive their inputs from, given that the necessary signals for the computation of positive reward prediction error, namely expected value, and outcome value, are not a feature of midbrain neurons. This is a surprisingly little addressed question (Schultz 2013, Schultz 2016b, Schultz 2016a). However, I have suggested that possible pathways originate in the orbitofrontal cortex and amygdala and influence the brainstem dopamine (and serotonin) neurons via pathways such as the ventral striatum to ventral pallidum to lateral habenula to rostrodorsal tegmental nucleus route or via the ventral striatum to ventral pallidum route (Rolls 2017a), as considered in Sections 2.2, 5.2.1 and Fig. 2.5 (see further Haber (2014).)

Despite these difficulties, the dopamine positive reward prediction error hypothesis has been built into models of learning in which the error signal is used to train synaptic connections in dopamine pathway recipient regions (such as presumably the striatum) (Waelti, Dickinson &

Schultz 2001, Dayan & Abbott 2001, Schultz 2013, Glimcher 2011b, Schultz 2016a). The error would be used in a reinforcement learning system to implement temporal difference learning (both of which are described by Dayan & Abbott (2001) and Rolls (2014a)). A possible effect of the dopamine to implement temporal difference learning would be for dopamine release to act via D1 receptors in the striatum to facilitate long-term synaptic potentiation (LTP) of the cortical glutamatergic excitatory inputs onto striatal neurons (see Schultz (2013)). This form of slow learning might help the striatum to learn stimulus-response habits (see Section 5.3). Consistently, we (Rolls, McCabe & Redoute 2008e), and many others (Garrison, Erdeniz & Done 2013), have found that activations in the ventral striatum are correlated with temporal difference reward/punishment prediction errors in a number of tasks.

Overall, although there is much evidence that some dopamine neurons encode a positive reward prediction error signal, there are difficulties with the hypothesis (Rolls 2014a). To the extent that this is the case, the dopamine system may be viewed in primates including humans, as one of the output systems of the orbitofrontal cortex (Fig. 2.5), which plays a role in training for example stimulus-response habit learning in the basal ganglia (Section 5.3).

5.3 The basal ganglia as an output system for emotional and motivational behaviour

5.3.1 Overview of the basal ganglia

The basal ganglia are evolutionarily old subcortical structures that provide a route for emotion-related parts of the brain, including the orbitofrontal cortex, amygdala, and anterior cingulate cortex, to produce habit-related stimulus-response behaviours (Fig. 3.1).

More generally, the striatum, which consists of the caudate nucleus, putamen, and ventral striatum / nucleus accumbens, receive from the nearest part of the cerebral cortex, and then converge further to a second stage of processing in the globus pallidus and substantia nigra (Figs. 5.5 and 5.6).

The principle of operation of both the striatum, and globus pallidus / substantia nigra is that the neurons directly inhibit each other, using the inhibitory transmitter GABA (gamma-amino-butyric acid). This is a simple and safe way to select outputs, with the two stage convergence (cortex to striatum; striatum to pallidum / substantia nigra) helping to make this possible by limiting the number of inputs to neurons at any stage of processing to $\approx 10,000$.

The dopamine inputs to the striatum may facilitate the appropriate mappings from input to output in this system.

Interestingly, the outputs of the basal ganglia are not directed down towards the brainstem motor areas, but instead project via the thalamus back up to the cortex, including motor cortical areas, but also other cortical areas (Fig. 5.5). The basal ganglia may thus be a more general system for allowing competition between the outputs of different cortical areas, to select mapping to a few outputs, to ensure consistency in the execution of movements.

In Parkinson's disease, the dopamine neurons gradually degenerate, and the linkage between cortical inputs and movements starts to fail.

More full evidence on the operation of the basal ganglia is provided elsewhere (Rolls 2014a, Rolls 2016c).

5.3.2 Systems-level architecture of the basal ganglia

The point-to-point connectivity of the basal ganglia as shown by experimental anterograde and retrograde neuroanatomical path tracing techniques in the primate is indicated in Figs. 5.5

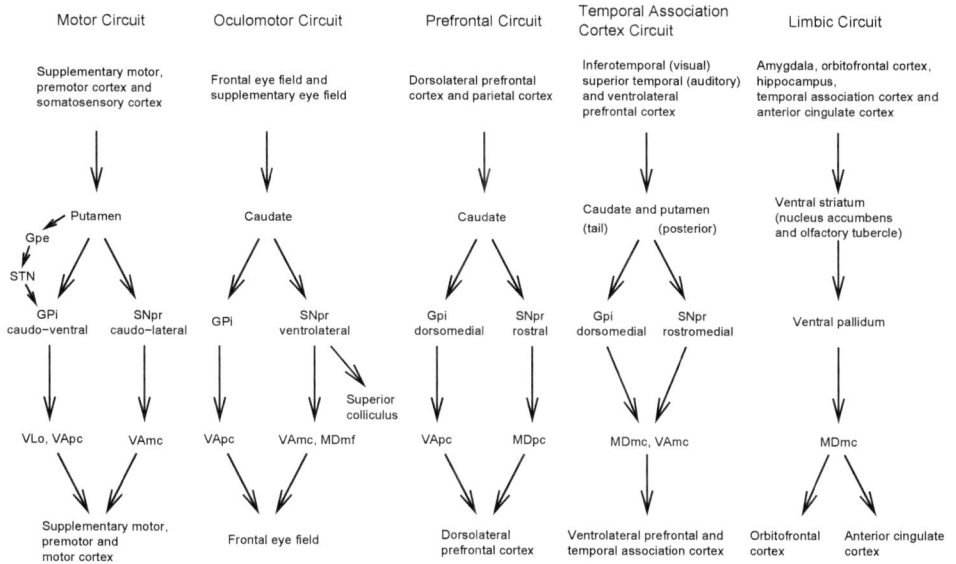

Fig. 5.5 A synthesis of some of the anatomical studies (see text) of the connections of the basal ganglia. GPe, Globus Pallidus, external segment; GPi, Globus Pallidus, internal segment; MD, nucleus medialis dorsalis; SNpr, Substantia Nigra, pars reticulata; VAmc, n. ventralis anterior pars magnocellularis of the thalamus; VApc, n. ventralis anterior pars compacta; VLo, n. ventralis lateralis pars oralis; VLm, n. ventralis pars medialis. An indirect pathway from the striatum via the external segment of the globus pallidus and the subthalamic nucleus (STN) to the internal segment of the globus pallidus is present for the first four circuits (left to right in the figure) of the basal ganglia.

and 5.6. The general connectivity is for cortical or limbic inputs to reach the striatum, which then projects to the globus pallidus and substantia nigra pars reticulata, which in turn project via the thalamus back to the cerebral cortex (DeLong & Wichmann 2010, Gerfen & Surmeier 2011, Buot & Yelnik 2012, Haber 2016). Within this overall scheme, there is a set of at least partially segregated parallel processing streams, as illustrated in Figs. 5.5 and 5.6 (Rolls & Johnstone 1992, Rolls 2014a, Rolls 2016c, Haber 2016, Bostan, Dum & Strick 2018, Heilbronner, Rodriguez-Romaguera, Quirk, Groenewegen & Haber 2016).

Of especial interest in the context of reward mechanisms in the brain, limbic and related structures such as the amygdala, orbitofrontal cortex, and hippocampus project to the ventral striatum (which includes the nucleus accumbens), which has connections through the ventral pallidum to the mediodorsal nucleus of the thalamus and thus to the prefrontal and cingulate cortices (Buot & Yelnik 2012, Julian, Keinath, Frazzetta & Epstein 2018, Haber 2016, Heilbronner et al. 2016, Heilbronner, Meyer, Choi & Haber 2018). It is notable that the projections from the amygdala and orbitofrontal cortex are not restricted to the nucleus accumbens, but also reach the adjacent ventral part of the head of the caudate nucleus (Amaral & Price 1984, Seleman & Goldman-Rakic 1985, Haber 2016, Heilbronner, Rodriguez-Romaguera, Quirk, Groenewegen & Haber 2016).

At striatal neurons of the direct pathway (from the striatum directly to the globus pallidus internal segment), dopamine has excitatory effects via the D1 receptor by eliciting or prolonging glutamate excitatory inputs. At striatal neurons in the indirect pathway (from the striatum via the external segment of the globus pallidus via the subthalamic nucleus to the internal segment of the globus pallidus, see Fig. 5.5), D2 receptor activation has inhibitory effects by reducing glutamate release and prolonging membrane down states (hyperpolarization). Both effects of dopamine tend to promote behavioural output (Gerfen & Surmeier 2011).

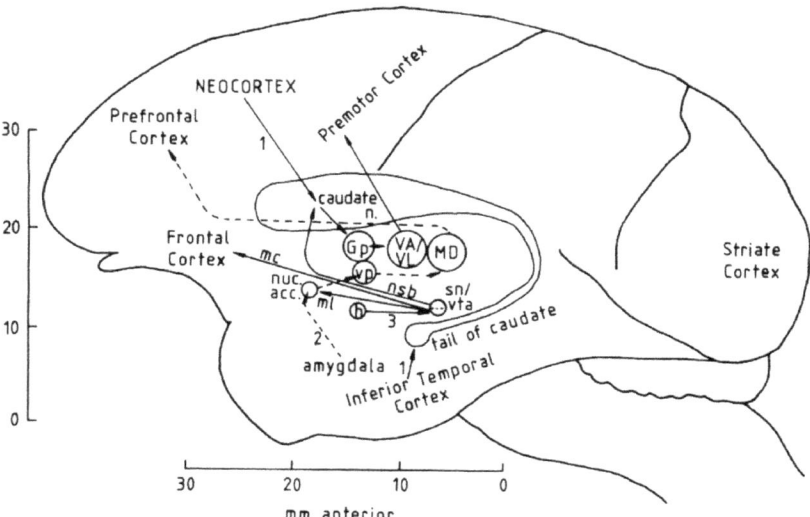

Fig. 5.6 Some of the striatal and connected regions in which the activity of single neurons is described shown on a lateral view of the brain of the macaque monkey. Gp, globus pallidus; h, hypothalamus; sn, substantia nigra, pars compacta (A9 cell group), which gives rise to the nigrostriatal dopaminergic pathway, or nigrostriatal bundle (nsb); vta, ventral tegmental area, containing the A10 cell group, which gives rise to the mesocortical dopamine pathway (mc) projecting to the frontal and cingulate cortices and to the mesolimbic dopamine pathway (ml), which projects to the nucleus accumbens (nuc acc). There is a route from the nucleus accumbens to the ventral pallidum (vp) which then projects to the mediodorsal nucleus of the thalamus (MD) which in turn projects to the prefrontal cortex. Correspondingly, the globus pallidus projects via the ventral anterior and ventrolateral (VA/VL) thalamic nuclei to cortical areas such as the premotor cortex.

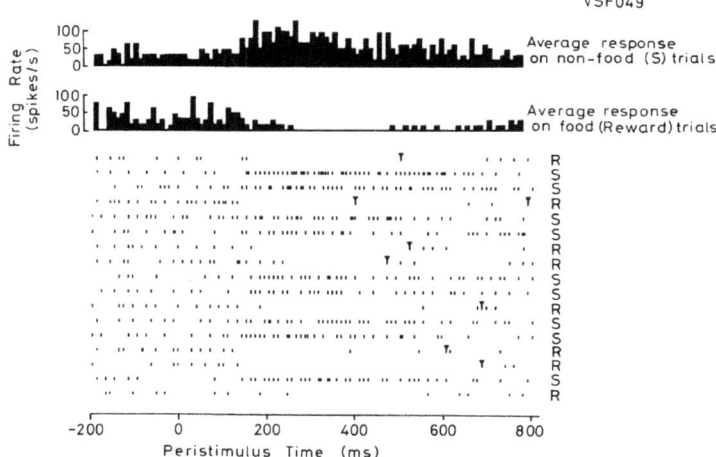

Fig. 5.7 Responses of a ventral striatal neuron in a visual discrimination task. The neuron reduced its firing rate to the S+ on food reward trials (R), and increased its firing rate to the S– on non-food trials (S) on which aversive saline was obtained if a lick was made. Rastergrams and peristimulus time histograms are shown. The inverted triangles show where lick responses were made on the food reward (R) trials. (Reprinted from Behavioural Brain Research, 55 (2), Graham V. Williams, Edmund T. Rolls, Christiana M. Leonard, and Chantal Stern, Neuronal responses in the ventral striatum of the behaving macaque, pp. 243–52, Copyright 1993, with permission from Elsevier.)

5.3.3 Neuronal activity in different parts of the striatum

We will focus first on neuronal activity in the **ventral striatum**, because it is particularly relevant to the processing of rewards by the basal ganglia. We again focus on neuronal research in monkeys, because the inputs from the orbitofrontal cortex are so different to those in rodents.

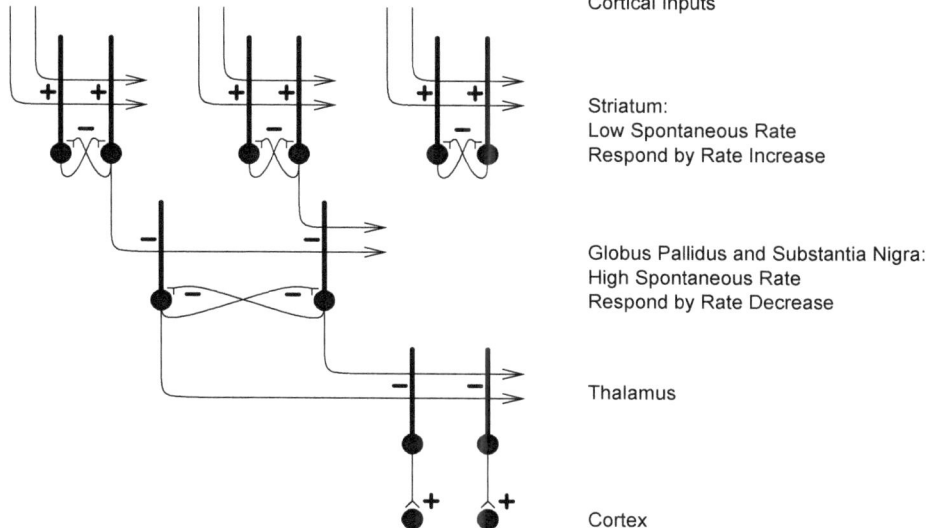

Fig. 5.8 Simple hypothesis of basal ganglia network architecture. A key aspect is that in both the striatum, and in the globus pallidus and substantia nigra pars reticulata, there are direct inhibitory connections (−) between the principal neurons, as shown. These synapses use GABA as a transmitter. Excitatory inputs to the striatum are shown as +. (Reproduced from Neural Networks and Brain Function by Edmund T. Rolls and Alessandro Treves, p. 220, Figure 9.14 © Edmund T. Rolls and Alessandro Treves, 1998. Reproduced by permission of Oxford University Press and The Authors.)

Some neurons in the macaque ventral striatum respond to rewarding visual stimuli in a visual discrimination task, but the responses are less clear than of neurons in the orbitofrontal cortex that projects into the ventral striatum. Other ventral striatal neurons responded to faces; to novel visual stimuli; to other visual stimuli; in relation to somatosensory stimulation and movement; or to cues that signalled the start of a task (Rolls & Williams 1987, Williams, Rolls, Leonard & Stern 1993).

Neurons in the **tail of the caudate nucleus** and adjoining putamen which receive from the inferior temporal visual cortex and the prestriate cortex (Kemp & Powell 1970, Saint-Cyr, Ungerleider & Desimone 1990) respond to visual stimuli, but habituate quite rapidly (Caan, Perrett & Rolls 1984). These neurons may be involved in detecting and orienting to new visual stimuli.

Neurons in the **postero-ventral putamen**, which receives from the inferior temporal visual cortex and the prefrontal cortex (Goldman & Nauta 1977, Van Hoesen, Yeterian & Lavizzo-Mourey 1981) had responses in a visual short-term memory task (delayed match-to-sample) task, responding for example in the delay period (Johnstone & Rolls 1990, Rolls & Johnstone 1992). They reflect the activity in the cortical areas that project into this part of the striatum.

Neurons in the **head of the caudate nucleus**, which receives from the prefrontal cortex (Kemp & Powell 1970, Haber 2016) had activity to many environmental stimuli, and frequently to cues that a task was about to start (Rolls, Thorpe & Maddison 1983b). These neurons may be involved in the preparation for movement.

The activity of many neurons in the anterior **putamen**, which receives from motor and somatosensory cortical areas, is related to movements (Rolls, Thorpe, Boytim, Szabo & Perrett 1984, DeLong & Wichmann 2010). There is a somatotopic organization of neurons in the putamen, with separate areas containing neurons responding to arm, leg, or orofacial movements. Some of these neurons respond only to active movements, and others to active and to passive movements. Many of these neurons respond in relation to mouth movements such as licking. Similar neurons are found in the substantia nigra, pars reticulata, to which the putamen projects (Mora, Mogenson & Rolls 1977).

The activity of neurons in different parts of the striatum is described in much more detail by Rolls (2014a) in *Emotion and Decision-Making Explained*, which is available online as a .pdf at https://www.oxcns.org.

5.3.4 How do the basal ganglia perform their computations?

This evidence, and much other evidence on the dendritic arrangements within the basal ganglia (Percheron, Yelnik & François 1984a, Percheron, Yelnik & François 1984b, Percheron, Yelnik, François, Fenelon & Talbi 1994, Yelnik 2002, Buot & Yelnik 2012), have been put together to formulate a hypothesis about the operation of the basal ganglia, with is sketched in Fig. 5.8 (Rolls 2014a, Rolls 2016c). The hypothesis is that the basal ganglia with multistage convergence, with learning of associated inputs onto striatal neurons, and mutual inhibition between the neurons provides a mechanism for selecting a few outputs to drive behaviour. In the context of reinforcing stimuli, this provides a basis for stimuli for any cortical area to be linked associatively, perhaps with the facilitation of dopamine, to link the stimuli to responses. This theory, and the evidence for it, is considered in detail elsewhere (Rolls 2014a) (available online as a .pdf at https://www.oxcns.org).

6 The orbitofrontal cortex and emotion

6.1 An introduction to emotion

The orbitofrontal cortex is important in emotion and motivation. A brief introduction to our understanding of emotion and motivation is provided in Section 6.1, to provide a conceptual basis for helping to understand some of the functions of the orbitofrontal cortex in emotion (Rolls 2014a, Rolls 2018b). Section 6.2 provides an approach to understanding rewards, punishers, and reinforcement contingencies, which are very important for understanding the functions of the orbitofrontal cortex. Section 6.4 compares the orbitofrontal cortex emotional route to action with the rational, reasoning, route to action, and considers how decisions are made between these two routes. Section 6.5 compares the functions of the orbitofrontal cortex with that of the evolutionarily older amygdala.

What are emotions? Why do we have emotions? What is their adaptive value? What are the brain mechanisms of emotion, and how can disorders of emotion be understood? Why does it feel like something to have an emotion? Why do emotions sometimes feel so intense? Here we consider answers to these questions.

We can similarly ask what motivates us: What is motivation? How is motivation controlled? How is motivation produced and regulated by the brain? What goes wrong in motivational disorders, for example in appetite disorders which produce overeating and obesity? How do these motivational control systems operate to ensure that we eat approximately the correct amount of food to maintain our body weight, or drink just enough to replenish our thirst? What are some of the underlying reasons for the different patterns of sexual behaviour found in different animals and humans? Why (and how) do we like some types of touch (e.g. a caress), and what is the relation of this to motivation? What brain processes underlie addiction? What is the relation between emotion, and motivational states such as hunger, appetite, and sexual behaviour? It turns out that the explanations for motivational behaviour are in many ways similar to those for emotional behaviour, and therefore they are also considered here.

Some of my approach to emotion (Rolls 2014a, Rolls 2018b) can be summarized in the following:

1. What produces emotions? The general answer I propose is reinforcing stimuli, that is rewards and punishers, as shown in Fig. 6.1.
2. What types of emotion are there? I propose that there are many different types of emotion that can be elicited to a different reinforcer (e.g. pain), as set out in Fig. 6.1, and that there are many different reinforcers, each of which can produce emotional states in the way illustrated in Fig. 6.1.
3. Why do we have emotions? The overall answer I propose is that emotions are evolutionarily adaptive as they provide an efficient way for genes to influence our behaviour to increase their reproductive fitness.
4. How do we have emotions? Part of the answer to this lies in the functions of the orbitofrontal cortex as described in this book, with the contribution of other brain regions described elsewhere (Rolls 2014a, Rolls 2018b).

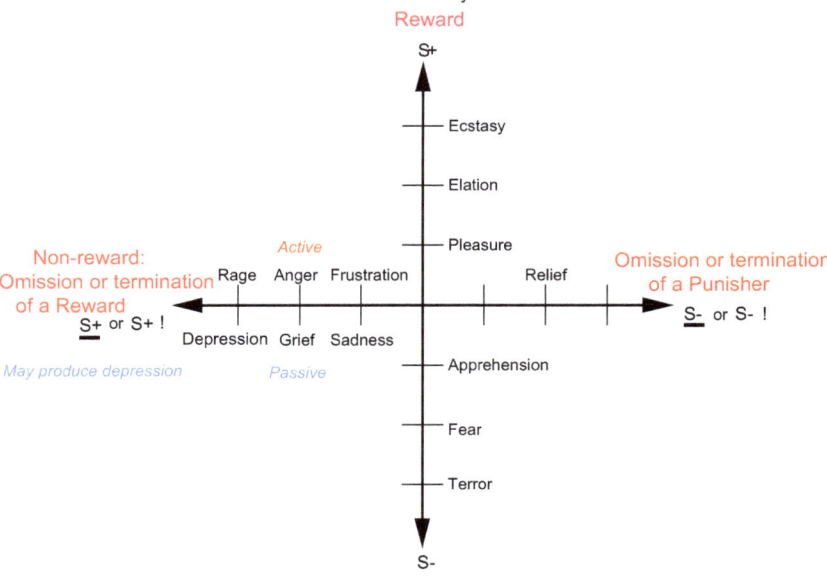

Fig. 6.1 Some of the emotions associated with different reinforcement contingencies are indicated. Intensity increases away from the centre of the diagram, on a continuous scale. The classification scheme created by the different reinforcement contingencies consists with respect to the action of (1) the delivery of a reward (S+), (2) the delivery of a punisher (S–), (3) the omission of a reward (S+) (extinction) or the termination of a reward (S+!) (time out), and (4) the omission of a punisher (S–) (avoidance) or the termination of a punisher (S–!) (escape). Note that the vertical axis describes emotions associated with the delivery of a reward (up) or punisher (down). The horizontal axis describes emotions associated with the non-delivery of an expected reward (left) or the non-delivery of an expected punisher (right). For the contingency of non-reward (horizontal axis, left) different emotions can arise depending on whether an active action is possible to respond to the non-reward, or whether no action is possible, which is labelled as the passive condition. In the passive condition, non-reward may produce depression. The diagram summarizes emotions that might result for one reinforcer as a result of different contingencies. Every separate reinforcer has the potential to operate according to contingencies such as these. This diagram does not imply a dimensional theory of emotion, but shows the types of emotional state that might be produced by a specific reinforcer. Each different reinforcer will produce different emotional states, but the contingencies will operate as shown to produce different specific emotional states for each different reinforcer.

5. What is motivation? Motivation is a state in which we want a goal (e.g. a food reward, or avoiding pain) and are willing to perform an action to obtain the goal.

6. What are moods? These are states in which the eliciting stimulus may not be clear, or may have disappeared some time ago.

7. How do we take decisions?

    One answer I provide is in terms of attractor networks, which are described in Section 3.13. They have the interesting property that they are influenced by randomness in the exact times at which neurons fire in the brain, which makes our decision-making a little non-deterministic and probabilistic. This randomness (or stochasticity) is evolutionarily adaptive, and contributes in other brain areas to original thought and creativity.

    Another answer is that humans, and perhaps closely related animals, have a second, reasoning, system for making decisions (Rolls 2014a, Rolls 2018b) (Section 6.4). This can make long-term decisions, which can be for the good of the individual, and not primarily for the good of the genes. These two properties make the two decision-making systems have quite different aims or goals, and this can lead to internal conflict in decision-making. I argue that these two systems are, generally across a large population, in balance; and that there may be considerable differences between individuals in their relative importance. I also argue that which system (the emotional or the rational) is used for any particular decision is influenced by the randomness (stochasticity) just

introduced.
8. Why do emotional states feel like something? This is part of the large problem of consciousness, which I address elsewhere (Rolls 2012c, Rolls 2014a, Rolls 2018b).
9. Why can emotions feel so strong in humans? I address this briefly here, and in more detail elsewhere (Rolls 2014a, Rolls 2018b).

Emotion and motivation are linked by the property that both involve rewards and punishers. Emotions can be thought of as states elicited by rewards or punishers. Motivation can be thought of as a state in which a goal is being sought, such as reward, or avoidance of a punisher. An example of a reward might be the food obtained when one has performed an action to obtain the food. An example of a motivational state might be hunger, when one wants to perform an action in order to obtain a food reward. These definitions and concepts are summarized next, and are further developed elsewhere (Rolls 2014a, Rolls 2018b).

To help clarify some of the fundamental ways in which emotion is linked to instrumental reinforcers, but not to all properties of stimuli that happen to be rewards or punishers, and as a guide to further research, it is useful to specify some important points about Rolls' theory of emotion (Rolls, 2014a). First, the theory specifies that it is instrumental reinforcers, which specify the goals for action, that produce emotions. The theory is set in an evolutionary, Darwinian context, for it holds that the specification by genes of a set of primary reinforcers (such as sweet taste when hungry, affiliative touch, pain, attachment, altruism) is an efficient way for genes to direct adaptive behaviour, and is much more efficient than specifying actions (such as climbing a tree when an apple is seen, reaching for the apple, and putting it in the mouth). By specifying the goals for action, the process allows the actual behaviour required to obtain the goal to be learned, providing great flexibility in the actions. The actual emotion that is produced by the reinforcer depends on the contingency (delivery of a reward or punisher; omission or termination of a reward or punisher); on the primary reinforcer; and on the particular secondary reinforcer (Rolls 2014a). The point made here is that it is by virtue of being a goal for action that instrumental reinforcers produce emotions. A stimulus that happens to be an instrumental reinforcer may be able to produce many other effects, and disrupting these other effects might not alter emotions. This is important when interpreting the effects of brain damage on emotion and reinforcers: it is only the goal-related aspect of the reinforcing stimulus that the theory holds is closely related to emotion (Rolls 2014a). An example comes from considering autonomic responses. An instrumental reinforcer such as sweet taste when hungry will produce autonomic responses such as salivation (and these can be classically conditioned). But the mechanisms and brain's circuitry for producing salivation, and more generally for classical (Pavlovian) conditioning (see Section 3.2 of Rolls (2014a)), may be quite different from the circuitry involved in specifying a stimulus as a goal for action, and performing action-outcome instrumental learning (where outcome refers to whether the reinforcer, the goal for action, is received). (This highlights how different Rolls' theory of emotion (Rolls 2014a, Rolls 2018b) is to that of Damasio (1994), who argues that emotions are related to autonomic feedback, and his theory is not based on the concept of emotions as being states elicited by instrumental reinforcers.) Evidence that autonomic effects are not required for emotions (Rolls 2014a) includes findings that patients with peripheral autonomic failure do not suffer from disrupted emotions (Heims, Critchley, Dolan, Mathias & Cipolotti 2004).

Reinforcing stimuli may produce many other effects (Rolls 2014a), including informational in which they may not be acting as a goal for an action (Murray & Izquierdo 2007); Pavlovian Instrumental Transfer in which a classically conditioned stimulus may enhance instrumental behaviour (Cardinal et al. 2002); and incentive effects in which reward devaluation outside the instrumental task may not immediately influence the goal value with respect to instrumental actions etc (Cardinal et al. 2002). In summary, we would expect a close link between the goal-related aspects of the reinforcing stimulus and emotion, but not necessarily between other effects produced by stimuli that happen to be instrumental reinforcers, or produce classically conditioned effects (see Section 3.2 of Rolls (2014a). It is important to appreciate this when assessing whether there are in fact any dissociations between brain mechanisms involved in emotion and brain mechanisms that are involved in instrumental learning where the stimulus acts as a goal for action as in action-outcome learning (cf. Murray & Izquierdo (2007)). In so far as classical (Pavlovian) conditioning can influence instrumental actions, for example in some of the ways described above, then this type of learning can play a role in emotion, and indeed the amygdala has been implicated in some of these classically conditioned effects on emotion (Cardinal et al. 2002) (see Section 6.5). Further, in so far as stimulus-reinforcer association learning (also known as stimulus-outcome learning, where the outcome is the reinforcer) is essential for defining the goals for action when the stimulus is associated by learning with a reinforcer, then this is very important in emotion, and neurons in the orbitofrontal cortex learn this type of association, and can reverse it rapidly, and this is a fundamental role that the orbitofrontal cortex plays in emotion. The use of these goals identified by associative learning for association with action to implement action-outcome learning is a process that takes place beyond the orbitofrontal cortex, in structures to which it projects such as the anterior cingulate cortex.

To make the point in everyday language, Rolls' theory of emotion (Rolls 2014a) holds that emotions are states elicited by goals (which are reinforcers). Does not this resonate with common understanding of emotions? Do we not have emotions when we attain our goals; and if we do not?

We may note that it is not an improvement to the theory to hold that the goal for which the animal or human works is the emotional state, for this does not provide an answer, but immediately leads to the questions: What is it that accounts for these emotional states? Why and how are emotions related to goals for action? How are emotional states selected for in evolution so that they are produced by something in the environment? That approach would not provide an explanation, but would just raise questions. It is much clearer to hold that instrumental reinforcers are selected in evolution to be the goals for action because they are a way for genes to specify useful goals in terms of survival value; and then to note that the states elicited by these instrumental reinforcers are emotional states (Rolls 2014a). Unless exceptions are found to this rule (that instrumental reinforcers in their goal-related effects produce emotional states, and that emotional states are produced by instrumental reinforcers in their goal-related effects), then this seems a powerful account of emotions (Rolls 2014a).

Second, action-outcome learning, not habit learning, even though the latter is instrumental, is what the theory holds is related to emotion (Rolls 2014a). If a rewarded behaviour is performed for a large number of trials, it becomes a habit and may be implemented by stimulus-response associations that are formed in brain regions such as the basal ganglia (Rolls 2014a). After such overlearning, the behaviour may be performed rather automatically and calmly, without much emotion, as in a well-learned active avoidance task. It is therefore argued that instrumental behaviour when performed in this automated way by a 'habit' system does not require the type of processing that is related to emotion. On the other hand, while the instrumental behaviour is being learned, associations are being formed between actions and outcomes, and the outcomes are being tested to see whether they meet the goals. Thus in action-outcome learning the goals are being explicitly processed and are instrumental reinforcers, and are being met or not, and it is in these conditions of goal-related events that the theory holds that emotions arise (Rolls 2014a).

Third, the instrumental reinforcer and the emotion correspond. If a food reward is not given, the emotional state will be different from when a social reinforcer is not given, or when a monetary reward is not given (Rolls 2014a). As there is some dissociation between brain systems involved in processing different instrumental reinforcers, the prediction is that a particular emotion will only be impaired if the relevant brain system involved in representing the goals or instrumental reinforcers involved in that particular emotion are impaired. It would of course be necessary to test cases where this correspondence of instrumental reinforcer and the emotion being measured applies in order to test whether instrumental reinforcers are linked to emotional states. It would be important to consider this when assessing the effects of lesions on emotion (cf. Murray & Izquierdo (2007).

Because of the importance of reward and punishment for emotion and motivation, and for understanding the functions of the orbitofrontal cortex, I define in Section 6.2 reward and punishment, and describe some of the types of learning that involve rewards and punishers. However, for those who wish in a first reading to skip the definitions in Section 6.2 (which are provided to ensure that there is a firm foundation for understanding emotion, motivation, and the functions of the orbitofrontal cortex), it may be useful simply to think of a reward as something for which an animal (which includes humans) will work, and a punisher as something that an animal will work to escape from or avoid.

Some stimuli are innately rewarding or punishing and are called primary reinforcers (for example no learning is necessary to respond to pain as aversive), while other stimuli are learned or secondary reinforcers (for example the sight of a chocolate cake is not innately rewarding, but may become a learned reinforcer, for which we may work, by the process of association learning between the sight of the cake and its taste, where the taste is a primary reward or reinforcer). This type of learning, which is important in emotion and motivation, is called stimulus–reinforcement association learning. (A better term is stimulus–reinforcer association learning, where reinforcer is being used to mean a stimulus that might be a reward or a punisher.)

6.2 Rewards and punishers, and learning about rewards and punishers: instrumental learning and stimulus–reinforcer association learning

A reward is something for which an animal (including of course a human) will work. A punisher is something that an animal will work to escape or avoid (or that will decrease the probability of actions on which it is contingent). In order to exclude simple reflex-like behaviour, the concept invoked here by the term 'work' is to perform an arbitrary behaviour (called an operant response) in order to obtain the reward or avoid the punisher. An example of an operant response might be putting money in a vending machine to obtain food, or for a rat pressing a lever to obtain food. In these cases, the food is the reward. Another example of an operant response might be moving from one place to another in order to escape from or avoid an aversive (punishing) stimulus such as a cold draught. If the aversive stimulus starts and then the response is made, this is referred to as *escape* from the punisher. If a warning stimulus (such as a flashing light) indicates that the punisher will be delivered unless the operant response is made, then the animal may learn to perform the operant response when the warning stimulus is given in order to *avoid* the punisher.

Because the definitions of reward and punisher make it a requirement that it must be at least possible to demonstrate learning of an arbitrary operant response (made to obtain the reward or to escape from or avoid the punisher), we see that learning is implicit in the definition of reward and punisher. (Merely swimming up a chemical gradient towards a source of food as occurs in single cell organisms is called a taxis; it does not require learning, and does not make the food qualify as a reward under the definition.) In that rewards and punishers do imply the ability to learn what to do to obtain the reward or escape from or avoid the punisher, we call rewards and punishers 'instrumental reinforcers', because they are reinforcers that are obtained when actions are instrumental when trying to obtain goals, the rewards.

This introduction leads to the definition of instrumental **reinforcers** as stimuli that if their occurrence, termination, or omission is made contingent upon the making of an action, alter the probability of the future emission of that action (as a result of the contingency (i.e. dependency) on the action). The alteration of the probability of an action (or behavioural response) is the measure that instrumental learning has taken place to obtain a goal. A positive reinforcer (such as food) increases the probability of emission of an action on which it is contingent; the process is termed **positive reinforcement**, and the outcome is a reward (such as food). A negative reinforcer (such as a painful stimulus) increases the probability of emission of an action which causes the negative reinforcer to be omitted (as in active avoidance) or terminated (as in escape), and the procedure is termed **negative reinforcement**. In contrast, **punishment** refers to procedures in which the probability of an action is decreased. Punishment thus describes procedures in which an action decreases in probability if it is followed by a painful stimulus, as in passive avoidance. Punishment can also be used to refer to a procedure involving the omission or termination of a reward ('extinction' and 'time out' respectively), both of which decrease the probability of actions (Gray 1975, Mackintosh 1983, Dickinson 1980, Lieberman 2000, Mazur 2012).

My argument is that an affectively positive or 'appetitive' stimulus (which produces a state of pleasure) acts operationally as a **reward**, which when delivered acts instrumentally as a positive reinforcer, or when not delivered (omitted or terminated) acts to decrease the probability of actions on which it is contingent. Conversely I argue that an affectively negative or aversive stimulus (which produces an unpleasant state) acts operationally as a **punisher**, which when delivered acts instrumentally to decrease the probability of actions on which it is contingent, or when not delivered (escaped from or avoided) acts as a negative reinforcer in that it then increases the probability of the action on which its non-delivery is contingent[9] (Rolls 2014a).

Reinforcers, that is rewards or punishers, may be unlearned or **primary reinforcers**, or learned or secondary reinforcers. An example of a primary reinforcer is pain, which is innately a punisher. The first time a painful stimulus is ever delivered, it will be escaped from, and no learning that it is aversive is needed. Similarly, the first time a sweet taste is delivered, it can act as a positive reinforcer, so it is a primary positive reinforcer or reward. Other stimuli become reinforcing by learning, because of their association with primary reinforcers, thereby becoming '**secondary reinforcers**'. For example, a (previously neutral) sound that regularly precedes an electric shock can become a secondary reinforcer. Animals will learn operant responses (actions) reinforced by the secondary reinforcer, for example jumping to a place where the secondary reinforcer is not present or terminates. Secondary reinforcers are thus important in enabling animals to avoid primary punishers such as pain.

There is a close relation of all these processes to emotion, for fear is an emotional state that might be produced by a sound that has previously been associated with an electric shock. Shock in this example is the primary punisher, and fear is the emotional state that occurs to the tone stimulus as a result of the learning of the stimulus (i.e. tone)–reinforcer (i.e. shock)

---

[9]Note that my definition of a punisher, which is similar to that of an aversive stimulus, is of a stimulus or event that can either decrease the probability of actions on which it is contingent, or increase the probability of actions on which its non-delivery is contingent. The term punishment is restricted to situations where the probability of an action is being decreased.

association. Another example of a secondary reinforcer is a visual stimulus associated with the taste of a food. For example, the first time we see a new type of food we do not treat the sight of the new visual stimulus as reinforcing, but if the stimulus has a good taste, the sight of the object becomes a positive secondary reinforcer, and we may choose the food when we see it in future by virtue of its association with a primary reinforcer. This type of learning is thus called '**stimulus–reinforcer association learning**'. (The operation is often referred to as stimulus–reinforcement association learning.) This type of learning is very important in many emotions, because it is as a result of this type of learning that many previously neutral stimuli come to elicit emotional responses, as in the example of fear above.

Unconditioned reinforcing stimuli often elicit autonomic responses. (Autonomic responses are those mediated through the autonomic nervous system, via the vagus and sympathetic nerves, which affect smooth muscle.) Examples include alterations of heart rate and of blood pressure which might be produced by a painful stimulus; and salivation which might be produced by the taste of food. Many endocrine (hormonal) responses are also mediated through the autonomic nervous system and so are autonomic responses, for example the release of adrenaline (epinephrine) from the adrenal gland during emotional excitement. Previously neutral stimuli, such as the sound in our previous example, can by pairing with unconditioned stimuli, such as shock in the previous example, come by learning the association, to produce learned autonomic responses. In the example the tone might by pairing with shock come to elicit a change in heart rate, and sweating. This type of learning is called **classical conditioning**, and also **Pavlovian conditioning** after Ivan Pavlov who performed many of the original studies of this type of learning, including learned salivation to the sound of a bell that predicted the taste of food. It is a type of learning that is very similar to stimulus–reinforcer association learning, except that in the case of classical conditioning the responses involved are autonomic and endocrine responses.

A key difference between **instrumental learning** and classical conditioning apart from the response systems involved lies in the contingencies that operate. In classical conditioning the animal has no control over whether the unconditioned stimulus is delivered (as in the experiments of Pavlov just described). In contrast, the whole notion of instrumental learning is that what the animal does is instrumental in determining whether the reinforcer (the goal) is obtained, or escaped from or avoided. Both types of learning are important in emotions because instrumental reinforcers produce emotional responses, but also typically produce autonomic responses that therefore typically occur during emotional states, and indeed mediate important effects of emotions such as preparing the body for action by increasing heart rate etc.

A more detailed description of the nature of classical (Pavlovian) conditioning and instrumental learning, and how both are related to emotion, is provided by Rolls (2014a).

Motivation refers to the state an animal is in when it is willing to work for a reward or to escape from or avoid a punisher. So for example we say that an animal is motivated to work for the taste of food, and in this case the motivational state is called hunger. The definition of motivation thus implies the capacity to perform any, arbitrary, operant response in order to obtain the reward or escape from or avoid the punisher. By implying an operant response, we exclude simple behaviours such as reflexes and taxes (such as swimming up a chemical gradient), as described above. By implying learning of any response to obtain a reward (or avoid a punisher), motivation thus focuses on behaviours in which a goal is defined. Motivation is one of the states that are involved in understanding brain design, related to the fundamental issue of how goals for behaviour are defined, and how an appropriate behaviour is selected, as described in this book and brought together into a theory elsewhere (Rolls 2014a, Rolls 2018b).

This treatment of rewards and punishers provides background to what is described in Chapter 3, for it clarifies the operations involved in the functions of the orbitofrontal cortex in expected reward value and outcome reward value, and in understanding how these processes are related to emotion. Indeed, emotions can be distinguished by their relationship to different reinforcement contingencies, as shown in Fig. 6.1. What is shown in this Figure relates to emotional states that may relate to any one reinforcer. As shown in Chapter 3, there are many different reinforcers, each operated on by the types of reinforcement contingency set out in Fig. 6.1, so the number of emotions that can be accounted for in this way is very large, as described fully elsewhere (Rolls 2014a, Rolls 2018b).

6.3 Individual differences in emotion, personality, and the orbitofrontal cortex

Given that there are individual differences in emotion, can these individual differences be related to the functioning of brain systems involved in affective behaviour such as the orbitofrontal and pregenual cingulate cortex? Part of the background is that differential sensitivity to reward, punishment, non-reward, and relief (see Fig. 6.1) may underlie differences in personality (Eysenck & Eysenck 1985, Gray 1970, Rolls 2014a, Rolls 2018b).

Some individuals, chocolate cravers, report that they crave chocolate more than non-cravers, and this is associated with increased liking of chocolate, increased wanting of chocolate, and eating chocolate more frequently than non-cravers (Rodriguez, Warren, Moreno, Cepeda-Benito, Gleaves, Del Carmen Fernandez & Vila 2007). In a test of whether these individual differences are reflected in the affective systems in the orbitofrontal cortex and pregenual cingulate cortex, Rolls & McCabe (2007) used fMRI to measure the response to the flavor of chocolate, to the sight of chocolate, and to their combination, in chocolate cravers vs non-cravers. SPM analyses showed that the sight of chocolate produced more activation in chocolate cravers than non-cravers in the medial orbitofrontal cortex and ventral striatum. For cravers vs non-cravers, a combination of a picture of chocolate with chocolate in the mouth produced a greater effect than the sum of the components (i.e. supralinearity) in the medial orbitofrontal cortex and pregenual cingulate cortex. Furthermore, the pleasantness ratings of the chocolate and chocolate-related stimuli had higher positive correlations with the fMRI BOLD signals in the pregenual cingulate cortex and medial orbitofrontal cortex in the cravers than in the non-cravers. Thus there were differences between cravers and non-cravers in their responses to the sensory components of a craved food in the orbitofrontal cortex, pregenual cingulate cortex, and ventral striatum, and in some of these regions the differences are related to the subjective pleasantness of the craved foods. An implication is that individual differences in brain responses to very pleasant foods help to understand the mechanisms that drive the liking for specific foods by indicating that some brain systems (but not others such as the insular taste cortex) respond more to the rewarding aspects of some foods, and thus influence and indeed even predict the intake of those foods (which was much higher in chocolate cravers than non-cravers) (Rolls & McCabe 2007).

Investigating another difference between individuals, it was found that reward sensitivity in different individuals (as measured by a behavioural activation scale) is correlated with activations in the orbitofrontal cortex and ventral striatum to pictures of appetizing vs disgusting food (Beaver, Lawrence, Ditzhuijzen, Davis, Woods & Calder 2006).

When cognitive labels (such as 'Rich delicious flavour') modulate humans' ratings of the pleasantness of flavor, it is possible that some individuals are more affected by this suggestion than others. We investigated this in relation to the study by Grabenhorst et al. (2008a) on cognitive effects on flavor by measuring the suggestibility of the subjects using parts of the SHSS (Stanford Hypnotic) Suggestibility Scale (Weitzenhoffer & Hilgard 1962). It was found that one of the most reliable measures in this scale, the moving hands apart test in which subjects are told that there is a force pushing the hands apart, was correlated with the magnitude of the effect of the cognitive label 'Rich delicious flavour' on the pleasantness rating of a standard flavor (r=0.71, df=9, p=0.023) in the subjects used in this study. An implication is that an underlying personality variable related to suggestibility is also related to cognitive effects on affective ratings (and thus emotion), with the brain region showing a large modulation of its BOLD response by the cognitive labels to these stimuli being the medial orbitofrontal cortex and pregenual cingulate cortex (Grabenhorst et al. 2008a).

In addition, as described elsewhere (Section 3.8), in the context that there are many types of impulsiveness (Dalley & Robbins 2017), we have argued that one mechanism promoting impulsiveness may be under-connectedness of the lateral orbitofrontal cortex non-reward system (Cheng, Rolls, Robbins, Gong, Liu, Lv, Du, Wen, Ma, Quinlan, Garavan, Artiges, Papadopoulos Orfanos, Smolka, Schumann, Kendrick & Feng 2019). Another mechanism that may promote impulsiveness is over-connectedness of the medial orbitofrontal cortex reward system (Cheng et al. 2019). Consistent with this, sensation-seeking is associated with increased functional connectivity of the medial orbitofrontal cortex with the anterior cingulate cortex (Wan, Rolls, Cheng & Feng 2019).

Further, as described in Section 3.16, those who smoke have low functional connectivity of the lateral orbitofrontal cortex, which may promote impulsiveness and the administration of nicotine which may act to increase activity generally in the brain, in that those who tend to smoke have low overall functional connectivity (Cheng, Rolls et al (2019)). Those who drink have high functional connectivity of the medial orbitofrontal cortex (Cheng et al. 2019), which may promote sensation-seeking (Wan et al. 2019). These results were obtained in a study with more than 2000 participants. These differences were related to personality, in that increased impulsivity was found in smokers, associated with decreased functional connectivity of the non-reward-related lateral orbitofrontal cortex; and increased impulsivity was found in high amount drinkers, associated with increased functional connectivity of the reward-related medial orbitofrontal cortex (Cheng et al. 2019).

6.4 Emotional orbitofrontal vs rational routes to action

The introduction to emotion above provides a firm conceptual framework for understanding why the orbitofrontal cortex is so important in emotion, as considered also in Emotion and Decision-Making Explained (Rolls 2014a). In the present section, I show that at least in humans, there are other routes to action that can be invoked in emotion-related situations in which the orbitofrontal cortex may take a role in emotion and action, but not necessarily the whole or only part.

6.4.1 Some of the different routes to action produced by emotion-related stimuli

Fig. 3.1 on page 18 shows two major routes to behaviour related to emotional stimuli. The first may involve the orbitofrontal cortex (and amygdala) projecting to the habit system (in which the basal ganglia are implicated), and projecting to a system for goal-directed action-outcome learning, in which the cingulate cortex is implicated. This route is sometimes described as operating implicitly, which implies without consciousness, though the issue of conscious feelings is described elsewhere (Rolls 2014a, Rolls 2018b).

The second route is described as involving a **reasoning system** that may use some form of language involving syntax (grammar) to plan several steps ahead. It is this second route on which I focus in this Section, for it enables actions to be performed for completely different goals than those specified by genes as primary reinforcers which can use the first route just described for output. This reasoning system is very important for understanding human emotion, because its decisions can be made in a completely different way, and do not necessarily lead to decisions that are consistent with those specified by the gene-defined reinforcers that are important in the first 'emotion-related' route to behavioural output. I argue in this Section that our reasoning system enables us to go beyond what 'Selfish Genes' might encourage (Dawkins 1976), and that when we use the term 'free will', it is to the rational system that we may wish to refer, together with the non-deterministic, probabilistic, nature of brain computation (Rolls 2012c, Rolls 2014a, Rolls 2016c).

I will give a simple example to make the point clear. Our genes may predispose us to like foods that are sweet and fatty (with modern supernormal examples ice cream and chocolate), and these may be rewarding to us because of the processes taking place in brain regions such as the orbitofrontal cortex and amygdala. But our reasoning system may know about discoveries in science and medicine that provide evidence that these foods may tend to promote obesity and poor health if eaten in quantity. So our reasoning system may enable us to override what our gene-based emotional system involving the orbitofrontal cortex urges, and instead to eat the healthy foods, for the potential advantage to the individual person of a healthy and long life.

6.4.2 Examples of some complex behaviours that may be performed implicitly

A starting point is that many actions can be performed relatively automatically, without apparent conscious intervention, that is implicitly.

An example sometimes given is driving a car for a short distance while the person may be thinking about something else.

Another example is the identification of a visual stimulus that can occur without conscious awareness if the stimulus is very short (as in backward masking) or weak (Rolls & Tovee 1994, Rolls 2003).

Another example is much of the sensory processing and actions that involve the dorsal stream of visual processing to the parietal cortex, such as a patient posting a letter through a letter box at the correct orientation even when the patient may not be aware of what the object is (Milner & Goodale 1995, Goodale 2004, Milner 2008) because of damage to the ventral visual stream which implements object recognition (Rolls 2016c).

Another example is blindsight, in which humans with damage to the visual cortex may be able to point to objects even when they are not aware of seeing an object (Weiskrantz 1997, Weiskrantz 1998, Weiskrantz 2009).

Similar evidence applies to emotions, some of the processing for which can occur without conscious awareness (De Gelder, Vroomen, Pourtois & Weiskrantz 1999, Phelps & LeDoux 2005, LeDoux 2008, LeDoux & Pine 2016, LeDoux et al. 2018).

Consistent with the hypothesis of multiple routes to action, only some of which involve conscious awareness, is the evidence that split-brain patients may not be aware of actions being performed by the 'non-dominant' hemisphere (Gazzaniga & LeDoux 1978, Gazzaniga 1988, Gazzaniga 1995).

Also consistent with multiple, including non-verbal, routes to action, patients with focal brain damage, for example to the orbitofrontal cortex, may perform actions, yet comment verbally that they should not be performing those actions (Rolls et al. 1994a, Hornak et al. 2003) (Section 4.2). In both these types of patient, confabulation may occur, in that a verbal account of why the action was performed may be given, and this may not be related at all to the environmental event that actually triggered the action (Gazzaniga & LeDoux 1978, Gazzaniga 1988, Gazzaniga 1995, Rolls, Hornak, Wade & McGrath 1994a).

6.4.3 A reasoning, rational, route to action

The second ('explicit') route in (at least) humans involves a computation with many 'if ... then' statements, to implement a plan to obtain a reward. In this case, the reward may actually be deferred as part of the plan, which might involve working first to obtain one reward, and only then to work for a second more highly valued reward, if this was thought to be overall an optimal strategy in terms of resource usage (e.g. time). In this case, syntax is required, because the many symbols (e.g. names of people) that are part of the plan must be correctly linked or bound. Such linking might be of the form: 'if A does this, then B is likely to do this, and this will cause C to do this ...'. The requirement of syntax for this type of planning implies that involvement of a syntactic system in the brain is required (see Fig. 3.1). **Thus the explicit language system in humans may allow working for deferred rewards by enabling use of a one-off, individual, plan appropriate for each situation.** This explicit system may allow immediate rewards to be deferred, as part of a long-term plan. This ability to defer immediate rewards and plan syntactically in this way for the long term may be an important way in which the explicit system extends the capabilities of the implicit emotion systems that respond more directly to rewards and punishers, or to rewards and punishers with fixed expectancies such as can be learned by reinforcement learning.

Consistent with the point being made about evolutionarily old emotion-based decision systems vs a recent rational system present in humans (and perhaps other animals with syntactic processing) is that humans trade off immediate costs/benefits against cost/benefits that are delayed by as much as decades, whereas non-human primates have not been observed to engage in unpreprogrammed delay of gratification involving more than a few minutes (Rachlin 1989, Kagel, Battalio & Green 1995, McClure, Laibson, Loewenstein & Cohen 2004, Rosati 2017).

Another building block for such planning operations in the brain may be the type of short-term memory in which the prefrontal cortex is involved. This short-term memory may be, for example in non-human primates, of where in space a response has just been made. A development of this type of short-term memory system in humans to enable multiple short-term memories to be held in place correctly, preferably with the temporal order of the different items in the short-term memory coded correctly, may be another building block for the multiple step 'if .... then' type of computation in order to form a multiple step plan. Such short-term memories are implemented in the (dorsolateral and inferior convexity) prefrontal cortex of non-human primates and humans (Goldman-Rakic 1996, Petrides 1996, Deco & Rolls 2003, Rolls 2016c), and may be part of the reason why prefrontal cortex damage impairs planning and executive function (Gilbert & Burgess 2008).

We may examine some of the advantages and behavioural functions that language, present as the most recently added layer to the above system (Fig. 3.1), would confer.

One major advantage would be the ability to plan actions through many potential stages and to evaluate the consequences of those actions without having to perform the actions. For this, the ability to form propositional statements, and to perform syntactic operations on the semantic representations of states in the world, would be important.

Also important in this system would be the ability to have second-order thoughts about the type of thought that I have just described (e.g. I think that she thinks that ..., involving 'theory of mind'), as this would allow much better modelling and prediction of others' behaviour, and therefore of planning, particularly planning when it involves others. Second-order thoughts are thoughts about thoughts. Higher-order thoughts refer to second-order, third-order, etc., thoughts about thoughts... This capability for higher-order thoughts would also enable reflection on past events, which would also be useful in planning [10].

In contrast, non-linguistic behaviour would be driven by learned reinforcement associations, learned rules etc., but not by flexible planning for many steps ahead involving a model of the world including others' behaviour.

It is important to state that the language ability referred to here is not necessarily human verbal language (though this would be an example). What it is suggested is important to multiple step planning is the syntactic manipulation of symbols, and it is this syntactic manipulation of symbols that is the sense in which language is defined and used here. The type of syntactic processing need not be at the natural language level (which implies a universal grammar), but could be at the level of mentalese (Rolls 2014a, Rolls 2004c, Fodor 1994, Rolls & Deco 2015b).

In summary, I understand **reasoning, and rationality**, to involve syntactic manipulations of symbols. Reasoning thus typically may involve multiple steps of 'if .. then' conditional statements, all executed as a one-off or one-time process (see below), and is very different from associatively learned conditional rules typically learned over many trials, such as 'if yellow, a left choice is associated with reward'.

6.4.4 The Selfish Gene vs The Selfish Phenotype

I have provided evidence in the earlier part of this section (6.4) that there are two main routes to decision-making and action. The first route selects actions by gene-defined goals for action, is closely associated with emotion, and involved brain systems such as the orbitofrontal cortex and cingulate cortex. The second route involves multistep planning and reasoning which requires syntactic processing to keep the symbols involved at each step separate from the symbols in different steps. (This second route is used by humans and perhaps by closely related animals.) Now the 'interests' of the first and second routes to decision-making and action are different. As argued convincingly by Richard Dawkins in *The Selfish Gene* (Dawkins 1976, Dawkins 1989), and by others (Hamilton 1964, Ridley 1993, Hamilton 1996), many behaviours occur in the interests of the survival of the genes, not of the individual (nor of the group), and much behaviour can be understood in this way. I have extended this approach by arguing that an important role for some genes in evolution is to define the goals for actions that will lead to better survival of those genes; that emotions are the states associated with these gene-defined goals; and that the defining of goals for actions rather that actions themselves is an efficient way for genes to operate, as it leaves flexibility of choice of action open until the animal is alive (Rolls 2014a). This provides great simplification of the genotype, as action details do not need to be specified, just rewarding and punishing stimuli, and also provides flexibility of action in the face of changing environments faced by the genes. Thus the interests that are implied when the first route to action (that typically involves the orbitofrontal and cingulate cortices) is chosen are those of the 'selfish genes', not those of the individual.

However, the second route to action allows, by reasoning, decisions to be taken that might not be in the interests of the genes, might be longer term decisions, and might be in the interests of the individual. An example might be a choice not to have children, but instead to devote oneself to science, medicine, music, or literature. The reasoning, rational,

---

[10] A thought may be defined briefly as an intentional mental state, that is a mental state that is about something. Thoughts include beliefs, and are usually described as being propositional (Rosenthal 2005). An example of a thought is "It is raining". A more detailed definition is as follows. A thought may be defined as an occurrent mental state (or event) that is intentional – that is a mental state that is about something – and also propositional, so that it is evaluable as true or false. Thoughts include occurrent beliefs or judgements. An example of a thought would be an occurrent belief that the earth moves around the sun / that Maurice's boat goes faster with two sails / that it never rains in southern California.)

system presumably evolved because taking longer-term decisions involving planning rather than choosing a gene-defined goal might be advantageous at least sometimes for genes. But an unforeseen consequence of the evolution of the rational system might be that the decisions would, sometimes, not be to the advantage of any genes in the organism. After all, evolution by natural selection operates utilizing genetic variation like a Blind Watchmaker (Dawkins 1986). In this sense, the interests when the second route to decision-making is used are at least sometimes those of the 'selfish phenotype'. Hence the decision-making referred to in this Section (6.4) is between a first system where the goals are gene-defined, and a second rational system in which the decisions may be made in the interests of the genes, or in the interests of the phenotype and not in the interests of the genes. Thus we may speak of the choice as sometimes being between the 'Selfish Genes' and the 'Selfish Phenes'.

Now what keeps the decision-making between the 'Selfish Genes' and the 'Selfish Phenes' more or less under control and in balance? If the second, rational, system chose too often for the interests of the 'Selfish Phene', the genes in that phenotype would not survive over generations. Having these two systems in the same individual will only be stable if their potency is approximately equal, so that sometimes decisions are made with the first route, and sometimes with the second route. If the two types of decision-making, then, compete with approximately equal potency, and sometimes one is chosen, and sometimes the other, then this is exactly the scenario in which stochastic processes in the decision-making mechanism are likely to play an important role in the decision that is taken. The same decision, even with the same evidence, may not be taken each time a decision is made, because of noise in the system.

The system itself may have some properties that help to keep the system operating well. One is that if the second, rational, system tends to dominate the decision-making too much, the first, gene-based emotional (orbitofrontal cortex) system might fight back over generations of selection, and enhance the magnitude of the reward value specified by the genes, so that emotions might actually become stronger as a consequence of them having to compete in the interests of the selfish genes with the rational decision-making process.

Another property of the system may be that sometimes the rational system cannot gain all the evidence that would be needed to make a rational choice. Under these circumstances the rational system might fail to make a clear decision, and under these circumstances, basing a decision on the gene-specified emotions involving the orbitofrontal cortex is an alternative. Indeed, Damasio (1994) argued that under circumstances such as this, emotions might take an important role in decision-making. In this respect, I agree with him, basing my reasons on the arguments above. He called the emotional feelings gut feelings, and, in contrast to me, hypothesized that actual feedback from the gut was involved. His argument seemed to be that if the decision was too complicated for the rational system, then send outputs to the viscera, and whatever is sensed by what the periphery sends back could be used in the decision-making, and would account for the conscious feelings of the emotional states. My reading of the evidence is that the feedback from the periphery is not necessary for the emotional decision-making, or for the feelings, nor would it be computationally efficient to put the viscera and more generally the periphery in the loop given that the information starts from the brain (Rolls 2014a).

Another property of operation is that the interests of the second, rational, system, although involving a different form of computation, should not be too far from those of the gene-defined emotional system, for the arrangement to be stable in evolution by natural selection. One way that this could be facilitated would be if the gene-based goals felt pleasant or unpleasant in the rational system, and in this way contributed to the operation of the second, rational, system. This is something that I propose is the case. This provides an account of why rewards feel good (Rolls 2014a).

6.4.5 Decision-making between the implicit and explicit systems

The question then arises of how decisions are made in animals such as humans that have both the implicit, direct reward-based, and the explicit, rational, planning systems (see Fig. 3.1). One particular situation in which the first, implicit, system may be especially important is when rapid reactions to stimuli with reward or punishment value must be made, for then the direct connections from structures such as the orbitofrontal cortex to the basal ganglia may allow rapid actions. Another is that when there may be too many factors to be taken into account easily by the explicit, rational, planning, system, then the implicit system may be used to guide action.

In contrast, when the implicit system continually makes errors, it would then be beneficial for the organism to switch from automatic, direct, action based on obtaining what the orbitofrontal cortex system decodes as being the most positively reinforcing choice currently available, to the explicit conscious control system which can evaluate with its long-term planning algorithms what action should be performed next. Indeed, it would be adaptive for the explicit system to be regularly assessing performance by the more automatic system, and to switch itself in to control behaviour quite frequently, as otherwise the adaptive value of having the explicit system would be less than optimal.

Another factor that may influence the balance between control by the implicit and explicit systems is the presence of pharmacological agents such as alcohol, which may alter the balance towards control by the implicit system, may allow the implicit system to influence more the explanations made by the explicit system, and may within the explicit system alter the relative value it places on caution and restraint vs commitment to a risky action or plan.

There may also be a flow of influence from the explicit, verbal system to the implicit system, in that the explicit system may decide on a plan of action or strategy, and exert an influence on the implicit system that will alter the reinforcement evaluations made by and the signals produced by the implicit system. An example of this might be that if a pregnant woman feels that she would like to escape a cruel mate, but is aware that she may not survive in the jungle, then it would be adaptive if the explicit system could suppress some aspects of her implicit behaviour towards her mate, so that she does not give signals that she is displeased with her situation[11]. Another example might be that the explicit system might, because of its long-term plans, influence the implicit system to increase its response to for example a positive reinforcer. One way in which the explicit system might influence the implicit system is by setting up the conditions in which, for example, when a given stimulus (e.g. person) is present, positive reinforcers are given, to facilitate stimulus–reinforcement association learning by the implicit system of the person receiving the positive reinforcers. Conversely, the implicit system may influence the explicit system, for example by highlighting certain stimuli in the environment that are currently associated with reward, to guide the attention of the explicit system to such stimuli.

However, it may be expected that there is often a conflict between these systems, in that the first, implicit, system is able to guide behaviour particularly to obtain the greatest immediate reinforcement, whereas the explicit system can potentially enable immediate rewards to be deferred, and longer-term, multistep, plans to be formed. This type of conflict will occur in animals with a syntactic planning ability, that is in humans and any other animals that have the ability to process a series of 'if ... then' stages of planning. This is a property of the human language system, and the extent to which it is a property of non-human primates is not yet

---

[11] In the literature on self-deception, it has been suggested that unconscious desires may not be made explicit in consciousness (or actually repressed), so as not to compromise the explicit system in what it produces (Alexander 1979, Trivers 1985, Nesse & Lloyd 1992).

fully clear. In any case, such conflict may be an important aspect of the operation of at least the human mind, because it is so essential for humans to decide correctly, at every moment, whether to invest in a relationship or a group that may offer long-term benefits, or whether to pursue immediate benefits directly (Nesse & Lloyd 1992).

Decision-making as implemented in neural networks in the brain is now becoming understood, and is described in Sections 3.13 and 9.3. As shown there, two attractor states, each one corresponding to a decision, compete in an attractor single network with the evidence for each of the decisions acting as biases to each of the attractor states. The non-linear dynamics, and the way in which noise due to the random spiking of neurons makes the decision-making probabilistic, makes this a biologically plausible model of decision-making consistent with much neurophysiological and fMRI data (Wang 2002, Rolls & Deco 2010, Deco, Rolls, Albantakis & Romo 2013, Rolls 2016c).

I propose (Rolls 2005, Rolls 2014a) that this model applies to taking decisions between the implicit (unconscious) and explicit (conscious) systems in emotional decision-making, where the two different systems could provide the biasing inputs λ_1 and λ_2 to the model. An implication is that noise will influence with probabilistic outcomes which system takes a decision, depending on the magnitude of the competing inputs from the emotional and rational systems.

When decisions are taken, sometimes confabulation may occur, in that a verbal account of why the action was performed may be given, and this may not be related at all to the environmental event that actually triggered the action (Gazzaniga & LeDoux 1978, Gazzaniga 1988, Gazzaniga 1995, Rolls 2014a, LeDoux 2008, Rolls 2012c). It is accordingly possible that sometimes in normal humans when actions are initiated as a result of processing in a specialized brain region such as the orbitofrontal cortex involved in some types of rewarded behaviour, the language system may subsequently elaborate a coherent account of why that action was performed (i.e. confabulate). This would be consistent with a general view of brain evolution in which, as areas of the cortex evolve, they are laid on top of existing circuitry connecting inputs to outputs, and in which each level in this hierarchy of separate input–output pathways may control behaviour according to the specialized function it can perform (Rolls 2016c). This hierarchical overlaying is an important concept for understanding emotion, the different brain systems involved in different aspects of emotion and decision-making, and the relation between the implicit and explicit systems (Rolls 2014a). When a new layer is added, previous layers may lose some of their importance, as appears to occur in the taste system in which in primates the subcortical processing from the brainstem nucleus of the solitary tract is lost; when the granular orbitofrontal cortex of primates becomes relatively more important than the amygdala; and when language areas are added on top of existing circuitry (Fig. 3.1) (Rolls 2016c).

6.5 Comparison between the functions of the orbitofrontal cortex and amygdala in emotion

A brain structure that has similar connections to the orbitofrontal cortex, the amygdala, but is much older in evolution, is described in this section, to help highlight what is special about the orbitofrontal cortex. It will be argued that with the great development of the orbitofrontal cortex in primates including humans, the orbitofrontal cortex becomes much more important in emotion and related functions in humans than the amygdala.

6.5.1 Overview of the functions of the amygdala in emotion

The amygdala is an evolutionarily old subcortical structure with parts of it present in amphibia and reptiles. This is in contrast with the orbitofrontal cortex, which develops greatly in primates including humans as shown in Fig. 1.3.

The connections of the amygdala are similar to those of the orbitofrontal cortex, as shown in Figs. 2.1 and 2.2, and the amygdala connections do involve many with the orbitofrontal cortex.

The amygdala does have neurons that respond to primary reinforcers such as the taste, flavour, and smell of food; touch; and aversive stimuli. The amygdala also has neurons that learn associations between visual and auditory stimuli, and primary reinforcers. However, this learning does not support rule-based one-trial reversal learning, so the amygdala is less good at this rapid emotion-related learning than the orbitofrontal cortex. The primate amygdala also contains a population of neurons specialized to respond to faces, and damage to the human amygdala can alter the ability to discriminate between different facial expressions, though this may be related to how faces are fixated.

Classically conditioned responses such as autonomic, freezing, and startle responses to auditory stimuli can depend on outputs from the amygdala to structures such as the hypothalamus and ventral striatum. Bilateral damage to the amygdala can produce a deficit in learning to associate visual and other stimuli with a primary (i.e. unlearned) reward or punisher. For example, monkeys with damage to the amygdala when shown foods and non-foods pick up both and place them in their mouths. When such visual or auditory discrimination learning is tested more formally, it is found that primates including humans with amygdala damage have difficulty in associating the sight or sound of a stimulus with whether it produces a reward, or is noxious and should be avoided. Sensory-specific satiety (the reduced choice of a food devalued by feeding to satiety) is impaired by damage to the amygdala (as is also the case for the orbitofrontal cortex).

In humans and other primates the amygdala does not appear to play such an important role in emotional and social behaviour as the orbitofrontal cortex, with the changes to emotion much more subtle after amygdala damage. Further, the deficits described after amygdala damage involve fear conditioning (with classical conditioning of for example autonomic responses and effects on startle especially studied), and somewhat subtle aspects of face expression processing. In evolution, the balance may have moved to the orbitofrontal cortex, which has evolved much more recently, and may allow more powerful computations, such as those involved in rapid reversal learning and rapid correction of behaviour, to be implemented, as described in Chapters 3 and 9.

Indeed, LeDoux, who has performed research on the amygdala, is, with colleagues, now suggesting that the amygdala may have little to do with subjective feelings of emotion (LeDoux et al. 2018). In contrast, the orbitofrontal cortex may be much more closely related to emotional feelings, in that activations in it are linearly related to subjective affective ratings of pleasantness, and damage to the orbitofrontal cortex impairs subjective emotional feelings, as described in Chapters 3 and 4.

A much fuller analysis of the functions of the amygdala in emotion in primates including humans is provided by Rolls (2014a), with further human studies described in Whalen & Phelps (2009). The rodent literature and how it has focussed on conditioned responses and not on emotional feelings is described more fully elsewhere (LeDoux 2012, LeDoux & Pine 2016, LeDoux et al. 2018).

6.5.2 The amygdala and the associative processes involved in emotion-related learning

The amygdala is implicated in some learning processes involved in emotion including some classically conditioned effects, but not in other learning processes involved in emotion. To clarify this, I briefly summarize some of these learning processes, with a much fuller analysis provided elsewhere (Cardinal, Parkinson, Hall & Everitt 2002, Rolls 2014a).

When a conditioned stimulus (CS) (such as a tone) is paired with a primary reinforcer or unconditioned stimulus (US) (such as a painful stimulus), then there are opportunities for a number of types of association to be formed.

Some of these involve 'classical conditioning' or 'Pavlovian conditioning', in which no action is performed that affects the contingency between the conditioned stimulus and the unconditioned stimulus. Typically an unconditioned response (UR), for example an alteration of heart rate, is produced by the US, and will come to be elicited by the CS as a conditioned response (CR). These responses are typically autonomic (such as the heart beating faster), or endocrine (for example the release of adrenaline (epinephrine in American usage) by the adrenal gland).

In addition, the organism may learn to perform an instrumental response with the skeletal muscles in order to alter the probability that the primary reinforcer will be obtained. In our example, the experimenter might alter the contingencies so that when the tone sounded, if the organism performed an action such as pressing a lever, then the painful stimulus could be avoided. This is confirmed to be instrumental learning if the response learned is arbitrary, for example performing the opposite response, such as raising the lever to avoid the painful stimulus.

In the instrumental learning situation there are still opportunities for many classically conditioned responses including emotional states such as fear to occur. For example, in Pavlovian–instrumental transfer, if a stimulus that predicts the arrival of sucrose as a result of Pavlovian conditioning is provided during an instrumental task such as working to obtain sucrose, the responding (e.g. lever pressing) can be enhanced. Further, approach to a food may be under Pavlovian rather than instrumental control. Finally, we must beware of the facts that after overtraining, habits may be formed in which stimuli may become inflexibly linked to responses, with the reward value of the goal no longer directly influencing behaviour, as shown by the fact that the response may continue for at least one trial after the goal has been devalued by for example feeding to satiety. This had led to some confusion in the literature (Berridge & Robinson 1998, Berridge, Robinson & Aldridge 2009), for when the goal controls the behaviour, wanting is driven by liking, and what happens during habits is not an exception, as habits are stimulus-response associations and have little to do with wanting or liking a goal (Rolls 2014a, Rolls 2013c).

6.5.3 Connections of the amygdala

The amygdala is a subcortical region in the anterior part of the temporal lobe. It receives massive projections in the primate from the overlying temporal lobe cortex (Van Hoesen 1981, Amaral, Price, Pitkanen & Carmichael 1992, Ghashghaei & Barbas 2002, Freese & Amaral 2009) (see Fig. 6.2). Via these inputs, the amygdala receives inputs about objects and faces that could become secondary reinforcers, as a result of pattern association in the amygdala with primary reinforcers. The amygdala also receives inputs that are potentially about primary reinforcers, e.g. taste inputs (from the insula, and from the secondary taste cortex in the orbitofrontal cortex), and somatosensory inputs, potentially about the rewarding or painful aspects of touch (from the somatosensory cortex via the insula). The amygdala

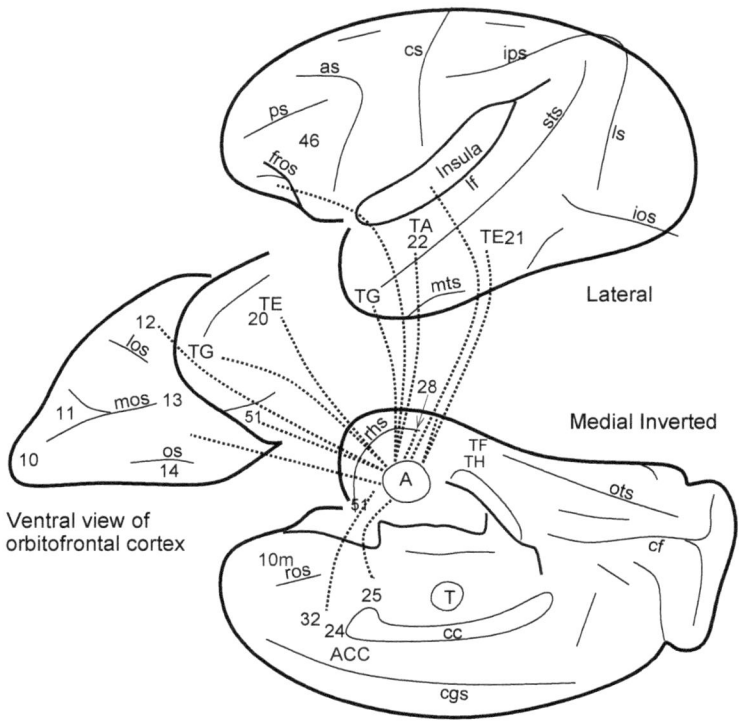

Fig. 6.2 Connections of the amygdala shown on lateral, ventral, and medial inverted views of the monkey brain. Abbreviations: as, arcuate sulcus; cc, corpus callosum; cf, calcarine fissure; cgs, cingulate sulcus; cs, central sulcus; ls, lunate sulcus; ios, inferior occipital sulcus; mos, medial orbital sulcus; os, orbital sulcus; ots, occipito-temporal sulcus; ps, principal sulcus; rhs, rhinal sulcus; sts, superior temporal sulcus; lf, lateral (or Sylvian) fissure (which has been opened to reveal the insula); A, amygdala; ACC, anterior cingulate cortex; INS, insula; T, thalamus; TE (21), inferior temporal visual cortex; TA (22), superior temporal auditory association cortex; TF and TH, parahippocampal cortex; TG, temporal pole cortex; 12, 13, 11, orbitofrontal cortex; 24, 32, parts of the anterior cingulate cortex; 25, subgenual cingulate cortex; 28, entorhinal cortex; 51, olfactory (prepyriform and periamygdaloid) cortex. The cortical connections shown provide afferents to the amygdala, but are reciprocated. (Modified from G. W. Van Hoesen, The differential distribution, diversity and sprouting of cortical projections to the amygdala in the rhesus monkey, in Y. Ben-Ari (ed.), The Amygdaloid Complex, pp. 77–90 © 1981 Elsevier, with permission.)

receives strong projections from the posterior orbitofrontal cortex (see Fig. 6.2, areas 12 and 13) where there are value representations, and from the anterior cingulate cortex (Carmichael & Price 1995a, Ghashghaei & Barbas 2002, Freese & Amaral 2009).

Although there are some inputs from early on in some sensory pathways, for example auditory inputs from the medial geniculate nucleus (LeDoux 1992, Pessoa & Adolphs 2010), this route is unlikely to be involved in most emotions, for which cortical analysis of the stimulus is likely to be required. Emotions are usually elicited to environmental stimuli analysed to the object level (including other organisms), and not to retinal arrays of spots or the frequency (tone) of a sound as represented in the cochlea.

Some of the outputs of the amygdala relevant to different types of response in rodents are shown in Fig. 6.3, and in addition there are backprojections to the neocortical areas that project to the amygdala.

6.5.4 Effects of amygdala lesions

6.5.4.1 Amygdala lesions in primates

Bilateral removal of the amygdala in monkeys produces striking behavioural changes which include tameness, a lack of emotional responsiveness, excessive examination of objects, often with the mouth, and eating of previously rejected items such as meat (Weiskrantz 1956). These behavioural changes comprise much of the Kluver–Bucy syndrome which is produced in monkeys by bilateral anterior temporal lobectomy (Kluver & Bucy 1939). In analyses of the bases of these behavioural changes, it has been observed that there are deficits in some types of learning. For example, Larry Weiskrantz (1956) found that bilateral ablation of the amygdala in the monkey produced a deficit on learning an active avoidance task. The monkeys failed to learn to make a response when a light signalled that shock would follow unless the response was made. He was perhaps the first to suggest that these monkeys had difficulty with forming associations between stimuli and reinforcers, when he suggested that "the effect of amygdalectomy is to make it difficult for reinforcing stimuli, whether positive or negative, to become established or to be recognized as such" (Weiskrantz 1956). In this avoidance task, associations between a stimulus and punishers were impaired.

It has been confirmed with the more selective type of neurotoxic amygdala lesion that non-foods as well as foods are picked up and eaten, and also that emotional responses to snakes and human intruders are impaired (Murray & Izquierdo 2007), but there are relatively minor changes in social behaviour (Amaral 2003, Bliss-Moreau, Moadab, Bauman & Amaral 2013), and this is consistent with the trend for the orbitofrontal cortex to become relatively more important in emotion and social behaviour in primates including humans. The amygdala is implicated by lesion studies in learning associations between visual stimuli and rewards, and devaluation by feeding to satiety is impaired too (Murray & Izquierdo 2007).

A difference between the effects of selective amygdala lesions and orbitofrontal cortex lesions in monkeys is that selective amygdala lesions have no effect on object reversal learning, whereas orbitofrontal cortex lesions do impair object reversal learning (Murray & Izquierdo 2007) (see further Section 4.1). Further, and consistently, orbitofrontal but not selective amygdala lesions impair instrumental extinction (i.e. they showed a large number of choices of the previously rewarded object when it was no longer rewarded) (Murray & Izquierdo 2007). This is consistent with the evidence described in Chapter 3 that the orbitofrontal cortex is important in rapid, one-trial, learning and reversal between visual stimuli and primary reinforcers using both associative and rule-based mechanisms, and its representations of outcome value, expected value, and negative reward prediction error (Thorpe, Rolls & Maddison 1983, Rolls 2014a, Rolls & Grabenhorst 2008). These contributions of the orbitofrontal cortex are facilitated by its neocortical architecture, which can operate using attractors that are important in many functions including short-term memory, attention, rule-based operation with switching, long-term memory, and decision-making which may help it to compute and utilize non-reward to reset value representations in the orbitofrontal cortex (Rolls 2014a).

6.5.4.2 Amygdala lesions in rats

In rats, there is also evidence that the amygdala is involved in behaviour to stimuli learned as being associated with reward as well as with punishers. We may summarize these investigations in the rat as follows. The central nuclei of the amygdala encode or express Pavlovian S–R (stimulus–response, CS–UR) associations (including conditioned suppression, conditioned orienting, conditioned autonomic and endocrine responses, and Pavlovian–instrumental transfer); and modulate perhaps by arousal the associability of representations stored elsewhere in the brain (Gallagher & Holland 1994, Gallagher & Holland 1992, Holland & Gallagher 1999). In contrast, the basolateral amygdala (BLA) encodes or retrieves the affective value of the predicted US, and can use this to influence action–outcome learning via pathways to brain regions such as the nucleus accumbens and prefrontal cortex including the orbitofrontal cortex (Cardinal et al. 2002). We shall see below that the nucleus accumbens is not involved in action–outcome learning itself, but does allow the affective states retrieved by the BLA to conditioned stimuli to influence instrumental behaviour by for example Pavlovian–instrumental transfer, and facilitating locomotor approach to food which appears to be in rats a Pavlovian process (Cardinal et al. 2002, Cardinal & Everitt 2004, Everitt & Robbins 2013, Rolls 2014a). This leaves parts of the prefrontal and cingulate cortices as strong candidates for action–outcome learning.

In a different model of fear-conditioning in the rat, Davis and colleagues (Davis 2006), have used the fear-potentiated startle test, in which the amplitude of the acoustic startle reflex is increased when elicited in the presence of a stimulus previously paired with shock. Lesions of either the central nucleus or the lateral and basolateral nuclei of the amygdala block the expression of fear-potentiated startle. These latter amygdala nuclei may be the site of plasticity for fear conditioning, because local infusion of the NMDA (N-methyl-d-aspartate) receptor antagonist AP5 (which blocks long-term potentiation, an index of synaptic plasticity) blocks the acquisition but not the maintenance of fear-potentiated startle (Davis 2006). These investigations have now been extended to primates, in which similar effects are found, with ibotenic acid-induced lesions of the amygdala preventing the acquisition of fear-potentiated startle, though, remarkably, not the expression of fear-potentiated startle when fear conditioning was carried out prior to the lesion (Davis, Antoniadis, Amaral & Winslow 2008).

Reconsolidation refers to a process in which after a memory has been stored, it may be weakened or lost if recall is performed during the presence of a protein synthesis inhibitor (Debiec, LeDoux & Nader 2002, Debiec, Doyere, Nader & LeDoux 2006). The implication that has been drawn is that whenever a memory is recalled, some reconsolidation process requiring protein synthesis may be needed. The computational utility of reconsolidation is considered by Rolls (2016c). Here, it is of interest that this applies to fear association mechanisms in the amygdala (Doyere, Debiec, Monfils, Schafe & LeDoux 2007), and drug-associated memories in the amygdala (Milton, Lee, Butler, Gardner & Everitt 2008). The findings have interesting implications for the treatment of fear-associated memories. For example, in humans old fear memories can be updated with non-fearful information provided during the reconsolidation window. As a consequence, fear responses are no longer expressed, an effect that can last at least a year and is selective only to reactivated memories without affecting other memories (Schiller, Monfils, Raio, Johnson, LeDoux & Phelps 2010), although success has so far been limited (Kroes, Schiller, LeDoux & Phelps 2016). Procedures that influence the extinction of fear memory may also be useful in the treatment of fear states (Davis 2011).

6.5.5 Neuronal activity in the primate amygdala to reinforcing stimuli

There is clear evidence that some neurons in the primate amygdala respond to stimuli that are potentially primary reinforcers. For example, Sanghera, Rolls & Roper-Hall (1979) found some amygdala neurons with taste responses. In an extensive study of 1416 macaque amygdala neurons, Kadohisa, Rolls & Verhagen (2005a) showed that a very rich and detailed representation of the stimulus (such as food) that is in the mouth is provided by neurons that respond to oral stimuli. An example of a macaque single amygdala orally-responsive neuron is shown in Fig. 6.4. The neuron had different responses to different tastes, different temperatures of what was in the mouth, and different viscosities, but had no response to the texture of fatty oils. Other amygdala neurons were selective for even one modality, responding for example only to the oral texture of fat (Kadohisa, Rolls & Verhagen 2005a). 3.1% of the recorded amygdala neurons responded to oral stimuli. Of the orally responsive neurons, some (39%) represent the viscosity of oral stimuli, tested using carboxymethyl-cellulose in the range 1–10,000 centiPoise. Other neurons (5%) responded to fat in the mouth by encoding its texture (shown by the responses of these neurons to a range of fats, and also to non-fat oils such as

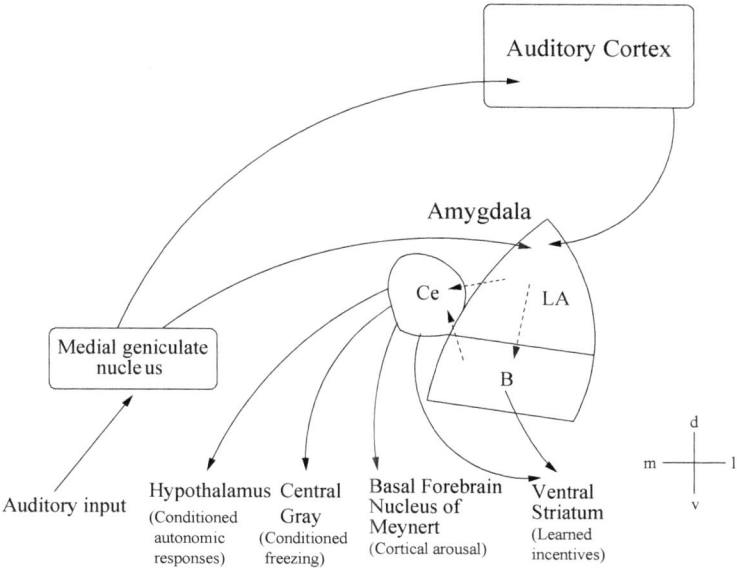

Fig. 6.3 The pathways for fear-conditioning to pure-tone auditory stimuli associated with footshock in the rat. The lateral amygdala (LA) receives auditory information directly from the medial part of the medial geniculate nucleus (the auditory thalamic nucleus), and from the auditory cortex. Intra-amygdala projections (directly and via the basal and basal accessory nuclei, B) end in the central nucleus (Ce) of the amygdala. Different output pathways from the central nucleus and the basal nucleus mediate different conditioned fear-related effects. d, dorsal; v, ventral; m, medial; l, lateral. (Reproduced from G. J. Quirk, J. L. Armony, J. C. Repa, X. F. Li, and J. E. LeDoux, Emotional memory: a search for sites of plasticity, Cold Spring Harbor Symposia on Quantitative Biology, 61, pp. 247–257, figure 1b © 1996, Cold Spring Harbor Laboratory Press.)

silicone oil $(Si(CH_3)_2O)_n$) and mineral oil (pure hydrocarbon), but no or small responses to the cellulose viscosity series or to the fatty acids linoleic acid and lauric acid). Some neurons (7%) responded to gritty texture (produced by microspheres suspended in carboxymethyl cellulose). Some neurons (41%) responded to the temperature of the liquid in the mouth. Some amygdala neurons responded to capsaicin, and some to fatty acids (but not to fats in the mouth). Some amygdala neurons respond to taste, texture and temperature unimodally, but others combine these inputs. An interesting difference is that in terms of best responses to different tastes, 57% of the orbitofrontal cortex taste neurons had their best responses to glucose, whereas 21% of the amygdala neurons had their best response to glucose (Kadohisa, Rolls & Verhagen 2005b). (More amygdala neurons had their best responses to sour (HCl) (18%) and monosodium glutamate (14%) (Kadohisa, Rolls & Verhagen 2005b).)

These results show that a very detailed representation of substances in the mouth, which are likely to be primary reinforcers, is present in the primate amygdala (Kadohisa, Rolls & Verhagen 2005a). Less is known about whether it is though the reinforcer value of the stimuli that is represented. It has been shown that satiety produces a rather modest (on average 58%) reduction in the responses of amygdala neurons to taste (Yan & Scott 1996, Rolls & Scott 2003), in comparison to the essentially complete reduction of responsiveness found in orbitofrontal cortex taste neurons (Rolls, Sienkiewicz & Yaxley 1989). Further, the representation in the amygdala of these oral stimuli does not appear to be on any simple hedonic basis, in that no direction in the multidimensional taste space in Fig. 7 of Kadohisa, Rolls & Verhagen (2005a) reflected the measured preference of the monkeys for the stimuli, nor were the response profiles of the neurons to the set of stimuli closely related to the preferences of the macaques for the stimuli (Kadohisa, Rolls & Verhagen 2005a). The failure to find very strong effects of satiety on the responsiveness of amygdala taste neurons (Yan & Scott 1996, Rolls & Scott 2003) mirrors the earlier finding of Sanghera, Rolls & Roper-Hall

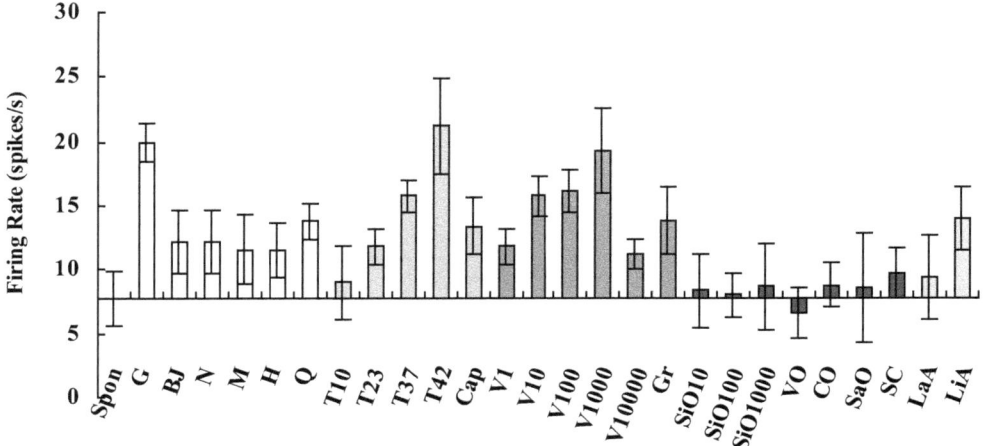

Fig. 6.4 The responses of an amygdala neuron (bo217) with differential responses to taste, temperature and viscosity. The neuron did not respond to fat texture. The mean ($\pm$ the standard error of the mean, sem) firing rate responses to each stimulus calculated in a 1 s period over 4–6 trials are shown. The spontaneous (Spon) firing rate is shown. G, N, M, H and Q are the taste stimuli. T10–T42 are the temperature stimuli. V1 - V10,000 are the CMC viscosity series with the viscosity in cP. The fat texture stimuli were SiO10, SiO100, SiO1000 (silicone oil with the viscosity indicated), vegetable oil (VO), coconut oil (CO) and safflower oil (SaO). BJ is fruit juice; Cap is 10 μM capsaicin; LaA is 0.1 mM lauric acid; LiA is 0.1 mM linoleic acid; Gr is the gritty stimulus. (Reprinted from Neuroscience, 132 (1), M. Kadohisa, J. V. Verhagen, and E. T. Rolls, The primate amygdala: Neuronal representations of the viscosity, fat texture, temperature, grittiness and taste of foods, pp. 33–48. doi.org/10.1016/j.neuroscience.2004.12.005 Copyright © 2005 IBRO. Published by Elsevier Ltd. All rights reserved.)

(1979) of inconsistent effects of feeding to satiety on the responses of amygdala visual neurons responding to the sight of food.

Recordings from single neurons in the amygdala of the monkey have shown that some neurons do respond to visual stimuli, consistent with the inputs from the temporal lobe visual cortex (Sanghera, Rolls & Roper-Hall 1979). Other neurons responded to auditory, gustatory, olfactory, or somatosensory stimuli, or in relation to movements. In tests of whether the neurons responded on the basis of the association of stimuli with reinforcers, it was found that approximately 20% of the neurons with visual responses had responses that occurred primarily to stimuli associated with reinforcers, for example to food and to a range of stimuli which the monkey had learned signified food in a visual discrimination task for food reward (Sanghera, Rolls & Roper-Hall 1979, Rolls 1981c, Wilson & Rolls 1993, Wilson & Rolls 2005, Rolls 2000c). Many of these neurons responded more to the positive discriminative stimulus (S+) than to the negative visual discriminative stimulus (S–) in the Go/NoGo visual discrimination task (Rolls 2000c, Wilson & Rolls 2005). However, none of these neurons (in contrast with some neurons in the orbitofrontal cortex) responded exclusively to rewarded stimuli, in that all responded at least partly to one or more neutral, novel, or aversive stimuli.

The degree to which the visual responses of these amygdala neurons are associated with reinforcers has been assessed in learning tasks. When the association between a visual stimulus and an instrumental reinforcer was altered by reversal (so that the visual stimulus formerly associated with juice reward became associated with aversive saline and vice versa), it was found that 10 of 11 neurons did not reverse their responses (and for the other neuron the evidence was not clear) (Sanghera, Rolls & Roper-Hall 1979, Rolls 1992a, Rolls 2000c).

Although more investigations would be useful, the evidence now available indicates that primate amygdala neurons do not alter their activity flexibly and rapidly (in one or even a few trials) in visual discrimination reversal learning (Rolls 1992a, Rolls 2000c, Rolls 2014a). What has been found in contrast is that neurons in the orbitofrontal cortex do show very rapid, often one-trial, reversal of their responses in visual discrimination reversal, and it therefore seems likely that the orbitofrontal cortex is especially involved when repeated relearning and re-assessment of stimulus–reinforcer associations are required, as described above, rather than initial learning, in which the amygdala may be involved. (It is noted that some other studies do not address the issue convincingly of rapid reversal, for they were not studying one-trial reversal with instrumental learning, but instead slow classical conditioning (Paton, Belova, Morrison & Salzman 2006, Morrison, Saez, Lau & Salzman 2011). However, more recent studies in that series are in fact consistent with the discoveries we have made that the orbitofrontal cortex updates reward value representations more rapidly and flexibly than the amygdala, in that neural responses to reward-predictive cues updated more rapidly in the orbitofrontal cortex than amygdala, and activity in the orbitofrontal cortex but not the amygdala was modulated by recent reward history (Saez, Saez, Paton, Lau & Salzman 2017).

Evidence that primate amygdala neurons encode reward value is that while monkeys chose between saving liquid reward with interest and spending the accumulated reward, some of the neurons reflected the accumulating value (Grabenhorst, Hernadi & Schultz 2012) and reflect whether a macaque will perform economic saving (Hernadi, Grabenhorst & Schultz 2015, Grabenhorst, Hernadi & Schultz 2016). Overall, there is thus evidence that some amygdala neurons reflect reward value, yet do not reverse their value-related responses rapidly (in the one trial shown by orbitofrontal cortex neurons), and the evidence from the effects of selective amygdala lesions (Murray & Izquierdo 2007) is consistent with this.

6.5.6 Responses of primate amygdala neurons to novel stimuli that are reinforcing

Wilson & Rolls (2005) (see Rolls (2000c)) discovered that some amygdala neurons with reward-related responses also responded to relatively novel visual stimuli. When the monkeys are given such relatively novel stimuli outside the task, they will reach out for and explore the objects, and in this respect the novel stimuli are reinforcing. Repeated presentation of the stimuli results in habituation of the neuronal response and of behavioural approach, if the stimuli are not associated with a primary reinforcer. It is thus suggested that the amygdala neurons described operate as filters that provide an output if a stimulus is associated with a positive reinforcer, or is positively reinforcing because of relative unfamiliarity, and that provide no output if a stimulus is familiar and has not been associated with a positive primary reinforcer or is associated with a punisher. The functions of this output may be to influence the interest shown in a stimulus, whether it is approached or avoided, whether an affective response occurs to it, and whether a representation of the stimulus is made or maintained (see Rolls (2014a)).

It is an important adaptation to the environment to explore relatively novel objects or situations, for in this way advantage due to gene inheritance can become expressed and selected for. This function appears to be implemented in the amygdala in this way. Lesions of the amygdala impair the operation of this mechanism, in that objects are approached and explored indiscriminately, relatively independently of whether they are associated with reinforcers (including punishers), or are novel or familiar (Rolls 2014a).

6.5.7 Neuronal responses in the amygdala to faces

Another interesting group of neurons in the amygdala responds primarily to faces (Rolls 1981c, Leonard, Rolls, Wilson & Baylis 1985). Each of these neurons responds to some

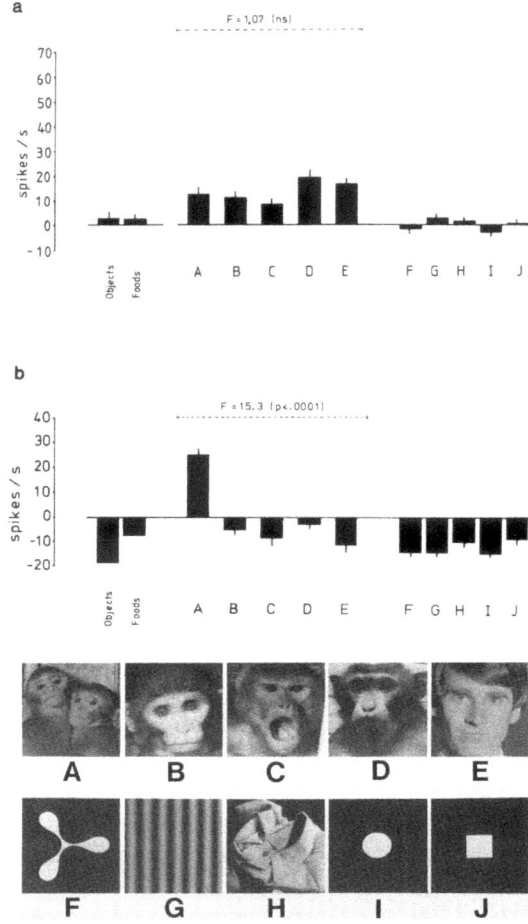

Fig. 6.5 The responses of two neurons (a,b) in the amygdala to a variety of monkey and human face stimuli (A–E), and to non-face stimuli (F–J, objects, and foods). Each bar represents the mean response above baseline with the standard error calculated over 4 to 10 presentations. The F ratio for an analysis of variance calculated over the face sets indicates that the neurons shown range from very selective between faces (neuron b, Y0809) to relatively non-selective (neuron A, Z0264). Some stimuli produced inhibition below the spontaneous firing rate. (Reprinted from Behavioural Brain Research, 15 (2), C. M. Leonard, E. T. Rolls, F. A. W. Wilson, and G. C. Baylis, Neurons in the amygdala of the monkey with responses selective for faces, pp. 159–76. Copyright © 1985 Published by Elsevier B.V.)

but not all of a set of faces, and thus across an ensemble could convey information about the identity of the face (see Fig. 6.5). These neurons are found especially in the basal accessory nucleus of the amygdala (Leonard, Rolls, Wilson & Baylis 1985), a part of the amygdala that develops markedly in primates (Amaral et al. 1992). Similar neurons have been further analysed (Gothard, Battaglia, Erickson, Spitler & Amaral 2007, Gothard, Mosher, Zimmerman, Putnam, Morrow & Fuglevand 2018), and, as with face-selective neurons in the orbitofrontal cortex (Rolls, Critchley, Browning & Inoue 2006a), some neurons respond to face identity, some to face expression, and some to combinations of identity and expression. In addition, some neurons in the primate amygdala respond during social interactions, some may respond preferentially to eyes (as do some neurons in the temporal lobe visual cortex (Perrett, Rolls & Caan 1982)), and their output may influence face expression (Brothers & Ring 1993, Gothard et al. 2018). Face-selective neurons have also been found now in the human amygdala (Rutishauser, Tudusciuc, Neumann, Mamelak, Heller, Ross, Philpott, Sutherling & Adolphs 2011, Rutishauser, Mamelak & Adolphs 2015).

6.5.8 Evidence from humans

In relation to neurons in the macaque amygdala with responses selective for faces and social interactions (Leonard, Rolls, Wilson & Baylis 1985, Gothard, Mosher, Zimmerman, Putnam, Morrow & Fuglevand 2018), a patient (DR) has been described who has bilateral damage to or disconnection of the amygdala, and has an impairment of face-expression matching and identification, but not of matching face identity or in discrimination (Young, Aggleton, Hellawell, Johnson, Broks & Hanley 1995, Young, Hellawell, Van de Wal & Johnson 1996). This patient is also impaired at detecting whether someone is gazing at the patient, another important social signal (Perrett et al. 1985). The same patient is also impaired at the auditory recognition of fear and anger (Scott, Young, Calder, Hellawell, Aggleton & Johnson 1997).

Adolphs, Tranel, Damasio & Damasio (1994) also found face expression but not face identity impairments in a patient (SM) with bilateral damage to the amygdala, and extended this to other patients (Adolphs, Tranel & Baron-Cohen 2002). The bilateral amygdala patient SM was especially impaired at recognizing the face expression of fear, and also rated expressions of fear, anger, and surprise as less intense than control subjects. It has been shown that SM's impairment stems from an inability to make normal use of information from the eye region of faces when judging emotions, which in turn is related to a lack of spontaneous fixations on the eyes during free viewing of faces (Adolphs, Gosselin, Buchanan, Tranel, Schyns & Damasio 2005), though this is mainly evident just for the first fixation (Kennedy & Adolphs 2011). Although SM fails to look normally at the eye region in all facial expressions, her selective impairment in recognizing fear is explained by the fact that the eyes are the most important feature for identifying this emotion. Indeed, SM's recognition of fearful faces became entirely normal when she was instructed explicitly to look at the eyes. This finding provides a mechanism to explain the amygdala's role in fear recognition, and points to new approaches for the possible rehabilitation of patients with defective emotion perception.

The changes in emotion in patients with amygdala lesions are much less marked than those in patients with orbitofrontal cortex damage, and special tests, analogous in some cases to those developed in rodent studies, are necessary to reveal deficits (Phelps & LeDoux 2005). For example, patients with amygdala lesions are impaired at learning conditioned skin conductance responses when a blue square is associated with a shock, and are also impaired in acquiring the same autonomic response to fear by verbally instructed learning or by observational learning (Phelps 2004, Phelps, O'Connor, Gatenby, Gore, Grillon & Davis 2001, Phelps 2006, Whalen & Phelps 2009). The human amygdala has been described as being important mainly for some fear responses to some stimuli, such as whether an individual backs off in a social encounter (Adolphs 2003, Adolphs et al. 2005, Phelps 2004, Schiller et al. 2010, Feinstein, Adolphs, Damasio & Tranel 2011). Interestingly, the amygdala was involved during aversive conditioning with primary reinforcers (electric shock) and less so with a secondary reinforcer (money), as suggested by both an fMRI analysis and a follow-up case study with a patient with bilateral amygdala damage (Delgado, Jou & Phelps 2011).

The important point has been made that the amygdala may be involved in some of the behavioral responses in humans related to emotion, but that the subjective emotional feeling conscious state may be unaltered by treatments that reverse some of these behavioral measures (LeDoux & Pine 2016, LeDoux et al. 2018). One implication is that the amygdala, at least in humans, may have quite restricted roles in emotion. In contrast, damage to the orbitofrontal cortex has major effects not only on emotional behaviour, but also on subjective, conscious, feelings of emotion in humans, as described in Chapter 4. Two conclusions follow. First, the orbitofrontal cortex, due to its great development and evolution in primates including humans, may be much more important in emotion than the amygdala (Rolls 2017b). Second, subjective emotional states are not necessarily closely related to at least some behavioral measures of emotion, consistent with the multiple routes to action concepts developed in Section 6.4 and more fully elsewhere (Rolls 2014a, Rolls 2018b). To emphasise what is an important point with many implications: some behavioral measures related to emotion in humans may not reflect or be closely related to subjective emotional state; and vice versa.

An interesting advance conceptually is provided by the finding that personality interacts with whether particular stimuli activate the human amygdala. For example, happy face expressions are more likely to activate the human amygdala in extraverts than in introverts (Canli, Sivers, Whitfield, Gotlib & Gabrieli 2002). In addition, positively affective pictures interact with extraversion to produce activation of the amygdala (Canli, Zhao, Desmond, Kang, Gross & Gabrieli 2001). This supports the conceptually important point that part of the basis of personality may be differential sensitivity to different rewards and punishers, and omission and termination of rewards and punishers (Rolls 2014a). It has additionally been found that negative pictures interact with neuroticism in producing differential activation of the human amygdala (Canli et al. 2001). Further, FFFS and BIS-related personality traits related to an anxiety-related 'Behavioural Inhibition System', and to a fear-related 'Fight, Flight, Freeze System', are positively correlated to activity in the amygdala in response to negative stimuli (Kennis, Rademaker & Geuze 2013).

7 The orbitofrontal cortex, depression, and other mental disorders

The main focus of this Chapter is on the roles of the orbitofrontal cortex in depression, but the relation of the orbitofrontal cortex to bipolar disorder, autism, attention-deficit hyperactivity disorder (ADHD), and obsessive-compulsive disorder are considered later in the Chapter.

7.1 Depression

Major depressive disorder is ranked by the World Health Organization as the leading cause of years-of-life lived with disability (Drevets 2007, Gotlib & Hammen 2009, Hamilton, Chen & Gotlib 2013). Major depressive episodes, found in both major depressive disorder and bipolar disorder, are pathological mood states characterized by persistently sad or depressed mood. Major depressive disorders are generally accompanied by: (1) altered incentive and reward processing, evidenced by lack of motivation, apathy, and anhedonia (lack of pleasure); (2) impaired modulation of anxiety and worry, manifested by generalized, social and panic anxiety, and oversensitivity to negative feedback; (3) inflexibility of thought and behaviour in association with changing reinforcement contingencies, apparent as ruminative thoughts of self-reproach, pessimism, and guilt, and inertia toward initiating goal-directed behaviour; (4) altered integration of sensory and social information, as evidenced by mood-congruent processing biases; (5) impaired attention and memory, shown as performance deficits on tests of attention set-shifting and maintenance, and autobiographical and short-term memory; and 6) visceral disturbances, including altered weight, appetite, sleep, and endocrine and autonomic function (Drevets 2007, Gotlib & Hammen 2009).

This Section describes depression, its brain mechanisms, and a new attractor-based theory of some of the brain mechanisms that are related to depression (Rolls 2016e).

7.1.1 The economic and social cost of depression

The economic cost of depression is enormous. For example, the cost to Europe of work-related depression was estimated to be €617 billion annually in 2013, and is rising (Matrix 2013). The total was made up of costs to employers resulting from absenteeism (€272 billion), loss of productivity (€242 billion), health care costs of €63 billion, and social welfare costs in the form of disability benefit payments (€39 billion).

In addition, there is a major personal burden to sufferers and their families of depression. Moreover, in most countries the number of people who suffer from depression during their lives falls within an 8-12% range, so that if the numbers of people who suffer from depression, and the effects on their families is included, the effects of advances in our understanding of depression will affect the lives of millions of people worldwide.

7.1.2 The triggers and causes of depression: non-reward systems

There are two main types of depression.

One is **reactive**, in which an event triggers depression. This is typically an event in which a reward or rewards are no longer available. An example might be a death in the family, in which a loved one is no longer present. Another might be losing a job, in which all the social and financial benefits of work may be withdrawn.

Some of the triggers of depression have been described in more detail (Rantala, Luoto, Krams & Karlsson 2018). They include:

1. Infection (during which sickness and depression might be adaptive by conserving metabolic resources for the use of the immune system to fight the infection). Although a contribution of activity in the immune system may contribute to depression (Bhattacharya, Derecki, Lovenberg & Drevets 2016), this on its own would not seem to account for all the symptoms of depression, such as low self-esteem, and anhedonia.

2. Long-term stress, in which steroid hormone levels may be increased (Gold 2015, McEwen, Gray & Nasca 2015). These steroid hormones, such as corticosterone, are adaptive in the short-term by preparing the body for action, but in the long term, can contribute to depression, and are associated with many changes in the brain, including a reduction of excitatory synaptic connections in some brain areas such as the hippocampus (McEwen et al. 2015). The stress may be produced in the first instance by non-reward or punishment, and this concept links research on stress to the approach to emotion and depression described in this book. The 'love and trust' hormone oxytocin is low in the periphery in depression, and may perhaps normally (when not depressed) help to counteract some of the effects of stress (McQuaid, McInnis, Abizaid & Anisman 2014).

3. Loneliness, which can be a non-reward and stressor in that humans benefit from social interactions in many ways (Rolls 2012c). Indeed, a solitary individual is more vulnerable to predators, hostile conspecifics and other forces of nature than individuals in social groups (Rantala et al. 2018).

4. Traumatic experience, such as injury, which can lead to stress.

5. Hierarchy conflict, in which successful competition between individuals may be adaptive (Rolls 2014a). Depression may function as a signal that an individual has given up after a hierarchy conflict; and may also lead to a change of behaviour as a response to non-reward.

6. Grief, as in the loss of a loved one. The grief may be the subjective state associated with the loss of the reward. The change produced by a loss of the reward may in evolutionary history be adaptive by stopping behaviour for the previously rewarded stimulus, and leading to new behaviour. Forty-two per cent of individuals whose spouse had passed away fulfilled the diagnostic criteria of clinical depression a month after the spouse's death (Rantala et al. 2018).

7. Romantic rejection, again a major non-reward, where the romantic attachment has the biological utility of leading to pair-bonding and successful reproduction in humans and birds, in which two parents promote gene fitness because the young are immature at birth (Rolls 2014a).

8. Postpartum (or peripartum) depression, which occurs in 10–15% of women in the six months following childbirth (Kuehner 2017). Postpartum depression may be adaptive in functioning as a signal to kin and the spouse that the mother requires more support.

9. The season, as in seasonal affective disorder (SAD), which may occur in the winter when the days are short. SAD is more common in people with evening chronotypes (Sandman, Merikanto, Maattanen, Valli, Kronholm, Laatikainen, Partonen & Paunio 2016), and light therapy, especially in the morning, is an effective treatment.

10. Chemicals, such as alcohol and cocaine, the repeated use of which can lead to depression (Rantala et al. 2018).

11. Somatic diseases.

12. Starvation, in which depression may conserve energy (Rantala et al. 2018); or obesity, in which inflammation may be associated with depression.

13. The prevalence of depression is twice as high in women as in men, and a number of factors or triggers may contribute to this (Kuehner 2017).

Although many of these states elicited by these triggers are adaptive in the sense of evolutionary biology (Rantala et al. 2018) (including in reducing risk-taking behaviour and impulsivity as shown below), some may not be adaptive in humans. Part of the reason for this, I suggest, is that many emotions may be stronger in humans than in our ancestors, because of the evolution of the reasoning system in humans, which enables planning and thinking for multiple steps ahead, which can reveal how great a loss has just occurred, as described in Section 6.4 and by Rolls (2018b). These stronger emotions in humans may take our emotional system out of the range of rewards, non-rewards, and punishers in which our non-language-using ancestors evolved (Rolls 2014a, Rolls 2018b).

A second main type of depression is when there may be no identifiable event or cause in the environment, but the depression just comes on. This is referred to as **endogenous** (internally generated) depression. The brain systems in this case for non-reward may be too sensitive and imbalanced, resulting in the brain entering a depressed state even without an identifiable external trigger. Different individuals may have different sensitivities to different types of reward and reward contingency, contributing to differences in personality (Rolls 2014a), and this is part of the way in which evolution works. But the result may be that some people are very sensitive to non-reward, and are for this reason more likely to become depressed. (Although the term 'endogenous depression' is less common now than in the past, the argument just provided does provide an approach to understanding why in some cases it may be difficult to identify the environmental cause of the depression, if the brain system in some individuals is very sensitive to non-reward, or even is triggered into an attractor state by internal noise in the brain as described in Section 3.13.)

The understanding of emotion described in Chapter 6 leads to a clear approach to understanding depression, which relates to most of the triggers described above. Depression is produced when expected rewards are not available as expected, shown on the non-reward axis in Fig. 6.1. With this non-reward contingency, if an action is possible, perhaps to obtain the reward or to prevent the situation re-occurring in future, then emotions such as anger and rage may be felt (the 'active' condition for non-reward in Fig. 6.1). If no action is possible, then sadness, grief, or depression may result (the 'passive' condition for non-reward in Fig. 6.1). Although most of the triggers of depression listed above may be related to the reinforcement contingency of non-reward (Rolls 2016e, Rolls 2018b), some triggers are related to changes in body state such as starvation or obesity, which may trigger the same brain mechanisms that respond to non-reward as part of an evolutionary adaptive strategy to deal with the current environment.

The brain-related and non-reward contingency approach taken here may be especially useful in the situation that the genetics of depression does not so far suggest a few important genes related to depression that might provide indications about possible treatments, but instead that there may be a large number of genes each of which makes a small contribution (Flint & Kendler 2014) requiring a polygenic approach (Bigdeli et al. (2017)).

a. Reversal   b. Stop-signal task

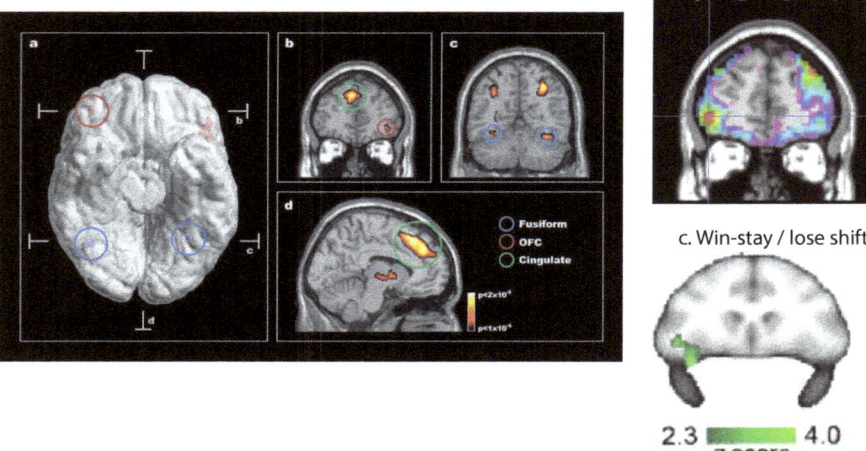

c. Win-stay / lose shift

Fig. 7.1 a. **The human lateral orbitofrontal cortex is activated by non-reward.** Activation of the lateral orbitofrontal cortex in a visual discrimination reversal task on reversal trials, when a face was selected but the expected reward was not obtained, indicating that the subject should select the other face in future to obtain the reward. a) A ventral view of the human brain with indication of the location of the two coronal slices (b,c) and the transverse slice (d). The activations with the red circle in the lateral orbitofrontal cortex (OFC, peaks at [42 42 -8] and [-46 30 -8]) show the activation on reversal trials compared to the non-reversal trials. For comparison, the activations with the blue circle show the fusiform face area produced just by face expressions, not by reversal, which are also indicated in the coronal slice in (c). b) A coronal slice showing the activation in the right orbitofrontal cortex on reversal trials. Activation is also shown in the supracallosal anterior cingulate region (Cingulate, green circle) that is also known to be activated by many punishing, unpleasant, stimuli (see Grabenhorst and Rolls (2011)). (From Neuroimage 20 (2), Morten L. Kringelbach and Edmund T. Rolls, Neural correlates of rapid reversal learning in a simple model of human social interaction, pp. 1371–83, doi.org/10.1016/S1053-8119(03)00393-8, Copyright © 2003 Elsevier Inc. All rights reserved.) **b. Activations in the human lateral orbitofrontal cortex are related to a signal to change behaviour in the stop-signal task.** In the task, a left or right arrow on a screen indicates which button to touch. However on some trials, an up-arrow then appears, and the participant must change the behavior, and stop the response. There is a larger response on trials on which the participant successfully changes the behavior and stops the response, as shown by the contrast stop-success - stop-failure, in the ventrolateral prefrontal cortex in a region including the lateral orbitofrontal cortex, with peak at [-42 50 -2] indicated by the cross-hairs, measured in 1709 participants. There were corresponding effects in the right lateral orbitofrontal cortex [42 52 -4]. Some activation in the dorsolateral prefrontal cortex in an area implicated in attention is also shown. (Modified from Deng, Rolls et al, 2017). **c. Bold signal in the macaque lateral orbitofrontal related to win-stay / lose-shift performance, that is, to reward reversal performance.** (Modified from Chau et al, 2015).

7.1.3 Brain systems that underlie depression

We start with the concept that brain systems involved in detecting non-reward are likely to be involved in depression (Fig. 6.1) (Rolls 2016e, Rolls 2018b). In the following, I summarize evidence that, on this basis, implicates the lateral orbitofrontal cortex in depression.

The orbitofrontal cortex contains a population of neurons that respond to non-reward and maintain their firing for many seconds after the non-reward, providing evidence that they have entered an attractor state that maintains a memory of the non-reward (Thorpe, Rolls & Maddison 1983, Rolls 2014a) (Section 3.8). An example of such a neuron is shown in Fig. 3.46 on page 76. These neurons signal that a reward is less than was expected, and are termed negative reward prediction error neurons because they respond to this type of prediction error (Section 3.8).

The human lateral orbitofrontal cortex is activated by non-reward (not obtaining an expected reward) during reward reversal (Kringelbach & Rolls 2003). This is illustrated in Fig. 7.1a, which shows activations in the lateral orbitofrontal cortex on reversal trials, that is when the human participant chose one person's face, and did not obtain the expected reward.

Activations in the lateral orbitofrontal cortex are also produced by a signal to stop a response that is now incorrect, which is another situation in which behaviour must change in order to be correct (Deng, Rolls et al. (2017), Fig. 7.1b). Orbitofrontal cortex activations in the stop-signal task have further been related to how impulsive the behaviour is (Whelan et al. (2012)). In this context, it has been suggested that impulsiveness may reflect how sensitive an individual is to non-reward or punishment (Rolls 2014a), with one reason for being impulsive that one may not be very sensitive to non-reward, and the non-rewarding consequences of one's actions. Further, we have shown that people with orbitofrontal cortex damage become more impulsive (Berlin et al. 2004, Berlin et al. 2005).

The lateral orbitofrontal cortex also responds to many punishing, unpleasant, stimuli (Grabenhorst & Rolls 2011, Rolls 2014a) (Fig. 3.54) including bad odour (Rolls, Kringelbach & De Araujo 2003c) and losing money (O'Doherty, Kringelbach, Rolls, Hornak & Andrews 2001a). Consistent with this human neuroimaging evidence and with the macaque neurophysiology (Thorpe, Rolls & Maddison 1983, Rolls 2014a), the macaque lateral orbitofrontal cortex is also activated by non-reward during a reversal task as shown by fMRI (Chau et al. 2015) (Fig. 7.1c).

Further evidence that the orbitofrontal cortex is involved in changing rewarded behaviour when non-reward is detected is that damage to the human orbitofrontal cortex impairs reward reversal learning, in that the previously rewarded stimulus is still chosen during reversal even when no reward is being obtained (Rolls, Hornak, Wade & McGrath 1994a, Hornak, O'Doherty, Bramham, Rolls, Morris, Bullock & Polkey 2004, Fellows & Farah 2003, Fellows 2011).

Now it is well established that not receiving expected reward, or receiving unpleasant stimuli or events, can produce depression (Beck 2008, Drevets 2007, Harmer & Cowen 2013, Price & Drevets 2012, Pryce, Azzinnari, Spinelli, Seifritz, Tegethoff & Meinlschmidt 2011, Eshel & Roiser 2010). A clear example is that if a member of the family dies, then this is the removal of reward (in that we would work to try to avoid this), and the result of the removal of the reward can be depression. More formally, in terms of learning theory, the omission or termination of a reward can give rise to sadness or depression, depending on the magnitude of the reward that is lost, if there is no action that can be taken to restore the reward (the 'passive' condition for non-reward in Fig. 6.1) (Rolls 2014a, Rolls 2018b). If an action can be taken, then frustration and anger may arise to the same reinforcement contingency (Rolls 2014a). This relates the current approach to the learned helplessness approach to depression, in which depression may arise because no actions can be taken to restore rewards (Forgeard, Haigh, Beck, Davidson, Henn, Maier, Mayberg & Seligman 2011, Pryce et al. 2011). A useful therapy for depression may be to help humans to re-appreciate how their actions can lead to rewards, in order to break the cycle of no longer trying to obtain rewards.

7.2 A non-reward attractor theory of depression

The finding that neurons in the lateral orbitofrontal cortex can respond for many seconds following non-reward provides evidence that they have entered an attractor state that maintains a memory of the non-reward (Thorpe, Rolls & Maddison 1983, Rolls 2014a) (Section 3.8). An example of such a neuron is shown in Fig. 3.46. Attractor networks are described in Sections 3.13 and 9.2, and by Rolls (2016c).

The theory has been proposed that in depression, this lateral orbitofrontal cortex non-reward / punishment attractor network system is more easily triggered, and maintains its attractor-related firing for longer (Rolls 2016e, Rolls 2017a, Rolls 2017c, Rolls 2018b). The greater attractor-related firing of the non-reward / punishment system triggers negative cognitive states held on-line in other cortical systems such as the language system and in the

Interaction of non-reward and language networks in depression

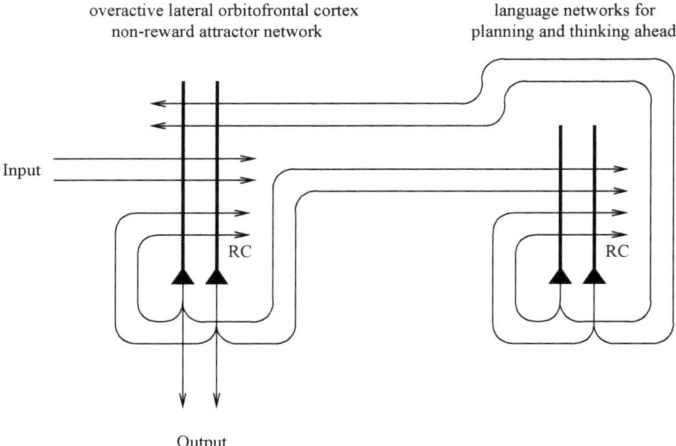

Fig. 7.2 Interaction of orbitofrontal cortex non-reward networks with language networks in depression. Illustration of how an overactive non-reward attractor network in the lateral orbitofrontal cortex could send excitatory information forward to networks for language and planning ahead; which could in turn send excitatory 'top-down' feedback back down to the orbitofrontal non-reward network to maintain its over-activity. It is suggested that such a system with mutual 'long loop' re-excitation contributes to the persistent ruminating thoughts in depression. (Modified from Rolls 2016e.)

dorsolateral prefrontal cortex which is implicated in attentional control. These other cortical systems then in turn have top-down effects on the orbitofrontal non-reward system that bias it in a negative direction (Rolls 2013a) (see Fig. 3.53), and thus increase the sensitivity of the lateral orbitofrontal cortex to non-reward and maintain its overactivity (Rolls 2016e) (Fig. 7.2). It is proposed that the interaction of non-reward and language / attentional brain systems of these types accounts for the ruminating and continuing depressive thoughts, which occur as a result of a positive feedback cycle between these types of brain system (Rolls 2016e).

Indeed, we have shown that cognitive states can have 'top-down' effects on affective representations in the orbitofrontal cortex (De Araujo, Rolls, Velazco, Margot & Cayeux 2005, Grabenhorst, Rolls & Bilderbeck 2008a, McCabe, Rolls, Bilderbeck & McGlone 2008, Rolls 2013a). Further, top-down selective attention can also influence affective representations in the orbitofrontal cortex (Rolls et al. 2008a, Grabenhorst & Rolls 2008, Ge et al. 2012, Luo, Ge, Grabenhorst, Feng & Rolls 2013, Rolls 2013a), and paying attention to depressive symptoms when depressed may in this way exacerbate the problems in a positive feedback way.

More generally, the presence of the cognitive ability to think ahead and see the implications of recent events that is afforded by language may be a computational development in the brain that exacerbates the vulnerability of the human brain to depression (Rolls 2014a, Rolls 2018b). For example, with language we can think ahead and see that perhaps the loss of an individual in one's life may be long-term, and this thought and its consequences for our future can become fully evident.

The theory is that one way in which depression could result from over-activity in this lateral orbitofrontal cortex system is if there is a major negatively reinforcing life event that produces reactive depression and activates this system, which then becomes self-re-exciting based on the cycle between the lateral orbitofrontal cortex non-reward / punishment attractor system and the cognitive / language system, which together operate as a systems-level attractor (Fig. 7.2). (The generic cortical architecture for such reciprocal feedforward and feedback excitatory effects is illustrated by Rolls (2016c).

The theory is that a second way in which depression might arise is if this lateral orbitofrontal cortex non-reward / punishment system is especially sensitive in some individuals. This might be related for example to genetic predisposition, or to the effects of stress (Gold 2015). In this case, the orbitofrontal system would over-react to normal levels of non-reward or punishment, and start the local attractor circuit in the lateral orbitofrontal cortex (Rolls 2016e, Rolls & Deco 2016), which in turn would activate the cognitive system, which would feed back to the over-reactive lateral orbitofrontal cortex system to maintain now a systems-level attractor with ruminating thoughts. This is described as a 'systems-level' attractor because it includes mutual excitations between different brain areas.

An important complementary part of the theory of depression is that the medial orbitofrontal cortex, implicated in reward processing, has reduced sensitivity to rewards or reduced functional connectivity, and that this contributes to the anhedonia and lack of motivation in depression (Rolls 2016e, Rolls 2018a, Rolls 2018b), with evidence for this described below (Xie et al. 2019, Ma 2015, Rolls et al. 2019a, Rolls, Cheng & Feng 2019b).

7.3 Evidence consistent with the non-reward attractor theory of depression

There is some evidence for altered structure and function of the lateral orbitofrontal cortex in depression (Drevets 2007, Ma 2015, Price & Drevets 2012). For example, reductions of grey-matter volume and cortex thickness have been demonstrated specifically in the posterolateral OFC (BA 47, caudal BA 11 and the adjoining BA 45), and also in the subgenual cingulate cortex (BA 24, 25) (Drevets 2007, Nugent, Milham, Bain, Mah, Cannon, Marrett, Zarate, Pine, Price & Drevets 2006). In depression, there is increased cerebral blood flow in areas that include the ventrolateral orbitofrontal cortex (which is a prediction of the theory), and also in regions such as the subgenual cingulate cortex and amygdala, and these increases appear to be related to the mood change, in that they become more normal when the mood state remits (Drevets 2007).

In the first brain-wide voxel-level resting state functional connectivity neuroimaging analysis of depression (with 421 patients with major depressive disorder and 488 controls), we have found that one major circuit with altered functional connectivity involved the medial orbitofrontal cortex BA 13, which had reduced functional connectivity in depression with memory systems in the parahippocampal gyrus and medial temporal lobe (Cheng, Rolls, Qiu, Liu, Tang, Huang, Wang, Zhang, Lin, Zheng, Pu, Tsai, Yang, Lin, Wang, Xie & Feng 2016) (Fig. 7.3). (Reduced functional connectivity is measured by a reduced correlation between the activity of two brain areas, and implies that they are communicating less effectively.) The lateral orbitofrontal cortex BA 47/12, involved in non-reward and punishing events, did not have this reduced functional connectivity with memory systems, so that there is an imbalance in depression towards decreased reward-related memory system functionality.

A second major circuit difference was that the lateral orbitofrontal cortex area BA 47/12 had higher functional connectivity with the precuneus, the angular gyrus, and the temporal visual cortex BA 21 in patients with major depressive disorder than in controls (Cheng et al. 2016) (Fig. 7.3). This enhanced functional connectivity of the non-reward/punishment system (BA 47/12) with the precuneus (involved in the sense of self and agency), and the angular gyrus (involved in language) is thus related to the explicit affectively negative sense of the self, and of self-esteem, in depression. Further investigations have provided more evidence for increased functional connectivity of the lateral orbitofrontal cortex with the precuneus (Cheng, Rolls, Qiu, Yang, Ruan, Wei, Zhao, Meng, Xie & Feng 2018c), posterior cingulate cortex (providing a route into memory) (Cheng et al. 2018b), and the anterior cingulate cortex (Rolls et al. 2018c), and in a completely different patient population these

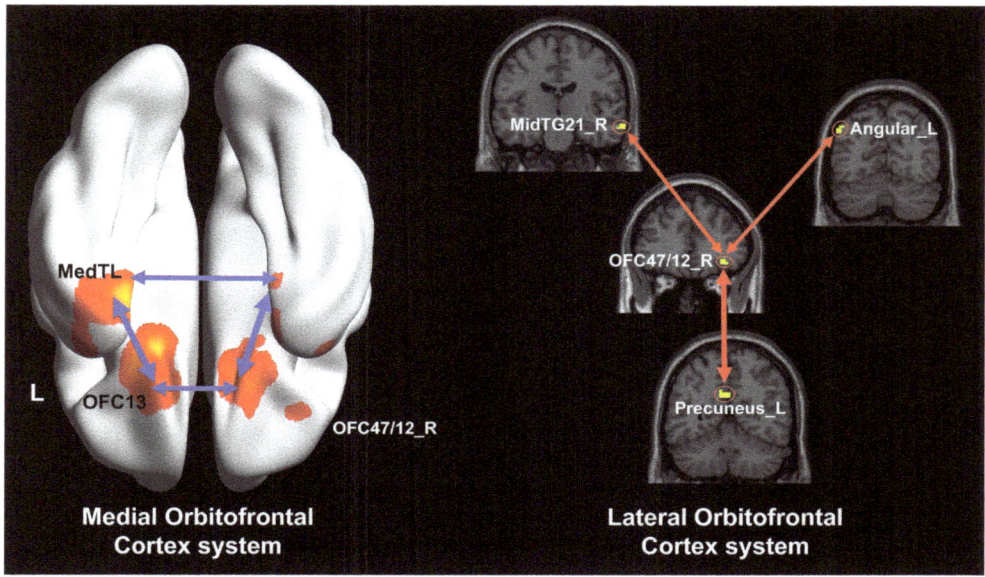

Fig. 7.3 Resting state functional connectivity in depression. The medial and lateral orbitofrontal cortex networks that show different functional connectivity in patients with depression. A decrease in functional connectivity is shown in blue, and an increase in red. MedTL – medial temporal lobe from the parahippocampal gyrus to the temporal pole; MidTG21R – middle temporal gyrus area 21 right; OFC13 – medial orbitofrontal cortex area 13; OFC47/12R – lateral orbitofrontal cortex area 47/12 right. The lateral orbitofrontal cortex cluster in OFC47/12 is visible on the ventral view of the brain anterior and lateral to the OFC13 clusters. (Modified from Cheng, Rolls et al, 2016.)

functional connectivities involving the lateral orbitofrontal cortex were correlated with the Depressive Problems score (Cheng, Rolls, Ruan & Feng 2018d), as described below.

The reduced functional connectivity of the medial orbitofrontal cortex, implicated in reward, with memory systems provides a new way of understanding how memory systems may be biased away from pleasant events in depression. The increased functional connectivity of the lateral orbitofrontal cortex, implicated in non-reward and punishment, with areas of the brain implicated in representing the self, language, and inputs from face and related perceptual systems provides a new way of understanding how unpleasant events and thoughts, and lowered self-esteem, may be exacerbated in depression (Cheng et al. 2016, Rolls et al. 2018a).

Because the lateral orbitofrontal cortex responds to many punishing and non-rewarding stimuli (Grabenhorst & Rolls 2011, Rolls 2014a, Rolls 2014b) that are likely to elicit autonomic/visceral responses, as does the supracallosal anterior cingulate cortex, and in view of connections from these areas to the anterior insula which is implicated in autonomic/visceral function (Critchley & Harrison 2013, Rolls 2016b), the anterior insula would also be expected to be overactive in depression, which it is (Drevets 2007, Hamilton et al. 2013, Ma 2015).

Treatments that can reduce depression such as a single dose of ketamine (Zanos & Gould 2018) (see further Section 7.7.2) may act in part by quashing the attractor state in the lateral orbitofrontal cortex at least temporarily. Evidence consistent with this is that the activity of the lateral orbitofrontal cortex is decreased by a single dose of ketamine (Lally, Nugent, Luckenbaugh, Niciu, Roiser & Zarate 2015). This NMDA receptor blocker may act at least in part by decreasing the high firing rate state of attractor networks by reducing transmission in the recurrent collateral excitatory connections between the neurons (Rolls 2016c, Rolls, Loh, Deco & Winterer 2008d, Rolls & Deco 2010, Rolls 2012a, Deco et al. 2013, Rolls & Deco 2015a). Given that a ketamine metabolite, hydroxynorketamine, may be related to the antidepressant effects of ketamine and may act via facilitating effects mediated by AMPA receptors (Zanos & Gould 2018), the effects of ketamine might be mediated by increasing the medial orbitofrontal cortex reward-related system (which tends to be reciprocally related to the lateral orbitofrontal non-reward system), or the functional connectivity of the medial orbitofrontal cortex reward system with the hippocampal system which is reduced in depression (Fig. 7.3). Electroconvulsive therapy may have antidepressant effects, may also knock the non-reward system out of its attractor state, and this may contribute to any antidepressant effect.

Electrical stimulation of the brain that may relieve depression (Hamani, Mayberg, Snyder, Giacobbe, Kennedy & Lozano 2009, Hamani, Mayberg, Stone, Laxton, Haber & Lozano 2011, Lujan, Chaturvedi, Choi, Holtzheimer, Gross, Mayberg & McIntyre 2013) may act in part by providing reward that reciprocally inhibits the non-reward system, and/or by interfering with the attractor state. Treatment with antidepressant drugs decreases the activity of this non-reward lateral orbitofrontal cortex system (Ma 2015).

Antidepressant drugs such as Selective Serotonin Reuptake Inhibitors (SSRIs) may treat depression by producing positive biases in the processing of emotional stimuli (Harmer & Cowen 2013), increasing brain responses to positive stimuli and decreasing responses to negative stimuli (Ma 2015). The reward and non-reward systems are likely to operate reciprocally, so that facilitating the reward system, or providing rewards, and thus activating the medial orbitofrontal cortex (O'Doherty, Kringelbach, Rolls, Hornak & Andrews 2001a, Grabenhorst & Rolls 2011, Rolls 2014a) (Fig. 3.54), may operate in part by inhibiting the overactivity in the lateral orbitofrontal cortex non-reward / punishment system (Rolls et al. 2018a).

Further, in research stimulated by the theory and results described here (Rolls 2016e, Cheng et al. 2016), it has been shown that transcranial magnetic stimulation of the lateral orbitofrontal cortex, which may disrupt its activity, helps in the treatment of depression (Feffer, Fettes, Giacobbe, Daskalakis, Blumberger & Downar 2018, Downar 2019), and that direct electrical stimulation of the orbitofrontal cortex can lift mood states (Rao et al. 2018).

7.4 Advances in understanding the functions of the orbitofrontal cortex in depression

7.4.1 Overview

We have seen evidence that implicates the orbitofrontal cortex in depression in Sections 7.2 and 7.3.

1. Sadness and depression can be caused by not receiving expected rewards, or by receiving punishers.
2. The lateral orbitofrontal cortex is implicated in detecting these reinforcement contingencies and thus in negative emotions, which are produced by these reward contingencies.
3. It has been proposed that the lateral orbitofrontal is overactive in depression, and continues its activity for long periods because of attractor networks implemented within the lateral orbitofrontal cortex, and by long-loop attractor networks between the lateral orbitofrontal cortex and reciprocally connected brain areas.
4. This theory of depression has been supported by functional neuroimaging studies that show increased functional connectivity of the lateral orbitofrontal cortex with other brain areas including the angular gyrus which is involved in language, which may contribute to continuing negative ruminating thoughts; and the precuneus which is involved in the sense of the self, and which may contribute to the low self-esteem that can occur in depression.

5. The medial orbitofrontal cortex is involved in reward processing, pleasure, and happiness, and has decreased connectivity with hippocampal memory systems in depression, which may contribute to the fewer happy memories present in depression.
6. These investigations have been supported by another investigation with participants from the general population in the USA, which showed that similar changes in functional connectivity were found in people who tended to have symptoms of depression (Cheng et al. 2018d).
7. These ideas have been supported by studies showing that transcranial magnetic stimulation of the lateral orbitofrontal cortex may help in the treatment of depression (Feffer et al. 2018, Downar 2019).
8. Thus the investigations described have implications not only for understanding depression better, but also for the treatment of depression.

In this section (7.4), recent advances in understanding the connectivity of brain systems related to depression are described, and many involve functional connectivity links with the orbitofrontal cortex. One of the measures used, functional connectivity, is measured by the correlation of the activity between two brain regions. If the correlation is high, then this implies that if the signal in one brain area increases, this is associated with an increase in the connected brain region. The implication of increased functional connectivity then is that two connected brain areas are 'talking to each other' strongly, and vice versa for decreased functional connectivity. An overview of some of the findings described in this section (7.4) follows, and a summary of some of the differences in functional connectivity in depression in voxel-level studies in large populations of participants are provided in Fig. 7.4 (Rolls et al. 2019b). This is in the context that a number of studies have provided evidence for different functional connectivity that may include the orbitofrontal cortex, anterior cingulate cortex, amygdala, and hippocampus, but that many of these studies have involved relatively small numbers of participants, and whole brain regions (Helm, Viol, Weiger, Tass, Grefkes, Del Monte & Schiepek 2018). The studies described next on which we focus have included large numbers of participants to provide robust results, and voxel-level analysis to enable separation of connectivity of nearby brain areas such as the medial and lateral orbitofrontal cortex (Rolls et al. 2019b).

In Sections 7.4.2 and 7.4.8 the evidence on the **orbitofrontal cortex** is extended by showing in a new population of individuals, from the USA, who have not been selected to have depression, that in this general population any tendency to have depressive symptoms is associated with similar changes in functional connectivity of the lateral orbitofrontal cortex found in patients (who were from China) diagnosed with depression (Cheng et al. 2018d). This is important validation of the theory that the orbitofrontal cortex is a key region with altered connectivity related to depression, and is consistent with the theory of depression proposed in Section 7.2. Section 7.4.2 also describes an activation study which shows that those at high risk of depression have high activation of the lateral orbitofrontal cortex in a non-reward condition; and are relatively insensitive to differences in reward in the medial orbitofrontal cortex (Xie et al. 2019), consistent with the theory of depression (Rolls 2016e, Rolls 2018a).

Another fascinating and new finding on a different group of people is that happiness and subjective well-being are correlated with decreased functional connectivity of the lateral orbitofrontal cortex (Liu, Ma, Rolls, Wei, Zhang, Chen, Meng, Qiu & Feng 2019). This is consistent with the hypothesis that increased non-rewarding processing (which is likely to be related to increased functional connectivity), including that related to sadness and depression, involves *increased* functional connectivity of the lateral orbitofrontal, for happiness is correlated with *decreased* lateral orbitofrontal cortex functional connectivity (Liu et al. 2019). Possible explanations are that people with high well-being are less affected by non-rewarding

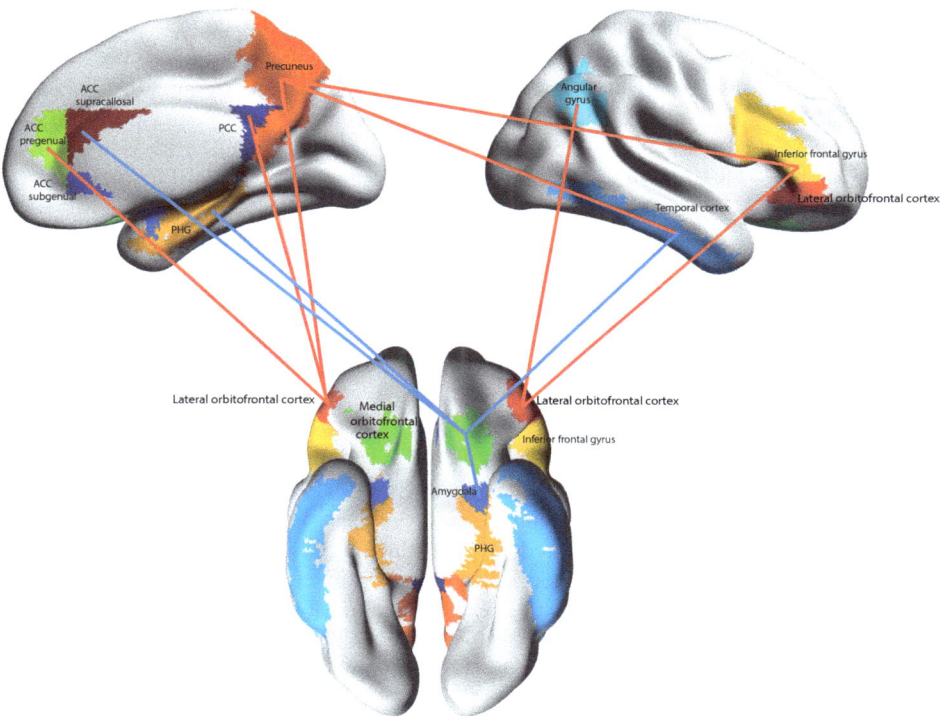

Fig. 7.4 Functional connectivity (FC) differences of the medial and lateral orbitofrontal cortex in major depressive disorder. Higher functional connectivity in depression is shown in red, and includes higher functional connectivity of the non-reward / punishment-related lateral orbitofrontal cortex with the precuneus, posterior cingulate cortex (PCC), pregenual anterior cingulate cortex (ACC), angular gyrus, and inferior frontal gyrus. Lower functional connectivity in depression is shown in blue, and includes lower functional connectivity of the medial orbitofrontal cortex with the parahippocampal gyrus memory system (PHG), amygdala, temporal cortex and supracallosal anterior cingulate cortex (ACC). The part of the medial orbitofrontal cortex in which voxels were found with lower functional connectivity in depression is indicated in green. The areas shown apart from that are as defined in the automated anatomical labelling atlas (AAL2) (Rolls et al., 2015), although the investigations that form the basis for the summary were at the voxel level. (After Rolls, Cheng and Feng, 2019b.)

events; and/or that considerable exposure to non-rewarding events may lead to increased in lateral orbitofrontal cortex connectivity.

In Section 7.4.3, the connections from the orbitofrontal cortex to one of the areas to which it projects, the **anterior cingulate cortex**, are considered (Rolls et al. 2018c). It is shown that the medial orbitofrontal, which is involved in processing reward value and pleasure, has high connectivity with the most anterior part of the anterior cingulate cortex (pregenual), which is also activated by rewards. The anterior cingulate cortex is implicated in learning which actions to take to obtain rewards, and the connectivity just described appears to be a way for rewards to reach the anterior cingulate cortex, so that rewards received can influence this type of action to (reward) outcome learning. Correspondingly, it is shown that the lateral orbitofrontal, which is involved in processing non-reward value and unpleasant stimuli, has high connectivity with the supracallosal part of the anterior cingulate cortex (just above the anterior part of the corpus callosum), which is also activated by non-reward and unpleasant stimuli. This provides a route for the costs of actions to be taken into account in learning which actions to take to maximise rewards and minimise the costs of the actions (see further Section 5.1).

It is also shown in Section 7.4.3 that in depression the anterior cingulate cortex has reduced connectivity with the orbitofrontal cortex, and also with temporal lobe areas involved in perception, the parahippocampal gyrus and hippocampus involved in memory, and motor areas. The concept is described that the anterior cingulate cortex, with its representations of rewards and punishers received from the orbitofrontal cortex and which is involved in interfacing these to action systems, appears to contribute to depression by disconnecting rewards and punishers from their action-related and other outputs. This would result is insensitivity to the effects of rewards and punishers, amotivational states, and feelings of helplessness (Rolls et al. 2018c).

Evidence is also described in Section 7.4.3 that a subcallosal part of the anterior cingulate cortex can be activated by negative stimuli, has increased activity in depression, and has been a target for deep brain stimulation to relieve depression (which might act by disrupting activity here), though this has not yet been validated in large-scale studies.

In Section 7.4.4 it is shown that the **posterior cingulate cortex** has significantly increased functional connectivity with the lateral orbitofrontal cortex in depression. The posterior cingulate cortex provides a gateway into the hippocampal memory system for spatial information including information about the self. These findings support the theory that the non-reward system in the lateral orbitofrontal cortex has increased effects on memory systems, which contribute to the rumination about sad memories and events in depression (Cheng et al. 2018b).

In Section 7.4.5, it is shown that in depression the **amygdala**, a brain region implicated in emotion, has reduced functional connectivity with the brain regions with which it is connected, including the orbitofrontal cortex (Cheng, Rolls, Qiu, Xie, Lyu, Li, Huang, Yang, Tsai, Lyu, Zhuang, Lin, Xie & Feng 2018a). A possible implication is that because the amygdala is somewhat disconnected in depression, it may be important to focus on other brain regions such as the lateral orbitofrontal cortex that have increased functional connectivity in depression, and may be more closely related to the strong emotional feelings of sadness in depression.

In Section 7.4.6 further evidence is provided that the **precuneus**, a medial parietal cortex region implicated in the sense of self and agency, has increased functional connectivity in depression with the lateral orbitofrontal cortex, a region implicated in non-reward and which is thereby implicated in depression (Cheng et al. 2018c). These findings support the theory that the non-reward system in the lateral orbitofrontal cortex has increased effects on areas in which the self is represented including the precuneus, resulting in the low self-esteem that may be present in depression (Rolls 2016e).

In Section 7.4.7 research is described that goes beyond functional connectivity to **effective connectivity** between different brain areas to measure directed influences of human brain regions on each other (Rolls et al. 2018a). Effective connectivity is conceptually very different, for it measures the effect of one brain region on another in a particular direction, and can in principle therefore provide information more closely related to the causal processes that operate in brain function, that is, how one brain region influences another. In the context of disorders of brain function, the effective connectivity may provide evidence on which brain regions may have altered function, and then influence other brain regions, by comparing effective connectivity in patients and control participants.

The results obtained with the use of effective connectivity are consistent with the hypotheses that some aspects of hippocampal processing, perhaps those related to unpleasant memories, are increased in depression (Rolls 2016e, Cheng et al. 2016); that the temporal cortex has increased effective connectivity to the precuneus which with its connectivity with memory systems and the lateral orbitofrontal cortex may contribute to low self-esteem and negative memories; that the influence of temporal lobe memory systems on specifically the medial orbitofrontal cortex is reduced in depression; and that this in turn may contribute to increased activity in the lateral orbitofrontal cortex non-reward system in depression (Rolls et al. 2018a).

All this new research supports the ideas presented in this Chapter that the orbitofrontal cortex is a key region for understanding how processing is different in depression. Increased connectivity of the lateral orbitofrontal cortex non-reward system in depression may contribute to the increased sadness in depression. The decreased functional connectivity of the medial orbitofrontal cortex reward system may contribute to the reduced happiness in depression. This makes further understanding of these brain areas important for understanding depression better, and potentially for treating depression better.

7.4.2 Orbitofrontal cortex

The human *medial orbitofrontal cortex* has activations related to many rewarding and subjectively pleasant stimuli (Rolls & Grabenhorst 2008, Grabenhorst & Rolls 2011, Rolls 2014a) (Fig. 3.54). In the sense that reward vs non-reward and punishment are reciprocally related in their effects in the medial vs lateral orbitofrontal cortex respectively (O'Doherty, Kringelbach, Rolls, Hornak & Andrews 2001a, Rolls 2014a, Xie, Jia, Rolls, Liu, Banaschewski, Barker, Bodke, Bromberg, C., Quinlan, Desrivieres, Flor, Grigis, Garavan, Gowland, Heinz, Hohmann, Ittermann, Martinot, Martinot, Nees, Papadopoulos Orfanos, Paus, Poustka, Frohner, Smolka, Walter, Whelan, Schumann, Feng & IMAGEN 2019), the anhedonia of depression can also be related to decreased functional connectivity of the medial orbitofrontal cortex in depression (Cheng et al. 2016, Rolls et al. 2019a), and to decreased effects of pleasant rewarding stimuli in the medial orbitofrontal cortex during depression, effects that can be restored by antidepressants (Ma 2015).

The *lateral orbitofrontal cortex / inferior frontal gyrus region* that responds to signals to inhibit a response in the stop-signal task (Deng et al. 2017) is implicated in impulsive behavior, with damage in this region increasing impulsive behavior (Aron et al. 2014). This is of potential importance, for treatment with antidepressants, which would be expected to reduce the over-activity in this ventrolateral prefrontal cortex region, might thereby increase impulsiveness relative to that in the depressed state. Indeed, it is an interesting hypothesis that impulsiveness might reflect under-activity in this ventrolateral prefrontal cortex region, and that depression produced by oversensitivity to non-reward and punishment might reflect over-activity in this lateral orbitofrontal cortex / ventrolateral prefrontal cortex region. In a certain sense, these types of behaviour might reflect opposite ends of a continuum of non-reward/punishment sensitivity. One end of the spectrum of sensitivity to non-reward could be impulsive behaviour (with too little sensitivity to non-reward and punishment); and the other end could be depression (with too much sensitivity to non-reward and punishment). The ventrolateral prefrontal cortex region refers here to a part of the lateral orbitofrontal cortex region BA12/47, and its continuation round the inferior prefrontal convexity to include parts of the inferior frontal gyrus, as found for the stop-signal task (Deng et al. 2017).

In an activation study using the monetary incentive delay task in 1140 19-year-old participants, it was found that the medial orbitofrontal cortex showed graded increasing activations for No win (0 points) to Small win (2 points) to Large win (10 points) conditions (Xie et al. 2019). Conversely, the lateral orbitofrontal cortex showed graded increases in activation for the Large win to Small win to No win conditions (Fig. 7.5). In a subgroup of 97 participants at a high risk of depression as assessed by the Adolescent Depression Rating Scale (Revah-Levy, Birmaher, Gasquet & Falissard 2007, Revah-Levy, Speranza, Barry, Hassler, Gasquet, Moro & Falissard 2011), there was higher activation in the lateral orbitofrontal in the No win condition (Xie et al. 2019). This is consistent with the theory that the lateral orbitofrontal cortex with its relation to non-reward is more sensitive in depression (or in this case, those at high risk of depression) to not receiving rewards (Rolls 2016e). Further, in the high risk group, the medial orbitofrontal cortex showed much less graded effects across the three increasing reward conditions (Xie et al. 2019). This is consistent with the theory that the

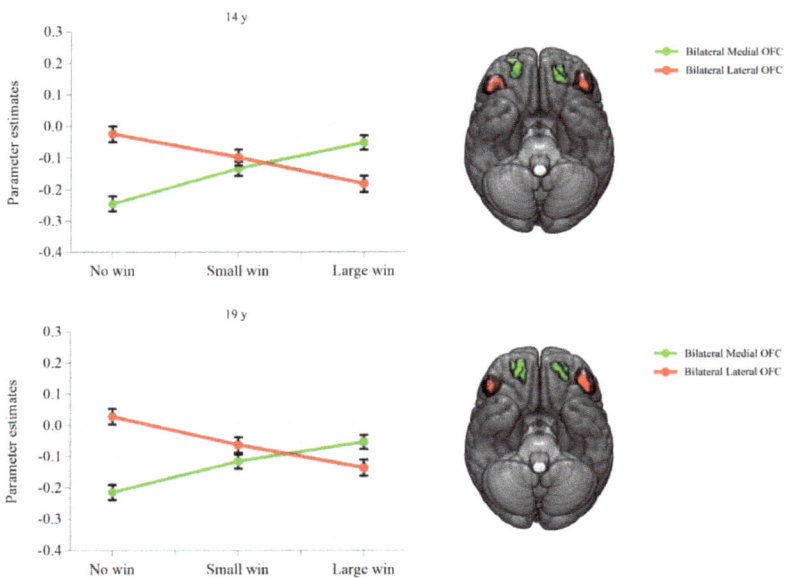

Fig. 7.5 The lateral orbitofrontal cortex region in which activations increased towards no reward (see below) in the monetary incentive delay task are shown in red in 1140 participants at age 19 and in the same participants at age 14. The conditions were Large win (10 points) to Small win (2 points) to No win (0 points) (at 19; sweets were used at 14). The medial orbitofrontal cortex region in which activations increased with increasing reward from No win to Small win to High win) is shown in green. The parameter estimates are shown from the activations for the whole group of 1140 participants (mean ± sem) with the lateral orbitofrontal in red and medial orbitofrontal cortex in green. In a subgroup at high risk of depression as shown by the Adolescent Depression Rating Scale, it was further found that there was a greater activation to the No win condition in the lateral orbitofrontal cortex; and the medial orbitofrontal cortex was less sensitive to the differences in reward value. (Modified from Xie, Jia, Rolls et al, 2019.)

medial orbitofrontal cortex with its relation to reward is less sensitive in depression (or in this case, those at high risk of depression) to receiving rewards, and may relate to the anhedonia and lack of motivation in depression (Rolls 2016e). Part of the interest of this investigation (Xie et al. 2019) is that it is an activation study, which complements the functional connectivity studies that provide consistent evidence for the theory of depression.

It is an interesting thought that these orbitofrontal cortex systems have evolved to have a distribution of efficacy that may serve to produce variation, so important in evolution by natural selection in different environments, in the tendency to initiate behaviour or not. Under-responsiveness of the lateral orbitofrontal cortex system might lead to individuals with risky, impulsive, behaviour. Over-responsiveness of the lateral orbitofrontal cortex may lead to behaviour very sensitive to non-reward, so that nothing risky is attempted, with at the end of the spectrum depressive behaviour being the outcome. The variation between individuals may reflect the fact that different behavioural strategies can have advantages; and that the genes may maintain this variation, as having variation may be useful for different environments.

Some of the recent findings on the brain functional connectivity differences related to depression have come from patients with depression from large datasets from China and Taiwan. A recent study with a completely different population of people has extended these results, by using participants drawn from the general population in the USA as part of the Human Connectome Project. In this investigation, participants were not selected on the basis of whether they were depressed, but part of the data collected in addition to the resting state fMRI scans consisted of the Adult Self-Report Depressive Problems score, a questionnaire which measures to what extent people may have depressive symptoms. In this general population, we found in a sample of 1017 participants (ages 22–35 years) that

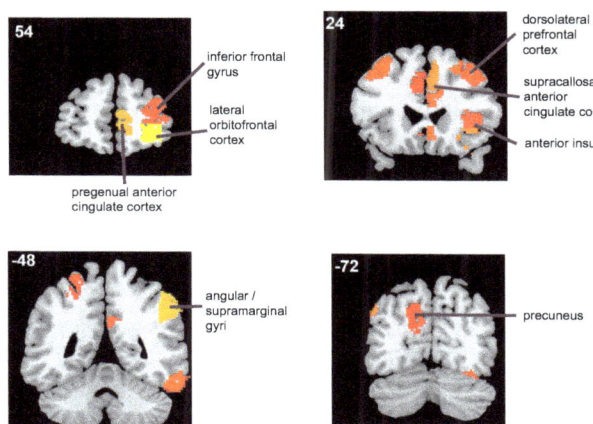

Fig. 7.6 Brain areas with functional connectivities related to the Adult Self-Report Depressive Problems scores from the analysis of Human Connectome Project data in individuals from the normal population. The significance value for the links to be included is p <0.005. The color (red through orange to yellow) reflects the number of correlated links in each of the 250 areas in the atlas by Shen et al (2013). Most of the functional connectivity links are positively correlated with the depression score. The anterior insula region is continuous with and just posterior to the lateral orbitofrontal cortex, and this anteroventral part of the insula is implicated in autonomic function. The number on each slice is the MNI Y coordinate. The right side of the brain is on the right of each image. (Adapted from JAMA Psychiatry, 75 (10), Wei Cheng, Edmund T. Rolls, Hongtao Ruan, and Jianfeng Feng, Functional Connectivities in the Brain That Mediate the Association Between Depressive Problems and Sleep Quality, pp. 1052–1061 Copyright © 2018, American Medical Association.)

the Adult Self-Report Depressive Problems score was positively correlated with functional connectivity involving areas such as the lateral orbitofrontal cortex and the adjacent inferior frontal gyrus, the dorsolateral prefrontal cortex (involved in working memory and attention), the anterior cingulate cortex, the angular gyrus, and the precuneus (implicated in the sense of self) (Fig. 7.6) (Cheng, Rolls, Ruan & Feng 2018d).

Part of the importance of this investigation (Cheng et al. 2018d) is that it provides strong support for a role of the lateral orbitofrontal cortex in depression. The findings were not on patients selected to have depression, but instead were on a general population in the USA in which a tendency to have depressive symptoms could be assessed, and indeed the correlations arose especially from the presence of 92 people who at some time had been diagnosed with depression. Yet very similar brain regions were identified in this investigation as having increased functional connectivity related to depressive symptoms, as in patients from China with a diagnosis of major depressive disorder. This important cross-validation provides support for the theory that the lateral orbitofrontal cortex is a key brain area that might be targeted in the search for treatments for depression (Rolls 2016e).

It is of interest that in the analysis of correlations of functional connectivities with depressive scores, the hippocampus / parahippocampal gyrus is not prominent in Fig. 7.6; that the angular gyrus is prominent; and that the medial orbitofrontal cortex is not prominent. Part of the importance of these new findings (Cheng et al. 2018d) is that they confirm in a completely different dataset the increased functional connectivity not only of the lateral orbitofrontal cortex, but also of the precuneus and angular gyrus found in patients with major depressive disorder (Cheng et al. 2016).

In a more recent study we focussed on functional connectivity in 125 unmedicated depressed people compared to 254 controls (Rolls, Cheng, Du, Wei, Qiu, Dai, Zhou, Xie & Feng 2019a). Functional connectivities between voxels in the lateral orbitofrontal cortex and the right inferior frontal gyrus, precuneus, posterior cingulate cortex, ventromedial prefrontal cortex, and the angular and middle frontal gyri were higher in unmedicated patients, and closer to controls in medicated patients. The lateral orbitofrontal cortex projects to the inferior frontal gyrus, and very interestingly higher functional connectivity was found in depression of voxels in the right inferior frontal gyrus with voxels in the lateral and medial orbitofrontal cortex, cingulate cortex, inferior and middle temporal gyrus and temporal pole, the angular gyrus, precuneus, hippocampus and middle and superior frontal gyrus. In medicated patients these functional connectivities of the inferior frontal gyrus were lower and towards those in controls.

It was proposed that one way in which the orbitofrontal cortex influences behaviour in depression is via the right inferior frontal gyrus, which projects in turn to premotor cortical areas. Consistent with the consequent hypothesis that the inferior frontal gyrus route may allow non-reward signals to have too great an effect to inhibit behaviour in depression, lesions of the right inferior frontal gyrus impair stopping in the stop-signal task, and produce impulsiveness (Aron et al. 2014). Also consistent with the hypothesis, successful stopping in the stop-signal task is associated with high activation of the inferior frontal gyrus and lateral orbitofrontal cortex (Deng et al. 2017).

In the same investigation (Rolls et al. 2019a), medial orbitofrontal cortex voxels had lower functional connectivity with temporal cortex areas, the parahippocampal gyrus, fusiform gyrus, and supplementary motor area, and medication did not result in these being closer to controls. This is consistent with the anhedonia of depression and reduced happy memories being related to these low functional connectivities of the medial orbitofrontal cortex with temporal lobe and memory systems. What is especially interesting is that these low functional connectivities are not normalized by treatment with antidepressant drugs (Rolls et al. 2019a), suggesting that a goal of future treatment for depression might be to increase the functionality of the medial orbitofrontal cortex.

In an activation study within the reinforcement learning framework, it was reported that positive reward prediction error in the medial orbitofrontal cortex was reduced in depression, and was correlated with anhedonia, but the learning was intact, in 28 drug naive patients with depression (Rothkirch, Tonn, Kohler & Sterzer 2017).

7.4.3 Anterior cingulate cortex

The supracallosal *anterior cingulate cortex* is activated by many aversive stimuli, and the pregenual cingulate cortex by many pleasant stimuli (Fig. 3.54) (Grabenhorst & Rolls 2011, Rolls 2014a). However, the anterior cingulate cortex appears to be involved in action-outcome learning, where the outcome refers to the reward or punisher for which an action is being learned (Rudebeck et al. 2008, Camille et al. 2011, Grabenhorst & Rolls 2011, Rushworth et al. 2011, Rushworth et al. 2012, Rolls 2014a) (Section 5.1). In contrast, the medial orbitofrontal cortex is implicated in reward-related processing and learning, and the lateral orbitofrontal cortex in non-reward and punishment-related processing and learning (Rolls 2014a). These involve stimulus-stimulus associations, where the second stimulus is a reward (or its omission), or a punisher (Rolls 2014a) (Chapter 6). Now given that emotions can be considered as states elicited by rewarding and punishing stimuli, and that moods such as depression can arise from prolonged non-reward or punishment (Rolls 2014a), the part of the brain that processes these stimulus-stimulus associations, the orbitofrontal cortex, is more likely to be involved in depression than the action-related parts of the cingulate cortex.

The *subgenual (or subcallosal) cingulate cortex* has also been implicated in depression, and electrical stimulation in that region may relieve depression (Mayberg 2003, Hamani et al. 2009, Hamani et al. 2011, Lozano, Giacobbe, Hamani, Rizvi, Kennedy, Kolivakis, Debonnel, Sadikot, Lam, Howard, Ilcewicz-Klimek, Honey & Mayberg 2012, Laxton, Neimat, Davis, Womelsdorf, Hutchison, Dostrovsky, Hamani, Mayberg & Lozano 2013a, Lujan et al. 2013) (although it has not been possible to confirm this in a double-blind study (Holtzheimer, Husain, Lisanby, Taylor, Whitworth, McClintock, Slavin, Berman, McKhann, Patil, Rittberg, Abosch,

Pandurangi, Holloway, Lam, Honey, Neimat, Henderson, DeBattista, Rothschild, Pilitsis, Espinoza, Petrides, Mogilner, Matthews, Peichel, Gross, Hamani, Lozano & Mayberg 2017)). However, the subgenual cingulate cortex is also implicated in autonomic function (Gabbott et al. 2003), and this could be related to some of the effects found in this area that are related to depression. Whether the subgenual cingulate cortex is activated because of inputs from the orbitofrontal cortex, or performs separate computations is not yet clear. Indeed, the orbitofrontal cortex has the inputs and representations required to compute non-reward, namely representations of expected value, and reward and punishment outcome value (Rolls 2014a) (Section 3.8), and it is not clear that the subgenual cingulate cortex has the information to perform that computation. Further, the possibility is considered that electrical stimulation of the subcallosal region, which includes parts of the ventromedial prefrontal cortex (Laxton et al. 2013a), that may relieve depression, may do so at least in part by activating connections involving the orbitofrontal cortex, other parts of the anterior cingulate cortex, and the striatum (Johansen-Berg et al. 2008, Hamani et al. 2009, Lujan et al. 2013).

In a recent study, the first fully voxel-level resting state functional-connectivity neuroimaging analysis of depression of the anterior cingulate cortex, with 282 patients with major depressive disorder and 254 controls, was performed (Rolls et al. 2018c). In the healthy controls, the medial orbitofrontal cortex was shown to have strong functional connectivity with the pregenual cingulate cortex, in both of which rewards are represented; and the lateral orbitofrontal cortex (and inferior frontal gyrus) was shown to have strong functional connectivity with the supracallosal, more dorsal, anterior cingulate cortex area, both of which are activated by unpleasant aversive stimuli (Rolls et al. 2018c) (Fig. 5.2; Section 5.1.2). In the group with major depressive disorder, voxels in the anterior cingulate cortex had significantly reduced functional connectivity with the orbitofrontal cortex, temporal lobe areas, the parahippocampal gyrus and hippocampus, and motor areas. The strengths of some of these functional connectivities were correlated with the Beck Depression Inventory and duration of illness measures of the depression, showing that these differences of functional connectivity were related to the depression.

In depression, overall the anterior cingulate cortex had significantly reduced functional connectivity with the orbitofrontal cortex, temporal lobe areas, the parahippocampal gyrus and hippocampus, and motor areas. The anterior cingulate cortex, with its representations of rewards and punishers received from the orbitofrontal cortex and which is involved in interfacing these to action systems, appears to contribute to depression by disconnecting rewards and punishers from their action-related and other outputs. This would result is insensitivity to the effects of rewards and punishers, amotivational states, and feelings of helplessness (Rolls et al. 2018c).

However, in addition in depression, increased functional connectivity was found between the lateral orbitofrontal cortex and the pregenual and subcallosal parts of the anterior cingulate cortex (Rolls et al. 2018c). This is consistent with the hypothesis that more non-reward information is being transmitted from the orbitofrontal cortex to the anterior cingulate cortex, and that this contributes to the depression (Rolls et al. 2018c).

7.4.4 Posterior cingulate cortex

The posterior cingulate cortex is a region with strong connectivity in primates with the entorhinal cortex and parahippocampal gyrus (areas TF and TH), and thus with the hippocampal memory system (Bubb et al. 2017, Vogt 2009, Rolls 2018a, Rolls & Wirth 2018) (Fig. 5.3 on page 149). The posterior cingulate cortex is an interesting region of convergence between ventral stream processing involved in the identification of objects, people, face expression, etc using visual, auditory, and tactile multimodal processing, and the dorsal stream process-

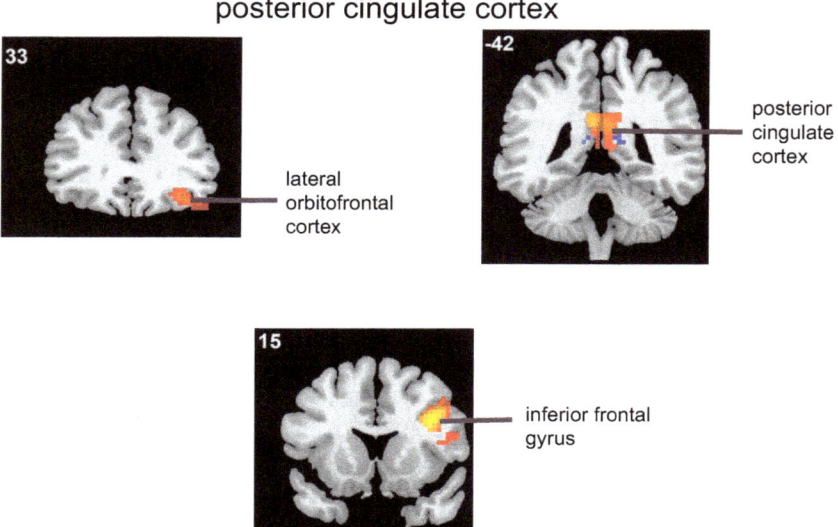

Fig. 7.7 Posterior cingulate cortex. Anatomical location of voxels with significantly different functional connectivity with the posterior cingulate cortex in depression in 125 unmedicated patients vs 254 controls obtained from the voxel-based Association Study (vAS). Red indicates voxels with an increase in functional connectivity in depression, and blue a decrease. Functional connectivity links between pairs of voxels are considered only if they are significantly different with $p < 0.0001$. The right of the brain is on the right of each slice. The Y values are in MNI coordinates. The analysis showed that the main differences in depression for the posterior cingulate cortex are an increase in functional connectivity of the posterior cingulate cortex with the lateral orbitofrontal cortex and a part of the inferior frontal gyrus. (Adapted from Wei Cheng, Edmund T. Rolls, Jiang Qiu, Xiongfei Xie, Dongtao Wei, Chu-Chung Huang, Albert C. Yang, Shih-Jen Tsai, Qi Li, Jie Meng, Ching-Po Lin, Peng Xie, and Jianfeng Feng, Increased functional connectivity of the posterior cingulate cortex with the lateral orbitofrontal cortex in depression, Translational Psychiatry, 8 (90), /doi.org/10.1038/s41398-018-0139-1 © 2018 Cheng, Rolls, Qiu, Xie, Wei, Huang, Yang, Tsai, Li, Meng, Lin, Xie, and Feng. This work is licensed under the Creative Commons Attribution 4.0 International License. It is attributed to the authors Cheng, Rolls, Qiu, Xie, Wei, Huang, Yang, Tsai, Li, Meng, Lin, Xie, and Feng.)

ing involved in spatial processing and action in space, providing access for both processing streams to the hippocampal memory system (Vogt 2009, Vogt & Pandya 1987, Vogt & Laureys 2009, Rolls 2018a, Rolls & Wirth 2018, Rolls 2019d). The posterior cingulate cortex also has connections with the orbitofrontal cortex (Vogt & Pandya 1987, Vogt & Laureys 2009) (Fig. 5.3). The posterior cingulate region (including the retrosplenial cortex) is consistently engaged by a range of tasks that examine episodic memory including autobiographical memory, and imagining the future; and also spatial navigation and scene processing (Leech & Sharp 2014, Auger & Maguire 2013). Self-reflection and self-imagery activate the ventral part of the posterior cingulate cortex (vPCC, the part with which we will be mainly concerned here) (Kircher et al. 2002, Kircher et al. 2000, Johnson et al. 2002, Sugiura et al. 2005).

To analyze the functioning of the posterior cingulate cortex (PCC) in depression, we performed the first fully voxel-level resting-state functional connectivity neuroimaging analysis of depression of the posterior cingulate cortex, with 336 patients with major depressive disorder and 350 controls (Cheng et al. 2018b). In the 350 controls, it was shown that the posterior cingulate cortex has high functional connectivity with the parahippocampal regions that are involved in memory.

In depression, the posterior cingulate cortex had significantly higher functional connectivity with the lateral orbitofrontal cortex, a region implicated in non-reward and which is thereby implicated in depression (Fig. 7.7). In patients receiving medication, the functional connectivity between the lateral orbitofrontal cortex and the posterior cingulate cortex was decreased back towards that in the controls. These findings support the theory that the non-reward system in the lateral orbitofrontal cortex has increased effects on memory systems, which contribute to the rumination about sad memories and events in depression (Cheng et al. 2018b).

The posterior cingulate cortex also had increased connectivity with BA 45 in the inferior frontal gyrus (Fig. 7.7) (Cheng et al. 2018b), a region involved in speech production which is closely related to the laryngeal motor area (Kumar, Croxson & Simonyan 2016). The increased connectivity between the posterior cingulate cortex system involved in the sense of self and in memory, and the inferior frontal gyrus BA45 speech / language system, may also contribute to the ruminating negative thoughts in depression. (Prefrontal and premotor areas can be active when the thoughts are about actions, even if the actions are not actually being made. In contrast, the primary motor cortex, area 4, is active only if the movements are actually being made (Passingham & Wise 2012).)

7.4.5 Amygdala

In addition to the insula, lateral orbitofrontal cortex, and supracallosal anterior cingulate cortex, which are all activated by unpleasant stimuli (Grabenhorst & Rolls 2011, Rolls 2014a), parts of the *amygdala* are activated by unpleasant stimuli, and parts by pleasant stimuli (Rolls 2014a), and amygdala activation has been related to depression (Harmer & Cowen 2013, Ma 2015, Price & Drevets 2012). However, the amygdala is less involved in non-reward, especially the rule-based reversal of which stimuli are classified as rewarding that is required in a rapid reward reversal task (Rolls 2014a). The orbitofrontal cortex is special in this, because the evidence is that it has attractor states than can be activated by non-reward (Thorpe, Rolls & Maddison 1983, Rolls 2014a), and these attractor states provide a basis for biasing the correct populations of neurons in the orbitofrontal cortex to implement the rapid one-trial reversal (Deco & Rolls 2005a, Rolls 2014a, Rolls & Deco 2016) (Chapter 3). Because the lateral orbitofrontal cortex has recurrent collaterals that can maintain attractor states, it is more likely to be involved in maintaining attractor states elicited by non-reward, including depression, than the amygdala (Rolls 2014a). The amygdala may therefore because of its responsiveness to punishing stimuli be related to depression, but may not be a structure that maintains its activity in an attractor state after non-reward, and during the mood state of depression.

To analyze the functioning of the amygdala in depression, we performed the first voxel-level resting state functional connectivity neuroimaging analysis of depression of voxels in the amygdala with all other voxels in the brain, with 336 patients with major depressive disorder and 350 controls (Cheng, Rolls, Qiu, Xie, Lyu, Li, Huang, Yang, Tsai, Lyu, Zhuang, Lin, Xie & Feng 2018a). Amygdala voxels had decreased functional connectivity with the medial orbitofrontal cortex (involved in reward); the lateral orbitofrontal cortex (involved in non-reward and punishment); temporal lobe areas (involved in visual and auditory perception), including the temporal pole, and inferior temporal gyrus; and the parahippocampal gyrus (involved in memory) (Figs. 7.8 and 7.9). The strengths of the functional connectivity of the amygdala voxels with the medial orbitofrontal cortex and temporal lobe voxels were correlated with the Beck Depression Inventory and duration of illness measures of the depression.

Parcellation analysis in 350 healthy controls based on voxel-level functional connectivity showed that the basal division of the amygdala has high functional connectivity with medial orbitofrontal cortex areas, and the dorsolateral part of the amygdala has especially strong functional connectivity with the lateral orbitofrontal cortex and its related ventral parts of the inferior frontal gyrus. In depression, the basal amygdala division had especially reduced functional connectivity with the medial orbitofrontal cortex which is involved in reward; and the dorsolateral amygdala subdivision had relatively reduced functional connectivity with the lateral orbitofrontal cortex which is involved in non-reward and punishment (Cheng

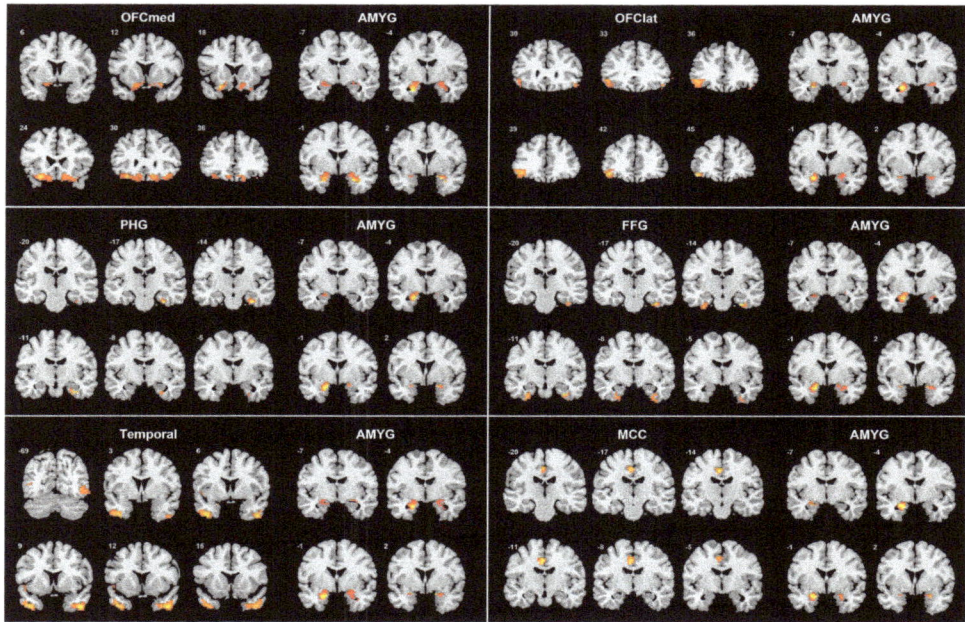

Fig. 7.8 The voxel-level functional connectivity for amygdala voxels that are significantly different in the depressed and the control group, separated by the automated anatomical atlas (AAL2) region in which the significant voxels were located. For each AAL2 area illustrated, the left six slices through that area at the MNI Y level indicated show the locations of the voxels with different functional connectivity with the amygdala. The right four slices at Y=-2, 1, 4, and 7 show the amygdala voxels with different functional connectivity in depressed patients compared to controls for that brain area. Measure of Association (MA) values are shown. Voxels with decreased functional connectivity are shown in blue, and with increased functional connectivity in red/yellow. Voxels are indicated where the functional connectivity with the paired region is p <0.05 (FDR corrected). OFCmed – medial orbitofrontal cortex; OFClat – lateral orbitofrontal cortex; PHG – parahippocampal gyrus; FFG – fusiform gyrus; Temporal – temporal cortical areas; MCC – middle cingulate cortex; FFG – fusiform gyrus. (Adapted from Wei Cheng, Edmund T Rolls, Jiang Qiu, Xiongfei Xie, Wujun Lyu, Yu Li, Chu-Chung Huang, Albert C Yang, Shih-Jen Tsai, Fajin Lyu, Kaixiang Zhuang, Ching-Po Lin, Peng Xie, and Jianfeng Feng, Functional connectivity of the human amygdala in health and in depression, Social Cognitive and Affective Neuroscience, 13 (6), pp. 557–568, Figure 2, https://doi.org/10.1093/scan/nsy032 © 2018 Cheng, Rolls, Qiu, Xie, Lyu, Li, Huang, Yang, Tsai, Lyu, Zhuang, Lin, Xie, and Feng. This work is licensed under the Creative Commons Attribution 4.0 International License. It is attributed to the authors Cheng, Rolls, Qiu, Xie, Lyu, Li, Huang, Yang, Tsai, Lyu, Zhuang, Lin, Xie, and Feng.)

et al. 2018a).

We can summarize these results (Fig. 7.9) (Cheng et al. 2018a) as follows. First, given that the amygdala has some roles in emotion (Aggleton 2000, Whalen & Phelps 2009, LeDoux 2012, Rolls 2014a), its reduced functional connectivity with the medial orbitofrontal cortex which is involved in reward and positive mood, may contribute to the lowering of mood by being somewhat disconnected from the orbitofrontal cortex in depression.

Second, the functional connectivity reductions of the amygdala with medial temporal lobe areas such as the parahippocampal, perirhinal and entorhinal cortex implicated in memory is similar to that of the medial orbitofrontal cortex, which has greatly reduced functional connectivity with the medial temporal lobe memory system (Cheng et al. 2016), and which with its role in reward may be related to the reduced processing of happy memories, and therefore an imbalance towards unhappy memories, in depression (Cheng et al. 2016, Rolls 2016e).

Third, some voxels in the amygdala had decreased functional connectivity with some temporal cortex areas including the inferior temporal gyrus, temporal pole, and fusiform gyrus, areas known to be involved in visual and multimodal processing (Rolls 2012d, Rolls 2016c). These decreases of these functional connectivities were correlated with the severity of the symptoms and the illness duration, and these functional connectivities were higher in medicated than unmedicated patients. This is thus strong evidence that the reduction of

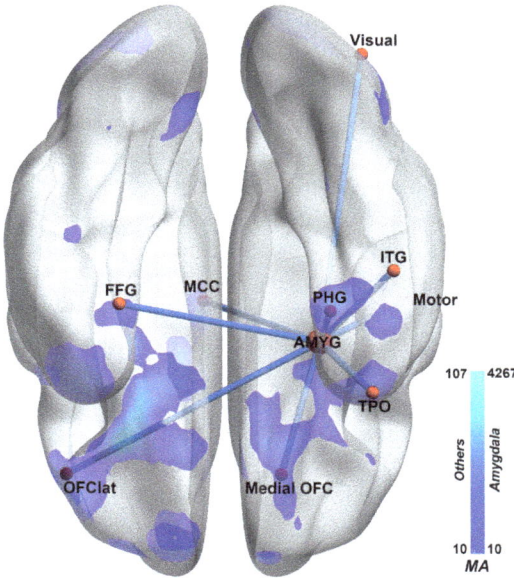

Fig. 7.9 Summary of amygdala functional connectivity differences in depression. The amygdala networks that show different functional connectivity in patients with depression. Ventral view of the brain. A decrease in functional connectivity is shown in blue, and an increase in red, at the voxel level, with the scale shown on the right calibrated using the measure of Association of each voxel (MA, see text). AMYG – amygdala; HIP – hippocampus; ITG – inferior temporal gyrus; MCC – Mid-cingulate cortex; Motor – pre- and post-central gyrus and Rolandic operculum; OFC– orbitofrontal cortex; PHG – parahippocampal area; FFG– fusiform gyrus; TPO– temporal pole; Visual – some occipital areas. Voxels with different functional connectivity from controls are shown by the blue shading, with decreases evident in depression. (Adapted from Wei Cheng, Edmund T Rolls, Jiang Qiu, Xiongfei Xie, Wujun Lyu, Yu Li, Chu-Chung Huang, Albert C Yang, Shih-Jen Tsai, Fajin Lyu, Kaixiang Zhuang, Ching-Po Lin, Peng Xie, and Jianfeng Feng, Functional connectivity of the human amygdala in health and in depression, Social Cognitive and Affective Neuroscience, 13 (6), pp. 557–568, Figure 2, https://doi.org/10.1093/scan/nsy032 © 2018 Cheng, Rolls, Qiu, Xie, Lyu, Li, Huang, Yang, Tsai, Lyu, Zhuang, Lin, Xie, and Feng. This work is licensed under the Creative Commons Attribution 4.0 International License. It is attributed to the authors Cheng, Rolls, Qiu, Xie, Lyu, Li, Huang, Yang, Tsai, Lyu, Zhuang, Lin, Xie, and Feng.)

connectivity between temporal cortex areas and the amygdala is important in depression. These temporal cortex areas may introduce inputs relevant to emotion to the amygdala, in that neurons in the primate inferior temporal visual cortex respond to faces (Perrett et al. 1982, Rolls 2011a, Rolls 2012d), and similar neurons are found in the amygdala (Leonard et al. 1985), linking these regions to emotional responses to faces. The hypothesis is that these temporal cortical areas provide important inputs to the amygdala, and that backprojections from the amygdala reach these areas and also earlier cortical including occipital visual areas (Rolls 2014a, Rolls 2016c, Amaral & Price 1984).

Fourth, some amygdala voxels had reduced functional connectivity with the middle cingulate cortex, involved in motor function, in depression (Cheng et al. 2018a). This pathway has been identified in macaques, and it has been suggested is involved in influences of amygdala face processing subsystems on emotional face expressions associated with social communication and emotional constructs such as fear, anger, happiness, and sadness (Morecraft, McNeal, Stilwell-Morecraft, Gedney, Ge, Schroeder & van Hoesen 2007). Interestingly, no effects were found relating the amygdala in depression to a different cingulate area involved in reward and pleasure, the anterior cingulate cortex. This again emphasizes the importance of the orbitofrontal cortex and the regions connected to it in depression (Rolls 2016e).

7.4.6 Precuneus

The precuneus is a medial parietal cortex region implicated in the sense of self and agency, and in autobiographical memory (Cavanna & Trimble 2006, Freton, Lemogne, Bergouignan,

Delaveau, Lehericy & Fossati 2014). In our fMRI investigation of functional connectivity in depression, we found that the lateral orbitofrontal cortex had increased functional connectivity in depression with some voxels in the precuneus and posterior cingulate cortex (Cheng et al. 2016). We therefore went on to analyze further the role of the precuneus in depression (Cheng, Rolls, Qiu, Yang, Ruan, Wei, Zhao, Meng, Xie & Feng 2018c), as described next.

The precuneus and the adjoining retrosplenial cortex (areas 29 and 30) are key regions related to spatial function, memory, and navigation (Bubb et al. 2017). The retrosplenial cortex provides connections to and receives connections from the hippocampal system, connecting especially with the parahippocampal gyrus areas TF and TH, and with the subiculum (Kobayashi & Amaral 2003, Kobayashi & Amaral 2007, Bubb et al. 2017) (Fig. 5.3). The precuneus can be conceptualized as providing access to the hippocampus for spatial and related information from the parietal cortex (given the rich connections between the precuneus and parietal cortex). Object information from the temporal lobe connects to and from the hippocampus via the perirhinal cortex (Rolls 2015d). This provides a basis for the hippocampus to associate together object and spatial information in the single network in the CA3 region of the hippocampus, to form an episodic memory with object and spatial components (Kesner & Rolls 2015). However, reward-related / emotional information may also be part of an episodic memory, and connections from the orbitofrontal cortex to the hippocampal system via the perirhinal and entorhinal cortex pathway are likely to be one route (Rolls 2014a, Rolls 2015d, Rolls 2016c, Rolls 2017c). Interestingly, the relatively strong functional connectivity between the precuneus and the lateral orbitofrontal cortex described here indicates that reward / punishment-related information also enters this part of the system (Fig. 5.3).

To further analyze the functioning of the precuneus in depression, we performed the first fully voxel-level resting state functional connectivity neuroimaging analysis of depression of the precuneus, with 282 patients with major depressive disorder and 254 controls (Cheng et al. 2018c). In 125 patients not receiving medication, voxels in the precuneus had significantly increased functional connectivity with the lateral orbitofrontal cortex, a region implicated in non-reward and which is thereby implicated in depression (Fig. 7.10). In patients receiving medication, the functional connectivity between the lateral orbitofrontal cortex and precuneus was decreased back towards that in the controls (Cheng et al. 2018c). These findings support the theory that the non-reward system in the lateral orbitofrontal cortex has increased effects on areas in which the self is represented including the precuneus, resulting in low self-esteem (Rolls 2016e).

Functional connectivity was also increased in depression between the precuneus and an inferior frontal gyrus region BA45 that probably is involved in speech production using the larynx and language (Kumar et al. 2016); the angular and supramarginal areas (involved in language); and the temporal cortex including the temporal pole (involved in perception) (Cheng et al. 2018c). The increased connectivity of the precuneus with angular and supramarginal cortical areas involved in language and the inferior frontal gyrus speech / language system may contribute to the negative ruminating thoughts about the self in depression (Cheng et al. 2018c) (Fig. 7.10.

In the 254 controls, it was shown that the precuneus has high functional connectivity with the parahippocampal and dorsolateral prefrontal regions that are involved in memory; and with the parietal cortex. This connectivity, also present in depression, may enable negative memories about the self to be recalled back from memory to influence current thinking (Cheng et al. 2018c).

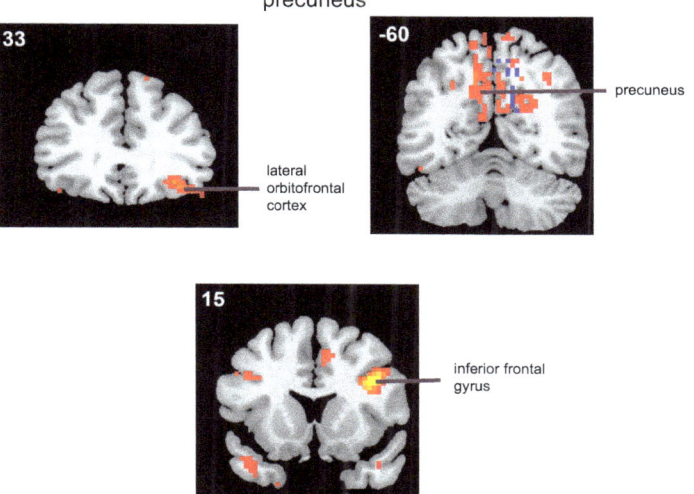

Fig. 7.10 Anatomical location of voxels with significantly different functional connectivity with the precuneus in depression in 125 unmedicated patients vs 254 controls obtained from the voxel-based Association Study (vAS). Red indicates voxels with an increase in functional connectivity in depression, and blue a decrease. Functional connectivity links between pairs of voxels are considered only if they are significantly different with FDR correction p <0.05.) The right of the brain is on the right of each slice. The Y values are in MNI coordinates. This shows that the main differences in depression that is unmedicated are an increase in functional connectivity between the precuneus and the lateral orbitofrontal cortex and an inferior frontal gyrus region. (Adapted from Biological Psychiatry: Cognitive Neuroscience and Neuroimaging, 3 (12), Wei Cheng, Edmund T. Rolls, Jiang Qiu, Deyu Yang, Hongtao Ruan, Dongtao Wei, Libo Zhao, Jie Meng, Peng Xie, and Jianfeng Feng, Functional Connectivity of the Precuneus in Unmedicated Patients With Depression, pp. 1040–1049, © 2018 Society of Biological Psychiatry. Published by Elsevier Inc. All rights reserved.)

7.4.7 Effective connectivity in depression

Resting state functional connectivity reflects correlations in the activity between brain areas. The concept is that if the correlations between two brain areas are higher, this may reflect stronger influences between them, including stronger transmission of information from one to the other (Deco & Kringelbach 2014, Cheng et al. 2016). Because the measure of functional connectivity is a correlation, it does not address the direction of the influence between two brain areas.

We have recently gone beyond functional connectivity to effective connectivity between different brain areas to measure directed influences of human brain regions on each other (Rolls et al. 2018a). Effective connectivity is conceptually very different, for it measures the effect of one brain region on another in a particular direction, and can in principle therefore provide information more closely related to the causal processes that operate in brain function, that is, how one brain region influences another. In the context of disorders of brain function, the effective connectivity may provide evidence on which brain regions may have altered function, and then influence other brain regions, by comparing effective connectivity in patients and controls participants. Effective connectivity can also provide a generative model and understanding of brain connectivity.

We utilized a new approach to the measurement of effective connectivity in which each brain area has a simple dynamical model, and known anatomical connectivity is used to provide constraints (Gilson, Moreno-Bote, Ponce-Alvarez, Ritter & Deco 2016). This helps the approach to measure the effective connectivity between the 94 automated anatomical atlas (AAL2) brain areas (Rolls et al. 2015a) using resting state functional magnetic resonance imaging. This approach also defines a Σ parameter for each brain area which reflects the variation (variance) of the signal in each brain area.

We found that effective connectivity directed to the medial orbitofrontal cortex from areas

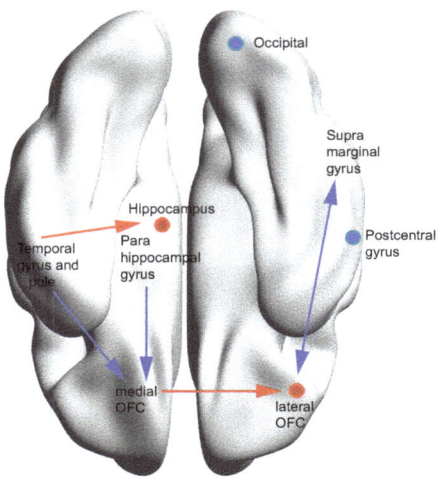

Fig. 7.11 Summary of the networks that show different effective connectivity in patients with depression, shown on a ventral view of the brain. A decrease in effective connectivity in patients with major depressive disorder is shown in blue, and an increase in red. In most cases there was a similar change in the effective connectivity in both directions in depression. The direction of the arrows shows though the direction of the stronger (termed forward) effective connectivity. Regions with an increased value of Σ, reflecting increased activity, are indicated by a red circle; and regions with a decreased value of Σ, are indicated by a blue circle. (Reprinted from Biological Psychiatry: Cognitive Neuroscience and Neuroimaging, 3(2), Edmund T. Rolls, Wei Cheng, Matthieu Gilson, Jiang Qiu, Zicheng Hu, Hongtao Ruan, Yu Li, Chu-Chung Huang, Albert C. Yang, Shih-Jen Tsai, Xiaodong Zhang, Kaixiang Zhuang, Ching-Po Lin, Gustavo Deco, Peng Xie, and Jianfeng Feng, Effective connectivity in depression, pp. 187–197, doi.org/10.1016/j.bpsc.2017.10.004 © 2017 Society of Biological Psychiatry. Published by Elsevier Inc. All rights reserved.)

including the parahippocampal gyrus, temporal pole, inferior temporal gyrus, and amygdala was decreased in depression (Rolls et al. 2018a) (Fig. 7.11). This is the forward direction for most of these links, i.e. the direction in which the directed connectivity is stronger (Rolls et al. 2018a, Rolls 2016c). This implies less strong positive driving influences of these input regions on the medial and middle orbitofrontal cortex, regions implicated in reward, and thus helps to elucidate part of the decreased feelings of happy states in depression (Rolls 2016e).

The lateral orbitofrontal cortex, an area implicated in non-reward and punishment, had an increased level of activity as reflected in Σ in the depressed group (Fig. 7.11). This was associated with increased effective connectivity from the medial orbitofrontal cortex directed to the lateral orbitofrontal cortex (Fig. 7.11). Given that the medial and lateral orbitofrontal cortex tend to have activations that are related reciprocally to each other, and that there is likely to be less reward-related activity in the medial orbitofrontal cortex in depression, this effective connectivity link may contribute to the increased activity in the lateral orbitofrontal cortex in depression.

The forward links from temporal cortical areas to the precuneus are increased in depression (and are close to significant after FDR correction), and this may relate to representations of the sense of self (Cavanna & Trimble 2006), which become more negative in depression (Rolls 2016e, Cheng et al. 2016, Cheng et al. 2018c).

A notable finding was that Σ was also increased in the right and left hippocampus of patients with depression, reflecting it is suggested some type of heightened memory-related processing. This is in the context that the effective connectivity directed from the temporal pole to the hippocampus is increased in depression (Fig. 7.11).

Together these differences of effective connectivity in depression (Rolls et al. 2018a) are consistent with the hypotheses that some aspects of hippocampal processing, perhaps those related to unpleasant memories, are increased in depression (Rolls 2016e, Cheng et al. 2016); that temporal cortex has increased effective connectivity to the precuneus which with its connectivity with memory systems and the lateral orbitofrontal cortex may contribute to low self-esteem and negative memories; that the influence of temporal lobe memory systems on specifically the medial orbitofrontal cortex is reduced in depression; and that this in turn may contribute to increased activity in the lateral orbitofrontal cortex non-reward system in depression (Rolls et al. 2018a).

The value of effective connectivity in understanding the operation of these systems in depression is that although the functional connectivity (which reflects correlations) between these areas has been shown to be reduced in depression (Cheng et al. 2016), it is only by using effective connectivity that we understand better the direction of the major influence between these brain regions (from the temporal lobe to the medial orbitofrontal cortex), and for example that this directed connectivity is reduced in depression (Rolls et al. 2018a).

7.4.8 Depression and poor sleep quality

Many individuals with depression report poor sleep quality (Becker, Jesus, Joao, Viseu & Martins 2017). What is the relation between depression and sleep? What are the brain systems that relate to depression and sleep quality? Understanding the answers to these questions may lead to better directed treatments for depression, and may improve sleep quality.

To advance understanding of the brain regions involved in sleep and depression, brain areas that mediate the effect of depression that underlies poor sleep quality were analyzed (Cheng et al. 2018d). The relation between functional connectivity (FC), depressive symptoms (the Adult Self-Report Depressive Problems scores) and poor sleep quality was measured in 1017 participants in the Human Connectome Project (HCP), with cross-validation of the sleep findings in 5342 participants from the UK Biobank.

181 functional connectivity links involving areas such as the precuneus, anterior cingulate cortex and the lateral orbitofrontal cortex related to sleep quality were identified. 39 of these sleep-related links were also related to the depressive scores. The brain areas with increased functional connectivity of these common links related to both sleep and depressive scores included the lateral orbitofrontal cortex; the dorsolateral prefrontal cortex; the anterior and posterior cingulate cortex; the insula; the parahippocampal gyrus and hippocampus; the amygdala; the temporal cortex; and the precuneus (Fig. 7.12). A mediation analysis showed that these functional connectivities in the brain contribute to the relation between depression and poor sleep quality.

The implication is that the increased functional connectivity between these brain regions provides a neural basis for how depression leads to poor sleep quality (Cheng et al. 2018d). This in turn has implications for the treatment of depression, and its effects on poor sleep quality (Cheng et al. 2018d).

Evidence was also found in this general population that the Depressive Problems scores were correlated with functional connectivities between areas that included the lateral orbitofrontal cortex, cingulate cortex; precuneus, angular gyrus, and temporal cortex (Cheng et al. 2018d) (Fig. 7.6). Part of the importance of this is that it provides strong support for a role of the lateral orbitofrontal cortex in depression. Our previous findings on functional and effective connectivity in depression (Cheng et al. 2016, Rolls et al. 2018a, Cheng et al. 2018c, Rolls et al. 2018c, Cheng et al. 2018b, Cheng et al. 2018a) were in hundreds of patients with major depressive disorder and controls in China. The findings in the present study (Cheng et al. 2018d) were not on patients selected to have depression, but instead were on a general population in the U.S.A. in which a tendency to have depressive problems could

216 | The orbitofrontal cortex, depression, and other mental disorders

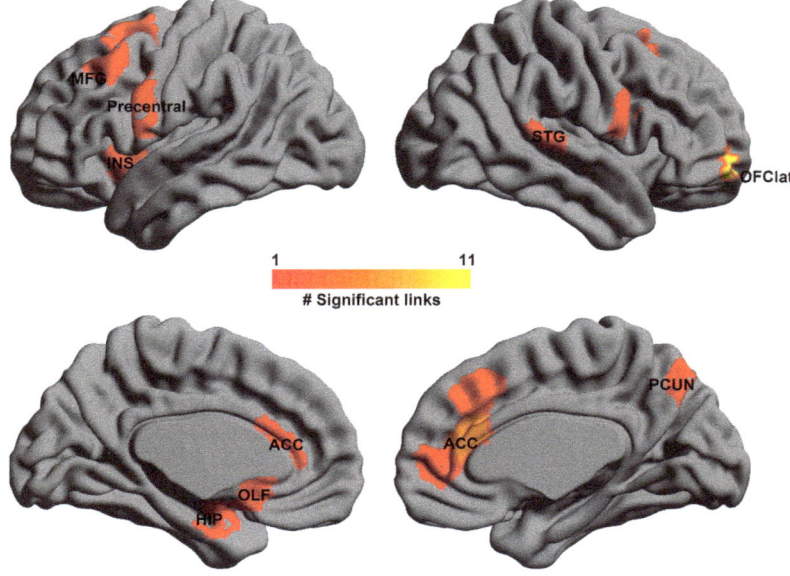

Fig. 7.12 The Shen atlas areas with functional connectivities related to sleep quality, and then selected to be also related to depression. There were 39 such links (significant with NBS correction, p <0.05). ACC – anterior cingulate cortex; HIP– hippocampus; INS – insula; MFG – middle frontal gyrus; OFClat – lateral orbitofrontal cortex; OLF – olfactory tubercle / ventral striatum; PCUN; precuneus; Precentral – precentral gyrus; STG – superior temporal gyrus. (Modified from JAMA Psychiatry, 75 (10), Wei Cheng, Edmund T. Rolls, Hongtao Ruan, and Jianfeng Feng, Functional Connectivities in the Brain That Mediate the Association Between Depressive Problems and Sleep Quality, pp. 1052–1061 Copyright © 2018, American Medical Association.)

be assessed. In fact, the correlations arose especially from the presence of 92 people who at some time had been diagnosed with depression. It is important cross-validation that very similar brain regions were identified in the present investigation as having increased functional connectivity related to depressive problems, including the lateral orbitofrontal cortex, precuneus and dorsolateral prefrontal cortex, as in our previous investigations.

This important cross-validation in a completely different population and in people not selected to have depression (Cheng et al. 2018d) provides support for the theory that the lateral orbitofrontal cortex is a key brain area that might be targeted in the search for treatments for depression (Rolls 2016e).

7.5 Possible subtypes of depression

There is growing interest in possible subtypes of depression, for it may be possible to treat different subtypes differently, for example by targeting different brain systems, or by different types of cognitive therapy (Downar, Blumberger, Rizvi, Daskalakis, Kennedy & Giacobbe 2019, Drysdale, Grosenick, Downar, Dunlop, Mansouri, Meng, Fetcho, Zebley, Oathes, Etkin, Schatzberg, Sudheimer, Keller, Mayberg, Gunning, Alexopoulos, Fox, Pascual-Leone, Voss, Casey, Dubin & Liston 2017).

One subtype may be related to anhedonia, a reduction in pleasure and in reward-related learning. This could be related to reduced functioning of the medial orbitofrontal cortex and related brain systems such as the ventral striatum. Pathological distortions of activity in this system (i.e. hypoactivity for conventional positive incentives and hyperactivity for negative incentives) may relate to this symptom of major depressive disorder: anhedonia. Patients with high anhedonia show a poor response to serotonergic antidepressants and to rTMS.

A second possible subtype may be related to prominent (almost compulsive) negative thoughts, and to increased anxiety and neuroticism. This subtype may include a tendency to counterproductive reappraisal of innocuous stimuli as hypothetically harmful or negative. There may also be suicidal ideation. This subtype could be related to increased sensitivity and persistence of networks in the lateral orbitofrontal cortex non-reward / punishment and related networks.

A third possible subtype may have reduced cognitive control and response inhibition, and increased impulsivity. Individuals in this subtype may for example have difficulty in resisting binge eating. The type of impulsivity is that reflected in delay discounting (in which there is impulsive choice of immediate rewards) and clinical measures (e.g. the Barratt impulsivity scale). This may be related to anterior cingulate cortex and related networks.

A fourth subtype may have anxiety as an accompaniment (Drysdale et al. 2017), and this subtype may be especially helped by rTMS of the lateral orbitofrontal cortex (Feffer et al. 2018).

7.6 Implications for treatments for depression

7.6.1 Brain-based treatments

This non-reward / punishment attractor network sensitivity theory of depression has implications for treatments. These implications can be understood and further explored in the context of investigations of the factors that influence the stability of attractor neuronal networks with integrate-and-fire neurons with noise introduced by the close to Poisson spiking times of the neurons (Wang 2002, Rolls 2016c, Deco, Rolls & Romo 2009, Rolls & Deco 2010, Deco et al. 2013, Loh, Rolls & Deco 2007, Rolls & Deco 2015a, Rolls 2016c).

One implication is that anti-anxiety drugs, by increasing inhibition, might reduce the stability of the high firing rate state of the non-reward attractor, thus acting to quash the depression-related attractor state.

A second implication is that it might be possible to produce agents that decrease the efficacy of NMDA receptors in the lateral orbitofrontal cortex, thereby reducing the stability of the depression-related attractor state. The evidence that there are genes that are selective for NMDA receptors for the neurons in different populations is that there are separate genetic knock-outs for NMDA receptors in the CA3 and CA1 regions of the hippocampus (Nakazawa, Quirk, Chitwood, Watanabe, Yeckel, Sun, Kato, Carr, Johnston, Wilson & Tonegawa 2002, Tonegawa, Nakazawa & Wilson 2003, Nakazawa, Sun, Quirk, Rondi-Reig, Wilson & Tonegawa 2003, Nakazawa, McHugh, Wilson & Tonegawa 2004).

The present theory suggests that searching for ways to influence the attractor networks in the lateral orbitofrontal cortex by decreasing the activity of neurons in this region may be of considerable interest. It should be noted that the present theory is a theory specifically of non-reward and punishment-related attractor networks in the lateral orbitofrontal cortex and related areas in relation to depression, and that alterations of attractor networks in other cortical areas may be related to other psychiatric disorders such as schizophrenia and obsessive-compulsive disorders (Rolls 2012a, Rolls 2016c).

In terms of the implications of the attractor-based aspect of the present theory, an important point is that the attractor dynamics must be kept stable in the face of the randomness or noise introduced into the system by the almost Poisson firing times of neurons for a given mean firing rate. For example, the spontaneous firing rate state of the non-reward attractor must be maintained stable when no non-reward inputs are present (or otherwise the non-reward attractor would jump into a high firing rate non-reward state for no external reason, contributing to depression). The inhibitory transmitter GABA may be important in maintaining this type of stability (Rolls & Deco 2010).

Moreover, the high firing rate state produced by non-reward must not reach too high a firing rate, as this would cause overstability of the non-reward / depression state. In a complementary way, if the high firing rate attractor state is insufficiently high, then that attractor state might be unstable, and the individual might be relatively insensitive to non-reward, not depressed, and impulsive because of not responding sufficiently to non-reward or punishment. The excitatory transmitter glutamate acting at NMDA or AMPA receptors may be important in setting the stability of the high firing rate attractor state. In this respect and in this sense, the tendency to become depressed or to be impulsive may be reciprocally related to each other.

Predictions for treatments follow from understanding these noisy attractor-based dynamics (Rolls & Deco 2010, Rolls 2016c) that are described in Section 3.13, and are considered next.

7.6.2 Behavioural treatments and cognitive therapy

The whole concept of attractor states (Section 3.13) has many implications for the treatment of depression, for rewards and other environmental changes and activities that tend to compete with the non-reward attractor state and quash it may be useful in the treatment of depression (Rolls 2016e, Rolls 2018b). These cognitive approaches might include diverting thought and attention away from the negative stimuli and influences that may contribute to the depression; and directing thought and attention towards rewards, which may help to quash the activity of the non-reward system by the reciprocal interactions between the brain systems involved in reward vs non-reward and punishment.

Particular implications of the attractor-based approach to depression include the following.

First, falling into an attractor state is an inherently non-linear process, and once in the attractor state, the system is stable and is difficult to perturb out of the attractor state, as shown in Section 3.13. An implication is that treatments will need to take this stability of attractor networks into account, and use effective perturbations to make the system move out of its stable attractor. These treatments might be at the purely behavioural or cognitive therapy level. The aim would be to help those with depression to understand some of the factors now thought to lead to depression, and to thereby help them to engage in behavioural changes that would knock the system out of its non-reward attractor. These might include strategies to prevent rumination by the patient deliberately interrupting sad ruminating thoughts, and engaging in activity that might involve performing very different behaviours that would compete with their non-reward attractor. This might involve tasks that require a lot of attention (perhaps activities such as sailing or golf), or that might involve obtaining rewards, which would tend to suppress the non-reward attractor because of the reciprocal relation between the medial orbitofrontal cortex reward system and the lateral orbitofrontal cortex non-reward/punishment system.

This strategy overlaps with the learned helplessness approach to depression, in which placing individuals for a prolonged period in which their actions do not lead to rewards results in the individuals not only obtaining a great deal of non-reward, but also learning to stop trying, as whatever is tried is ineffective (hence the term 'learned helplessness') (Seligman 1978). Setting up situations in which the individuals learn how to obtain rewards again is a beneficial treatment in this situation.

Second, there are multiple attractor loops, each one of which may contribute to the stability of the depressed state, and each one of which may need correction. For example, in Fig. 7.3 we see that in addition to the local attractor network in the lateral orbitofrontal cortex, there is increased functional connectivity between the lateral orbitofrontal cortex and the angular gyrus, which is involved in language (Cheng et al. 2016). This latter is a long loop attractor (implemented by reciprocal backprojections as well as forward connections between cortical areas (Rolls 2016c)), and may have different factors and time-courses that control its activity, such as what one is thinking about with one's syntactic system. In this example, either the short or the long loop might trigger the non-reward system back into its non-reward attractor state, and this needs to be taken account of in behavioural or cognitive treatment. One interesting aspect of this example is that because the syntactic system operates as a single information processing channel (Rolls & Deco 2015b, Rolls 2016c), filling it with positive thoughts would make it difficult to perform multiple step thinking about negative thoughts. This is relevant to the point made above about taking steps to prevent rumination in depression. It may for example be useful to introduce individuals to the idea that constantly returning to stimuli that relate to non-reward, such as the grave of a loved one, while in many ways admirable, may retrigger grief and possibly depression, unless active steps are taken to make something positive out of the situation.

Third, it is important to understand that both depression and non-impulsiveness may be related to non-reward, and that depressed people will, as part of an evolutionarily adaptive strategy, tend not to take risks. This may be important to at least understand when individuals are making financial or economic decisions, so that they can take this into account.

Fourth, noise in the brain caused by the stochastic spiking times of neurons is an important aspect of attractor dynamics, and could contribute to depression, which might occur without an external event causing it (Section 3.13).

Fifth, attractor networks in the brain bias each other and implement top-down attention by this computational process (Rolls 2016c). This again tends to enhance the stability of non-reward networks, because when in the non-reward state, this will tend to bias sensory and memory systems towards sad perceptions and sad memory recall.

Sixth, there are different types of non-reward. Not receiving an expected food reward leaves one adaptively in a state in which trying to obtain the food reward is a goal for action. Not receiving an expected social reward leaves one adaptively in a state in which trying to obtain the social reward is a goal for action. An implication is that understanding what the trigger is for the depression, the type of non-reward or punisher, is likely to be important in treating the depression behaviourally or cognitively.

Seventh, it is argued that different individuals have different sensitivities to different types of reward, non-reward, and punisher, and that this provides a basis for differences in personality (Rolls 2014a). It is argued that this is part of the way in which evolution works, by altering individuals' sensitivities to these goals (Rolls 2012c). This concept in turn should lead us to approach problems such as depression with the understanding that we are dealing with a high-dimensional space of specific rewards, non-rewards, and punishers, different dimensions of which may make different contributions to depression in different individuals.

Now, some of the behavioural and cognitive strategies outlined above have been developed in the context of cognitive therapy for depression, pioneered by Aaron Beck (Beck 1979, Beck 2008, Disner, Beevers, Haigh & Beck 2011). Cognitive behaviour therapy for depression has a great deal of success, and this is helpful information, for it indicates that behavioural and cognitive treatments using the attractor mechanism-based approach described here will lead in turn to well-founded treatments based on this more detailed understanding. In fact, the brain-based attractor approach to depression makes the underlying mechanisms much more explicit, and this it is hoped will lead to better explanations to patients of what may be causing their depression, as well as to better cognitive and behavioural as well as brain-based treatments.

7.7 Pharmacological treatments for depression

7.7.1 Serotonin (5HT)

A number of antidepressant medications increase serotonin (5-hydroxy-tryptamine, 5HT) signalling in the brain by inhibiting serotonin reuptake from the synaptic cleft, thus increasing the efficacy of the 5HT. They include selective serotonin reuptake inhibitors (SSRIs) such as fluoxetine (Prozac), serotonin norepinephrine reuptake inhibitors (SNRIs), and some tricyclic antidepressants such as imipramine which blocks the reuptake of 5-HT (5-hydroxy-tryptamine, serotonin), NA (noradrenaline), and DA (dopamine), in that order of potency. (They inhibit the presynaptic transporters with that order of efficacy (Soares & Young 2016), and blocking the reuptake increases the concentration in the synapse of the 5HT.)

The SSRI drugs may take several weeks to reduce the depression, although some effects are faster, such as effects on whether face expressions are sad (Harmer & Cowen 2013). One reason that the rapid increase of concentration of 5-HT produced by most of the antidepressant drugs does not work rapidly appears to be that there are 5-HT$_{1A}$ autoreceptors on the 5-HT cell bodies in the raphe nucleus (and also on the post-synaptic neurons), and when these are activated by the elevated 5-HT, the potassium conductance is increased, producing hyperpolarization of the 5-HT neurons, which decreases their firing, counteracting any influence of the potentially elevated 5-HT concentrations produced by most antidepressant drugs. It may be that this autoreceptor-mediated negative feedback becomes attenuated with a time course of weeks, and then the antidepressant drugs start to influence depression (see e.g. Celada, Puig, Armagos-Bosch, Adell & Artigas (2004)). Indeed, adaptation of these autoreceptors occurred through a desensitization process over the course of 2–3 weeks of SSRIs administration, allowing the recovery of 5-HT neurons to their normal firing rate in the presence of reuptake inhibition of 5-HT, thus overall increasing 5HT-influenced transmission (Ghasemi, Phillips, Fahimi, McNerney & Salehi 2017). Also, the blockade of 5-HT$_{2A}$ receptors by some atypical antipsychotic drugs may improve the clinical effects of SSRIs, perhaps by an action on the prefrontal cortex (Celada et al. 2004).

However, approximately 33% of patients with major depressive disorder do not respond to treatment with commonly used SSRIs, so at least some subtypes or aspects of depression may not be related to serotonin (Yohn, Gergues & Samuels 2017).

Serotonin neurons, whose cell bodies are in the raphe nucleus in the brainstem, have widespread projections throughout the brain, and where serotonin effects relate to antidepressant effects is not yet established. In animal models of depression, there is evidence that there is decreased neurogenesis in the dentate gyrus which is part of the hippocampal system, that antidepressants increase neurogenesis in the dentate gyrus, and that antidepressants have some of their behavioral effects in animal models only if this system is intact (Yohn et al. 2017). The significance of this for understanding depression or bipolar disorder is difficult to ascertain, for the hippocampus is mainly involved in memory, and not in emotion and mood (Rolls 2015d, Kesner & Rolls 2015, Rolls 2016c). Perhaps these differences in the hippocampus are related to the altered memory function in at least depression, with increased rumination of memories associated with different functional connectivity of the hippocampus and related systems in depression (Cheng et al. 2016, Cheng et al. 2018b). For example, the posterior cingulate cortex, which provides a route for information to reach the hippocampus, has increased functional connectivity with the lateral orbitofrontal cortex in depression (Cheng et al. 2018b), as described above.

A somewhat unaddressed issue is where the serotonin neurons in the raphe receive inputs from that might produce depression in the first place. In this context, it has now been suggested that reward and non-reward areas of the brain such as the orbitofrontal cortex and amygdala do provide a source of relevant inputs to the 5-HT neurons, via brain regions such as the habenula and ventral striatum (Rolls 2017a) (Fig. 2.5). The suggestion is that the orbitofrontal cortex and amygdala systems involved in reward and non-reward can operate via a lateral hypothalamic area / lateral preoptic area (POA) to influence the Lateral Habenula, medial part, which in turn can influence the 5-HT (serotonin) neurons in the raphe nuclei. Many antidepressant drugs may influence this cortical to brainstem pathway by influencing the effects of the 5-HT neurons, which terminate in many brain areas. The hippocampal influence via the septal nuclei and diagonal band of Broca may enable reward context to access the same Lateral Habenula, medial part, to 5-HT-neuron system (de Araujo et al. 2012, Rolls 2015a). The medial habenula also receives septal inputs, and projects to the interpeduncular nucleus, and thereby to 5-HT neurons (and probably dopamine neurons) (Fig. 2.5) (Proulx et al. 2014, Loonen & Ivanova 2016).

These connections are shown in the context of some of the pathways involved in reward-related processes and emotion shown on the lateral view of the brain of the macaque monkey in the upper part of Fig. 2.5 (Rolls 2017a). Connections from the primary taste and olfactory cortices to the orbitofrontal cortex and amygdala are shown. Connections are also shown in the 'ventral visual system' from the visual cortical areas V1 to V2, V4, the inferior temporal visual cortex, etc., with some connections reaching the amygdala and orbitofrontal cortex. In addition, connections from the somatosensory cortical areas BA 1, 2, and 3 that reach the orbitofrontal cortex directly and via the insular cortex, and that reach the amygdala via the insular cortex, are shown.

Corresponding pathways that provide a route for reward and emotion-related information to reach the dopamine neurons in the midbrain are also shown in Fig. 2.5. The orbitofrontal cortex, amygdala (and probably anterior cingulate cortex and subgenual cingulate cortex) systems involved in reward and non-reward can operate via a basal ganglia route (striatum, ventral pallidum, and globus pallidus / bed nucleus of the stria terminalis) to influence the Lateral Habenula, lateral part, which in turn via the GABAergic Rostromedial Tegmental nucleus can influence dopamine neurons in the Substantia Nigra pars compacta and ventral Tegmental Area (SNc and VTA). This provides a route for reward, non-reward, and reward prediction error signals of largely cortical origin to influence the dopamine neurons. Details of some of these anatomical connections are provided elsewhere (Proulx et al. 2014, Loonen & Ivanova 2016).

Consistent with these points (Rolls 2017a), in the lateral habenula, neurons that respond to signaled low reward value or to punishment have been described (Matsumoto & Hikosaka 2009b), and so have neurons that reflect negative reward prediction error (Bromberg-Martin & Hikosaka 2011). Similar neurons are found in the globus pallidus glutamatergic excitatory habenula-projecting neurons, providing evidence that the necessary computations are not performed in the lateral habenula (Stephenson-Jones et al. 2016).

7.7.2 Ketamine

A notable recent discovery is that ketamine, a N-methyl-D-aspartate (NMDA) receptor antagonist, in subanaesthetic doses, produces rapid (within hours) antidepressant responses in patients who are resistant to typical antidepressants, and that the effects may last for two weeks or longer (Zanos & Gould 2018, Iadarola, Niciu, Richards, Vande Voort, Ballard, Lundin, Nugent, Machado-Vieira & Zarate 2015, Maltbie, Kaundinya & Howell 2017, Zanos, Moaddel, Morris, Georgiou, Fischell, Elmer, Alkondon, Yuan, Pribut, Singh, Dossou, Fang, Huang, Mayo, Wainer, Albuquerque, Thompson, Thomas, Zarate & Gould 2016, Krystal, Abdallah, Sanacora, Charney & Duman 2019). Clinically, ketamine may be useful with a single dose, or doses may be repeated. The short-term effects of ketamine include blocking excitatory NMDA receptors on cortical pyramidal cells which reduces the excitatory effect produced by the excitatory transmitter glutamate; and blocking excitatory receptors on GABA inhibitory neurons, which will tend to decrease GABAergic neuron firing, resulting in a potential increase in pyramidal cell firing. However, ketamine produces further effects, such as inducing synaptogenesis on excitatory neurons, increased glutamate transmission, reversing the synaptic deficits caused by chronic stress, and effects of a ketamine metabolite hydroxynorketamine (Duman & Aghajanian 2012, Ghasemi et al. 2017, Zorumski, Izumi & Mennerick 2016, Abdallah, Adams, Kelmendi, Esterlis, Sanacora & Krystal 2016, Aleksandrova, Phillips & Wang 2017, Zanos & Gould 2018, Krystal et al. 2019). Given that the medial and lateral orbitofrontal cortex are differently involved in depression, refinement of these studies to these especially relevant brain areas may be productive. Another way in which ketamine may be effective in depression is by reducing inflammatory processes, which are sometimes related to depression (Ghasemi et al. 2017).

Stress is a factor that can lead to depression, and some antidepressants including ketamine enhance neurotrophic factors such as BDNF (brain-derived neurotrophic factor), which may help to reduce the damaging effects of prolonged stress (Yohn et al. 2017, Ghasemi et al. 2017).

To understand exactly how antidepressant drugs have their therapeutic effects, it is important to know how they act not just generally in neural tissue, but on particular brain areas and systems. For example, the evidence described above suggests that decreasing the functioning of the lateral orbitofrontal cortex (involved in non-reward), and increasing the functioning of the medial orbitofrontal cortex (involved in reward), may be useful in the treatment of depression, yet these brain regions are just a small distance apart, so measurements that relate to drug effects in particular brain areas may be important in understanding and developing new antidepressant treatments.

Indeed, one potentially fruitful link would be to develop drugs that have potency particularly for some of the brain areas now known to be involved in emotion, such as the lateral vs medial orbitofrontal cortex, amygdala, and cingulate cortex. Another potentially fruitful link is to investigate with neuroimaging the brain changes that occur in depression and in the treatment of depression with antidepressants, to gain further evidence in humans about the brain systems involved in depression, and potentially, with the use of transmitter-specific techniques available with positron emission tomography (PET), to continue to investigate neuropharmacological and neurochemical aspects of depression in humans, as well as the effects of deep brain stimulation (see Section 4.2).

7.8 Mania and bipolar disorder

So far in this Chapter, we have been considering unipolar depression.

Bipolar disorder includes recurrent periods of mania and depression. The severity of the mania is greatest in bipolar I disorder, moderate in bipolar II disorder, and lower in cyclothymia. During mania, behaviors may include increased energy, grandiosity, less sleep, risk preference / impulsivity, euphoria, aggression, high reward seeking, hypersexuality, and hyperactivity (Anderson, Haddad & Scott 2012, Soares & Young 2016). During depression there may be anhedonia, risk aversion, increased sleep, reduced libido, reduced energy, feeling tired, feeling helpless, and a greater risk of suicide (Anderson et al. 2012, Soares & Young 2016).

The incidence of bipolar disorder is 1–2%. The heritability is fairly high (80–90%), but the disease is polygenic, with many genes each contributing a little (Anderson et al. 2012, Soares & Young 2016).

7.8.1 Mania, increased responsiveness to reward, and decreased responsiveness to non-reward

What is the relation between mania and depression? Could it be that in mania, there is something that in terms of reward/non-reward systems, is almost the opposite of depression? Might there be in mania *increased sensitivity to reward, and decreased sensitivity to non-reward / punishment*? The latter might manifest itself as increased impulsiveness in mania. That is a suggestion that might be considered to be the opposite of what has been described for depression in the previous part of this Chapter.

It turns out that there is support for this hypothesis. It indeed appears that the risk for mania is characterized by a hypersensitivity to goal- and reward-relevant cues (Nusslock, Young & Damme 2014). This hypersensitivity can lead to an excessive increase in approach-related affect and motivation during life events involving rewards or goal striving and attainment. In the extreme, this excessive increase in reward-related affect is reflected in manic symptoms, such as pursuit of rewarding activities without attention to risks, elevated or irritable mood, decreased need for sleep, increased psychomotor activation, and extreme self-confidence. Some evidence consistent with the hypothesis is that patients with bipolar I disorder and their relatives showed greater activation of the medial orbitofrontal cortex in response to reward delivery (Wessa, Kanske & Linke 2014). Also, reduced deactivation of the medial orbitofrontal cortex (where rewards are represented) during reward reversal might reflect a reduced error signal in bipolar disorder patients and their relatives in the lateral orbitofrontal cortex. (The activation of the lateral orbitofrontal cortex by non-reward in healthy individuals is illustrated in Fig. 7.1.) This type of responsiveness has been found to be very different in mania, with apparently decreasing activations in the lateral orbitofrontal cortex during expectation of increasing loss, the opposite of what is found in healthy participants (Bermpohl, Kahnt, Dalanay, Hagele, Sajonz, Wegner, Stoy, Adli, Kruger, Wrase, Strohle, Bauer & Heinz 2010) which we discovered in the orbitofrontal cortex (O'Doherty, Kringelbach, Rolls, Hornak & Andrews 2001a). In this context, of potentially reduced sensitivity or even abnormal function of the lateral orbitofrontal cortex non-reward system in mania, it is relevant that manic bipolar patients continue to pursue immediate rewards despite negative consequences (Wessa et al. 2014). Further, impulsivity in mania is pervasive, encompassing deficits in attention and behavioral inhibition. In addition, impulsivity is greater if the illness is severe (with for example frequent episodes, substance use disorders, and suicide attempts) (Swann 2009). The significance of this is that impulsivity may reflect decreased sensitivity to non-reward, which is represented by activations in the lateral orbitofrontal cortex, where non-reward is represented (see above).

Thus mania may reflect a state in which there is decreased sensitivity of non-reward systems and hence increased impulsiveness due to reduced sensitivity of the lateral orbitofrontal cortex, and at the same time, increased sensitivity to reward reflected in activations in the medial orbitofrontal cortex and pregenual cingulate cortex. Although these medial and lateral orbitofrontal cortex systems may show reciprocally related activations within an individual, with for example increasing activations in the medial orbitofrontal cortex to increasing monetary gains and decreasing activations in the lateral orbitofrontal cortex, and vice versa to increasing monetary loss (O'Doherty et al. 2001a), the reward and non-reward systems could be, and indeed are likely to, have their sensitivity set by independent genes, providing a basis for some patients to be depressed, and others to show both mania and depression. Indeed, Rolls' theory of emotion (Rolls 2014a) (Chapter 6) would go beyond this, and suggest that the sensitivity to many different rewards (e.g. food when hungry, water when thirsty, pleasant touch, sensitivity to reputation), and correspondingly to many different non-rewards, may be set by genes somewhat independently. This provides a relation to personality (Rolls 2014a), with the implication that people with depression may be particularly sensitive to certain non-rewards or punishers, and people with mania may be particularly sensitive to particular rewards. This has important implications for therapy, which might be well-directed towards particular sensitivities to particular non-rewards and particular rewards in different individuals.

7.8.2 Attractor networks, mania, increased responsiveness to reward, and decreased responsiveness to non-reward

The question then arises of the extent to which attractor network operations contribute to mania.

In terms of responses to inputs that increase the expectancy of reward, a short-term attractor system, probably in the orbitofrontal cortex, is likely to be present, to bridge any temporal interval between the expected reward signal and the actual outcome. This could in principle be oversensitive in mania. When the reward, the outcome, is delivered, it might also be useful to have a short-term attractor, to help reset a rule attractor for which stimulus is currently rewarding. However, it would be maladaptive if these reward-expectancy or reward-outcome attractors normally operated for more than perhaps 10 s, for this would tend to break the important contingency between input stimuli and outcomes. In addition to these short-term attractors, there also needs to be a longer term attractor process to reflect mood state, which typically operates on a much longer time scale. This might again be an attractor (with separate competing attractors for different mood states), and this attractor might be re-activated by the longer loop through the language / planning system, which by recalling a recent reward might calculate the long-term benefits, helping to keep the mood state prolonged. This whole 'long-loop' attractor might also be more sensitive in mania.

Given that there is increased impulsiveness in mania, it is also a possibility that the lateral orbitofrontal cortex non-reward attractor network system is less responsive in mania, for lack of responsiveness to non-reward is expected to lead to impulsive behaviour, behaviour that is not restrained by non-reward or punishment. Given that there is some reciprocity between activations in the medial and lateral orbitofrontal cortex (O'Doherty et al. 2001a, Rolls et al. 2018a), it is a possibility that simultaneous low responsiveness of a lateral orbitofrontal cortex non-reward system, and high responsiveness of a medial orbitofrontal cortex reward system, are both contributors to the mania of bipolar disorder.

These are interesting concepts for future empirical exploration.

7.8.3 Other aspects of bipolar disorder

Bipolar disorder involves successive periods of mania and depression. The causes of the cycling between these states is not very clear. However, the circadian rhythm is disrupted in bipolar disorder, with a shortened sleep time, and a more rapid onset of rapid-eye movement (dreaming) sleep. Further, melatonin production, which is high at night, is more suppressed by light in bipolar patients than in controls (Soares & Young 2016). At least some individuals with bipolar disorder have differences in the clock genes that control circadian rhythms (Soares & Young 2016). Whereas light therapy may be used in depression (and is effective especially early in the morning), dark therapy may be used in mania (Soares & Young 2016).

The treatments used for bipolar disorder include those used to treat depression, for in the depressed phase the risk of suicide is increased. Antidepressants such as the SSRIs increase the synaptic efficacy of serotonin, as described in Section 7.7. Treatments such as these may be used in the depressed phase of bipolar disorder (Soares & Young 2016).

In the manic phase, 'mood stabilizers' such as lithium and valproate may be prescribed (Soares & Young 2016). Both may act by enhancing the activity of GABA (inhibitory) neurons and decreasing excitatory neuron activity (Soares & Young 2016).

There are differences in the hippocampal system in bipolar disorder. There is evidence for decreased (GABA) inhibitory neuron efficacy in hippocampal CA3, associated with altered gene expression, and also with a reduced number of GABA neurons (Benes & Subburaj 2016). The significance of this for understanding bipolar disorder is difficult to ascertain, for, as noted above, the hippocampus is mainly involved in memory, and not in emotion and mood (Rolls 2015d, Kesner & Rolls 2015, Rolls 2016c). Perhaps these differences in the hippocampus are related to the altered memory function in at least depression, with increased rumination of memories associated with different functional connectivity of the hippocampus and related systems in depression (Cheng et al. 2016, Cheng et al. 2018b).

7.9 Autism

Autism spectrum disorder (ASD) is a complex developmental disorder that is characterized by difficulties in social communication and social interaction; and restricted and repetitive behavior, interests, or activities (Lai, Lombardo & Baron-Cohen 2014). Recently, a great deal of attention has been focused on the delineation of neural systems for brain-behavior relationships in ASD given that $\approx 1\%$ of children are being diagnosed with this disorder (Kim, Leventhal, Koh, Fombonne, Laska, Lim, Cheon, Kim, Kim, Lee, Song & Grinker 2011). At the brain circuit level, most of what we understand about autism and its biological abnormalities during the resting state comes from fMRI studies targeting changes in a small number of brain regions (Minshew & Keller 2010, Müller, Shih, Keehn, Deyoe, Leyden & Shukla 2011, Maximo, Cadena & Kana 2014). These studies have suggested abnormality in connectivity between a group of related and partly overlapping brain systems characterized as the default mode network (Assaf, Jagannathan, Calhoun, Miller, Stevens, Sahl, O'Boyle, Schultz & Pearlson 2010, Lynch, Uddin, Supekar, Khouzam, Phillips & Menon 2013), social brain circuits (Gotts, Simmons, Milbury, Wallace, Cox & Martin 2012, Kennedy & Adolphs 2012), self-representation circuitry (Lombardo, Chakrabarti, Bullmore, Sadek, Pasco, Wheelwright, Suckling, Consortium & Baron-Cohen 2010), reward circuitry (Dichter, Felder, Green, Rittenberg, Sasson & Bodfish 2012a, Dichter, Richey, Rittenberg, Sabatino & Bodfish 2012b), the salience network (Uddin, Supekar, Lynch, Khouzam, Phillips, Feinstein, Ryali & Menon 2013), a motor control network (Kenet, Orekhova, Bharadwaj, Shetty, Israeli, Lee, Agam, Elam, Joseph, Hamalainen & Manoach 2012), and an imitation network (Shih, Shen, Ottl, Keehn, Gaffrey & Muller 2010). The conclusions drawn from these studies are based on either seed-based analysis, independent component analysis (ICA), or parcellation-based analysis and these have some limitations (Cheng et al. 2015).

To overcome some of these limitations, we performed the first voxel-level pair-wise whole brain comparison of resting state functional connectivity differences between 418 people with autism and 509 matched typically developing individuals (Cheng, Rolls, Gu, Zhang & Feng 2015). We identified a key system in the middle temporal gyrus / superior temporal sulcus (STS) region that has reduced cortical functional connectivity, and which is implicated in face expression processing involved in social behavior. This system has reduced functional connectivity with the ventromedial prefrontal cortex which, as shown in this book, is implicated in emotion and social communication. The middle temporal gyrus system is also implicated in theory of mind processing. We also identified in autism a second key system in the precuneus / superior parietal lobule region with reduced functional connectivity which is implicated in spatial functions including of oneself, and of the spatial environment. It was proposed that these two types of functionality, face expression-related, and of one's self and the environment, are important components of the computations involved in theory of mind, whether of oneself or of others, and that reduced connectivity within and between these regions including the orbitofrontal cortex may make a major contribution to the symptoms of autism.

7.10 Attention-deficit / hyperactivity disorder

Attention-deficit/hyperactivity disorder (ADHD) is a common dimensional and heritable neurodevelopmental disorder which is characterized by pervasive features of inattention, impulsiveness and hyperactivity (Thapar, Cooper, Eyre & Langley 2013). It affects approximately 5% of children and adolescents and causes significant morbidity in adults (Faraone, Asherson, Banaschewski, Biederman, Buitelaar, Ramos-Quiroga, Rohde, Sonuga-Barke, Tannock & Franke 2015). Subjects with ADHD frequently show deficits of sustained attention and timing functions, motor response and cognitive inhibition (Coghill, Seth & Matthews 2014), which are attributed to impairments in fronto-striato-cerebellar and frontoparietal brain circuits (Arnsten & Rubia 2012).

Impulsivity is associated with ADHD. There are many types of impulsiveness (Dalley & Robbins 2017). Risky choice is related to the medial orbitofrontal cortex and ventromedial prefrontal cortex and anterior cingulate cortex. Reflection impulsivity and impulsive choice are related to the ventrolateral prefrontal and lateral orbitofrontal cortex. Stopping impulsivity is related to the right inferior frontal gyrus, anterior medial prefrontal cortex and the supplementary motor areas (Dalley & Robbins 2017).

The stop-signal reaction time (SSRT) is generally lengthened in patients with ADHD (indicating difficulty in the stop-signal task) (Rubia, Alegria, Cubillo, Smith, Brammer & Radua 2014). In a study of 2,000 adolescents (Whelan, Conrod, Poline, Lourdusamy, Banaschewski, Barker, Bellgrove, Buchel, Byrne, Cummins, Fauth-Buhler, Flor, Gallinat, Heinz, Ittermann, Mann, Martinot, Lalor, Lathrop, Loth, Nees, Paus, Rietschel, Smolka, Spanagel, Stephens, Struve, Thyreau, Vollstaedt-Klein, Robbins, Schumann, Garavan & Consortium 2012), participants with subclinical measures of ADHD-like behaviour, as measured by interviews and rating scales for the diagnosis of ADHD, had reduced activity on successful stop trials bilaterally in the inferior frontal gyrus, as well as in the basal ganglia. Another study showed that the two common measures of impulsivity, delay discounting and SSRT, were not correlated in a large juvenile multicentre sample of patients with ADHD, but that together they accounted for much of the variance discriminating children with ADHD and unaffected control participants (Solanto, Abikoff, Sonuga-Barke, Schachar, Logan, Wigal, Hechtman, Hinshaw & Turkel 2001).

Alterations in motivated behavior are also a hallmark of attention-deficit/hyperactivity disorder, and consistent with this, activations to expected rewards were greater in the orbitofrontal cortex of adolescents with ADHD (Tegelbeckers, Kanowski, Krauel, Haynes, Breitling, Flechtner & Kahnt 2018).

7.11 Compulsivity

'Compulsivity' may be defined as the performance of repetitive, unwanted and functionally impairing overt or covert behaviours without adaptive function, performed in a habitual or stereotyped fashion, either according to rigid rules or as a means of avoiding perceived negative consequences (Robbins, Vaghi & Banca 2019). Probably the most known mental disorder characterized by compulsivity is obsessive-compulsive disorder (OCD). But compulsivity is also a key feature in addictive disorders, Tourette's syndrome, impulse control disorders in

Parkinson's disease, and the so-called obsessive-compulsive and related disorders (OCRDs), such as trichotillomania and body dysmorphic disorder (van den Heuvel, van Wingen, Soriano-Mas, Alonso, Chamberlain, Nakamae, Denys, Goudriaan & Veltman 2016).

It has been suggested that there are three circuits for obsessive-compulsive disorder, as follows (Milad & Rauch 2012). An affective circuit, connecting the ventromedial prefrontal cortex and anterior cingulate cortex with the nucleus accumbens and the thalamus, is relevant for affective and reward processing. A dorsal cognitive circuit, connecting dorsolateral prefrontal cortex, the caudate nucleus and the thalamus, is crucial for executive functions such as working memory and planning. A ventral cognitive circuit, connecting anterolateral orbitofrontal cortex, anterior part of the putamen and thalamus, is involved in motor preparation and response inhibition.

Very interestingly, using a probabilistic reward reversal learning task of the type shown to activate the lateral orbitofrontal cortex (O'Doherty, Kringelbach, Rolls, Hornak & Andrews 2001a, Kringelbach & Rolls 2003) and shown to be impaired by damage to the orbitofrontal cortex (Hornak et al. 2003), it has been shown that impaired reversal learning in obsessive-compulsive disorder is associated with hypoactivation of the lateral orbitofrontal cortex, both in patients with obsessive-compulsive disorder and unaffected relatives (Chamberlain, Menzies, Hampshire, Suckling, Fineberg, del Campo, Aitken, Craig, Owen, Bullmore, Robbins & Sahakian 2008, Robbins et al. 2019). This reduced sensitivity to non-reward due to reduced function of the lateral orbitofrontal cortex may be one way in which impulsiveness can be produced, and it is interesting that this can be involved in obsessive-compulsive disorder, at least of some types.

Gradually over time a specific functional shift may occur from impulsivity to compulsivity, and from goal-directed to habitual behavior, associated with an anatomical shift from more emotional parts of the striatum (ventral striatum) to the more response or habit-related dorsal striatum (Fineberg, Apergis-Schoute, Vaghi, Banca, Gillan, Voon, Chamberlain, Cinosi, Reid, Shahper, Bullmore, Sahakian & Robbins 2018, Robbins et al. 2019).

This evidence thus suggests that, although there are many types of compulsive behaviour, at least some involve initially impulsivity related to under-functioning of the lateral orbitofrontal cortex, perhaps connecting via inferior frontal gyrus areas on the right, which can become locked into a response-related behaviour involving connections to the dorsal, habit-related, striatum.

8 The rodent orbitofrontal cortex

8.1 Evolutionary trends

As described in Chapter 1, the prefrontal cortex has undergone great development in primates (Passingham & Wise 2012, Pandya, Seltzer, Petrides & Cipolloni 2015), partly for the reason that new prefrontal areas are required as new areas are added to the posterior sensory processing hierarchies. Further, one part of the prefrontal cortex, the orbitofrontal cortex, is very little developed in rodents, yet is one of the major brain areas involved in emotion and motivation in primates including humans (Rolls 2014a). Indeed, it has been argued that the granular prefrontal cortex is a primate innovation, and the implication of the argument is that any areas that might be termed orbitofrontal cortex in rats (Schoenbaum et al. 2009) are homologous only to the agranular parts of the primate orbitofrontal cortex (shaded mid grey in Fig. 1.3), that is to areas 13a, 14c, and the agranular insular areas labelled Ia in Fig. 1.3 (Wise 2008, Passingham & Wise 2012). It follows from that argument that for most areas of the orbitofrontal and medial prefrontal cortex in humans and macaques (those shaded light grey in Fig. 1.3), special consideration must be given to research in macaques and humans (Rolls 2014a, Rolls 2017b). As shown in Fig. 1.3, there may be no cortical area in rodents that is homologous to most of the primate including human orbitofrontal cortex (Preuss 1995, Wise 2008, Passingham & Wise 2012).

Before considering the rodent 'orbitofrontal cortex' in the rest of this Chapter, we consider first some evolutionary trends that enable differences between the primate and rodent orbitofrontal cortex to be better appreciated.

8.1.1 Evolution of the taste and flavour system

8.1.1.1 Principles

The development of some cortical areas has been so great in primates that even evolutionarily old systems such as the taste system appear to have been rewired, compared with that of rodents, to place much more emphasis on cortical processing, taking place in areas such as the orbitofrontal cortex (Rolls & Scott 2003, Scott & Small 2009, Small & Scott 2009, Rolls 2014a, Rolls 2016b) (Fig. 2.2).

In primates, the reward value of a taste is represented in the orbitofrontal cortex in that the responses of orbitofrontal taste neurons are modulated by hunger in just the same way as is the reward value or palatability of a taste. In particular, it has been shown that orbitofrontal cortex taste neurons stop responding to the taste of a food with which a monkey is fed to satiety, and that this parallels the decline in the acceptability of the food (see Fig. 3.5) (Rolls et al. 1989). In contrast, the representation of taste in the primary taste cortex of primates (Scott, Yaxley, Sienkiewicz & Rolls 1986, Yaxley, Rolls & Sienkiewicz 1990) is not modulated by hunger (Rolls, Scott, Sienkiewicz & Yaxley 1988, Yaxley, Rolls & Sienkiewicz 1988). Thus in the primary taste cortex of primates (and at earlier stages of taste processing including the nucleus of the solitary tract), the reward value of taste is not represented, and instead the identity of the taste is represented (Rolls 2016b, Rolls 2016f) (see Section 8.1.1.2). The importance of cortical processing of taste in primates, first for identity and intensity in the primary taste

Evolutionary trends | 229

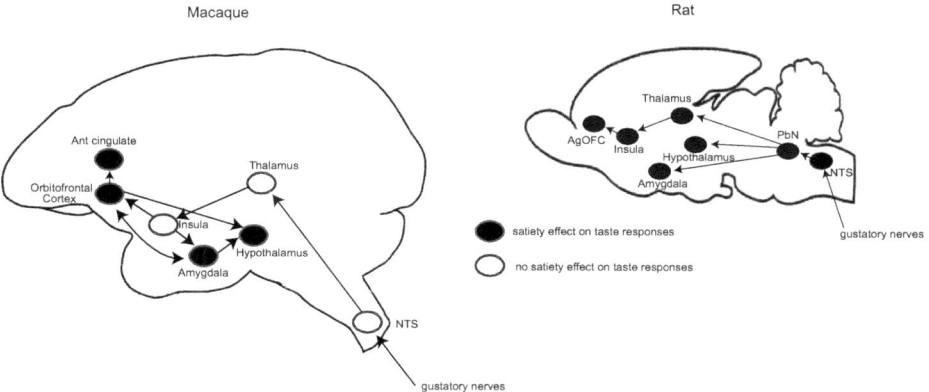

Fig. 8.1 Taste pathways in the macaque and rat. In the macaque, gustatory information reaches the nucleus of the solitary tract (NTS), which projects directly to the taste thalamus (ventral posteromedial nucleus, pars parvocellularis, VPMpc) which then projects to the taste cortex in the anterior insula (Insula). The insular taste cortex then projects to the orbitofrontal cortex and amygdala. The orbitofrontal cortex projects taste information to the anterior cingulate cortex. Both the orbitofrontal cortex and the amygdala project to the hypothalamus (and to the ventral striatum). In macaques, feeding to normal self-induced satiety does not decrease the responses of taste neurons in the NTS or taste insula (and by inference not VPMpc) (see text). In the rat, in contrast, the NTS projects to a pontine taste area, the parabrachial nucleus (PbN). The PbN then has projections directly to a number of subcortical structures, including the hypothalamus, amygdala, and ventral striatum, thus bypassing thalamo-cortical processing. The PbN in the rat also projects to the taste thalamus (VPMpc), which projects to the rat taste insula. The taste insula in the rat then projects to an agranular orbitofrontal cortex (AgOFC), which probably corresponds to the most posterior part of the primate OFC, which is agranular. (In primates, most of the orbitofrontal cortex is granular cortex, and the rat may have no equivalent to this. In the rat, satiety signals such as gastric distension and satiety-related hormones decrease neuronal responses in the NTS (see text), and by inference therefore in the other brain areas with taste-related responses, as indicated in the Figure.)

cortex, and then for reward value in the orbitofrontal cortex, is that both types of representation need to be interfaced to visual and other processing that requires cortical computation. For example, it may have adaptive value to be able to represent exactly what taste is present, and to link it by learning to the sight and location of the source of the taste, even when hunger and reward is not being produced, so that the source of that taste can be found in future, when it may have reward value.

In line with cortical processing to dominate the processing of taste in primates, there is no modulation of taste responsiveness at or before the primary taste cortex, and the pathways for taste are directly from the nucleus of the solitary tract in the brainstem to the taste thalamus and then to the taste cortex (Figs. 2.2 and 8.1). In contrast, in rodents such as the rat, the nucleus of the solitary tract connects to a pontine taste area, the parabrachial nucleus, that is not present in primates (Rolls & Scott 2003, Scott & Small 2009, Small & Scott 2009, Rolls 2016b). The rodent pontine taste area then not only has connections to the thalamus and thus to the cortex, but also has direct connections to many subcortical areas important in appetite control, including the amygdala and hypothalamus (Section 8.1.1.2). Moreover, in rodents, satiety reduces the responsiveness of neurons in the nucleus of the solitary tract to the taste of food by approximately 30%, so that taste processing in rodents is from the first synapse in the brain confounded by reward value, by hedonics (Rolls 2016b). That makes the taste system of rodents very difficult to understand functionally for different functions are not separated (taste identity and intensity vs hedonics), and makes the taste system of rodents a poor one with which to understand primate including human taste reward processing. This evidence emphasizes the importance of understanding the evidence from primates including humans, even in a system such as the taste system that one might think is evolutionarily so old (Section 8.1.1.2).

8.1.1.2 Taste processing in rodents

There are major differences in the neural processing of taste in rodents and primates (Rolls & Scott 2003, Small & Scott 2009, Scott & Small 2009, Rolls 2015b, Rolls 2016b) (Fig. 8.1). In rodents (and also in primates) taste information is conveyed by cranial nerves 7, 9 and 10 to the rostral part of the nucleus of the solitary tract (NTS) (Norgren 1990, Norgren & Leonard 1971, Norgren & Leonard 1973). However, although in primates the NTS projects to the taste thalamus and thus to the cortex (Fig. 2.2), in rodents the majority of NTS taste neurons responding to stimulation of the taste receptors of the anterior tongue project to the ipsilateral medial aspect of the pontine parabrachial nucleus (PbN), the rodent 'pontine taste area' (Small & Scott 2009, Cho, Li & Smith 2002). The remainder project to adjacent regions of the medulla. From the PbN the rodent gustatory pathway bifurcates into two pathways; 1) a ventral 'affective' projection to the hypothalamus, central gray, ventral striatum, bed nucleus of the stria terminalis and amygdala and 2) a dorsal 'sensory' pathway, which first synapses in the thalamus and then the agranular and dysgranular insular gustatory cortex (Norgren 1990, Norgren & Leonard 1971, Norgren 1974, Norgren 1976, Kosar, Grill & Norgren 1986). These regions, in turn, project back to the PbN to "sculpt the gustatory code" and guide complex feeding behaviours (Norgren 1990, Norgren 1976, Li & Cho 2006, Li, Cho & Smith 2002, Lundy & Norgren 2004, Di Lorenzo 1990, Scott & Small 2009, Small & Scott 2009).

It may be noted that there is strong evidence to indicate that the PbN gustatory relay is absent in the human and the nonhuman primate (Small & Scott 2009, Scott & Small 2009). First, second-order gustatory projections that arise from rostral NTS appear not to synapse in the PbN and instead join the central tegmental tract and project directly to the taste thalamus in primates (Beckstead, Morse & Norgren 1980, Pritchard, Hamilton & Norgren 1989). Second, despite several attempts, no one has successfully isolated taste responses in the monkey PbN (Norgren (1990); Small & Scott (2009) who cite Ralph Norgren, personal communication and Tom Pritchard, personal communication). Third, in monkeys the projection arising from the PbN does not terminate in the region of ventral basal thalamus that contains gustatory responsive neurons (Pritchard et al. 1989).

A further difference of rodent taste processing from that of primates is that physical and chemical signals of satiety have been shown to reduce the taste responsiveness of neurons in the nucleus in the solitary tract, and the pontine taste area, of the rat, with decreases in the order of 30%, as follows (Rolls & Scott 2003, Scott & Small 2009). Gastric distension by air or with 0.3 M NaCl suppress responses in the NTS, with the greatest effect on glucose (Gleen & Erickson 1976). Intravenous infusions of 0.5 g/kg glucose (Giza & Scott 1983), 0.5 U/kg insulin (Giza & Scott 1987a), and 40 μg/kg glucagon (Giza, Deems, Vanderweele & Scott 1993) all cause reductions in taste responsiveness to glucose in the NTS. The intraduodenal infusion of lipids causes a decline in taste responsiveness in the PBN, with the bulk of the suppression borne by glucose cells (Hajnal, Takenouchi & Norgren 1999). The loss of signal that would otherwise be evoked by hedonically positive tastes implies that the pleasure that sustains feeding is reduced, making termination of a meal more likely (Giza, Scott & Vanderweele 1992). Further, if taste activity in NTS is affected by the rat's nutritional state, then intensity judgements in rats should change with satiety. There is evidence that they do. Rats with conditioned aversions to 1.0 M glucose show decreasing acceptance of glucose solutions as their concentrations approach 1.0 M. This acceptance gradient can be compared between euglycemic rats and those made hyperglycemic through intravenous injections (Scott & Giza 1987). Hyperglycemic rats showed greater acceptance at all concentrations from 0.6 to 2.0 M glucose, indicating that they perceived these stimuli to be less intense than did conditioned rats with no glucose load (Giza & Scott 1987b).

The implication is that taste, and the closely related olfactory and visual processing that contribute to food reward value and expected value, are much more difficult to understand in rodents than in primates, partly because there is less segregation of 'what' (identity and intensity) from hedonic processing in rodents, partly because of the more serial hierarchical processing in primates (Fig. 2.2), and partly because in primates there has been great development of the granular orbitofrontal cortex which may help to support the rule-based switching of behaviour important for rapidly reversing stimulus-reward associations and behaviour.

8.1.2 Evolution of the temporal lobe cortex

Another reason for focusing interest on the primate brain is that there has been great development of the visual system in primates (Pandya, Seltzer, Petrides & Cipolloni 2015), and this itself has had important implications for the types of sensory stimuli that are processed by brain systems involved in emotion and motivation. One example is the importance of face identity and face expression decoding, which are both important in primate emotional behaviour, and indeed provide an important part of the foundation for much primate social behaviour (Rolls 2011a, Rolls 2014a, Rolls 2018b).

8.2 Divisions and functions of the rodent orbitofrontal cortex

The rat orbitofrontal cortex is located in the dorsal bank of the rhinal sulcus, and is divided into the medial orbital area (MO), ventral orbital area (VO), ventrolateral orbital area (VLO), lateral orbital area (LO), dorsolateral orbital area (DLO), and agranular insular (AI) areas Figs. 8.2 and 1.3c (Ongur & Price 2000, Izquierdo 2017, Rempel-Clower 2007). Although all prefrontal regions are agranular in the rat brain, these sectors of rat OFC are thought to be homologous to approximately one-third of the monkey caudal orbitomedial pre-frontal cortex because these regions share similar positioning and connectivity to subcortical structures (Price 2007). A comparison of the anatomical connections of different parts of the macaque and rodent orbitofrontal has been performed to provide 'connectivity-based inferences about homologies' across these species (Heilbronner et al. 2016).

An overview of the functions of different parts of the rat orbitofrontal cortex is shown in Fig. 8.2, and the account provided here follows a helpful meta-analysis by Izquierdo (2017).

Large lesions that damage MO, VO, LO, DLO, and AI produce a behavioral rigidity effect across paradigms ranging from the stop signal reaction time task (Eagle, Baunez, Hutcheson, Lehmann, Shah & Robbins 2008), 5-choice serial reaction time task (Chudasama, Passetti, Rhodes, Lopian, Desai & Robbins 2003), left-right lever (spatial) reversals (Boulougouris, Dalley & Robbins 2007), and reversal of reward contingencies associated with visual stimuli presented on touchscreens (Chudasama & Robbins 2003, Izquierdo, Brigman, Radke, Rudebeck & Holmes 2017) (see Izquierdo (2017)). More selective lesion effects are considered next.

It has been shown that LO is selectively involved in reversal learning (both deterministic and probabilistic), but not discrimination learning (Dalton, Wang, Phillips & Floresco 2016, Amodeo, McMurray & Roitman 2017). For example, medial OFC inactivation impaired probabilistic learning during the first discrimination, increased perseverative responding and reduced sensitivity to positive and negative feedback, suggestive of a deficit in incorporating information about previous action outcomes to guide subsequent behavior. Lateral OFC inactivation preferentially impaired performance during reversal phases. In contrast, prelimbic inactivation caused an apparent improvement in performance by increasing the number of

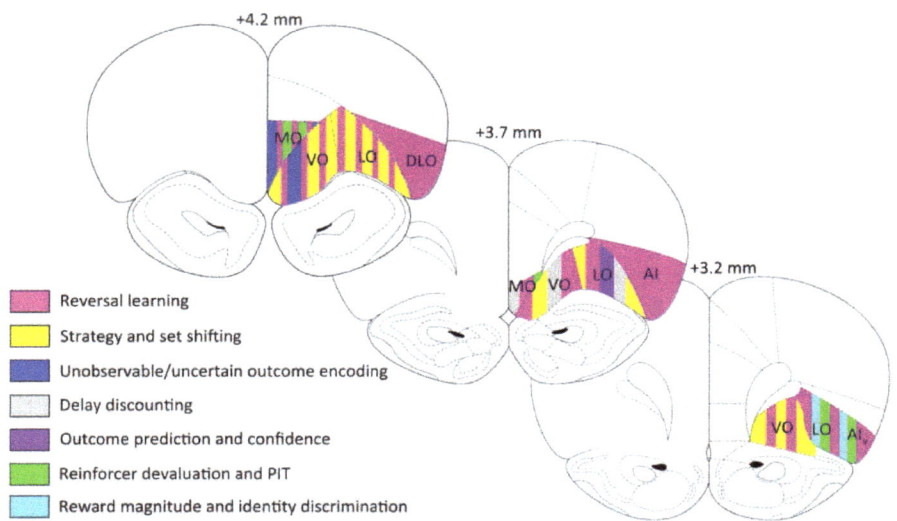

Fig. 8.2 Coronal sections depicting functional heterogeneity within rat OFC. Behavioral task effects are mapped onto coronal sections of rat OFC. Numerals on top of each section indicate the AP distance (in millimeters) from bregma. (Reproduced from Alicia Izquierdo, Functional heterogeneity within rat orbitofrontal cortex in reward learning and decision making, The Journal of Neuroscience, 37 (44), pp. 10529–10540, Figure 2, doi.org/10.1523/JNEUROSCI.1678-17.2017 ⓒ 2017 The Society for Neuroscience.).

reversals completed. This was associated with enhanced sensitivity to recently rewarded actions and reduced sensitivity to negative feedback. Infralimbic inactivation had no effect, whereas the anterior cingulate appeared to play a permissive role in this form of reversal learning (Dalton et al. 2016). Impaired reversal performance following LO inactivation also occurs in the context of Pavlovian responding, not just instrumental responding. LO also has a role in delay discounting: increasing preference for small, immediate over large, delayed rewards. The involvement of LO in delay discounting depends on whether there are explicit cues to signal delays to reward (see Izquierdo (2017)).

Claims that the rodent orbitofrontal cortex is not involved in reversal learning (Stalnaker, Cooch & Schoenbaum 2015) have not adequately dealt with the point that the type of one-trial rule-based rapid reversal learning that is important in primates including humans (see Chapters 3 and 4) may not take place in rodents.

The available evidence suggests that MO has an important role in risk and probability discounting, and in supporting value choices when outcomes are either ambiguous or changing in value. One way in which MO may support all these functions is by contributing a representation (e.g., memory) of reward value for use in guiding actions. This may be achieved by stable neuronal ensemble activity in this region (see Izquierdo (2017)).

VO and VLO may support reward learning and performance over increasing delays (i.e., delay discounting), the learning of the variance of value distributions over time (i.e., learning of risk), and the conditions (context or state) in which outcomes are expected. All these functions likely support the stabilization of expectations necessary for appropriate behavioral responses to changing or surprising events. These are similar to the functions of MO, yet there is appreciably more emphasis on cue-guided learning in VO and VLO studies, a trend that continues as one moves more laterally through rat OFC. VO may be particularly important in learning about value under conditions of delay uncertainty. Neurons in VLO signal an expected outcome (Steiner & Redish 2012), a missed outcome (when encountering a high-cost choice after skipping a low-cost choice used as a test of regret) (Steiner & Redish 2014), and neuronal firing in VLO is engaged when stimulus-outcome contingencies become stable with experience (Riceberg & Shapiro 2017). This is a difference with MO, where changes are a more important feature than stability (see Izquierdo (2017)).

Murray, Wise & Rhodes (2011) provided an overview of some similarities and differences between reward-related processing in primates and rodents, in the context that the rodent appears not to have areas homologous to most areas of the primate orbitofrontal cortex (Wise 2008), as rodents have only agranular orbitofrontal cortex (Fig. 1.3). Their discussion extends beyond the rat agranular orbitofrontal cortex to other frontal areas, including the following.

The prelimbic (PL) cortex lies along the medial wall of the rat frontal cortex (Fig. 1.3c). The prelimbic cortex appears to be important specifically in situations involving competition between associations guiding instrumental behavior. Evidence from prelimbic cortex lesions indicates that it is required for the encoding of response-outcome (R-O) (or action-outcome) associations during learning. This means that the prelimbic cortex plays an important role in maintaining control of instrumental behavior in favor of goal-directed R-O associations over competing habit-based stimulus-response (S-R) associations.

The infralimbic (IL) cortex lies along the medial wall of the frontal cortex and, in rats, is located immediately ventral to the PL cortex (Fig. 1.3c). IL is involved in habit formation by stimulus-response associations. This system is insensitive to devaluation, showing that this infralimbic system is involved in stimulus-response learning and not goal-dependent action-outcome learning (Killcross & Coutureau 2003b). The infralimbic cortex is also implicated in discrimination reversal learning (Chudasama & Robbins 2003) and extinction.

8.3 Neuronal activity in the rodent orbitofrontal cortex

Schoenbaum, Chiba & Gallagher (2000) tested whether rodent olfactory neurons show reversal. They recorded the activity in the orbitofrontal cortex of rats performing an odor discrimination task. Initially, rats were trained to sample an odor at the start of a trial. Presentation of one odor indicated that the rat would be rewarded at a well delivering sucrose solution, while presentation of another odor indicated that the rat would not be rewarded in that trial. Across this initial phase of learning, neurons in the orbitofrontal cortex gradually showed discrimination between the rewarded and unrewarded odors, where one ensemble of neurons exhibited high firing rates for the rewarded odor, and another ensemble exhibited equally high firing rates for the unrewarded odor (indicating a coding of stimulus-reward associations rather than of value). The contingencies were then reversed so that the previously rewarded odor was now unrewarded, and vice versa. Under these circumstances, a large proportion of rat OFC neurons encoding the odors in the initial phase stopped responding. Instead, new neurons were recruited, which encoded the new odor-outcome relationships.

There are some neurons like this in the macaque orbitofrontal cortex, where they are termed conditional reward neurons, and they are found for visual as well as olfactory discrimination reversal (Thorpe, Rolls & Maddison 1983, Rolls, Critchley, Mason & Wakeman 1996a) (Sections 3.6.3 and 3.3, Table 3.1). However many visual and olfactory neurons in the primate orbitofrontal cortex show full reversal of their firing when the reward association of a visual or olfactory stimulus is reversed (Thorpe et al. 1983, Rolls et al. 1996a) (Sections 3.6.3 and 3.3, Table 3.1). Moreover, the reversal for visual stimuli can be rule-based, that is, non-associative. This evidence thus suggests that the rodent and primate orbitofrontal cortex operate very differently.

Neuronal activity has also been compared in the rat medial and lateral orbitofrontal cortex (Lopatina, Sadacca, McDannald, Styer, Peterson, Cheer & Schoenbaum 2017). They examined how neurons from each area represented information about differently valued trial types, defined by the cue-outcome pairings, versus how those same neurons represented information about similar epochs between these different trial types, such as the stimulus sample, delay, and reward consumption epochs. The analysis provided evidence that ensembles in the lateral orbitofrontal cortex group states according to trial epoch, whereas those in the medial orbitofrontal cortex organize the same states by trial type.

In another study, it has been shown that rodent orbitofrontal neurons signal reward predictions, not reward prediction errors (Stalnaker, Liu, Takahashi & Schoenbaum 2018), and that is consistent with what has so far been found in macaques.

In another study, it has been shown that food reward and social reward activate different neuronal populations in the mouse orbitofrontal cortex (Jennings, Kim, Marshel, Raffiee, Ye, Quirin, Pak, Ramakrishnan & Deisseroth 2019). For comparison, in primates exquisite selectivity of orbitofrontal cortex neurons to different types of food reward (taste, smell, texture including fat texture, and the sight of food) has been shown, as has great selectivity of orbitofrontal cortex neurons to the sight of different socially relevant stimuli, including face identity, face expression, face gesture, social role of the individual, rank in the dominance hierarchy, and vocalization expression (see Chapter 3).

8.4   A state space representation in the rodent orbitofrontal cortex?

It has been suggested that the orbitofrontal cortex provides a cognitive map of state space[12] that could describe its role in value-based decision-making (Wilson, Takahashi, Schoenbaum & Niv 2014, Sharpe, Stalnaker, Schuck, Killcross, Schoenbaum & Niv 2019). According to this view, the orbitofrontal cortex represents previous stimuli, actions and other sensory features that occur in association with outcomes in a multidimensional array and thus supports reinforcement learning implemented elsewhere in the brain. That suggestion is based on findings in rodents (Wilson et al. 2014).

That suggestion does not fit the primate, including human, findings on the orbitofrontal cortex. These findings, described in Chapters 3 and 4 show that the primate orbitofrontal cortex contains representations of reward value, and is involved in learning and rapidly updating reward value representations, but does not have major representations of actions (Thorpe, Rolls & Maddison 1983, Rolls 2017c, Padoa-Schioppa & Assad 2006, Rolls 2014a, Grattan & Glimcher 2014). Moreover, the evidence described in this book shows that the primate including human orbitofrontal cortex performs reward-related learning very rapidly, and indeed provides expected value and reward outcome signals to subcortical regions including the striatum and habenula and thus to the dopamine system implicated in slow reinforcement learning of for example habits (Rolls 2017a, Rolls 2014a, Rolls 2016c, Rolls 2018b) (Fig. 2.5; Sections 5.2 and 5.3).

If the state-space hypothesis about the rodent orbitofrontal cortex is correct, then that provides further evidence for major differences in the rodent vs primate including human orbitofrontal cortex.

One point made by Wilson et al. (2014) is that the rodent orbitofrontal cortex may take into account non-observable information. That of course is the case for the primate orbitofrontal cortex, as shown by the rule-based one-trial visual discrimination reversal found in primates and primate orbitofrontal cortex neurons (Thorpe et al. 1983, Rolls et al. 1996a) (Sections 3.6.3

---

[12] A state-space representation is a mathematical model of a physical system as a set of input, output and state variables related by differential equations or difference equations. State variables are variables whose values evolve through time in a way that depends on the values they have at any given time and also depends on the externally imposed values of input variables. Output variables' values depend on the values of the state variables.

and 3.3). In this case, the rule, about which stimulus is currently rewarded, is held on-line in memory, and the reversal can therefore be a non-associative process, in which the information about what is rewarded is not contained in the stimulus being currently presented. That is, it is argued, one of the major properties of the cerebral cortex, that it can hold information on-line in short-term memory, and can base choices on 'non-observable' information (Rolls 2016c).

8.5 Synthesis

The rodent 'orbitofrontal cortex' is very different from the primate including human orbitofrontal cortex.

The rodent orbitofrontal cortex contains only agranular cortex, which corresponds to only a small region of the primate orbitofrontal cortex, posteriorly (Fig. 1.3) (Wise 2008, Passingham & Wise 2012)). Indeed, the human orbitofrontal cortex, most of which is granular (i.e. has a well-developed layer 4) is a part of the human brain that has expanded most during evolution (Spatz 1966).

The connectivity of the rodent reward systems including the orbitofrontal cortex is so different from that of primates that the principles of operation appear to be very different. One example is the taste system, which in primates proceeds mainly via thalamo-cortical processing through a primary taste cortex in the insula to the orbitofrontal cortex, whereas instead rodents have a pontine taste area which projects taste information to many subcortical areas. Moreover, in rodents, reward value as indicated in devaluation (satiety) studies involves reward processing even far peripherally in the first central relay, the nucleus of the solitary tract, making it a complex system as reward and identity processing about what the taste is are entangled with each other. A second example is that with the great development of the temporal lobe in primates, visual processing becomes highly elaborated and transmits information about face identity and face expression to the orbitofrontal cortex, where it can be used in emotional and social behaviour appropriate for different individuals given the face expression and gestures (including face view) of each individual. A third example is that because the visual representation in primates includes processing to the level of view-invariant representations of objects and faces, reward value-related learning in the orbitofrontal cortex is efficient, for after a value association is made to one view, it generalizes to other views or transforms (Rolls 2016c).

Although reward value is represented in the rodent (agranular) orbitofrontal cortex, so also apparently are behavioural responses, which makes the rodent orbitofrontal cortex very different to the primate orbitofrontal cortex. The primate orbitofrontal cortex appears to specialize in reward (and of course punishment and non-reward) value representations, but not in interfacing these value representations to actions (which occurs in the primate cingulate cortex) or to responses (which occurs in the striatum and other parts of the basal ganglia). In contrast, in rodents, the orbitofrontal cortex seems much more heterogeneous with behavioural responses also represented in it, and again, the system is more complex because different computations are apparently intermingled in the same brain region.

Although reward reversal learning is studied in rodents, it does not so far appear to be of the same powerful type as the rule-based system present in primates, which allows switching to a different stimulus even previously associated with punishment when no reward is received when it was expected by a behavioral choice on a single trial. This type of rapid, rule-based, reversal provides a foundation for rapid changes in social behaviour whenever feedback is received, and a similar rule-based system is not known to be present in rodents. This is consistent with the great development of cortical processing for these functions provided by the primate orbitofrontal cortex, given that the cortex provides a computational basis in its attractor networks for holding information online, and therefore producing behaviour that depends on 'hidden' internal states, rather than being more dominated by sensory input (Rolls 2016c).

9 Orbitofrontal cortex computations in a systems-level perspective

This chapter describes some of the computational approaches that are useful to understand the functions of the orbitofrontal cortex. The networks and mechanisms are described in more detail in *Cerebral Cortex: Principles of Operation* (Rolls 2016c), the Appendices of which are available online (https://www.oxcns.org).

Section 9.1 describes the operation of pattern association networks which might be used in the orbitofrontal cortex to associate the sight of a stimulus with its taste.

Section 9.2 describes the operation of autoassociation or attractor networks which might be used in the orbitofrontal cortex to maintain a rule online by continuing neuronal firing.

Section 9.3 describes the operation of the integrate-and-fire attractor network used to model probabilistic decision-making as described in Section 3.13.

Section 9.4 describes a neurophysiological and computational model for stimulus-reinforcer association learning and reversal in the orbitofrontal cortex.

Section 9.5 describes a theory and model of how non-reward neurons are produced in the orbitofrontal cortex.

9.1 Pattern association memory

A fundamental operation of most nervous systems is to learn to associate a first stimulus with a second that occurs at about the same time, and to retrieve the second stimulus when the first is presented. The first stimulus might be the sight of food, and the second stimulus the taste of food. After the association has been learned, the sight of food would enable its taste to be retrieved. In classical conditioning, the taste of food might elicit an unconditioned response of salivation, and if the sight of the food is paired with its taste, then the sight of that food would by learning come to produce salivation. Pattern associators are thus used where the outputs of the visual system interface to learning systems in the orbitofrontal cortex and amygdala that learn associations between the sight of objects and their taste or touch in stimulus–reinforcer association learning (see Chapter 3).

Pattern association is also used throughout the cerebral (neo)cortical areas, as it is the architecture that describes the backprojection connections from one cortical area to the preceding cortical area (Rolls 2016c). Pattern association thus contributes to implementing top-down influences in attention, including the effects of attention from higher to lower cortical areas.

9.1.1 Architecture and operation

The essential elements necessary for pattern association, forming what could be called a prototypical pattern associator network, are shown in Fig. 9.1. What we have called the second or unconditioned stimulus pattern is applied through unmodifiable synapses generating an input to each neuron, which, being external with respect to the synaptic matrix we focus on, we can call the external input e_i for the ith neuron. [We can also treat this as a vector, **e**, as indicated in the legend to Fig. 9.1. Vectors and simple operations performed with them

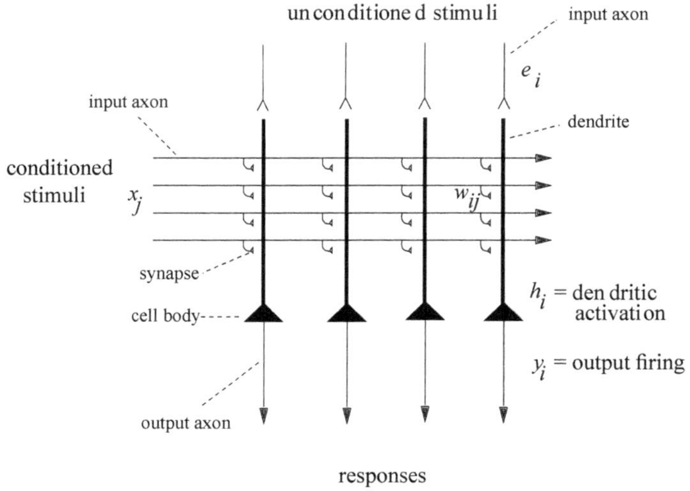

Fig. 9.1 A pattern association memory. An unconditioned stimulus has activity or firing rate e_i for the ith neuron, and produces firing y_i of the ith neuron. An unconditioned stimulus may be treated as a vector, across the set of neurons indexed by i, of activity $\mathbf{e}$. The firing rate response can also be thought of as a vector of firing $\mathbf{y}$. The conditioned stimuli have activity or firing rate x_j for the jth axon, which can also be treated as a vector $\mathbf{x}$.

are summarized by Rolls (2016c). This unconditioned stimulus is dominant in producing or forcing the firing of the output neurons (y_i for the ith neuron, or the vector $\mathbf{y}$)]. At the same time, the first or conditioned stimulus pattern consisting of the set of firings on the horizontally running input axons in Fig. 9.1 (x_j for the jth axon) (or equivalently the vector $\mathbf{x}$) is applied through modifiable synapses w_{ij} to the dendrites of the output neurons. The synapses are modifiable in such a way that if there is presynaptic firing on an input axon x_j paired during learning with postsynaptic activity on neuron i, then the strength or weight w_{ij} between that axon and the dendrite increases. This simple learning rule is often called the Hebb rule, after Donald Hebb who in 1949 formulated the hypothesis that if the firing of one neuron was regularly associated with another, then the strength of the synapse or synapses between the neurons should increase[13]. After learning, presenting the pattern $\mathbf{x}$ on the input axons will activate the dendrite through the strengthened synapses. If the cue or conditioned stimulus pattern is the same as that learned, the postsynaptic neurons will be activated, even in the absence of the external or unconditioned input, as each of the firing axons produces through a strengthened synapse some activation of the postsynaptic element, the dendrite. The total activation h_i of each postsynaptic neuron i is then the sum of such individual activations. In this way, the 'correct' output neurons, that is those activated during learning, can end up being the ones most strongly activated, and the second or unconditioned stimulus can be effectively recalled. The recall is best when only strong activation of the postsynaptic neuron produces firing, that is if there is a threshold for firing, just like real neurons. The advantages of this are evident when many associations are stored in the memory, as will soon be shown.

Next we introduce a more precise description of the above by writing down explicit mathematical rules for the operation of the simple network model of Fig. 9.1, which will help us to understand how pattern association memories in general operate. (In this description

---

[13]In fact, the terms in which Hebb put the hypothesis were a little different from an association memory, in that he stated that if one neuron regularly comes to elicit firing in another, then the strength of the synapses should increase. He had in mind the building of what he called cell assemblies. In a pattern associator, the conditioned stimulus need not produce before learning any significant activation of the output neurons. The connection strengths must simply increase if there is associated pre- and postsynaptic firing when, in pattern association, most of the postsynaptic firing is being produced by a different input.

we introduce simple vector operations, and, for those who are not familiar with these, refer the reader to Rolls (2016c).) We have denoted above a conditioned stimulus input pattern as **x**. Each of the axons has a firing rate, and if we count or index through the axons using the subscript j, the firing rate of the first axon is x_1, of the second x_2, of the jth x_j, etc. The whole set of axons forms a vector, which is just an ordered (1, 2, 3, etc.) set of elements. The firing rate of each axon x_j is one element of the firing rate vector **x**. Similarly, using i as the index, we can denote the firing rate of any output neuron as y_i, and the firing rate output vector as **y**. With this terminology, we can then identify any synapse onto neuron i from neuron j as w_{ij} (see Fig. 9.1). In this book, the first index, i, always refers to the receiving neuron (and thus signifies a dendrite), while the second index, j, refers to the sending neuron (and thus signifies a conditioned stimulus input axon in Fig. 9.1). We can now specify the learning and retrieval operations as follows:

9.1.1.1 Learning

The firing rate of every output neuron is forced to a value determined by the unconditioned (or external or forcing stimulus) input e_i. In our simple model this means that for any one neuron i,

$$y_i = \mathrm{f}(e_i) \qquad (9.1)$$

which indicates that the firing rate is a function of the dendritic activation, taken in this case to reduce essentially to that resulting from the external forcing input (see Fig. 9.1). The function f is called the activation function (see Rolls (2016c)), and its precise form is irrelevant, at least during this learning phase. For example, the function at its simplest could be taken to be linear, so that the firing rate would be just proportional to the activation.

The Hebb rule can then be written as follows:

$$\delta w_{ij} = \alpha y_i x_j \qquad (9.2)$$

where δw_{ij} is the change of the synaptic weight w_{ij} that results from the simultaneous (or conjunctive) presence of presynaptic firing x_j and postsynaptic firing or activation y_i, and α is a learning rate constant that specifies how much the synapses alter on any one pairing.

The Hebb rule is expressed in this multiplicative form to reflect the idea that both presynaptic and postsynaptic activity must be present for the synapses to increase in strength. The multiplicative form also reflects the idea that strong pre- and postsynaptic firing will produce a larger change of synaptic weight than smaller firing rates. It is also assumed for now that before any learning takes place, the synaptic strengths are small in relation to the changes that can be produced during Hebbian learning. We will see that this assumption can be relaxed later when a modified Hebb rule is introduced that can lead to a reduction in synaptic strength under some conditions.

9.1.1.2 Recall

When the conditioned stimulus is present on the input axons, the total activation h_i of a neuron i is the sum of all the activations produced through each strengthened synapse w_{ij} by each active neuron x_j. We can express this as

$$h_i = \sum_{j=1}^{C} x_j w_{ij} \qquad (9.3)$$

where $\sum_{j=1}^{C}$ indicates that the sum is over the C input axons (or connections) indexed by j to each neuron.

The multiplicative form here indicates that activation should be produced by an axon only if it is firing, and only if it is connected to the dendrite by a strengthened synapse. It also indicates that the strength of the activation reflects how fast the axon x_j is firing, and how strong the synapse w_{ij} is. The sum of all such activations expresses the idea that summation (of synaptic currents in real neurons) occurs along the length of the dendrite, to produce activation at the cell body, where the activation h_i is converted into firing y_i. This conversion can be expressed as

$$y_i = f(h_i) \tag{9.4}$$

where the function f is again the activation function. The form of the function now becomes more important. Real neurons have thresholds, with firing occurring only if the activation is above the threshold. Whatever the exact shape of the activation function, some non-linearity is an advantage, for it enables small activations produced by interfering memories to be minimized, and it can enable neurons to perform logical operations, such as to fire or respond only if two or more sets of inputs are present simultaneously (Rolls 2016c).

9.1.2 Properties

9.1.2.1 Generalization

During recall, pattern associators generalize, and produce appropriate outputs if a recall cue vector $\mathbf{x}_r$ is similar to a vector that has been learned already. This occurs because the recall operation involves computing the dot (inner) product of the input pattern vector $\mathbf{x}_r$ with the synaptic weight vector $\mathbf{w}_i$, so that the firing produced, y_i, reflects the similarity of the current input to the previously learned input pattern $\mathbf{x}$. (Generalization will occur to input cue or conditioned stimulus patterns $\mathbf{x}_r$ that are incomplete versions of an original conditioned stimulus $\mathbf{x}$, although the term completion is usually applied to the autoassociation networks described in Section 9.2.)

This is an extremely important property of pattern associators, for input stimuli during recall will rarely be absolutely identical to what has been learned previously, and automatic generalization to similar stimuli is extremely useful, and has great adaptive value in biological systems.

9.1.2.2 Graceful degradation or fault tolerance

If the synaptic weight vector $\mathbf{w}_i$ (or the weight matrix, which we can call $\mathbf{W}$) has synapses missing (e.g. during development), or loses synapses, then the activation h_i or $\mathbf{h}$ is still reasonable, because h_i is the dot product (correlation) of $\mathbf{x}$ with $\mathbf{w}_i$. The result, especially after passing through the activation function, can frequently be perfect recall. The same property arises if for example one or some of the conditioned stimulus (CS) input axons are lost or damaged. This is a very important property of associative memories, and is not a property of conventional computer memories, which produce incorrect data if even only 1 storage location (for 1 bit or binary digit of data) of their memory is damaged or cannot be accessed. This property of graceful degradation is of great adaptive value for biological systems.

9.2 Autoassociation or attractor memory

Autoassociative memories, or attractor neural networks, store memories, each one of which is represented by a pattern of neural activity. The memories are stored in the recurrent synaptic connections between the neurons of the network, for example in the recurrent collateral

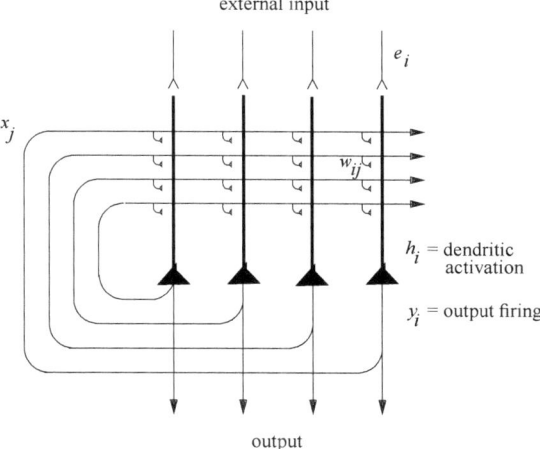

Fig. 9.2 The architecture of an autoassociative neural network.

connections between cortical pyramidal cells. Autoassociative networks can then recall the appropriate memory from the network when provided with a fragment of one of the memories. This is called completion. Many different memories can be stored in the network and retrieved correctly. A feature of this type of memory is that it is content addressable; that is, the information in the memory can be accessed if just the contents of the memory (or a part of the contents of the memory) are used. This is in contrast to a conventional computer, in which the address of what is to be accessed must be supplied, and used to access the contents of the memory. Content addressability is an important simplifying feature of this type of memory, which makes it suitable for use in biological systems. The issue of content addressability will be amplified below.

An autoassociation memory can be used as a short-term memory, in which iterative processing round the recurrent collateral connection loop keeps a representation active by continuing neuronal firing (Rolls 2016c).

9.2.1 Architecture and operation

The prototypical architecture of an autoassociation memory is shown in Fig. 9.2. The external input e_i is applied to each neuron i by unmodifiable synapses. This produces firing y_i of each neuron, or a vector of firing on the output neurons **y**. Each output neuron i is connected by a recurrent collateral connection to the other neurons in the network, via modifiable connection weights w_{ij}. This architecture effectively enables the output firing vector **y** to be associated during learning with itself. Later on, during recall, presentation of part of the external input will force some of the output neurons to fire, but through the recurrent collateral axons and the modified synapses, other neurons in **y** can be brought into activity. This process can be repeated a number of times, and recall of a complete pattern may be perfect. Effectively, a pattern can be recalled or recognized because of associations formed between its parts. This of course requires distributed representations.

Next we introduce a more precise and detailed description of the above, and describe the properties of these networks. Ways to analyze formally the operation of these networks are introduced in Appendix A4 of Rolls & Treves (1998), by Amit (1989), and by Rolls (2016c).

9.2.1.1 Learning

The firing of every output neuron i is forced to a value y_i determined by the external input e_i. Then a Hebb-like associative local learning rule is applied to the recurrent synapses in the

network:
$$\delta w_{ij} = \alpha y_i y_j. \tag{9.5}$$
It is notable that in a fully connected network, this will result in a symmetric matrix of synaptic weights, that is the strength of the connection from neuron 1 to neuron 2 will be the same as the strength of the connection from neuron 2 to neuron 1 (both implemented via recurrent collateral synapses).

It is a factor that is sometimes overlooked that there must be a mechanism for ensuring that during learning y_i does approximate e_i, and must not be influenced much by activity in the recurrent collateral connections, otherwise the new external pattern e will not be stored in the network, but instead something will be stored that is influenced by the previously stored memories. It is thought that in some parts of the brain, such as the hippocampus, there are processes that help the external connections to dominate the firing during learning (Rolls 2016c, Rolls 2018a).

9.2.1.2 Recall

During recall, the external input e_i is applied, and produces output firing, operating through the non-linear activation function described below. The firing is fed back by the recurrent collateral axons shown in Fig. 9.2 to produce activation of each output neuron through the modified synapses on each output neuron. The activation h_i produced by the recurrent collateral effect on the ith neuron is, in the standard way, the sum of the activations produced in proportion to the firing rate of each axon y_j operating through each modified synapse w_{ij}, that is,

$$h_i = \sum_j y_j w_{ij} \tag{9.6}$$

where $\sum_j$ indicates that the sum is over the C input axons to each neuron, indexed by j.

The output firing y_i is a function of the activation produced by the recurrent collateral effect (internal recall) and by the external input (e_i):

$$y_i = \mathrm{f}(h_i + e_i) \tag{9.7}$$

The activation function should be non-linear, and may be for example binary threshold, linear threshold, sigmoid, etc. The threshold at which the activation function operates is set in part by the effect of the inhibitory neurons in the network (not shown in Fig. 9.2). The connectivity is that the pyramidal cells have collateral axons that excite the inhibitory interneurons, which in turn connect back to the population of pyramidal cells to inhibit them by a mixture of shunting (divisive) and subtractive inhibition using GABA (gamma-amino-butyric acid) terminals (Rolls 2016c). There are many fewer inhibitory neurons than excitatory neurons (in the order of 5–10%) and of connections to and from inhibitory neurons (Rolls 2016c) and partly for this reason the inhibitory neurons are considered to perform generic functions such as threshold setting, rather than to store patterns by modifying their synapses. The non-linear activation function can minimize interference between the pattern being recalled and other patterns stored in the network, and can also be used to ensure that what is a positive feedback system remains stable. The network can be allowed to repeat this recurrent collateral loop a number of times. Each time the loop operates, the output firing becomes more like the originally stored pattern, and this progressive recall is usually complete within 5–15 iterations.

9.2.2 Introduction to the analysis of the operation of autoassociation networks

With complete connectivity in the synaptic matrix, and the use of a Hebb rule, the matrix of synaptic weights formed during learning is symmetric. The learning algorithm is fast, 'one-shot', in that a single presentation of an input pattern is all that is needed to store that pattern.

During recall, a part of one of the originally learned stimuli can be presented as an external input. The resulting firing is allowed to iterate repeatedly round the recurrent collateral system, gradually on each iteration recalling more and more of the originally learned pattern. Completion thus occurs. If a pattern is presented during recall that is similar but not identical to any of the previously learned patterns, then the network settles into a stable recall state in which the firing corresponds to that of the previously learned pattern. The network can thus generalize in its recall to the most similar previously learned pattern. The activation function of the neurons should be non-linear, since a purely linear system would not produce any categorization of the input patterns it receives, and therefore would not be able to effect anything more than a trivial (i.e. linear) form of completion and generalization.

Recall can be thought of in the following way, relating it to what occurs in pattern associators. The external input $\mathbf{e}$ is applied, produces firing $\mathbf{y}$, which is applied as a recall cue on the recurrent collaterals as $\mathbf{y}^T$. (The notation $\mathbf{y}^T$ signifies the transpose of $\mathbf{y}$, which is implemented by the application of the firing of the neurons $\mathbf{y}$ back via the recurrent collateral axons as the next set of inputs to the neurons.) The activity on the recurrent collaterals is then multiplied by the synaptic weight vector stored during learning on each neuron to produce the new activation h_i which reflects the similarity between $\mathbf{y}^T$ and one of the stored patterns. Partial recall has thus occurred as a result of the recurrent collateral effect. The activations h_i after thresholding (which helps to remove interference from other memories stored in the network, or noise in the recall cue) result in firing y_i, or a vector of all neurons $\mathbf{y}$, which is already more like one of the stored patterns than, at the first iteration, the firing resulting from the recall cue alone, $\mathbf{y} = \mathrm{f}(\mathbf{e})$. This process is repeated a number of times to produce progressive recall of one of the stored patterns.

Autoassociation networks operate by effectively storing associations between the elements of a pattern. Each element of the pattern vector to be stored is simply the firing of a neuron. What is stored in an autoassociation memory is a set of pattern vectors. The network operates to recall one of the patterns from a fragment of it. Thus, although this network implements recall or recognition of a pattern, it does so by an association learning mechanism, in which associations between the different parts of each pattern are learned. These memories have sometimes been called autocorrelation memories (Kohonen 1977), because they learn correlations between the activity of neurons in the network, in the sense that each pattern learned is defined by a set of simultaneously active neurons. Effectively each pattern is associated by learning with itself. This learning is implemented by an associative (Hebb-like) learning rule.

The system formally resembles spin glass systems of magnets analyzed quantitatively in statistical mechanics. This has led to the analysis of (recurrent) autoassociative networks as dynamical systems made up of many interacting elements, in which the interactions are such as to produce a large variety of basins of attraction of the dynamics. Each basin of attraction corresponds to one of the originally learned patterns, and once the network is within a basin it keeps iterating until a recall state is reached that is the learned pattern itself or a pattern closely similar to it. (Interference effects may prevent an exact identity between the recall state and a learned pattern.) This type of system is contrasted with other, simpler, systems of magnets (e.g. ferromagnets), in which the interactions are such as to produce only a limited number of related basins, since the magnets tend to be, for example, all aligned with each other. The states reached within each basin of attraction are called attractor states, and the analogy between autoassociator neural networks and physical systems with multiple attractors was drawn by Hopfield (1982) in a very influential paper. He was able to show that the recall state can be thought of as the local minimum in an energy landscape, where the energy would be defined as

$$E = -\frac{1}{2} \sum_{i,j} w_{ij}(y_i - <y>)(y_j - <y>). \tag{9.8}$$

This equation can be understood in the following way. If two neurons are both firing above their mean rate (denoted by $<y>$), and are connected by a weight with a positive value, then the firing of these two neurons is consistent with each other, and they mutually support each other, so that they contribute to the system's tendency to remain stable. If across the whole network such mutual support is generally provided, then no further change will take place, and the system will indeed remain stable. If, on the other hand, either of our pair of neurons was not firing, or if the connecting weight had a negative value, the neurons would not support each other, and indeed the tendency would be for the neurons to try to alter ('flip' in the case of binary units) the state of the other. This would be repeated across the whole network until a situation in which most mutual support, and least 'frustration', was reached. What makes it possible to define an energy function and for these points to hold is that the matrix is symmetric (see Hopfield (1982), Hertz, Krogh & Palmer (1991), Amit (1989)).

Physicists have generally analyzed a system in which the input pattern is presented and then immediately removed, so that the network then 'falls' without further assistance (in what is referred to as the unclamped condition) towards the minimum of its basin of attraction. A more biologically realistic system is one in which the external input is left on contributing to the recall during the fall into the recall state. In this clamped condition, recall is usually faster, and more reliable, so that more memories may be usefully recalled from the network. The approach using methods developed in theoretical physics has led to rapid advances in the understanding of autoassociative networks, and its basic elements are described in Appendix A4 of Rolls & Treves (1998), and by Hertz, Krogh & Palmer (1991) and Amit (1989).

9.2.3 Properties

The internal recall in autoassociation networks involves multiplication of the firing vector of neuronal activity by the vector of synaptic weights on each neuron. This inner product vector multiplication allows the similarity of the firing vector to previously stored firing vectors to be provided by the output (as effectively a correlation), if the patterns learned are distributed. As a result of this type of 'correlation computation' performed if the patterns are distributed, many important properties of these networks arise, including pattern completion (because part of a pattern is correlated with the whole pattern), and graceful degradation (because a damaged synaptic weight vector is still correlated with the original synaptic weight vector). Some of these properties are described next.

9.2.3.1 Completion

Perhaps the most important and useful property of these memories is that they complete an incomplete input vector, allowing recall of a whole memory from a small fraction of it. The memory recalled in response to a fragment is that stored in the memory that is closest in pattern similarity (as measured by the dot product, or correlation). Because the recall is iterative and progressive, the recall can be perfect.

This property and the associative property of pattern associator neural networks are very similar to the properties of human memory. This property may be used when we recall a part of a recent memory of a past episode from a part of that episode.

9.2.3.2 Generalization

The network generalizes in that an input vector similar to one of the stored vectors will lead to recall of the originally stored vector, provided that distributed encoding is used. The principle by which this occurs is similar to that described for a pattern associator.

9.2.3.3 Graceful degradation or fault tolerance

If the synaptic weight vector $\mathbf{w}_i$ on each neuron (or the weight matrix) has synapses missing (e.g. during development), or loses synapses (e.g. with brain damage or ageing), then the activation h_i (or vector of activations $\mathbf{h}$) is still reasonable, because h_i is the dot product (correlation) of $\mathbf{y}^T$ with $\mathbf{w}_i$. The same argument applies if whole input axons are lost. If an output neuron is lost, then the network cannot itself compensate for this, but the next network in the brain is likely to be able to generalize or complete if its input vector has some elements missing, as would be the case if some output neurons of the autoassociation network were damaged.

9.2.3.4 Speed

The recall operation is fast on each neuron on a single iteration, because the pattern $\mathbf{y}^T$ on the axons can be applied simultaneously to the synapses $\mathbf{w}_i$, and the activation h_i can be accumulated in one or two time constants of the dendrite (e.g. 10–20 ms). If a simple implementation of an autoassociation net such as that described by Hopfield (1982) is simulated on a computer, then 5–15 iterations are typically necessary for completion of an incomplete input cue $\mathbf{e}$. This might be taken to correspond to 50–200 ms in the brain, rather too slow for any one local network in the brain to function. However, it has been shown that if the neurons are treated not as McCulloch–Pitts neurons which are simply 'updated' at each iteration, or cycle of timesteps (and assume the active state if the threshold is exceeded), but instead are analyzed and modelled as 'integrate-and-fire' neurons in real continuous time, then the network can effectively 'relax' into its recall state very rapidly, in one or two time constants of the synapses (see Treves (1993), Battaglia & Treves (1998), Appendix A5 of Rolls & Treves (1998), and Rolls (2016c)). This corresponds to perhaps 20 ms in the brain.

One factor in this rapid dynamics of autoassociative networks with brain-like 'integrate-and-fire' membrane and synaptic properties is that with some spontaneous activity, some of the neurons in the network are close to threshold already before the recall cue is applied, and hence some of the neurons are very quickly pushed by the recall cue into firing, so that information starts to be exchanged very rapidly (within 1–2 ms of brain time) through the modified synapses by the neurons in the network. The progressive exchange of information starting early on within what would otherwise be thought of as an iteration period (of perhaps 20 ms, corresponding to a neuronal firing rate of 50 spikes/s) is the mechanism accounting for rapid recall in an autoassociative neuronal network made biologically realistic in this way. Further analysis of the fast dynamics of these networks if they are implemented in a biologically plausible way with 'integrate-and-fire' neurons is provided in Appendix A5 of Rolls & Treves (1998), and by Treves (1993). *The general approach applies to other networks with recurrent connections, not just autoassociators, and the fact that such networks can operate much faster than it would seem from simple models that follow discrete time dynamics is probably a major factor in enabling these networks to provide some of the building blocks of brain function.*

Learning is fast, 'one-shot', in that a single presentation of an input pattern $\mathbf{e}$ (producing $\mathbf{y}$) enables the association between the activation of the dendrites (the post-synaptic term h_i) and the firing of the recurrent collateral axons $\mathbf{y}^T$, to be learned. Repeated presentation with small variations of a pattern vector is used to obtain the properties of prototype extraction, extraction of central tendency, and noise reduction, because these arise from the averaging process produced by storing very similar patterns in the network.

9.2.3.5 Local learning rule

The simplest learning used in autoassociation neural networks, a version of the Hebb rule, is (as in equation 9.5)

$$\delta w_{ij} = \alpha y_i y_j.$$

The rule is a local learning rule in that the information required to specify the change in synaptic weight is available locally at the synapse, as it is dependent only on the presynaptic firing rate y_j available at the synaptic terminal, and the postsynaptic activation or firing y_i available on the dendrite of the neuron receiving the synapse. This makes the learning rule biologically plausible, in that the information about how to change the synaptic weight does not have to be carried to every synapse from a distant source where it is computed. As with pattern associators, since firing rates are positive quantities, a potentially interfering correlation is induced between different pattern vectors. This can be removed by subtracting the mean of the presynaptic activity from each presynaptic term, using a type of long-term depression. This can be specified as

$$\delta w_{ij} = \alpha y_i (y_j - z) \qquad (9.9)$$

where α is a learning rate constant. This learning rule includes (in proportion to y_i) increasing the synaptic weight if $(y_j - z) > 0$ (long-term potentiation), and decreasing the synaptic weight if $(y_j - z) < 0$ (heterosynaptic long-term depression). This procedure works optimally if z is the average activity $<y_j>$ of an axon across patterns.

Evidence that a learning rule with the general form of equation 9.5 is implemented in at least some parts of the brain comes from studies of long-term potentiation, described by Rolls (2016c). One of the important potential functions of heterosynaptic long-term depression is its ability to allow in effect the average of the presynaptic activity to be subtracted from the presynaptic firing rate (see Appendix A3 of Rolls & Treves (1998), and Rolls & Treves (1990)).

9.2.3.6 Capacity

One measure of storage capacity is to consider how many orthogonal patterns could be stored, as with pattern associators. If the patterns are orthogonal, there will be no interference between them, and the maximum number p of patterns that can be stored will be the same as the number N of output neurons in a fully connected network. Although in practice the patterns that have to be stored will hardly be orthogonal, this is not a purely academic speculation, since it was shown how one can construct a synaptic matrix that effectively orthogonalizes any set of (linearly independent) patterns (Kohonen 1977, Kohonen 1989, Personnaz, Guyon & Dreyfus 1985, Kanter & Sompolinsky 1987). However, this matrix cannot be learned with a local, one-shot learning rule, and therefore its interest for autoassociators in the brain is limited. The more general case of random non-orthogonal patterns, and of Hebbian learning rules, is considered next. However, it is important to reduce the correlations between patterns to be stored in an autoassociation network to not limit the capacity (Marr 1971, Kohonen 1977, Kohonen 1989, Kohonen, Oja & Lehtio 1981, Sompolinsky 1987, Rolls & Treves 1998), and in the brain mechanisms to perform pattern separation are frequently present (Rolls 2016d), including granule cells, as shown in many places in that book.

With non-linear neurons used in the network, the capacity can be measured in terms of the number of input patterns **y** (produced by the external input **e**, see Fig. 9.2) that can be stored in the network and recalled later whenever the network settles within each stored pattern's basin of attraction. The first quantitative analysis of storage capacity (Amit, Gutfreund & Sompolinsky 1987) considered a fully connected Hopfield (1982) autoassociator model, in which units are binary elements with an equal probability of being 'on' or 'off' in each pattern, and the number C of inputs per unit is the same as the number N of output units. (Actually it is equal to $N - 1$, since a unit is taken not to connect to itself.) Learning is taken to occur by clamping the desired patterns on the network and using a modified Hebb rule, in which the mean of the presynaptic and postsynaptic firings is subtracted from the firing on any one learning trial (this amounts to a covariance learning rule, and is described more fully in Appendix A4 of Rolls & Treves (1998)). With such fully distributed random patterns, the number of patterns that can be learned is (for C large) $p \approx 0.14C = 0.14N$, hence well below what could be achieved with orthogonal patterns or with an 'orthogonalizing' synaptic matrix. Many variations of this 'standard' autoassociator model have been analyzed subsequently.

Treves & Rolls (1991) have extended this analysis to autoassociation networks that are much more biologically relevant in the following ways. First, some or many connections between the recurrent collaterals and the dendrites are missing (this is referred to as diluted connectivity, and results in a non-symmetric synaptic connection matrix in which w_{ij} does not equal w_{ji}, one of the original assumptions made in order to introduce the energy formalism in the Hopfield model). Second, the neurons need not be restricted to binary threshold neurons, but can have a threshold linear activation function (see Rolls (2016c)). This enables the neurons to assume real continuously variable firing rates, which are what is found in the brain (Rolls & Tovee 1995, Treves, Panzeri, Rolls, Booth & Wakeman 1999). Third, the representation need not be fully distributed (with half the neurons 'on', and half 'off'), but instead can have a small proportion of the neurons firing above the spontaneous rate, which is what is found in parts of the brain such as the hippocampus that are involved in memory (see Treves & Rolls (1994), and Chapter 6 of Rolls & Treves (1998)). Such a representation is defined as being sparse, and the sparseness a of the representation can be measured, by extending the binary notion of the proportion of neurons that are firing, as

$$a = \frac{(\sum\limits_{i=1}^{N} y_i/N)^2}{\sum\limits_{i=1}^{N} y_i^2/N} \qquad (9.10)$$

where y_i is the firing rate of the ith neuron in the set of N neurons. Treves & Rolls (1991) have shown that such a network does operate efficiently as an autoassociative network, and can store (and recall correctly) a number of different patterns p as follows

$$p \approx \frac{C^{\text{RC}}}{a \ln(\frac{1}{a})} k \qquad (9.11)$$

where C^{RC} is the number of synapses on the dendrites of each neuron devoted to the recurrent collaterals from other neurons in the network, and k is a factor that depends weakly on the detailed structure of the rate distribution, on the connectivity pattern, etc., but is roughly in the order of 0.2–0.3.

The main factors that determine the maximum number of memories that can be stored in an autoassociative network are thus the number of connections on each neuron devoted to the recurrent collaterals, and the sparseness of the representation. For example, for $C^{\text{RC}} = 12,000$ and $a = 0.02$, p is calculated to be approximately $36,000$. This storage capacity can be realized, with little interference between patterns, if the learning rule includes some form of heterosynaptic long-term depression that counterbalances the effects of associative long-term potentiation (Treves & Rolls (1991); see Appendix A4 of Rolls & Treves (1998)). It should be noted that the number of neurons N (which is greater than C^{RC}, the number of recurrent collateral inputs received by any neuron in the network from the other neurons in the network) is not a parameter that influences the number of different memories that can be stored in the network. The implication of this is that increasing the number of neurons (without increasing the number of connections per neuron) does not increase the number of different patterns that can be stored (see Rolls & Treves (1998) Appendix A4), although it may enable simpler encoding of the firing patterns, for example more orthogonal encoding, to be used. This latter point, and setting up a cortical network without many pairs of neurons with more than one recurrent collateral connection between them, may account in part for why there are generally in the brain more neurons in a recurrent network than there are connections per neuron (Rolls 2016c, Rolls 2012e).

The non-linearity inherent in the NMDA receptor-based Hebbian plasticity present in the brain may help to make the stored patterns more sparse than the input patterns, and this may be especially beneficial in increasing the storage capacity of associative networks in the brain by allowing participation in the storage of especially those relatively few neurons with high firing rates in the exponential firing rate distributions typical of neurons in sensory systems (Rolls 2016c).

9.2.4 Use of autoassociation networks in the brain

Because of its 'one-shot' rapid learning, and ability to complete, this type of network is well suited for episodic memory storage, in which each episode must be stored and recalled later from a fragment, and kept separate from other episodic memories. It does not take a long time (the 'many epochs' of backpropagation networks) to train this network, because it does not have to 'discover the structure' of a problem. Instead, it stores information in the form in which it is presented to the memory, without altering the representation. An autoassociation network may be used for this function in the CA3 region of the hippocampus (Rolls 2018a, Rolls 2016c).

An autoassociation memory can also be used as a short-term memory, in which iterative processing round the recurrent collateral loop keeps a representation active until another input cue is received. This may be used to implement many types of short-term memory in the brain (Rolls 2016c).

An autoassociation or attractor network may also be used in decision-making, as described in Sections 3.13 and 9.3.

9.3 An integrate-and-fire implementation of an attractor network for decision-making

In this section the mathematical equations that describe the spiking activity and synapse dynamics in the integrate-and-fire simulations of decision-making described in Section 3.13 (Rolls et al. 2010b, Rolls et al. 2010c) and in other related models (Deco & Rolls 2003, Deco, Rolls & Horwitz 2004, Deco & Rolls 2005a, Deco & Rolls 2005d, Deco & Rolls 2005c, Deco & Rolls 2006, Loh, Rolls & Deco 2007, Rolls, Loh & Deco 2008c, Insabato, Pannunzi, Rolls & Deco 2010, Deco, Rolls & Romo 2010, Rolls & Deco 2011, Webb, Rolls, Deco & Feng 2011, Rolls & Webb 2012, Rolls, Webb & Deco 2012, Martinez-Garcia, Rolls, Deco & Romo 2011, Rolls, Dempere-Marco & Deco 2013, Rolls & Deco 2015b, Rolls & Deco 2015a, Rolls & Deco 2015a, Rolls & Deco 2016) are set out, in order to show in more detail how an integrate-and-fire simulation is implemented. The equations follow in general the formulation described by Brunel & Wang (2001), though each simulation describes its own architecture to be simulated and neurocomputational questions to be addressed, with additional dynamics introduced where described to implement synaptic facilitation and/or synaptic adaptation (Rolls 2016c).

Each neuron is described by an integrate-and-fire model. The subthreshold membrane potential $V(t)$ of each neuron evolves according to the following equation:

$$C_\mathrm{m}\frac{dV(t)}{dt} = -g_\mathrm{m}(V(t) - V_\mathrm{L}) - I_\mathrm{syn}(t) \tag{9.12}$$

where $I_\mathrm{syn}(t)$ is the total synaptic current flow into the cell, V_L is the resting potential, C_m is the membrane capacitance, and g_m is the membrane conductance. When the membrane potential $V(t)$ reaches the threshold V_thr a spike is generated, and the membrane potential is reset to V_reset. The neuron is unable to spike during the first τ_ref which is the absolute refractory period.

The total synaptic current is given by the sum of glutamatergic excitatory components (NMDA and AMPA) and inhibitory components (GABA). The external excitatory contributions (ext) from outside the network are produced through AMPA receptors ($I_\mathrm{AMPA,ext}$), while the excitatory recurrent synapses (rec) within the network act through AMPA and NMDA receptors ($I_\mathrm{AMPA,rec}$ and $I_\mathrm{NMDA,rec}$). The total synaptic current is therefore given by:

$$I_\mathrm{syn}(t) = I_\mathrm{AMPA,ext}(t) + I_\mathrm{AMPA,rec}(t) + I_\mathrm{NMDA,rec}(t) + I_\mathrm{GABA}(t) \tag{9.13}$$

where

$$I_\mathrm{AMPA,ext}(t) = g_\mathrm{AMPA,ext}(V(t) - V_\mathrm{E})\sum_{j=1}^{N_\mathrm{ext}} s_j^\mathrm{AMPA,ext}(t) \tag{9.14}$$

$$I_\mathrm{AMPA,rec}(t) = g_\mathrm{AMPA,rec}(V(t) - V_\mathrm{E})\sum_{j=1}^{N_E} w_j s_j^\mathrm{AMPA,rec}(t) \tag{9.15}$$

$$I_\mathrm{NMDA,rec}(t) = \frac{g_\mathrm{NMDA,rec}(V(t) - V_\mathrm{E})}{(1 + [\mathrm{Mg}^{++}]\exp(-0.062V(t))/3.57)}\sum_{j=1}^{N_E} w_j s_j^\mathrm{NMDA,rec}(t) \tag{9.16}$$

$$I_\mathrm{GABA}(t) = g_\mathrm{GABA}(V(t) - V_\mathrm{I})\sum_{j=1}^{N_I} s_j^\mathrm{GABA}(t) \tag{9.17}$$

In the preceding equations the reversal potential of the excitatory synaptic currents $V_\mathrm{E} = 0$ mV and of the inhibitory synaptic currents $V_\mathrm{I} = -70$ mV. The different form for the NMDA receptor-activated channels implements the voltage-dependence of NMDA receptors. This voltage-dependency, and the long time constant of the NMDA receptors, are important in the effects produced through NMDA receptors (Brunel & Wang 2001, Wang 1999). The synaptic strengths w_j are specified in the papers by Rolls and Deco cited above, and depend on the architecture being simulated. The fractions of open channels s are given by:

$$\frac{ds_j^\mathrm{AMPA,ext}(t)}{dt} = -\frac{s_j^\mathrm{AMPA,ext}(t)}{\tau_\mathrm{AMPA}} + \sum_k \delta(t - t_j^k) \tag{9.18}$$

$$\frac{ds_j^\mathrm{AMPA,rec}(t)}{dt} = -\frac{s_j^\mathrm{AMPA,rec}(t)}{\tau_\mathrm{AMPA}} + \sum_k \delta(t - t_j^k) \tag{9.19}$$

$$\frac{ds_j^\mathrm{NMDA,rec}(t)}{dt} = -\frac{s_j^\mathrm{NMDA,rec}(t)}{\tau_\mathrm{NMDA,decay}} + \alpha x_j(t)(1 - s_j^\mathrm{NMDA,rec}(t)) \tag{9.20}$$

$$\frac{dx_j(t)}{dt} = -\frac{x_j(t)}{\tau_\mathrm{NMDA,rise}} + \sum_k \delta(t - t_j^k) \tag{9.21}$$

$$\frac{ds_j^{\text{GABA}}(t)}{dt} = -\frac{s_j^{\text{GABA}}(t)}{\tau_{\text{GABA}}} + \sum_k \delta(t - t_j^k) \tag{9.22}$$

where the sums over k represent a sum over spikes emitted by presynaptic neuron j at time t_j^k. The value of $\alpha = 0.5$ ms^{-1}.

Typical values of the conductances for pyramidal neurons are: $g_{\text{AMPA,ext}}$=2.08, $g_{\text{AMPA,rec}}$=0.052, $g_{\text{NMDA,rec}}$=0.164, and g_{GABA}=0.67 nS; and for interneurons: $g_{\text{AMPA,ext}}$=1.62, $g_{\text{AMPA,rec}}$=0.0405, $g_{\text{NMDA,rec}}$=0.129 and g_{GABA}=0.49 nS.

The fixed parameters of the model of decision-making are shown in Table 9.1, and not only provide information about the values of the parameters used in the simulations, but also enable them to be compared to experimentally measured values.

Table 9.1 Parameters used in the integrate-and-fire simulations

N_E	800
N_I	200
r	0.1
w_+	2.2
w_I	1.015
N_{ext}	800
ν_{ext}	2.4 kHz
C_m (excitatory)	0.5 nF
C_m (inhibitory)	0.2 nF
g_m (excitatory)	25 nS
g_m (inhibitory)	20 nS
V_L	−70 mV
V_{thr}	−50 mV
V_{reset}	−55 mV
V_E	0 mV
V_I	−70 mV
$g_{\text{AMPA,ext}}$ (excitatory)	2.08 nS
$g_{\text{AMPA,rec}}$ (excitatory)	0.104 nS
g_{NMDA} (excitatory)	0.327 nS
g_{GABA} (excitatory)	1.25 nS
$g_{\text{AMPA,ext}}$ (inhibitory)	1.62 nS
$g_{\text{AMPA,rec}}$ (inhibitory)	0.081 nS
g_{NMDA} (inhibitory)	0.258 nS
g_{GABA} (inhibitory)	0.973 nS
$\tau_{\text{NMDA,decay}}$	100 ms
$\tau_{\text{NMDA,rise}}$	2 ms
τ_{AMPA}	2 ms
τ_{GABA}	10 ms
α	0.5 ms^{-1}

9.4 A neurophysiological and computational basis for stimulus–reinforcer association learning and reversal in the orbitofrontal cortex

A model for how very rapid, one-trial, reversal could be implemented in the orbitofrontal cortex (Deco & Rolls 2005a) is described in this section.

A first approach to the reversal is as follows, and can be understood by referring to Fig. 9.1 on page 237. Consider a neuron with unconditioned responses to taste in the orbitofrontal cortex. When a particular visual stimulus, say a triangle, was associated with the taste of glucose, the active synaptic connections for this visual (conditioned) stimulus would have shown long-term synaptic potentiation on to the taste neuron, which would respond to the sight of the triangle. During reversal, the same visual stimulus, the triangle, would again activate the same synaptic afferents to the neuron, but that neuron would be inactive when the taste of saline was given. Active presynaptic inputs and a low level of postsynaptic activation is the condition for homosynaptic long-term synaptic depression (LTD, see Rolls (2016c), which would then occur, resulting in a decline of the response of the neuron to the triangle. At the same time, visual presentation of a square would now be associated with the taste of glucose, which would activate the postsynaptic neuron, leading now to long-term potentiation of afferents on to that neuron made active by the sight of the square.

Although reversal might be implemented in the way just described by having long-term synaptic depression for synapses that represented the reward-associated stimulus before the reversal, and long-term potentiation of the new stimulus that after reversal is associated with reward, this would require one-trial LTP and one-trial homosynaptic LTD to account for one-trial stimulus–reward reversal (Thorpe, Rolls & Maddison 1983, Rolls, Critchley, Mason & Wakeman 1996a, Rolls 2000a). Moreover, the mechanism would not account for reversal learning set, the process by which during repeated reversal learning, performance gradually improves until reversal can occur in one trial. Even more, the mechanism would not account for the fact that after reversal learning set has been acquired, when the contingency is reversed, the animal makes a response to the current S+ expecting to get reward, but instead obtains the punisher. On the very first subsequent trial on which the pre-reversal S– is shown, the animal will perform a response to it expecting now to get reward, *even though the post-reversal S+ has not since the reversal been associated with reward to produce LTP for the post-reversal S+*. (This is in fact illustrated in Fig. 3.46 on page 76.) To implement this very rapid stimulus–reinforcer association reversal, a different mechanism is therefore needed. The mechanism can not rely on associative processes, but instead on a rule-based process, which requires the current rule to be held in mind, in short-term memory. This, and non-reward neurons that maintain their firing for many seconds as illustrated in Fig. 3.46, may be developments provided for by the evolution of granular orbitofrontal cortex areas in primates (see Section 1.2).

A model for how the very rapid, one-trial, reversal could be implemented has been developed (see Deco & Rolls (2005a) for a full description). The model uses a short-term memory autoassociation attractor network with associatively modifiable synaptic connections to hold the neurons representing the current rule active (see Fig. 9.3). Rule one might correspond to 'stimulus 1 (e.g. a triangle) is associated with reward, and stimulus 2 (e.g. a square) is associated with punishment'. Rule 2 might correspond to the opposite contingency. A small, very biologically plausible, modification of the standard one-layer autoassociation network is that there is a small amount of adaptation in the recurrent collateral synapses that keep the neurons representing the current rule firing. Now consider the case when the neurons representing rule one are firing. How does the rule module reverse? The proposal is that when

252 | Orbitofrontal cortex computations in a systems-level perspective

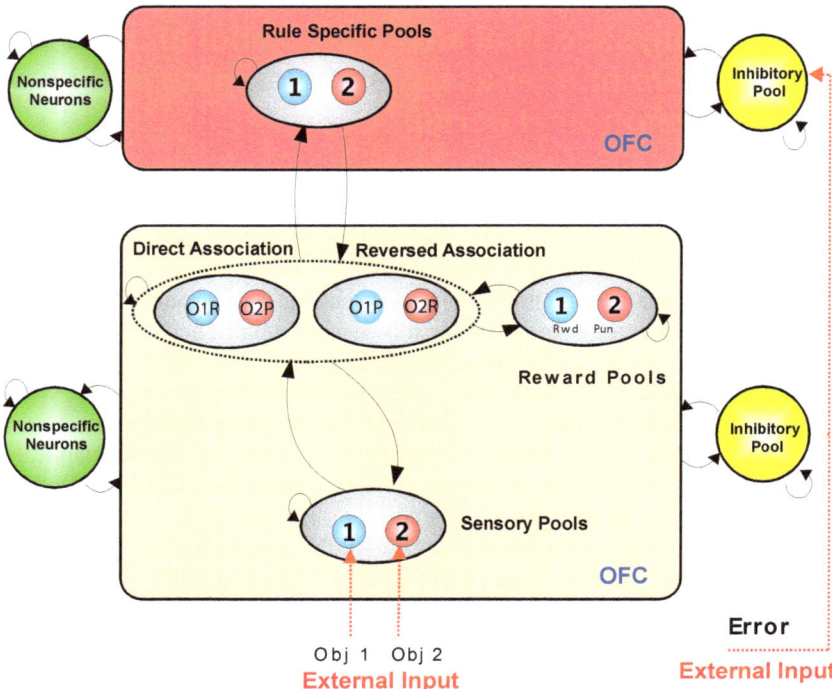

Fig. 9.3 Cortical architecture of the reward reversal model. There is a rule module (top) and a sensory – intermediate neuron – reward module (below). Neurons within each module are fully connected, and form attractor states. The sensory – intermediate neuron – reward module consists of three hierarchically organized levels of attractor network, with stronger synaptic connections in the forward than the backprojection direction. The intermediate level of the sensory – intermediate neuron – reward module contains neurons that respond to combinations of an object and its association with reward or punishment, e.g. object 1–reward (O1R, in the direct association set of pools), and object 1–punishment (O1P in the reversed association set of pools). These intermediate level neurons have the properties of 'conditional reward neurons' described in Section 3.6 and illustrated in Fig. 3.24, and provide a function for such conditional reward neurons. The rule module acts as a biasing input to bias the competition between the object–reward combination neurons at the intermediate level of the sensory – intermediate neuron – reward module. The whole model is implemented with integrate-and-fire neurons. (This material was originally published in Cerebral Cortex, 15 (1), Synaptic and spiking dynamics underlying reward reversal in the orbitofrontal cortex, G. Deco and E. T. Rolls, pp. 15–30 © 2005 Oxford University Press.)

the non-reward or error neurons described above (Section 3.8) fire, this additional set of firing neurons destabilizes the rule attractor module, by for example producing extra firing of the inhibitory neurons in the orbitofrontal cortex, which in turn inhibit the excitatory neurons in the rule autoassociation network, thus quenching its attractor state. This error input to the rule attractor network is shown in Fig. 9.3. After neuronal firing in the network has stopped and the error signal, which may last for 10 s as illustrated in Fig. 3.46 on page 76, is no longer present, then firing gradually can build up again in the rule attractor network. (This build-up may be assisted by non-specific inputs from other neurons in the area, as illustrated in Deco & Rolls (2005a).) However, with the competitive processes operating within the rule attractor network between the populations of neurons representing rule 1 and those representing rule 2, and the fact that the neurons or synapses that are part of the rule 1 attractor are partly adapted, the neurons that win the competition and become active are those representing rule 2, and the rule attractor has reversed its state. This process is illustrated in Fig. 9.4, and takes one trial. Reversal learning set takes a number of reversals to acquire because the correct attractors for the relevant rules, and their connections to other 'mapping' neurons, have to be learned.

To achieve the correct 'mapping' from stimuli to their reinforcer association, and thus emotional state, the rule neurons bias the competition in a mapping module, illustrated in Fig. 9.3. The mapping module has sensory input neurons, intermediate 'conditional reward' neurons (of the type described in Section 3.6 and illustrated in Fig. 3.24) which respond to

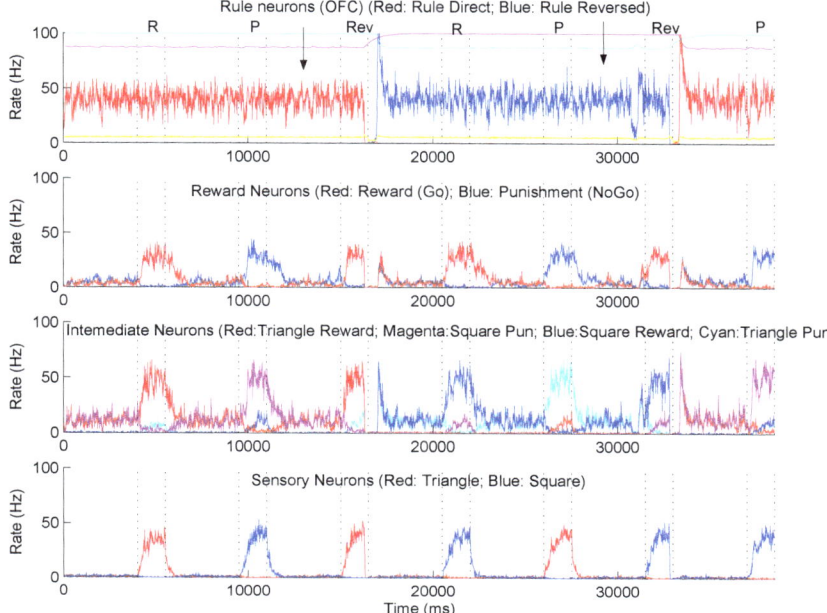

Fig. 9.4 Reward reversal model: Temporal evolution of the averaged population activity for all neural pools (sensory, intermediate (stimulus–reward), and Reward/Punishment) in the stimulus – intermediate – reward module and the rule module, during the execution and the reversal of the Go/NoGo visual discrimination task with a pseudorandom trial sequence after Thorpe, Rolls and Maddison (1983) and Rolls, Critchley, Mason and Wakeman (1996). Bottom row: the sensory neuronal populations, one of which responds to Object 1, a triangle (red), and the other to Object 2, a square (blue). The intermediate conditional stimulus–reward and stimulus–punishment neurons respond to for example Object 1 (Triangle) when it is associated with reward (Rw) (e.g. on trial 1, corresponding to O1R in Fig. 9.3), or to Object 2 (Square) when it is associated with punishment (Pun) (e.g. on trial 2, O2P). The top row shows the firing rate activity in the rule module, with the thin line at the top of this graph showing the mean probability of release P_{rel} of transmitter from the synapses of each population of neurons. The arrows show when the contingencies reversed. R: Reward trial; P: Punishment Trial; Rev: Reversal trial, i.e. the first trial after the reward contingency was reversed when Reward was expected but Punishment was obtained. The intertrial interval was 4 s. The yellow line shows the average activity of the inhibitory neurons. (See text for further details.) (This material was originally published in Cerebral Cortex, 15 (1), Synaptic and spiking dynamics underlying reward reversal in the orbitofrontal cortex, G. Deco and E. T. Rolls, pp. 15–30 © 2005 Oxford University Press.)

combinations of stimuli and whether they are currently associated with reward (or for other neurons to a punisher), and output neurons which represent the reinforcement association of the stimulus currently being viewed. (In the case described there are four populations or pools of neurons at the intermediate level, two for the direct rewarding context: object 1-rewarding, object 2-punishing, and two for the reversal condition: object 1-punishing, object 2-rewarding.) These intermediate pools or populations of neurons respond to combinations of the sensory stimuli and the expected reward, e.g. to object 1 and an expected reward (glucose obtained after licking), and are the conditional reward neurons described in Section 3.6 and illustrated in Fig. 3.24 on page 49. The sensory – intermediate – reward module thus consists of three hierarchically organized levels of attractor network, with stronger synaptic connections in the forward direction from input to output than the backprojection direction. The rule module acts as a biasing input to bias the competition between the object–reward combination neurons at the intermediate level of the sensory – intermediate – reward module. This biasing is achieved because rule 1 has associatively strengthened connections to object 1–rewarding and object 2–punishing neurons. (The whole network could be set up by simple associative learning operating to strengthen connections made with low probability between different neurons that are conjunctively active during the task in the network – see Deco & Rolls (2005a).)

Thus when object 1, e.g. the triangle, is being presented and rule one for direct mapping is in the rule module and biasing the intermediate neurons of the sensory – intermediate – reward module, then the intermediate neurons that fire are the object 1-reward neurons (O1R in Fig. 9.3), and these in turn through associative connections activate the reward neurons (Rwd in Fig. 9.3) at the third, reward/punishment, level of the hierarchy. If on the other hand object 1, e.g. the triangle, is being presented and rule two for reversed mapping is in the rule module and biasing the intermediate neurons of the sensory – intermediate – reward module, then the intermediate neurons that fire are the object 1–punishment (O1P) neurons, and these in turn through associative connections activate the punishment neurons (Pun) at the third, reward/punishment, level of the hierarchy. This model can thus account for one-trial reversal learning, and provides an account for the presence of the conditional reward and conditional punishment neurons found by Thorpe, Rolls & Maddison (1983) and Rolls, Critchley, Mason & Wakeman (1996a) in the orbitofrontal cortex (Section 3.6).

It is an important part of the architecture that at the intermediate level of the sensory – intermediate – reward module one set of neurons fire if an object being presented is currently associated with reward, and a different set if the object being presented is currently associated with punishment. This representation means that these neurons can be used for different functions, such as the elicitation of emotional or autonomic responses, which can occur for example to particular stimuli associated with particular reinforcers (Rolls 1999a). For example, particular emotions might arise if a particular cognitively processed input such as a particular person is associated with a particular type of reinforcer or reinforcement contingency.

It is also an interesting part of the architecture that associative synaptic modifiability (LTP, and LTD if present) is needed only to set up the functional architecture of the network while the reversal learning set is being acquired. However, once the correct synaptic connections have been set up to implement the architecture illustrated in Fig. 9.3, then no further synaptic modifiability is needed each time reversal occurs, as reversal is achieved just by the error signal quenching the current rule attractor, and the attractor for the other rule then starting up because its synapses are not adapted. This is an interesting prediction of the model. If tested by NMDA receptor blockers, which can block LTP, then it would be important to ensure that non-specific factors produced by the NMDA blockade such as less overall activity in the network, and the stabilizing effects of the long time constants of NMDA receptors, do not contribute to any result obtained. For this reason, use of a procedure for impairing synaptic modifiability other than NMDA receptor blockade would be useful in testing this prediction.

The network just described uses biased competition from a rule module to bias the mapping from sensory stimuli to the representation of a reward vs a punisher. An analogous rule network reversed in the same way by error signals quenching the current rule attractor, can be used to reverse the mapping from stimuli via intermediate stimulus–response neurons to response neurons, and thus to switch the stimulus-to-motor response being mapped in a model of conditional response learning (Deco & Rolls 2003, Deco & Rolls 2005a). While reward rule neurons have not been described yet for the orbitofrontal cortex, neurons which may correspond to stimulus–response rule neurons have been found in the dorsolateral prefrontal cortex (Wallis, Anderson & Miller 2001).

This model also provides a computational account of why the orbitofrontal cortex may play a more important role in rapid reversal learning than the amygdala. The account is based on the fact that a feature of cortical architecture is a highly developed set of local (within 1–2 mm) recurrent collateral excitatory associatively modifiable connections between pyramidal cells (Rolls & Deco 2002, Rolls & Treves 1998). These provide the basis for short-term memory attractor networks, and thus the basis for the rule attractor model which is at the heart of my suggestion for how rapid reversal learning is implemented (Deco & Rolls 2005a). In contrast, the amygdala is thought to have a much less well developed set of recurrent collateral excitatory connections, and thus may not be able to implement rapid reversal learning in the way described using competition biased by a rule module. Instead, the amygdala would need to rely on synaptic relearning as described in the first approach above, and this would be likely to be a slower process, and would certainly not lead to correct choice of the new S+ the first time it is presented after a punishment trial when the reversal contingency changes. Of course, in addition it is possible that the rapidity of LTP, and the efficacy of LTD, both of which would also facilitate rapid reversal, may be enhanced in the orbitofrontal cortex compared to the amygdala. Thus, the cortical neuronal reversal mechanism in the orbitofrontal cortex may be effectively a faster implementation in two ways than what is implemented in the amygdala. The cortical (in this case orbitofrontal cortex) mechanism may have evolved particularly to enable rapid updating by received reinforcers in social and other situations in primates. This hypothesis, that the orbitofrontal cortex, as a rapid learning mechanism, effectively provides an additional route for some of the functions performed by the amygdala, and is very important when this stimulus–reinforcer learning must be rapidly readjusted, has been developed elsewhere (Rolls 1990a, Rolls 1992a, Rolls 1996b, Rolls 1999a, Rolls 2000c, Rolls 2005).

Another feature of the rule attractor model of rapid reversal learning (Deco & Rolls 2005a) is that it does utilize a set of coupled attractor networks in the orbitofrontal cortex. Consistent with this, Hikosaka & Watanabe (2000) have shown that a short-term memory for reward, such as the flavour of a food, is represented by continuing firing in orbitofrontal cortex neurons in a reward delayed match-to-sample short-term memory task. This could be implemented by associatively modified synaptic connections between taste reward neurons (see Chapter 3) in the orbitofrontal cortex.

Although the mechanism has been described so far for visual-to-taste association learning, this is because neurophysiological experiments on this are most direct. It is likely, given the evidence from the effects of lesions, that taste is only one type of primary reinforcer about which such learning occurs in the orbitofrontal cortex, and is likely to be an example of a much more general type of stimulus–reinforcer learning system. Some of the evidence for this is that humans with orbitofrontal cortex damage are impaired at visual discrimination reversal when working for a reward that consists of points (Rolls, Hornak, Wade & McGrath 1994a) or money (Hornak, Bramham, Rolls, Morris, O'Doherty, Bullock & Polkey 2003) (see Section 4.2). Moreover, as described above, there is now evidence that the representation of the affective aspects of touch are represented in the human orbitofrontal cortex (Rolls, O'Doherty, Kringelbach, Francis, Bowtell & McGlone 2003d, McCabe, Rolls, Bilderbeck & McGlone 2008), and learning about what stimuli are associated with this class of primary reinforcer is also likely to be an important aspect of the stimulus–reinforcer association learning performed by the orbitofrontal cortex.

9.5 A theory and model of non-reward neural mechanisms in the orbitofrontal cortex

Single neurons in the primate orbitofrontal cortex respond when an expected reward is not obtained, and behavior must change. The human lateral orbitofrontal cortex is activated when non-reward, or loss occurs. The neuronal computation of this negative reward prediction error is fundamental for the emotional changes associated with non-reward, and with changing behavior. A mechanism for this computation has been proposed (Rolls & Deco 2016), as follows.

A single attractor network has a Reward population (or pool) of neurons that is activated by Expected Reward, and maintain their firing until, after a time, synaptic depression reduces the firing rate in this neuronal population. If a Reward Outcome is not received, the decreasing

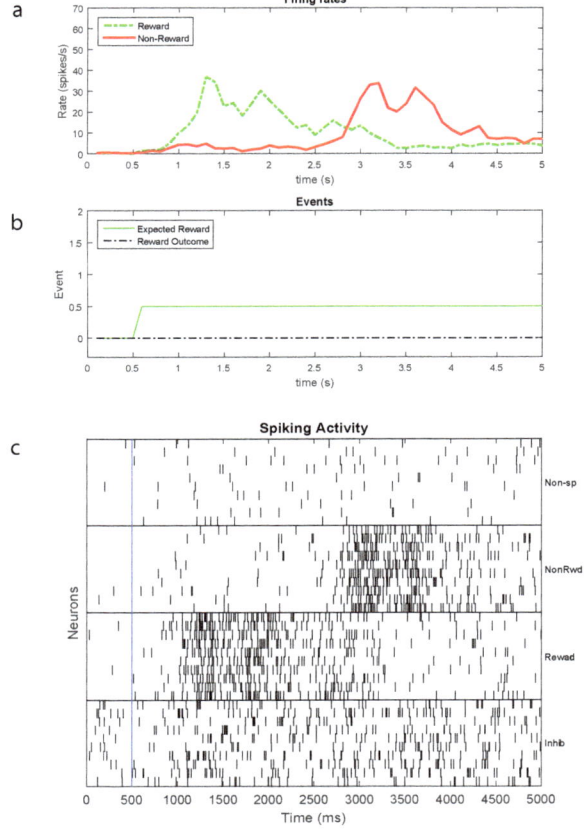

Fig. 9.5 The operation of the network when an Expected Reward is not obtained (extinction). a. The firing rates of the Reward population of neurons and the Non-Reward population of neurons during a 5 s trial. b. After a period of spontaneous activity from 0 until 0.5 s, the Expected Reward input was applied to the reward attractor population of neurons, and maintained at that level for the remainder of the trial. No Reward Outcome input was received. c. Rastergrams showing for each of the four populations of neurons, Non-Specific, Non-Reward, Reward, and Inhibitory, the spiking of ten neurons chosen at random from each population. Each small vertical line represents a spike from a neuron. Each horizontal row shows the spikes of one neuron. The different neurons are from the same trial. (Modified from Rolls and Deco 2016.)

firing in the Reward neurons releases the inhibition implemented by inhibitory neurons, and this results in a second population of Non-Reward neurons to start and continue firing encouraged by the spiking-related noise in the network. This is illustrated in the integrate-and-fire simulation shown in Fig. 9.5.

If a Reward Outcome is received, this keeps the Reward attractor active, and this through the inhibitory neurons prevents the Non-Reward attractor neurons from being activated. If an Expected Reward has been signalled, and the Reward Attractor neurons are active, their firing can be directly inhibited by a Non-Reward Outcome, and the Non-Reward neurons become activated because the inhibition on them is released (Rolls & Deco 2016).

The neuronal mechanisms in the orbitofrontal cortex for computing negative reward prediction error are important, for this system may be over-reactive in depression, under-reactive in impulsive behavior, and may influence the dopaminergic 'prediction error' neurons.

10 Synthesis: the Roles of the Orbitofrontal Cortex

10.1 Synthesis

In this Chapter, I draw together some of the points made in this book, to provide a synthesis of the functions of the orbitofrontal cortex. Important in this synthesis are the roles of the orbitofrontal cortex in the systems-level organisation of the brain.

10.1.1 The orbitofrontal cortex is the first stage of processing to represent reward value

The orbitofrontal cortex is the first region in the primate brain where outputs of the ventral processing systems that define what object is present in the visual, auditory, taste, and olfactory modalities become represented in terms of the reward value of the objects (Fig. 2.2 and Chapter 3).

To be clear: the valence of objects, reward vs punishment, is not represented in cortical processing streams before the orbitofrontal cortex, as shown by reward reversal experiments, and supported by devaluation investigations. It is not an exception that if a stimulus is paired with reward vs just a neutral stimulus, there may be some effect on processing in cortical areas before the orbitofrontal cortex, for there may be non-specific attentional and arousal-related effects, but this is not the same as saying that the reward vs punishment value including its valence or sign is represented before the orbitofrontal cortex in primates.

10.1.2 The orbitofrontal cortex represents the reward value of particular stimuli with different neuronal populations

The representation of reward value in the orbitofrontal cortex is often the reward value of a particular stimulus. One example of this is that many orbitofrontal cortex neurons respond to different combinations of taste, olfactory, oral texture, and visual stimuli, providing a rich representation of different stimuli in the orbitofrontal cortex (Chapter 3). It is the reward value of each stimulus that is represented, as shown by sensory-specific satiety devaluation experiments. Another example is provided by the conditional reward neurons in the orbitofrontal cortex, for they respond to one stimulus when it is rewarded but not when it is associated with punishment; and do not respond to other stimuli when they are associated with reward (Section 3.6.3).

10.1.3 The orbitofrontal cortex represents expected value, outcome value, and negative reward prediction error

These crucial variables for decision-making and neuroeconomic performance are represented and computed in the orbitofrontal cortex (Chapter 3).

10.1.4 The orbitofrontal cortex represents neuroeconomic value

Representations of neuroeconomic value are present in the primate orbitofrontal cortex, in that representations reflect for example both the quantity available, the probability, and the reward value of the good (Section 3.12).

10.1.5 Activations in the orbitofrontal cortex are often linearly related to the conscious subjective pleasantness (or unpleasantness) of stimuli

The great deal of evidence that activations in the orbitofrontal cortex are linearly related to the subjective pleasantness (or unpleasantness) of stimuli (Chapter 3) provides evidence that the orbitofrontal cortex is involved in conscious subjective experience, though the orbitofrontal cortex may of course be providing the inputs to other brain system involved in conscious subjective feelings (see Rolls (2014a) and Rolls (2018b)). Further evidence that orbitofrontal cortex processing is related to conscious emotional experience is that subjective emotional experience is changed in patients with damage to the orbitofrontal cortex (Hornak et al. 2003) (Chapter 4). Conscious emotional feelings may be less closely related to amygdala function (LeDoux et al. 2018, LeDoux & Pine 2016).

10.1.6 Face expression and face identity are both represented in the orbitofrontal cortex, and both are important for social interactions

The temporal lobe cortex, in the macaque cortex in the superior temporal sulcus and in the human middle temporal gyrus, performs much analysis of face expression and face gesture and dynamics (Section 3.6.6.10), which is then projected to the orbitofrontal cortex (Rolls et al. 2006a) (Section 3.6.5), where it is used in social interactions (Chapter 4). Dynamical changes, such as face and head gesture (e.g. turning the head and making eye contact, or the opposite), are an important part of this system (Section 3.6.5) (Rolls et al. 2006a).

10.1.7 The orbitofrontal cortex implements one-trial rule-based reward reversal

A key computational capacity of the orbitofrontal cortex is one-trial object-reward associations, which are rule-based (Sections 3.6, 9.4 and 9.5). This enables very rapid changes in behaviour when there is the slightest evidence that the current reinforcement contingencies are changing, and this is very likely to be important in primate social behaviour, in which sensitivity to social / rewarding feedback can be very important. This type of one-trial rule-based learning appears not to occur in rodents.

10.1.8 A common scale of reward value, but not a common currency

Empirical evidence and theoretical arguments show that different rewards are represented on a common scale, because this provides an appropriate input to an attractor decision-making network (Sections 3.12 and 3.12.2). Conversion to a common currency would not be adaptive, because the decision-making system needs to keep the particular reward that has won in the competition active, while goal-directed action can be performed to obtain the reward. A common currency would not specify the winning reward and goal for action (Section 3.12.2).

10.1.9 Relative and absolute value may both be represented in the orbitofrontal cortex

Absolute value is important for consistent long-term choice and transitive preferences. Relative value is useful for short-term choice, for example on a particular trial or a block of trials. Both may be represented in the orbitofrontal cortex (Section 3.12.3).

10.1.10 Top-down cognition and attention, even from the level of language, exert effects on the orbitofrontal cortex, and bias it

It is remarkable that word-level information can have a top-down cognitive and attentional biasing effect on value representations in the orbitofrontal, showing that even language can have an effect to bias emotions and emotional decision-making (Sections 3.9 and 3.10).

10.1.11 Decision-making in the ventromedial prefrontal cortex, VMPFC

Whereas much of the orbitofrontal cortex represents value on a continuous scale, in a more anterior part which may be part of medial prefrontal cortex area 10 and which may be described as the ventromedial prefrontal cortex, choice decision-making between stimuli of different reward value are made (Section 3.13).

10.1.12 Decision confidence is represented in the ventromedial prefrontal cortex, VMPFC

The fMRI signal from the decision-making area in the VMPFC reflects the confidence in a decision which is reflected in the difference between the decision variables, even before an outcome has been revealed. It is shown that this is a property of an attractor decision-making network (Section 3.13).

10.1.13 Decision-making in the orbitofrontal cortex reflects noise introduced by the Poisson nature of neuronal firing

This is a property of an attractor decision-making network with real spiking neurons, and evidence for this is provided by the fMRI signals on error trials (Rolls et al. 2010c) (Section 3.13).

10.1.14 Net value needs to be provided as the input to an attractor decision-making network

Net value, that is reward value minus negative or cost attributes, needs to be provided as the input to an attractor decision-making network. The reason for this is that a choice decision-making network would not inherently be able to relate the costs and rewards specific to each choice to each other – there would be a binding problem (Section 3.12).

10.1.15 The orbitofrontal cortex is a key brain area in emotion

Evidence for this, and a theory of why and how the orbitofrontal cortex is involved in emotion in relation to its roles in processing rewards and punishers, is described in Chapter 6.

10.1.16 The orbitofrontal cortex does not represent actions or behavioural responses

The orbitofrontal cortex contains representations of sensory stimuli in terms of their reward value (Chapter 3), but does not contain neurons that respond to actions or behavioural responses (Section 3.6.4). The cingulate cortex does interface actions to outcomes (Chapter 5.1), and the striatum interfaces stimuli to responses (Section 5.3).

10.1.17 The orbitofrontal cortex projects value information to several brain systems

Once reward value (and this includes neurons that respond to punishers) is encoded by the firing of orbitofrontal cortex neurons, this value-related information is projected to a number of cortical areas.

10.1.17.1 Anterior cingulate cortex

One is the anterior cingulate cortex, where the outcome value can be used to guide the learning of action-outcome associations (Section 5.1). Projections from the anterior cingulate cortex also reach the parahippocampal gyrus, where reward-related information can join information from dorsal stream pathways to enter the hippocampal memory system (Fig. 5.3 on page 149).

10.1.17.2 Posterior cingulate cortex

A second region that receives value-related information directly from the orbitofrontal cortex is the posterior cingulate cortex, which also receives from the anterior cingulate cortex (Fig. 5.3) (Section 5.1). The posterior cingulate cortex thus provides a dorsal route for reward-related information to reach the hippocampal memory system (Fig. 5.3).

The posterior cingulate cortex also potentially enables reward-related information to influence some areas of the parietal cortex with connections with the posterior cingulate cortex (Rolls 2019d, Whitlock 2017).

The posterior cingulate cortex also receives information from the parietal cortex about actions (Whitlock 2017), which are typically performed in a spatial context, and which then in the midcingulate areas (Vogt 2016) can be combined with reward outcome information from the orbitofrontal cortex projections to the anterior cingulate cortex to implement action-outcome learning (Fig. 5.3) (Rolls 2019a, Rolls 2019d).

10.1.17.3 Striatum

Another output of the orbitofrontal cortex (and the anterior cingulate cortex) is to the ventral striatum (nucleus accumbens and olfactory tubercle), from where it can influence regions such as the habenula and then the dopamine and serotonin-containing neurons in the brainstem (Fig. 2.5 and Chapter 6).

The ventral striatum appears to represent positive reward prediction error (at least as shown by human fMRI, see Section 10.2), which is also represented in the firing of dopamine neurons (Schultz 2016a). However, a little appreciated fact is that the dopamine neurons cannot fire in relation to positive reward prediction error signals unless they receive information about expected rewards and reward outcomes or the error signals that can be computed from them, and it is proposed that the orbitofrontal cortex (together with the amygdala) of primates is the source of reward-related information that is finally received by the dopamine neurons (Rolls 2017a) (Fig. 2.5 and Section 5.2). Consistent with this, it has been reported at the fMRI level that activations in the medial orbitofrontal cortex are related to positive reward prediction error (Rothkirch et al. 2017).

The dopamine positive reward prediction error signals are likely to be utilized in the striatum to learn stimulus-response, habit, associations (Section 5.2).

However, dopamine projections do reach the orbitofrontal cortex, and it is known that psychomotor stimulants such as amphetamine do activate the orbitofrontal cortex (Voellm et al. 2004). Indeed, the orbitofrontal cortex may be important in several types of addiction, including smoking and drinking (Section 3.16).

10.1.17.4 The right inferior frontal gyrus

The right inferior frontal gyrus may provide a route to action for the orbitofrontal cortex, given the connections to the inferior frontal gyrus from the lateral orbitofrontal cortex, the effects of lesions of the right inferior frontal gyrus in impairing response inhibition (in the stop-signal task) and increasing impulsiveness (Aron et al. 2014), activation of the inferior frontal gyrus in the same task (Deng et al. 2017), and increased functional connectivity of the inferior frontal gyrus in depression (Rolls et al. 2019a) (Section 7.4.2).

10.1.18 The orbitofrontal cortex develops greatly during evolution in primates and humans, and appears to overshadow the amygdala in emotion in primates including humans

Evidence for this is provided in Chapter 6 and Fig. 1.3.

10.1.19 The rodent orbitofrontal cortex is much less developed than the primate including human orbitofrontal cortex

The rodent orbitofrontal cortex is much less developed than the primate orbitofrontal cortex, with only an agranular part, homologous it is thought to the most posterior part of the primate orbitofrontal cortex (Fig. 1.3). Further, even the anatomical connections of for example the taste system and how these relate to the orbitofrontal cortex are very different in rodents (Chapter 8).

10.1.20 In addition to the orbitofrontal cortex reward value-based system for taking decisions, there is also a rational, reasoning route

The orbitofrontal cortex is especially important in value-based decisions where the values often represent reinforcers built in to animals that frequently operate in the interests of the selfish genes. However, there is in addition a rational, reasoning, route to action which can make decisions in the interests of the individual, or perfectly altruistically, as described in Section 6.4.

10.1.21 The orbitofrontal cortex is a key brain area in depression

Evidence for this, and a theory of why and how the orbitofrontal cortex is involved in depression, is described in Chapter 7.

10.1.22 The orbitofrontal cortex and addiction

Dopamine projections reach the orbitofrontal cortex, and it is known that psychomotor stimulants such as amphetamine activate the orbitofrontal cortex (Voellm et al. 2004). Indeed, the orbitofrontal cortex may be important in several types of addiction (Section 3.16).

Another example is smoking, in which there is low functional connectivity of the lateral orbitofrontal cortex, which may promote impulsiveness and the administration of nicotine which may act to increase activity generally in the brain, in that those who tend to smoke have low overall functional connectivity (Cheng et al. 2019) (Section 3.16).

Another example is drinking, in which there is high functional connectivity of the medial orbitofrontal cortex (Cheng et al. 2019), which may promote sensation-seeking (Wan et al. 2019) (Section 3.16).

10.2 The orbitofrontal cortex: future directions

The primate including human orbitofrontal cortex is, based on the research described in this book, a key brain system in reward processing, emotion, decision-making, and social behaviour. What are some key issues for the future?

Further work is needed on the orbitofrontal cortex negative reward prediction error neurons described in Section 3.8 (Thorpe et al. 1983). These neurons often respond to even a simple manipulation, such as withdrawing a reward that was about to be given. To what extent do they enter attractor states of continuing firing, which could be used to influence behaviour, and which could be related to depression (Chapter 7)? Do some of these neurons bridge delays of many seconds if a next trial is delayed for that long? What proportion of orbitofrontal cortex neurons respond to non-reward? Are they more likely to be found in the macaque lateral orbitofrontal cortex, as suggested by an fMRI investigation (Chau et al. 2015)?

Further work is needed on rule-encoding neurons that would be useful for holding online the current rule in a reversal task, or more generally in any situation in which a top-down influence on emotion must be maintained (Sections 3.6 and 9.4). Such neurons might be in the orbitofrontal cortex itself, or might be in areas implicated in short-term memory such as the dorsolateral prefrontal cortex.

The lateral orbitofrontal cortex area 12/47 extends round the inferior frontal convexity, where it abuts the inferior frontal gyrus, areas in the AAL2 atlas (Rolls et al. 2015a) which include the triangular part anteriorly (BA 45) and the opercular part posteriorly (BA 44). On the left this is part of Broca's area, and the lateral orbitofrontal cortex is held back from extending too far into the inferior frontal gyrus. On the right, the lateral orbitofrontal cortex may extend further round the inferior convexity. The right inferior frontal convexity area is implicated in the stop-signal task (Aron et al. 2014, Deng et al. 2017), and some types of impulsive behaviour, and has different functional connectivity in depression (Rolls et al. 2019a) (Chapter 7). It will be of interest to understand the relations between the lateral orbitofrontal cortex and the inferior frontal gyrus, especially on the right, much more. This is considered in Chapter 4, but much remains to be discovered about this ventrolateral prefrontal cortex (VLPFC) region. Is the right inferior frontal gyrus a region that receives information from the lateral orbitofrontal cortex, and provides a route for this to influence plans?

The posterior border of the lateral orbitofrontal cortex adjoins the most anterior part of the insula. It will be of interest to understand better what happens at this border, and the connections between the lateral orbitofrontal cortex and the anterior insula. This part of the insula is implicated in autonomic function (Rolls 2014a, Rolls 2016b), and the lateral orbitofrontal cortex is expected to drive autonomic function via connectivity to this part of the insula. However, it will be of interest to know whether this part of the insula performs any functions more closely related to emotion etc, or is primarily a slave to the orbitofrontal cortex and amygdala for autonomic output. Is it likely for example that this part of the insula projects visceral signals to the orbitofrontal cortex? The dorsal part of the anterior insula is a primary taste cortical area (Rolls 2014a, Rolls 2016b) (Section 3.2.5).

The posterior border of the medial orbitofrontal cortex adjoins the olfactory tubercle, which is part of the ventral striatum, and which receives inputs from the orbitofrontal cortex. In our investigations of depression, the olfactory tubercle often has similar functional connectivity to the medial orbitofrontal cortex (Rolls et al. 2018b). It will be of interest to investigate further what happens at this border, and whether this part of the ventral striatum may be different from the orbitofrontal cortex in representing positive reward prediction error.

It would be useful to investigate the hypothesis that the functions of the lateral orbitofrontal cortex and inferior frontal gyrus might be in a sense the opposite in depression (caused by overactivity and/or high functional connectivity (Rolls 2016e, Cheng et al. 2016, Rolls et al. 2019a)), and in impulsiveness and an inability to stop behaviour normally (produced by damage to the right inferior frontal gyrus (Aron et al. 2014)). There are many types of impulsivity (Dalley & Robbins 2017), and in terms of brain systems, at least the following could be considered. First, impulsivity may arise if there is a failure to re-evaluate reward value during reversal, related to the lateral orbitofrontal cortex. Second, there is perhaps a more response-related type of impulsiveness when the inferior frontal gyrus route to premotor areas in impaired. Third, there may be an action-related type of impulsiveness that may be related to the cingulate cortex if it is damaged.

We need further evidence on whether net value, that is reward value minus the negative properties or costs, is represented in the orbitofrontal cortex, for this is the representation that is needed to provide the decision variables for a reward-related attractor decision-making system that evaluates and compares two rewards (Section 3.12). Indeed, detailed neuronal studies in primates related to attractor network models of decision-making would be valuable to complement the fMRI-level investigations (Rolls et al. 2010b, Rolls et al. 2010c) (Section 3.13.3).

We need a computational model of how the cingulate cortex implements action-outcome learning, taking the benefits and costs of each potential action into account (Section 5.1).

fMRI evidence about whether the human orbitofrontal cortex represents positive reward prediction error is ambivalent, with one study reporting that it is not present (Hare, O'Doherty, Camerer, Schultz & Rangel 2008), and another study reporting positive reward prediction error in the medial orbitofrontal cortex (Rothkirch et al. 2017). Neuronal recording studies have not as far as I know established that orbitofrontal cortex neurons respond to positive reward prediction error in primates. However, in human fMRI, positive reward prediction error is reported in the ventral striatum (Hare et al. 2008), but this has not been reported at the neuronal level in primates, despite a number of studies (Schultz, Apicella, Scarnati & Ljungberg 1992, Schultz 2016b). Given that it is argued that the orbitofrontal cortex is the source of the expected reward and reward outcome signals needed for the computation of positive reward prediction error (Rolls 2017a) and connects to the dopamine neurons via the ventral striatum/ventral pallidum and habenula (Haber 2014, Rolls 2017a), it is of interest to know where on this pathway single neurons represent positive reward prediction error, and how it is computed. It is known that lateral habenula neurons decrease their firing rates for positive reward prediction error, and increase their firing rates for negative reward prediction error (Proulx et al. 2014, Matsumoto & Hikosaka 2007), so the habenula is on the pathway. For comparison, negative reward prediction error is computed in the orbitofrontal cortex (Thorpe et al. 1983, Kringelbach & Rolls 2003), and that could be a source of the signal that results in dopamine neurons decreasing their firing rates when an expected reward is not obtained (via the ventral striatum / habenula route).

Given the evidence described here that the lateral orbitofrontal may be overactive or overconnected in depression, and that the medial orbitofrontal cortex may be underactive or underconnected in depression (Chapter 7), it will be very useful to search for pharmaceutical agents that will target these regions specifically, as possible new treatments useful for depression.

We need better understanding of functional divisions of the primate orbitofrontal cortex, for lesion studies may not always have targeted functionally relevant regions (Chapter 4). We also need better parcellation of the human orbitofrontal cortex and inferior frontal gyrus, for the relations between different parts of these and depression appear to be important (Chapter 7 and Rolls et al. (2019a)).

Appendix 1 Glossary

A.1 General

An **affective state** is a term used to describe an emotional state (Chapter 6). It may have a connotation of subjective experience.

An **Attractor network** is formed by a set of neurons with positive connections between the neurons. Different subsets of neurons have especially strong connections between themselves, with each subset representing one memory or decision. Negative feedback inhibitory neurons implement competition between the neurons so that typically only one subset wins the competition. If an input is received that is close to one of the stored memories or decisions, then the network is attracted towards and recalls one of the stored memories. These networks, and how they are involved in **decision-making** are described in Section 3.13. An attractor network in the brain may store as many as 10,000 memories, if there are 10,000 connections to a neuron from the other neurons in the network. The operation of these networks with equations and quantitative analyses is described by Rolls (2016c).

Effective connectivity measures the effect of one brain area on another, that is a directed effect. The measure of activity is typically the BOLD signal, and the measurement involves comparing the signals in successive time-steps, with the underlying idea that if a first brain area has activity just before a second brain area, then the first brain area may be having a directed effect on a second brain area. In the cortex, there are typically connections in both directions between two cortical areas, and we sometimes refer to the direction as forward for the stronger connectivity, because in cortical hierarchies, the forward connectivity is generally stronger, as described by Rolls (2016c).

An **emotion** can be described operationally as a state elicited by an instrumental reinforcer (Chapter 6).

Fitness is the reproductive potential of genes. Through the process of natural selection and reproduction, fit genes are selected for the next generation.

Functional connectivity measures the correlation between the measure of activity (typically the BOLD signal) in two brain regions. A high functional connectivity implies that two brain areas are relatively strongly connected functionally. The relation might be produced by one area influencing the other, by the two areas influencing each other, or by a common input from another brain area. Functional connectivity does not imply that there is necessarily a direct anatomical connection, for the effects could be mediated through other brain areas.

Functional magnetic resonance imaging (fMRI) measures a blood oxygenation level dependent **(BOLD) signal**. When neural activity in a brain area increases, the blood flow increases, and this change of blood flow can be measured by the change in the amount of deoxyhaemoglobin (which is paramagnetic) in a brain region. The spatial resolution is in the order of 3 mm and so reflects the activity of hundreds of thousands of neurons, and the temporal resolution is in the order of several seconds.

Functional neuroimaging measures the activity of the brain either while the participant is resting, or during a task. The methods commonly used include functional magnetic resonance imaging of the brain (fMRI), positron emission tomography (PET), and magnetoencephalography (MEG).

A **pattern association network** learns the association between an input pattern (such as the sight of food) and the stimulus to be recalled (such as the taste of food). It can be used to compute **expected value**. This type of network is illustrated in Fig. 9.1, and is described quantitatively by Rolls (2016c).

A reward **prediction error** is positive if the **reward outcome** (e.g. the taste of food) is greater than the **expected value** (e.g. what is expected from the sight of food). Dopamine neurons appear to encode this error, useful in **reinforcement learning** (see Section 5.2). A reward **prediction error** is negative if the reward outcome (e.g. the taste of food) is less than the expected value (e.g. what is expected from the sight of food). This is sometimes referred to as **non-reward**. Some neurons in the orbitofrontal cortex encode negative reward prediction error, as described in Section 3.8, and may be related to depression, as described in Chapter 7.

Reward value refers to the value of a good, and is a term used in neuroeconomics and decision-making (Glimcher & Fehr 2013, Rolls 2014a). It can be measured by how much one would pay for the good, which might be a food, or how hard one would work to obtain the food. Stimuli with high reward value are rated as subjectively pleasant, and there is often a linear relation between the activation of the orbitofrontal cortex and the pleasantness of the stimulus (Chapter 3).

A.2 Learning theory terms

Instrumental reinforcers are stimuli that, if their occurrence, termination, or omission is made contingent upon the making of an action, alter the probability of the future emission of that action (Gray 1975, Mackintosh 1983, Dickinson 1980, Lieberman 2000, Mazur 2012, Rolls 2014a). Rewards and punishers are instrumental reinforcing stimuli. The notion of an action here is that an arbitrary action, e.g. turning right vs turning left, will be performed in order to obtain the reward or avoid the punisher, so that there is no pre-wired connection between the response and the reinforcer. Some stimuli are **primary (unlearned) reinforcers** (e.g., the taste of food if the animal is hungry, or pain); while others may become reinforcing by learning, because of their association with such primary reinforcers, thereby becoming '**secondary reinforcers**'. This type of learning may thus be called '**stimulus–reinforcer association learning**', and occurs via a stimulus–stimulus associative learning process.

A **positive reinforcer** (such as food) increases the probability of emission of an action on which it is contingent, the process is termed **positive reinforcement**, and the outcome is a **reward** (such as food).

A **negative reinforcer** (such as a painful stimulus) increases the probability of emission of an action that causes the negative reinforcer to be omitted (as in **active avoidance**) or terminated (as in **escape**), and the procedure is termed **negative reinforcement**.

Punishment refers to procedures in which the probability of an action is decreased. Punishment thus describes procedures in which an action decreases in probability if it is followed by a painful stimulus, as in **passive avoidance**. Punishment can also be used to refer to a procedure involving the omission or termination of a reward ('**extinction**' and '**time out**' respectively), both of which decrease the probability of responses (Gray 1975, Mackintosh 1983, Dickinson 1980, Lieberman 2000, Mazur 2012, Rolls 2014a).

A **punisher** when delivered acts instrumentally to decrease the probability of actions on which it is contingent, or when not delivered (escaped from or avoided) acts as a negative reinforcer in that it then increases the probability of the action on which its non-delivery is contingent. Note that my definition of a punisher, which is similar to that of an aversive stimulus, is of a stimulus or event that can either decrease the probability of actions on which it is contingent, or increase the probability of actions on which its non-delivery is contingent. The term **punishment** is restricted to situations where the probability of an action is being decreased.

Emotions are states elicited by instrumental reinforcers, where the states have the set of functions described in Chapter 6 and by Rolls (2014a). My argument is that an affectively positive or 'appetitive' stimulus (which produces a state of pleasure) acts operationally as a **reward**, which when delivered acts instrumentally as a positive reinforcer, or when not delivered (omitted or terminated) acts to decrease the probability of responses on which it is contingent. Conversely I argue that an affectively negative or aversive stimulus (which produces an unpleasant state) acts operationally as a **punisher**, which when delivered acts instrumentally to decrease the probability of actions on which it is contingent, or when not delivered (escaped from or avoided) acts as a negative reinforcer in that it then increases the probability of the action on which its non-delivery is contingent[14].

Classical conditioning or **Pavlovian conditioning**. When a **conditioned stimulus (CS)** (such as a tone) is paired with a primary reinforcer or **unconditioned stimulus (US)** (such as a painful stimulus), then there are opportunities for a number of types of association to be formed. Some of these involve 'classical conditioning' or 'Pavlovian conditioning', in which no action is performed that affects the contingency between the conditioned stimulus and the unconditioned stimulus. Typically an **unconditioned response (UR)**, for example an alteration of heart rate, is produced by the US, and will come to be elicited by the CS as a **conditioned response (CR)**. These responses are typically autonomic (such as the heart beating faster), or endocrine (for example the release of adrenaline (epinephrine in American usage) by the adrenal gland). In addition, the organism may learn to perform an instrumental response with the skeletal muscles in order to alter the probability that the primary reinforcer will be obtained. In our example, the experimenter might alter the contingencies so that when the tone sounded, if the organism performed a response such as pressing a lever, then the painful stimulus could be avoided. In the instrumental learning situation there are still

---

[14]Note that my definition of a punisher, which is similar to that of an aversive stimulus, is of a stimulus or event that can either decrease the probability of actions on which it is contingent, or increase the probability of actions on which its non-delivery is contingent. The term punishment is restricted to situations where the probability of an action is being decreased.

opportunities for many classically conditioned responses, including emotional states such as fear, to occur. The associative processes involved in classical conditioning, and the influences that these processes may have on instrumental performance, are described in Section 6.5.2.

Motivated behaviour occurs when an animal will perform an instrumental (i.e. arbitrary operant) response to obtain a reward or to escape from or avoid a punisher. If this criterion of an arbitrary operant response is not met, and only a fixed response can be performed, then the term **drive** can be used to describe the state of the animal when it will work to obtain or escape from the stimulus.

Long-term potentiation (LTP) is the increase in synaptic strength that can occur during learning. It is typically associative, depending on conjunctive presynaptic activity and postsynaptic depolarization.

Long-term depression (LTP) is the decrease in synaptic strength that can occur during learning. It is typically associative, occurring when the presynaptic activity is low and the postsynaptic depolarization is high (heterosynaptic long-term depression), or when the presynaptic activity is high, and the postsynaptic activity is only moderate (homosynaptic long-term depression).

References

Abbott LF, Rolls ET, & Tovee MJ (1996). Representational capacity of face coding in monkeys. *Cerebral Cortex* 6: 498–505.
Abdallah CG, Adams TG, Kelmendi B, Esterlis I, Sanacora G, & Krystal JH (2016). Ketamine's mechanism of action: A path to rapid-acting antidepressants. *Depression and Anxiety* 33: 689–697.
Abeles M (1991). *Corticonics: Neural Circuits of the Cerebral Cortex*. Cambridge University Press, Cambridge.
Adolphs R (2003). Cognitive neuroscience of human social behavior. *Nature Reviews Neuroscience* 4: 165–178.
Adolphs R, Tranel D, Damasio H, & Damasio AR (1994). Impaired recognition of emotion in facial expressions following bilateral damage to the human amygdala. *Nature* 372: 669–672.
Adolphs R, Tranel D, & Baron-Cohen S (2002). Amygdala damage impairs recognition of social emotions from facial expressions. *Journal of Cognitive Neuroscience* 14: 1–11.
Adolphs R, Gosselin F, Buchanan TW, Tranel D, Schyns P, & Damasio AR (2005). A mechanism for impaired fear recognition after amygdala damage. *Nature* 433: 68–72.
Aggelopoulos NC & Rolls ET (2005). Natural scene perception: inferior temporal cortex neurons encode the positions of different objects in the scene. *European Journal of Neuroscience* 22: 2903–2916.
Aggelopoulos NC, Franco L, & Rolls ET (2005). Object perception in natural scenes: encoding by inferior temporal cortex simultaneously recorded neurons. *Journal of Neurophysiology* 93: 1342–1357.
Aggleton JP, editor (2000). *The Amygdala, A Functional Analysis*. Oxford University Press, Oxford, 2nd edn.
Ahveninen J, Huang S, Nummenmaa A, Belliveau JW, Hung AY, Jaaskelainen IP, Rauschecker JP, Rossi S, Tiitinen H, & Raij T (2013). Evidence for distinct human auditory cortex regions for sound location versus identity processing. *Nat Commun* 4: 2585.
Ainslie G (1992). *Picoeconomics*. Cambridge University Press, Cambridge.
Al Omran Y & Aziz Q (2014). The brain-gut axis in health and disease. *Adv Exp Med Biol* 817: 135–53.
Aleksandrova LR, Phillips AG, & Wang YT (2017). Antidepressant effects of ketamine and the roles of ampa glutamate receptors and other mechanisms beyond nmda receptor antagonism. *J Psychiatry Neurosci* 42: 222–229.
Alexander RD (1979). *Darwinism and Human Affairs*. University of Washington Press, Seattle.
Amaral DG (2003). The amygdala, social behavior, and danger detection. *Annals of the New York Academy of Sciences* 1000: 337–347.
Amaral DG & Price JL (1984). Amygdalo-cortical projections in the monkey (Macaca fascicularis). *Journal of Comparative Neurology* 230: 465–496.
Amaral DG, Price JL, Pitkanen A, & Carmichael ST (1992). Anatomical organization of the primate amygdaloid complex. In Aggleton JP, editor, *The Amygdala*, chap. 1, 1–66. Wiley-Liss, New York.
Amit DJ (1989). *Modelling Brain Function*. Cambridge University Press, New York.
Amit DJ, Gutfreund H, & Sompolinsky H (1987). Statistical mechanics of neural networks near saturation. *Annals of Physics (New York)* 173: 30–67.
Amodeo LR, McMurray MS, & Roitman JD (2017). Orbitofrontal cortex reflects changes in response-outcome contingencies during probabilistic reversal learning. *Neuroscience* 345: 27–37.
Amunts K & Zilles K (2012). Architecture and organizational principles of broca's region. *Trends Cogn Sci* 16: 418–26.
Anderson AK, Christoff K, Stappen I, Panitz D, Ghahremani DG, Glover G, Gabrieli JD, & Sobel N (2003). Dissociated neural representations of intensity and valence in human olfaction. *Nature Neuroscience* 6: 196–202.
Anderson IM, Haddad PM, & Scott J (2012). Bipolar disorder. *BMJ* 345: e8508.
Anderson SW, Bechara A, Damasio H, Tranel D, & Damasio AR (1999). Impairment of social and moral behaviour related to early damage in human prefrontal cortex. *Nature Neuroscience* 2: 1032–1037.
Angeletos GM, Laibson D, Repetto A, Tobacman J, & Weinberg S (2001). The hyperbolic buffer stock model: calibration, simulation, and empirical evaluation. *Journal of Economic Perspectives* 15: 47–68.
Arnsten AF & Rubia K (2012). Neurobiological circuits regulating attention, cognitive control, motivation, and emotion: disruptions in neurodevelopmental psychiatric disorders. *J Am Acad Child Adolesc Psychiatry* 51: 356–67.
Arnsten AF, Wang M, & Paspalas CD (2015). Dopamine's actions in primate prefrontal cortex: Challenges for treating cognitive disorders. *Pharmacol Rev* 67: 681–96.
Aron AR, Fletcher PC, Bullmore ET, Sahakian BJ, & Robbins TW (2003). Stop-signal inhibition disrupted by damage to inferior frontal gyrus in humans. *Nature Neuroscience* 6: 115–116.

Aron AR, Robbins TW, & Poldrack RA (2014). Inhibition and the right inferior frontal cortex: one decade on. *Trends in Cognitive Sciences* 18: 177–85.

Assaf M, Jagannathan K, Calhoun VD, Miller L, Stevens MC, Sahl R, O'Boyle JG, Schultz RT, & Pearlson GD (2010). Abnormal functional connectivity of default mode sub-networks in autism spectrum disorder patients. *Neuroimage* 53: 247–56.

Auger SD & Maguire EA (2013). Assessing the mechanism of response in the retrosplenial cortex of good and poor navigators. *Cortex* 49: 2904–2913.

Azzi JC, Sirigu A, & Duhamel JR (2012). Modulation of value representation by social context in the primate orbitofrontal cortex. *Proc Natl Acad Sci U S A* 109: 2126–31.

Baddeley RJ, Abbott LF, Booth MJA, Sengpiel F, Freeman T, Wakeman EA, & Rolls ET (1997). Responses of neurons in primary and inferior temporal visual cortices to natural scenes. *Proceedings of the Royal Society B* 264: 1775–1783.

Balleine BW & Dickinson A (1998). The role of incentive learning in instrumental outcome revaluation by sensory-specific satiety. *Animal Learning and Behavior* 26: 46–59.

Barat E, Wirth S, & Duhamel JR (2018). Face cells in orbitofrontal cortex represent social categories. *Proceedings of the National Academy of Sciences (USA)* 115: E11158–E11167.

Barbaro N & Shackelford TK (2015). Book review: Nether no more: Bringing genital evolution to the forefront. *Evolutionary Psychology* 13: 262–265.

Barbas H (1988). Anatomic organization of basoventral and mediodorsal visual recipient prefrontal regions in the rhesus monkey. *Journal of Comparative Neurology* 276: 313–342.

Barbas H (1993). Organization of cortical afferent input to the orbitofrontal area in the rhesus monkey. *Neuroscience* 56: 841–864.

Barbas H (1995). Anatomic basis of cognitive–emotional interactions in the primate prefrontal cortex. *Neuroscience and Biobehavioral Reviews* 19: 499–510.

Barbas H (2007). Specialized elements of orbitofrontal cortex in primates. *Annals of the New York Academy of Sciences* 1121: 10–32.

Barbas H & Pandya DN (1989). Architecture and intrinsic connections of the prefrontal cortex in the rhesus monkey. *Journal of Comparative Neurology* 286: 353–375.

Barbas H, Zikopoulos B, & Timbie C (2011). Sensory pathways and emotional context for action in primate prefrontal cortex. *Biological Psychiatry* 69: 1133–1139.

Barlow HB (1972). Single units and sensation: a neuron doctrine for perceptual psychology. *Perception* 1: 371–394.

Barry DN, Chadwick MJ, & Maguire EA (2018). Nonmonotonic recruitment of ventromedial prefrontal cortex during remote memory recall. *PLoS Biol* 16: e2005479.

Battaglia F & Treves A (1998). Stable and rapid recurrent processing in realistic autoassociative memories. *Neural Computation* 10: 431–450.

Baylis GC, Rolls ET, & Leonard CM (1985). Selectivity between faces in the responses of a population of neurons in the cortex in the superior temporal sulcus of the monkey. *Brain Research* 342: 91–102.

Baylis GC, Rolls ET, & Leonard CM (1987). Functional subdivisions of temporal lobe neocortex. *Journal of Neuroscience* 7: 330–342.

Baylis LL & Gaffan D (1991). Amygdalectomy and ventromedial prefrontal ablation produce similar deficits in food choice and in simple object discrimination learning for an unseen reward. *Experimental Brain Research* 86: 617–622.

Baylis LL & Rolls ET (1991). Responses of neurons in the primate taste cortex to glutamate. *Physiology and Behavior* 49: 973–979.

Baylis LL, Rolls ET, & Baylis GC (1994). Afferent connections of the orbitofrontal cortex taste area of the primate. *Neuroscience* 64: 801–812.

Beaver JD, Lawrence AD, Ditzhuijzen Jv, Davis MH, Woods A, & Calder AJ (2006). Individual differences in reward drive predict neural responses to images of food. *Journal of Neuroscience* 26: 5160–5166.

Bechara A, Damasio AR, Damasio H, & Anderson SW (1994). Insensitivity to future consequences following damage to human prefrontal cortex. *Cognition* 50: 7–15.

Bechara A, Tranel D, Damasio H, & Damasio AR (1996). Failure to respond autonomically to anticipated future outcomes following damage to prefrontal cortex. *Cerebral Cortex* 6: 215–225.

Bechara A, Damasio H, Tranel D, & Damasio AR (1997). Deciding advantageously before knowing the advantageous strategy. *Science* 275: 1293–1295.

Bechara A, Damasio H, Tranel D, & Anderson SW (1998). Dissociation of working memory from decision making within the human prefrontal cortex. *Journal of Neuroscience* 18: 428–437.

Bechara A, Damasio H, Damasio AR, & Lee GP (1999). Different contributions of the human amygdala and ventromedial prefrontal cortex to decision making. *Journal of Neurosience* 19: 5473–5481.

Bechara A, Damasio H, Tranel D, & Damasio AR (2005). The Iowa Gambling Task and the somatic marker hypothesis: some questions and answers. *Trends in Cognitive Sciences* 9: 159–162.

Beck AT (1979). *Cognitive Therapy of Depression*. Guilford Press.

Beck AT (2008). The evolution of the cognitive model of depression and its neurobiological correlates. *American*

Journal of Psychiatry 165: 969–977.
Becker NB, Jesus SN, Joao K, Viseu JN, & Martins RIS (2017). Depression and sleep quality in older adults: a meta-analysis. *Psychol Health Med* 22: 889–895.
Beckstead RM, Morse JR, & Norgren R (1980). The nucleus of the solitary tract in the monkey: projections to the thalamus and brainstem nuclei. *Journal of Comparative Neurology* 190: 259–282.
Benabou R & Pycia M (2002). Dynamic inconsistency and self-control: a planner–doer interpretation. *Economics Letters* 77: 419–424.
Benes FM & Subburaj S (2016). Circuitry-specific hypermetabolism in the hippocampus of bipolar patients. In Soares JC & Young AH, editors, *Bipolar Disorders*, chap. 7, 70–89. Cambridge University Press, Cambridge, 3rd edn.
Berlin H & Rolls ET (2004). Time perception, impulsivity, emotionality, and personality in self-harming borderline personality disorder patients. *Journal of Personality Disorders* 18: 358–378.
Berlin H, Rolls ET, & Kischka U (2004). Impulsivity, time perception, emotion, and reinforcement sensitivity in patients with orbitofrontal cortex lesions. *Brain* 127: 1108–1126.
Berlin H, Rolls ET, & Iversen SD (2005). Borderline Personality Disorder, impulsivity, and the orbitofrontal cortex. *American Journal of Psychiatry* 58: 234–245.
Bermpohl F, Kahnt T, Dalanay U, Hagele C, Sajonz B, Wegner T, Stoy M, Adli M, Kruger S, Wrase J, Strohle A, Bauer M, & Heinz A (2010). Altered representation of expected value in the orbitofrontal cortex in mania. *Human Brain Mapping* 31: 958–969.
Bernoulli D (1738). Learning the value of information in an uncertain world. *Econometrica (1954)* 22: 22–36.
Berridge KC & Kringelbach ML (2015). Pleasure systems in the brain. *Neuron* 86: 646–64.
Berridge KC & Robinson TE (1998). What is the role of dopamine in reward: hedonic impact, reward learning, or incentive salience? *Brain Research Reviews* 28: 309–369.
Berridge KC, Robinson TE, & Aldridge JW (2009). Dissecting components of reward: 'liking', 'wanting', and learning. *Current Opinion in Pharmacology* 9: 65–73.
Bhattacharya A, Derecki NC, Lovenberg TW, & Drevets WC (2016). Role of neuro-immunological factors in the pathophysiology of mood disorders. *Psychopharmacology (Berl)* 233: 1623–36.
Bigdeli TB, Ripke S, Peterson RE, Trzaskowski M, Bacanu SA, Abdellaoui A, Andlauer TF, Beekman AT, Berger K, Blackwood DH, Boomsma DI, Breen G, Buttenschon HN, Byrne EM, Cichon S, Clarke TK, Couvy-Duchesne B, Craddock N, de Geus EJ, Degenhardt F, Dunn EC, Edwards AC, Fanous AH, Forstner AJ, Frank J, Gill M, Gordon SD, Grabe HJ, Hamilton SP, Hardiman O, Hayward C, Heath AC, Henders AK, Herms S, Hickie IB, Hoffmann P, Homuth G, Hottenga JJ, Ising M, Jansen R, Kloiber S, Knowles JA, Lang M, Li QS, Lucae S, MacIntyre DJ, Madden PA, Martin NG, McGrath PJ, McGuffin P, McIntosh AM, Medland SE, Mehta D, Middeldorp CM, Milaneschi Y, Montgomery GW, Mors O, Muller-Myhsok B, Nauck M, Nyholt DR, Nothen MM, Owen MJ, Penninx BW, Pergadia ML, Perlis RH, Peyrot WJ, Porteous DJ, Potash JB, Rice JP, Rietschel M, Riley BP, Rivera M, Schoevers R, Schulze TG, Shi J, Shyn SI, Smit JH, Smoller JW, Streit F, Strohmaier J, Teumer A, Treutlein J, Van der Auwera S, van Grootheest G, van Hemert AM, Volzke H, Webb BT, Weissman MM, Wellmann J, Willemsen G, Witt SH, Levinson DF, Lewis CM, Wray NR, Flint J, Sullivan PF, & Kendler KS (2017). Genetic effects influencing risk for major depressive disorder in china and europe. *Transl Psychiatry* 7: e1074.
Bisley JW & Goldberg ME (2010). Attention, intention, and priority in the parietal lobe. *Annual Review of Neuroscience* 33: 1–21.
Bjorklund A & Lindvall O (1986). Catecholaminergic brainstem regulatory systems. In Mountcastle VB, Bloom FE, & Geiger SR, editors, *Handbook of Physiology: The Nervous System*, vol. 4, Intrinsic systems of the Brain, 155–236. American Psychological Society, Bethesda.
Bliss-Moreau E, Moadab G, Bauman MD, & Amaral DG (2013). The impact of early amygdala damage on juvenile rhesus macaque social behavior. *J Cogn Neurosci* 25: 2124–40.
Blood AJ & Zatorre RJ (2001). Intensely pleasureable responses to music correlate with activity of brain regions implicated in reward and emotion. *Proceedings of the National Academy of Sciences USA* 98: 11818–11823.
Blood AJ, Zatorre RJ, Bermudez P, & Evans AC (1999). Emotional responses to pleasant and unpleasant music correlate with activity in paralimbic brain regions. *Nature Neuroscience* 2: 382–387.
Blumberg J & Kreiman G (2010). How cortical neurons help us see: visual recognition in the human brain. *The Journal of Clinical Investigation* 120: 3054–3063.
Bonnici HM & Maguire EA (2018). Two years later - revisiting autobiographical memory representations in vmpfc and hippocampus. *Neuropsychologia* 110: 159–169.
Booth DA (1985). Food-conditioned eating preferences and aversions with interoceptive elements: learned appetites and satieties. *Annals of the New York Academy of Sciences* 443: 22–37.
Booth MCA & Rolls ET (1998). View-invariant representations of familiar objects by neurons in the inferior temporal visual cortex. *Cerebral Cortex* 8: 510–523.
Bostan AC, Dum RP, & Strick PL (2018). Functional anatomy of basal ganglia circuits with the cerebral cortex and the cerebellum. *Prog Neurol Surg* 33: 50–61.
Boulougouris V, Dalley JW, & Robbins TW (2007). Effects of orbitofrontal, infralimbic and prelimbic cortical

lesions on serial spatial reversal learning in the rat. *Behav Brain Res* 179: 219–28.
Boussaoud D, Desimone R, & Ungerleider LG (1991). Visual topography of area TEO in the macaque. *Journal of Computational Neurology* 306: 554–575.
Bressler SL, Tang W, Sylvester CM, Shulman GL, & Corbetta M (2008). Top-down control of human visual cortex by frontal and parietal cortex in anticipatory visual spatial attention. *Journal of Neuroscience* 28: 10056–10061.
Brevers D, Cleeremans A, Verbruggen F, Bechara A, Kornreich C, Verbanck P, & Noel X (2012). Impulsive action but not impulsive choice determines problem gambling severity. *PLoS ONE* 7: e50647.
Bromberg-Martin ES & Hikosaka O (2011). Lateral habenula neurons signal errors in the prediction of reward information. *Nat Neurosci* 14: 1209–16.
Bromberg-Martin ES, Matsumoto M, & Hikosaka O (2010). Dopamine in motivational control: rewarding, aversive, and alerting. *Neuron* 68: 815–834.
Brosch M, Selezneva E, & Scheich H (2011). Representation of reward feedback in primate auditory cortex. *Front Syst Neurosci* 5: 5.
Brothers L & Ring B (1993). Mesial temporal neurons in the macaque monkey with responses selective for aspects of social stimuli. *Behavioural Brain Research* 57: 53–61.
Brunel N & Wang XJ (2001). Effects of neuromodulation in a cortical network model of object working memory dominated by recurrent inhibition. *Journal of Computational Neuroscience* 11: 63–85.
Brunel N & Wang XJ (2003). What determines the frequency of fast network oscillations with irregular neural discharges? I. Synaptic dynamics and excitation-inhibition balance. *Journal of Neurophysiology* 90: 415–430.
Bubb EJ, Kinnavane L, & Aggleton JP (2017). Hippocampal - diencephalic - cingulate networks for memory and emotion: An anatomical guide. *Brain Neurosci Adv* 1.
Buck L & Axel R (1991). A novel multigene family may encode odorant receptors: a molecular basis for odor recognition. *Cell* 65: 175–187.
Buck L & Bargmann CI (2013). Smell and taste: the chemical senses. In Kandel E, Schwartz JH, Jessell TH, Siegelbaum SA, & Hudspeth AJ, editors, *Principles of Neural Science*, chap. 32, 712–742. McGraw-Hill, New York, 5th edn.
Buckholtz JW, Treadway MT, Cowan RL, Woodward ND, Benning SD, Li R, Ansari MS, Baldwin RM, Schwartzman AN, Shelby ES, Smith CE, Cole D, Kessler RM, & Zald DH (2010). Mesolimbic dopamine reward system hypersensitivity in individuals with psychopathic traits. *Nature Neuroscience* 13: 419–421.
Buot A & Yelnik J (2012). Functional anatomy of the basal ganglia: limbic aspects. *Revue Neurologique (Paris)* 168: 569–575.
Bush G, Luu P, & Posner MI (2000). Cognitive and emotional influences in anterior cingulate cortex. *Trends in Cognitive Sciences* 4: 215–222.
Bush G, Vogt BA, Holmes J, Dales AM, Greve D, Jenike MA, & Rosen BR (2002). Dorsal anterior cingulate cortex: a role in reward-based decision making. *Proceedings of the National Academy of Sciences USA* 99: 523–528.
Butter CM (1969). Perseveration in extinction and in discrimination reversal tasks following selective prefrontal ablations in Macaca mulatta. *Physiology and Behavior* 4: 163–171.
Butter CM & Snyder DR (1972). Alterations in aversive and aggressive behaviors following orbitofrontal lesions in rhesus monkeys. *Acta Neurobiologica Experimentalis* 32: 525–565.
Butter CM, McDonald JA, & Snyder DR (1969). Orality, preference behavior, and reinforcement value of non-food objects in monkeys with orbital frontal lesions. *Science* 164: 1306–1307.
Butter CM, Snyder DR, & McDonald JA (1970). Effects of orbitofrontal lesions on aversive and aggressive behaviors in rhesus monkeys. *Journal of Comparative Physiology and Psychology* 72: 132–144.
Caan W, Perrett DI, & Rolls ET (1984). Responses of striatal neurons in the behaving monkey. 2. Visual processing in the caudal neostriatum. *Brain Research* 290: 53–65.
Cabanac M (1992). Pleasure: the common currency. *Journal of Theoretical Biology* 155: 173–200.
Cai X & Padoa-Schioppa C (2012). Neuronal encoding of subjective value in dorsal and ventral anterior cingulate cortex. *Journal of Neuroscience* 32: 3791–3808.
Cai X & Padoa-Schioppa C (2019). Neuronal evidence for good-based economic decisions under variable action costs. *Nat Commun* 10: 393.
Camille N, Tsuchida A, & Fellows LK (2011). Double dissociation of stimulus-value and action-value learning in humans with orbitofrontal or anterior cingulate cortex damage. *Journal of Neuroscience* 31: 15048–15052.
Canli T, Zhao Z, Desmond JE, Kang E, Gross J, & Gabrieli JD (2001). An fMRI study of personality influences on brain reactivity to emotional stimuli. *Behavioral Neuroscience* 115: 33–42.
Canli T, Sivers H, Whitfield SL, Gotlib IH, & Gabrieli JD (2002). Amygdala response to happy faces as a function of extraversion. *Science* 296: 2191.
Cardinal N & Everitt BJ (2004). Neural and psychological mechanisms underlying appetitive learning: links to drug addiction. *Current Opinion in Neurobiology* 14: 156–162.
Cardinal RN, Parkinson JA, Hall J, & Everitt BJ (2002). Emotion and motivation: the role of the amygdala, ventral striatum, and prefrontal cortex. *Neuroscience and Biobehavioral Reviews* 26: 321–352.
Carmichael ST & Price JL (1994). Architectonic subdivision of the orbital and medial prefrontal cortex in the

macaque monkey. *Journal of Comparative Neurology* 346: 366–402.
Carmichael ST & Price JL (1995a). Limbic connections of the orbital and medial prefrontal cortex in macaque monkeys. *Journal of Comparative Neurology* 363: 615–641.
Carmichael ST & Price JL (1995b). Sensory and premotor connections of the orbital and medial prefrontal cortex of macaque monkeys. *Journal of Comparative Neurology* 363: 642–664.
Carmichael ST & Price JL (1996). Connectional networks within the orbital and medial prefrontal cortex of macaque monkeys. *Journal of Comparative Neurology* 371: 179–207.
Carmichael ST, Clugnet MC, & Price JL (1994). Central olfactory connections in the macaque monkey. *Journal of Comparative Neurology* 346: 403–434.
Cavanna AE & Trimble MR (2006). The precuneus: a review of its functional anatomy and behavioural correlates. *Brain* 129: 564–583.
Celada P, Puig MV, Armagos-Bosch M, Adell A, & Artigas F (2004). The therapeutic role of 5-HT_{1A} and 5-HT_{2A} receptors in depression. *Journal of Psychiatry and Neuroscience* 29: 252–265.
Chamberlain SR, Menzies L, Hampshire A, Suckling J, Fineberg NA, del Campo N, Aitken M, Craig K, Owen AM, Bullmore ET, Robbins TW, & Sahakian BJ (2008). Orbitofrontal dysfunction in patients with obsessive-compulsive disorder and their unaffected relatives. *Science* 321: 421–2.
Chandrashekar J, Hoon MA, Ryba NJ, & Zuker CS (2006). The receptors and cells for mammalian taste. *Nature* 444: 288–294.
Chang L & Tsao DY (2017). The code for facial identity in the primate brain. *Cell* 169: 1013–1028 e14.
Chang SW, Gariepy JF, & Platt ML (2013). Neuronal reference frames for social decisions in primate frontal cortex. *Nat Neurosci* 16: 243–50.
Chau BK, Sallet J, Papageorgiou GK, Noonan MP, Bell AH, Walton ME, & Rushworth MF (2015). Contrasting roles for orbitofrontal cortex and amygdala in credit assignment and learning in macaques. *Neuron* 87: 1106–1118.
Chaudhari N & Roper SD (2010). The cell biology of taste. *Journal of Cell Biology* 190: 285–296.
Chaudhari N, Landin AM, & Roper S (2000). A metabolic glutamate receptor variant functions as a taste receptor. *Nature Neuroscience* 3: 113–119.
Cheng W, Rolls ET, Gu H, Zhang J, & Feng J (2015). Autism: reduced connectivity between cortical areas involved in face expression, theory of mind, and the sense of self. *Brain* 138: 1382–1398.
Cheng W, Rolls ET, Qiu J, Liu W, Tang Y, Huang CC, Wang X, Zhang J, Lin W, Zheng L, Pu J, Tsai SJ, Yang AC, Lin CP, Wang F, Xie P, & Feng J (2016). Medial reward and lateral non-reward orbitofrontal cortex circuits change in opposite directions in depression. *Brain* 139: 3296–3309.
Cheng W, Rolls ET, Qiu J, Xie X, Lyu W, Li Y, Huang CC, Yang AC, Tsai SJ, Lyu F, Zhuang K, Lin CP, Xie P, & Feng J (2018a). Functional connectivity of the human amygdala in health and in depression. *Soc Cogn Affect Neurosci* 13: 557–568.
Cheng W, Rolls ET, Qiu J, Xie X, Wei D, Huang CC, Yang AC, Tsai SJ, Li Q, Meng J, Lin CP, Xie P, & Feng J (2018b). Increased functional connectivity of the posterior cingulate cortex with the lateral orbitofrontal cortex in depression. *Transl Psychiatry* 8: 90.
Cheng W, Rolls ET, Qiu J, Yang D, Ruan H, Wei D, Zhao L, Meng J, Xie P, & Feng J (2018c). Functional connectivity of the precuneus in unmedicated patients with depression. *Biol Psychiatry Cogn Neurosci Neuroimaging* 3: 1040–1049.
Cheng W, Rolls ET, Ruan H, & Feng J (2018d). Functional connectivities in the brain that mediate the association between depressive problems and sleep quality. *JAMA Psychiatry* 75: 1052–1061.
Cheng W, Rolls ET, Robbins TW, Gong W, Liu Z, Lv W, Du J, Wen H, Ma L, Quinlan EB, Garavan H, Artiges E, Papadopoulos Orfanos D, Smolka MN, Schumann G, Kendrick K, & Feng J (2019). Decreased brain connectivity in smoking contrasts with increased connectivity in drinking. *Elife* 8: e40765.
Chib VS, Rangel A, Shimojo S, & O'Doherty JP (2009). Evidence for a common representation of decision values for dissimilar goods in human ventromedial prefrontal cortex. *Journal of Neuroscience* 29: 12315–12320.
Childress AR, Mozley PD, McElgin W, Fitzgerald J, Reivich M, & O'Brien CP (1999). Limbic activation during cue-induced cocaine craving. *American Journal of Psychiatry* 156: 11–18.
Cho YK, Li CS, & Smith DV (2002). Gustatory projections from the nucleus of the solitary tract to the parabrachial nuclei in the hamster. *Chemical Senses* 27: 81–90.
Chudasama Y & Robbins TW (2003). Dissociable contributions of the orbitofrontal and infralimbic cortex to pavlovian autoshaping and discrimination reversal learning: further evidence for the functional heterogeneity of the rodent frontal cortex. *J Neurosci* 23: 8771–80.
Chudasama Y, Passetti F, Rhodes SE, Lopian D, Desai A, & Robbins TW (2003). Dissociable aspects of performance on the 5-choice serial reaction time task following lesions of the dorsal anterior cingulate, infralimbic and orbitofrontal cortex in the rat: differential effects on selectivity, impulsivity and compulsivity. *Behav Brain Res* 146: 105–19.
Ciaramelli E (2008). The role of ventromedial prefrontal cortex in navigation: a case of impaired wayfinding and rehabilitation. *Neuropsychologia* 46: 2099–105.
Clark L, Cools R, & Robbins TW (2004). The neuropsychology of ventral prefrontal cortex: decision-making and

reversal learning. *Brain and Cognition* 55: 41–53.
Clark L, Bechara A, Damasio H, Aitken MR, Sahakian BJ, & Robbins TW (2008). Differential effects of insular and ventromedial prefrontal cortex lesions on risky decision-making. *Brain* 131: 1311–22.
Coghill DR, Seth S, & Matthews K (2014). A comprehensive assessment of memory, delay aversion, timing, inhibition, decision making and variability in attention deficit hyperactivity disorder: advancing beyond the three-pathway models. *Psychol Med* 44: 1989–2001.
Cooper JR, Bloom FE, & Roth RH (2003). *The Biochemical Basis of Neuropharmacology*. Oxford University Press, Oxford, 8th edn.
Corbetta M & Shulman GL (2002). Control of goal-directed and stimulus-driven attention in the brain. *Nature Reviews Neuroscience* 3: 201–215.
Courtiol E & Wilson DA (2017). The olfactory mosaic: Bringing an olfactory network together for odor perception. *Perception* 46: 320–332.
Craig AD, Chen K, Bandy D, & Reiman EM (2000). Thermosensory activation of insular cortex. *Nature Neuroscience* 3: 184–190.
Critchley H, Daly E, Phillips M, Brammer M, Bullmore E, Williams S, Van Amelsvoort T, Robertson D, David A, & Murphy D (2000). Explicit and implicit neural mechanisms for processing of social information from facial expressions: a functional magnetic resonance imaging study. *Hum Brain Mapp* 9: 93–105.
Critchley HD & Harrison NA (2013). Visceral influences on brain and behavior. *Neuron* 77: 624–638.
Critchley HD & Rolls ET (1996a). Responses of primate taste cortex neurons to the astringent tastant tannic acid. *Chemical Senses* 21: 135–145.
Critchley HD & Rolls ET (1996b). Olfactory neuronal responses in the primate orbitofrontal cortex: analysis in an olfactory discrimination task. *Journal of Neurophysiology* 75: 1659–1672.
Critchley HD & Rolls ET (1996c). Hunger and satiety modify the responses of olfactory and visual neurons in the primate orbitofrontal cortex. *Journal of Neurophysiology* 75: 1673–1686.
Croxson PL, Walton ME, O'Reilly JX, Behrens TE, & Rushworth MF (2009). Effort-based cost-benefit valuation and the human brain. *Journal of Neuroscience* 29: 4531–4541.
Dalley JW & Robbins TW (2017). Fractionating impulsivity: neuropsychiatric implications. *Nat Rev Neurosci* 18: 158–171.
Dalton GL, Wang NY, Phillips AG, & Floresco SB (2016). Multifaceted contributions by different regions of the orbitofrontal and medial prefrontal cortex to probabilistic reversal learning. *J Neurosci* 36: 1996–2006.
Damasio AR (1994). *Descartes' Error: Emotion, Reason, and the Human Brain*. Grosset/Putnam, New York.
Damasio H, Grabowski T, Frank R, Galaburda AM, & Damasio AR (1994). The return of Phineas Gage: clues about the brain from the skull of a famous patient. *Science* 264: 1102–1105.
Davis M (2006). Neural systems involved in fear and anxiety measured with fear-potentiated startle. *American Psychologist* 61: 741–756.
Davis M (2011). NMDA receptors and fear extinction: implications for cognitive behavioral therapy. *Dialogues in Clinical Neuroscience* 13: 463–474.
Davis M, Antoniadis EA, Amaral DG, & Winslow JT (2008). Acoustic startle reflex in rhesus monkeys: a review. *Reviews in Neuroscience* 19: 171–185.
Dawkins MS (1986). *Unravelling Animal Behaviour*. Longman, Harlow, 1st edn.
Dawkins R (1976). *The Selfish Gene*. Oxford University Press, Oxford.
Dawkins R (1989). *The Selfish Gene*. Oxford University Press, Oxford, 2nd edn.
Dayan P & Abbott LF (2001). *Theoretical Neuroscience*. MIT Press, Cambridge, MA.
de Araujo IE, Ferreira JG, Tellez LA, Ren X, & Yeckel CW (2012). The gut-brain dopamine axis: a regulatory system for caloric intake. *Physiol Behav* 106: 394–9.
de Araujo IE, Lin T, Veldhuizen MG, & Small DM (2013). Metabolic regulation of brain response to food cues. *Curr Biol* 23: 878–83.
De Araujo IET & Rolls ET (2004). Representation in the human brain of food texture and oral fat. *Journal of Neuroscience* 24: 3086–3093.
De Araujo IET, Kringelbach ML, Rolls ET, & Hobden P (2003a). Representation of umami taste in the human brain. *Journal of Neurophysiology* 90: 313–319.
De Araujo IET, Kringelbach ML, Rolls ET, & McGlone F (2003b). Human cortical responses to water in the mouth, and the effects of thirst. *Journal of Neurophysiology* 90: 1865–1876.
De Araujo IET, Rolls ET, Kringelbach ML, McGlone F, & Phillips N (2003c). Taste-olfactory convergence, and the representation of the pleasantness of flavour in the human brain. *European Journal of Neuroscience* 18: 2059–2068.
De Araujo IET, Rolls ET, Velazco MI, Margot C, & Cayeux I (2005). Cognitive modulation of olfactory processing. *Neuron* 46: 671–679.
De Gelder B, Vroomen J, Pourtois G, & Weiskrantz L (1999). Non-conscious recognition of affect in the absence of striate cortex. *NeuroReport* 10: 3759–3763.
Debiec J, LeDoux JE, & Nader K (2002). Cellular and systems reconsolidation in the hippocampus. *Neuron* 36: 527–538.

Debiec J, Doyere V, Nader K, & LeDoux JE (2006). Directly reactivated, but not indirectly reactivated, memories undergo reconsolidation in the amygdala. *Proceedings of the National Academy of Sciences USA* 103: 3428–3433.

Deco G & Kringelbach ML (2014). Great expectations: using whole-brain computational connectomics for understanding neuropsychiatric disorders. *Neuron* 84: 892–905.

Deco G & Rolls ET (2002). Object-based visual neglect: a computational hypothesis. *European Journal of Neuroscience* 16: 1994–2000.

Deco G & Rolls ET (2003). Attention and working memory: a dynamical model of neuronal activity in the prefrontal cortex. *European Journal of Neuroscience* 18: 2374–2390.

Deco G & Rolls ET (2004). A neurodynamical cortical model of visual attention and invariant object recognition. *Vision Research* 44: 621–644.

Deco G & Rolls ET (2005a). Synaptic and spiking dynamics underlying reward reversal in the orbitofrontal cortex. *Cerebral Cortex* 15: 15–30.

Deco G & Rolls ET (2005b). Attention, short term memory, and action selection: a unifying theory. *Progress in Neurobiology* 76: 236–256.

Deco G & Rolls ET (2005c). Neurodynamics of biased competition and cooperation for attention: a model with spiking neurons. *Journal of Neurophysiology* 94: 295–313.

Deco G & Rolls ET (2005d). Sequential memory: a putative neural and synaptic dynamical mechanism. *Journal of Cognitive Neuroscience* 17: 294–307.

Deco G & Rolls ET (2006). A neurophysiological model of decision-making and Weber's law. *European Journal of Neuroscience* 24: 901–916.

Deco G, Rolls ET, & Horwitz B (2004). 'What' and 'where' in visual working memory: a computational neurodynamical perspective for integrating fMRI and single-neuron data. *Journal of Cognitive Neuroscience* 16: 683–701.

Deco G, Rolls ET, & Romo R (2009). Stochastic dynamics as a principle of brain function. *Progress in Neurobiology* 88: 1–16.

Deco G, Rolls ET, & Romo R (2010). Synaptic dynamics and decision-making. *Proceedings of the National Academy of Sciences* 107: 7545–7549.

Deco G, Rolls ET, Albantakis L, & Romo R (2013). Brain mechanisms for perceptual and reward-related decision-making. *Progress in Neurobiology* 103: 194–213.

Deen B, Koldewyn K, Kanwisher N, & Saxe R (2015). Functional organization of social perception and cognition in the superior temporal sulcus. *Cereb Cortex* 25: 4596–609.

Dehaene S, Dehaene-Lambertz G, & Cohen L (1998). Abstract representations of numbers in the animal and human brain. *Trends in Neurosciences* 21: 355–361.

Delgado MR, Jou RL, & Phelps EA (2011). Neural systems underlying aversive conditioning in humans with primary and secondary reinforcers. *Frontiers in Neuroscience* 5: 71.

DeLong M & Wichmann T (2010). Changing views of basal ganglia circuits and circuit disorders. *Clinical EEG and Neuroscience* 41: 61–67.

Deng WL, Rolls ET, Ji X, Robbins TW, Banaschewski T, Bokde A, Bromberg U, Buechel C, Desrivieres S, Conrod P, Flor H, Frouin V, Gallinat J, Garavan H, Gowland P, Heinz A, Ittermann B, Martinot JL, Lemaitre H, Nees F, Papadopoulos Orfanos D, Poustka L, Smolka MN, Walter H, Whelan R, Schumann G, Feng J, & the Imagen consortium (2017). Separate neural systems for behavioral change and for emotional responses to failure during behavioral inhibition. *Human Brain Mapping* 38: 3527–3537.

Derbyshire SWG, Vogt BA, & Jones AKP (1998). Pain and Stroop interference tasks activate separate processing modules in anterior cingulate cortex. *Experimental Brain Research* 118: 52–60.

Desimone R & Duncan J (1995). Neural mechanisms of selective visual attention. *Annual Review of Neuroscience* 18: 193–222.

Di Lorenzo PM (1990). Corticofugal influence on taste responses in the parabrachial pons of the rat. *Brain Research* 530: 73–84.

Diamond A (2007). Consequences of variations in genes that affect dopamine in prefrontal cortex. *Cereb Cortex* 17 Suppl 1: i161–70.

Dichter GS, Felder JN, Green SR, Rittenberg AM, Sasson NJ, & Bodfish JW (2012a). Reward circuitry function in autism spectrum disorders. *Soc Cogn Affect Neurosci* 7: 160–72.

Dichter GS, Richey JA, Rittenberg AM, Sabatino A, & Bodfish JW (2012b). Reward circuitry function in autism during face anticipation and outcomes. *J Autism Dev Disord* 42: 147–60.

Dickinson A (1980). *Contemporary Animal Learning Theory*. Cambridge University Press, Cambridge.

Diehl MM & Romanski LM (2014). Responses of prefrontal multisensory neurons to mismatching faces and vocalizations. *J Neurosci* 34: 11233–43.

Disner SG, Beevers CG, Haigh EA, & Beck AT (2011). Neural mechanisms of the cognitive model of depression. *Nat Rev Neurosci* 12: 467–77.

Dolan RJ, Fink GR, Rolls ET, Booth M, Holmes A, Frackowiak RSJ, & Friston KJ (1997). How the brain learns to see objects and faces in an impoverished context. *Nature* 389: 596–599.

Douglas RJ, Markram H, & Martin KAC (2004). Neocortex. In Shepherd GM, editor, *The Synaptic Organization of the Brain*, chap. 12, 499–558. Oxford University Press, Oxford, 5th edn.

Downar J (2019). Orbitofrontal cortex: A 'non-rewarding' new treatment target in depression? *Curr Biol* 29: R59–R62.

Downar J, Blumberger DM, Rizvi SJ, Daskalakis ZJ, Kennedy H, & Giacobbe P (2019). Targeting the neural subtypes of depression .

Doyere V, Debiec J, Monfils MH, Schafe GE, & LeDoux JE (2007). Synapse-specific reconsolidation of distinct fear memories in the lateral amygdala. *Nature Neuroscience* 10: 414–416.

Drevets WC (2007). Orbitofrontal cortex function and structure in depression. *Annals of the New York Academy of Sciences* 1121: 499–527.

Drysdale AT, Grosenick L, Downar J, Dunlop K, Mansouri F, Meng Y, Fetcho RN, Zebley B, Oathes DJ, Etkin A, Schatzberg AF, Sudheimer K, Keller J, Mayberg HS, Gunning FM, Alexopoulos GS, Fox MD, Pascual-Leone A, Voss HU, Casey BJ, Dubin MJ, & Liston C (2017). Resting-state connectivity biomarkers define neurophysiological subtypes of depression. *Nat Med* 23: 28–38.

Duman RS & Aghajanian GK (2012). Synaptic dysfunction in depression: potential therapeutic targets. *Science* 338: 68–72.

D'Urso G, Dell'Osso B, Rossi R, Brunoni AR, Bortolomasi M, Ferrucci R, Priori A, de Bartolomeis A, & Altamura AC (2017). Clinical predictors of acute response to transcranial direct current stimulation (tdcs) in major depression. *J Affect Disord* 219: 25–30.

Eagle DM, Baunez C, Hutcheson DM, Lehmann O, Shah AP, & Robbins TW (2008). Stop-signal reaction-time task performance: role of prefrontal cortex and subthalamic nucleus. *Cereb Cortex* 18: 178–88.

Eisenberger NI & Lieberman MD (2004). Why rejection hurts: a common neural alarm system for physical and social pain. *Trends in Cognitive Neuroscience* 8: 294–300.

Elliffe MCM, Rolls ET, & Stringer SM (2002). Invariant recognition of feature combinations in the visual system. *Biological Cybernetics* 86: 59–71.

Eshel N & Roiser JP (2010). Reward and punishment processing in depression. *Biological Psychiatry* 68: 118–124.

Eslinger P & Damasio A (1985). Severe disturbance of higher cognition after bilateral frontal lobe ablation: patient EVR. *Neurology* 35: 1731–1741.

Everitt BJ & Robbins TW (2013). From the ventral to the dorsal striatum: Devolving views of their roles in drug addiction. *Neuroscience and Biobehavioural Reviews* 37: 1946–1954.

Everitt BJ, Belin D, Economidou D, Pelloux Y, Dalley JW, & Robbins TW (2008). Review. neural mechanisms underlying the vulnerability to develop compulsive drug-seeking habits and addiction. *Philosopjical Transactions of the Royal Society London B Biological Sciences* 363: 3125–3135.

Everitt BJ, Giuliano C, & Belin D (2018). Addictive behaviour in experimental animals: prospects for translation. *Philos Trans R Soc Lond B Biol Sci* 373.

Eysenck HJ & Eysenck SBG (1985). *Personality and Individual Differences: a Natural Science Approach*. Plenum, New York.

Faraone SV, Asherson P, Banaschewski T, Biederman J, Buitelaar JK, Ramos-Quiroga JA, Rohde LA, Sonuga-Barke EJ, Tannock R, & Franke B (2015). Attention-deficit/hyperactivity disorder. *Nat Rev Dis Primers* 1: 15020.

Farrow TF, Zheng Y, Wilkinson ID, Spence SA, Deakin JF, Tarrier N, Griffiths PD, & Woodruff PW (2001). Investigating the functional anatomy of empathy and forgiveness. *NeuroReport* 12: 2433–2438.

Feffer K, Fettes P, Giacobbe P, Daskalakis ZJ, Blumberger DM, & Downar J (2018). 1hz rtms of the right orbitofrontal cortex for major depression: Safety, tolerability and clinical outcomes. *Eur Neuropsychopharmacol* 28: 109–117.

Feierstein CE, Quirk MC, Uchida N, Sosulski DL, & Mainen ZF (2006). Representation of spatial goals in rat orbitofrontal cortex. *Neuron* 51: 495–507.

Feinstein JS, Adolphs R, Damasio A, & Tranel D (2011). The human amygdala and the induction and experience of fear. *Current Biology* 21: 34–38.

Fellows LK (2007). The role of orbitofrontal cortex in decision making: a component process account. *Annalls of the New York Academy of Sciences* 1121: 421–430.

Fellows LK (2011). Orbitofrontal contributions to value-based decision making: evidence from humans with frontal lobe damage. *Annals of the New York Academy of Sciences* 1239: 51–58.

Fellows LK & Farah MJ (2003). Ventromedial frontal cortex mediates affective shifting in humans: evidence from a reversal learning paradigm. *Brain* 126: 1830–1837.

Fellows LK & Farah MJ (2005). Different underlying impairments in decision-making after ventromedial and dorsolateral frontal lobe damage in humans. *Cerebral Cortex* 15: 58–63.

Fineberg NA, Apergis-Schoute AM, Vaghi MM, Banca P, Gillan CM, Voon V, Chamberlain SR, Cinosi E, Reid J, Shahper S, Bullmore ET, Sahakian BJ, & Robbins TW (2018). Mapping compulsivity in the dsm-5 obsessive compulsive and related disorders: Cognitive domains, neural circuitry, and treatment. *Int J Neuropsychopharmacol* 21: 42–58.

Fiorillo CD, Tobler PN, & Schultz W (2003). Discrete coding of reward probability and uncertainty by dopamine neurons. *Science* 299: 1898–1902.

Fisher C & Freiwald WA (2015). Contrasting specializations for facial motion within the macaque face-processing system. *Curr Biol* 25: 261–266.
Flint J & Kendler KS (2014). The genetics of major depression. *Neuron* 81: 1214.
Fodor JA (1994). *The Elm and the Expert: Mentalese and its Semantics*. MIT Press, Cambridge, MA.
Forgeard MJ, Haigh EA, Beck AT, Davidson RJ, Henn FA, Maier SF, Mayberg HS, & Seligman ME (2011). Beyond depression: Towards a process-based approach to research, diagnosis, and treatment. *Clinical Psychology (New York)* 18: 275–299.
Fox CR & Poldrack RA (2009). Prospect theory and the brain. In Glimcher PW, Camerer CF, Fehr E, & Poldrack RA, editors, *Neuroeconomics. Decision Making and the Brain*, chap. 11, 145–173. Academic Press, London.
Francis S, Rolls ET, Bowtell R, McGlone F, O'Doherty J, Browning A, Clare S, & Smith E (1999). The representation of pleasant touch in the brain and its relationship with taste and olfactory areas. *NeuroReport* 10: 453–459.
Franco L, Rolls ET, Aggelopoulos NC, & Treves A (2004). The use of decoding to analyze the contribution to the information of the correlations between the firing of simultaneously recorded neurons. *Experimental Brain Research* 155: 370–384.
Franco L, Rolls ET, Aggelopoulos NC, & Jerez JM (2007). Neuronal selectivity, population sparseness, and ergodicity in the inferior temporal visual cortex. *Biological Cybernetics* 96: 547–560.
Frederick S, Loewenstein T, & O'Donoghue (2002). Time discounting and time preference: a critical review. *Journal of Economic Literature* 40: 351–401.
Freeman WJ & Watts JW (1950). *Psychosurgery in the Treatment of Mental Disorders and Intractable Pain*. Thomas, Springfield, IL, 2nd edn.
Freese JL & Amaral DG (2009). Neuroanatomy of the primate amygdala. In Whalen PJ & Phelps EA, editors, *The Human Amygdala*, chap. 1, 3–42. Guilford, New York.
Freiwald WA & Tsao DY (2010). Functional compartmentalization and viewpoint generalization within the macaque face-processing system. *Science* 330: 845–51.
Freiwald WA, Tsao DY, & Livingstone MS (2009). A face feature space in the macaque temporal lobe. *Nat Neurosci* 12: 1187–96.
Freton M, Lemogne C, Bergouignan L, Delaveau P, Lehericy S, & Fossati P (2014). The eye of the self: precuneus volume and visual perspective during autobiographical memory retrieval. *Brain Struct Funct* 219: 959–68.
Frey S & Petrides M (2002a). Orbitofrontal cortex and memory formation. *Neuron* 36: 171–176.
Frey S & Petrides M (2002b). Orbitofrontal cortex and memory formation. *Neuron* 36: 171–6.
Frey S & Petrides M (2003). Greater orbitofrontal activity predicts better memory for faces. *European Journal of Neuroscience* 17: 2755–8.
Frey S, Kostopoulos P, & Petrides M (2000). Orbitofrontal involvement in the processing of unpleasant auditory information. *European Journal of Neuroscience* 12: 3709–3712.
Friston KJ, Buechel C, Fink GR, Morris J, Rolls ET, & Dolan RJ (1997). Psychophysiological and modulatory interactions in neuroimaging. *Neuroimage* 6: 218–229.
Fujisawa TX & Cook ND (2011). The perception of harmonic triads: an fMRI study. *Brain Imaging Behav* 5: 109–125.
Fulton JF (1951). *Frontal Lobotomy and Affective Behavior. A Neurophysiological Analysis*. W. W. Norton, New York.
Furl N, Hadj-Bouziane F, Liu N, Averbeck BB, & Ungerleider LG (2012). Dynamic and static facial expressions decoded from motion-sensitive areas in the macaque monkey. *Journal of Neuroscience* 32: 15952–15962.
Fuster JM (2015). *The Prefrontal Cortex*. Academic Press, London, 5th edn.
Gabbott PL, Warner TA, Jays PR, & Bacon SJ (2003). Areal and synaptic interconnectivity of prelimbic (area 32), infralimbic (area 25) and insular cortices in the rat. *Brain Research* 993: 59–71.
Gallagher M & Holland PC (1992). Understanding the function of the central nucleus: is simple conditioning enough? In Aggleton JP, editor, *The Amygdala: Neurobiological Aspects of Emotion, Memory, and Mental Dysfunction*, 307–321. Wiley-Liss, New York.
Gallagher M & Holland PC (1994). The amygdala complex: multiple roles in associative learning and attention. *Proceedings of the National Academy of Sciences USA* 91: 11771–11776.
Garcia-Cabezas MA & Barbas H (2017). Anterior cingulate pathways may affect emotions through orbitofrontal cortex. *Cereb Cortex* 27: 4891–4910.
Garrison J, Erdeniz B, & Done J (2013). Prediction error in reinforcement learning: a meta-analysis of neuroimaging studies. *Neurosci Biobehav Rev* 37: 1297–310.
Gazzaniga MS (1988). Brain modularity: towards a philosophy of conscious experience. In Marcel AJ & Bisiach E, editors, *Consciousness in Contemporary Science*, chap. 10, 218–238. Oxford University Press, Oxford.
Gazzaniga MS (1995). Consciousness and the cerebral hemispheres. In Gazzaniga MS, editor, *The Cognitive Neurosciences*, chap. 92, 1392–1400. MIT Press, Cambridge, MA.
Gazzaniga MS & LeDoux J (1978). *The Integrated Mind*. Plenum, New York.
Ge T, Feng J, Grabenhorst F, & Rolls ET (2012). Componential Granger causality, and its application to identifying the source and mechanisms of the top-down biased activation that controls attention to affective vs sensory processing. *Neuroimage* 59: 1846–1858.

Georges-François P, Rolls ET, & Robertson RG (1999). Spatial view cells in the primate hippocampus: allocentric view not head direction or eye position or place. *Cerebral Cortex* 9: 197–212.
Gerfen CR & Surmeier DJ (2011). Modulation of striatal projection systems by dopamine. *Annual Reviews of Neuroscience* 34: 441–466.
Ghasemi M, Phillips C, Fahimi A, McNerney MW, & Salehi A (2017). Mechanisms of action and clinical efficacy of nmda receptor modulators in mood disorders. *Neurosci Biobehav Rev* 80: 555–572.
Ghashghaei HT & Barbas H (2002). Pathways for emotion: interactions of prefrontal and anterior temporal pathways in the amygdala of the rhesus monkey. *Neuroscience* 115: 1261–1279.
Gilbert SJ & Burgess PW (2008). Executive function. *Curr Biol* 18: R110–4.
Gilson M, Moreno-Bote R, Ponce-Alvarez A, Ritter P, & Deco G (2016). Estimation of directed effective connectivity from fmri functional connectivity hints at asymmetries in the cortical connectome. *PLoS Computational Biology* 12: e1004762.
Giza BK & Scott TR (1983). Blood glucose selectively affects taste-evoked activity in rat nucleus tractus solitarius. *Physiology and Behaviour* 31: 643–650.
Giza BK & Scott TR (1987a). Intravenous insulin infusions in rats decrease gustatory-evoked responses to sugars. *American Journal of Physiology* 252: R994–R1002.
Giza BK & Scott TR (1987b). Blood glucose level affects perceived sweetness intensity in rats. *Physiology and Behaviour* 41: 459–464.
Giza BK, Scott TR, & Vanderweele DA (1992). Administration of satiety factors and gustatory responsiveness in the nucleus tractus solitarius of the rat. *Brain Research Bulletin* 28: 637–639.
Giza BK, Deems RO, Vanderweele DA, & Scott TR (1993). Pancreatic glucagon suppresses gustatory responsiveness to glucose. *American Journal of Physiology* 265: R1231–7.
Glascher J, Adolphs R, Damasio H, Bechara A, Rudrauf D, Calamia M, Paul LK, & Tranel D (2012). Lesion mapping of cognitive control and value-based decision making in the prefrontal cortex. *Proceedings of the National Academy of Sciences U S A* 109: 14681–14686.
Gleen JF & Erickson RP (1976). Gastric modulation of gustatory afferent activity. *Physiology and Behaviour* 16: 561–568.
Glimcher P (2003). The neurobiology of visual-saccadic decision making. *Annual Review of Neuroscience* 26: 133–179.
Glimcher P (2004). *Decisions, Uncertainty, and the Brain*. MIT Press, Cambridge, MA.
Glimcher P (2011a). *Foundations of Neuroeconomic Analysis*. Oxford University Press, Oxford.
Glimcher PW (2011b). Understanding dopamine and reinforcement learning: the dopamine reward prediction error hypothesis. *Proceedings of the National Academy of Sciences U S A* 108 Suppl 3: 15647–15654.
Glimcher PW & Fehr E (2013). *Neuroeconomics: Decision-Making and the Brain*. Academic Press, New York, 2nd edn.
Glimcher PW, Camerer CF, Fehr E, & Poldrack RA, editors (2009). *Neuroeconomics. Decision Making and the Brain*. Academic Press, London.
Gold PW (2015). The organization of the stress system and its dysregulation in depressive illness. *Molecular Psychiatry* 20: 32–47.
Goldman PS & Nauta WJH (1977). An intricately patterned prefronto-caudate projection in the rhesus monkey. *Journal of Comparative Neurology* 171: 369–386.
Goldman-Rakic PS (1996). The prefrontal landscape: implications of functional architecture for understanding human mentation and the central executive. *Philosophical Transactions of the Royal Society B* 351: 1445–1453.
Goleman D (1995). *Emotional Intelligence*. Bantam, New York.
Goodale MA (2004). Perceiving the world and grasping it: dissociations between conscious and unconscious visual processing. In Gazzaniga MS, editor, *The Cognitive Neurosciences III*, 1159–1172. MIT Press, Cambridge, MA.
Goodglass H & Kaplan E (1979). Assessment of cognitive deficit in brain-injured patient. In Gazzaniga MS, editor, *Handbook of Behavioural Neurobiology*, vol. 2, Neuropsychology, 3–22. Plenum, New York.
Gothard KM, Battaglia FP, Erickson CA, Spitler KM, & Amaral DG (2007). Neural responses to facial expression and face identity in the monkey amygdala. *Journal of Neurophysiology* 97: 1671–1683.
Gothard KM, Mosher CP, Zimmerman PE, Putnam PT, Morrow JK, & Fuglevand AJ (2018). New perspectives on the neurophysiology of primate amygdala emerging from the study of naturalistic social behaviors. *Wiley Interdiscip Rev Cogn Sci* 9.
Gotlib IH & Hammen CL (2009). *Handbook of Depression*. Guilford Press, New York.
Gottfried JA, O'Doherty J, & Dolan RJ (2003). Encoding predictive reward value in human amygdala and orbitofrontal cortex. *Science* 301: 1104–1107.
Gotts SJ, Simmons WK, Milbury LA, Wallace GL, Cox RW, & Martin A (2012). Fractionation of social brain circuits in autism spectrum disorders. *Brain* 135: 2711–25.
Grabenhorst F & Rolls ET (2008). Selective attention to affective value alters how the brain processes taste stimuli. *European Journal of Neuroscience* 27: 723–729.
Grabenhorst F & Rolls ET (2009). Different representations of relative and absolute subjective value in the human

brain. *Neuroimage* 48: 258–268.
Grabenhorst F & Rolls ET (2010). Attentional modulation of affective vs sensory processing: functional connectivity and a top down biased activation theory of selective attention. *Journal of Neurophysiology* 104: 1649–1660.
Grabenhorst F & Rolls ET (2011). Value, pleasure, and choice systems in the ventral prefrontal cortex. *Trends in Cognitive Sciences* 15: 56–67.
Grabenhorst F & Rolls ET (2014). The representation of oral fat texture in the human somatosensory cortex. *Human Brain Mapping* 35: 2521–2530.
Grabenhorst F, Rolls ET, Margot C, da Silva M, & Velazco MI (2007). How pleasant and unpleasant stimuli combine in the brain: odor combinations. *Journal of Neuroscience* 27: 13532–13540.
Grabenhorst F, Rolls ET, & Bilderbeck A (2008a). How cognition modulates affective responses to taste and flavor: top-down influences on the orbitofrontal and pregenual cingulate cortices. *Cerebral Cortex* 18: 1549–1559.
Grabenhorst F, Rolls ET, & Parris BA (2008b). From affective value to decision-making in the prefrontal cortex. *European Journal of Neuroscience* 28: 1930–1939.
Grabenhorst F, D'Souza A, Parris BA, Rolls ET, & Passingham RE (2010a). A common neural scale for the subjective value of different primary rewards. *Neuroimage* 51: 1265–1274.
Grabenhorst F, Rolls ET, Parris BA, & D'Souza A (2010b). How the brain represents the reward value of fat in the mouth. *Cerebral Cortex* 20: 1082–1091.
Grabenhorst F, Hernadi I, & Schultz W (2012). Prediction of economic choice by primate amygdala neurons. *Proceedings of the National Academy of Sciences U S A* 109: 18950–18955.
Grabenhorst F, Hernadi I, & Schultz W (2016). Primate amygdala neurons evaluate the progress of self-defined economic choice sequences. *Elife* 5: e18731.
Graham HN (1992). Green tea composition, consumption and polyphenol chemistry. *Preventative Medicine* 21: 334–350.
Grattan LE & Glimcher PW (2014). Absence of spatial tuning in the orbitofrontal cortex. *PLoS One* 9: e112750.
Gray JA (1970). The psychophysiological basis of introversion-extraversion. *Behaviour Research and Therapy* 8: 249–266.
Gray JA (1975). *Elements of a Two-Process Theory of Learning*. Academic Press, London.
Gross CG, Bender DB, & Gerstein GL (1979). Activity of inferior temporal neurons in behaving monkeys. *Neuropsychologia* 17: 215–229.
Gross CG, Desimone R, Albright TD, & Schwartz EL (1985). Inferior temporal cortex and pattern recognition. *Experimental Brain Research* Suppl. 11: 179–201.
Grossberg S (1988). Non-linear neural networks: principles, mechanisms, and architectures. *Neural Networks* 1: 17–61.
Guest S, Grabenhorst F, Essick G, Chen Y, Young M, McGlone F, de Araujo I, & Rolls ET (2007). Human cortical representation of oral temperature. *Physiology and Behavior* 92: 975–984.
Haber SN (2014). The place of dopamine in the cortico-basal ganglia circuit. *Neuroscience* 282: 248–57.
Haber SN (2016). Corticostriatal circuitry. *Dialogues Clin Neurosci* 18: 7–21.
Haber SN & Knutson B (2010). The reward circuit: linking primate anatomy and human imaging. *Neuropsychopharmacology* 35: 4–26.
Haid D, Widmayer P, Voigt A, Chaudhari N, Boehm U, & Breer H (2013). Gustatory sensory cells express a receptor responsive to protein breakdown products (GPR92). *Histochemistry and Cell Biology* 140: 137–145.
Hajnal A, Takenouchi K, & Norgren R (1999). Effect of intraduodenal lipid on parabrachial gustatory coding in awake rats. *Journal of Neuroscience* 19: 7182–7190.
Hamani C, Mayberg H, Snyder B, Giacobbe P, Kennedy S, & Lozano AM (2009). Deep brain stimulation of the subcallosal cingulate gyrus for depression: anatomical location of active contacts in clinical responders and a suggested guideline for targeting. *Journal of Neurosurgery* 111: 1209–1215.
Hamani C, Mayberg H, Stone S, Laxton A, Haber S, & Lozano AM (2011). The subcallosal cingulate gyrus in the context of major depression. *Biological Psychiatry* 69: 301–308.
Hamilton JP, Chen MC, & Gotlib IH (2013). Neural systems approaches to understanding major depressive disorder: an intrinsic functional organization perspective. *Neurobiology of Disease* 52: 4–11.
Hamilton WD (1964). The genetical evolution of social behaviour. *Journal of Theoretical Biology* 7: 1–52.
Hamilton WD (1996). *Narrow Roads of Gene Land*. W. H. Freeman, New York.
Han W, Tellez LA, Perkins MH, Perez IO, Qu T, Ferreira J, Ferreira TL, Quinn D, Liu ZW, Gao XB, Kaelberer MM, Bohorquez DV, Shammah-Lagnado SJ, de Lartigue G, & de Araujo IE (2018). A neural circuit for gut-induced reward. *Cell* 175: 665–678 e23.
Hare TA, O'Doherty J, Camerer CF, Schultz W, & Rangel A (2008). Dissociating the role of the orbitofrontal cortex and the striatum in the computation of goal values and prediction errors. *J Neurosci* 28: 5623–30.
Harlow JM (1848). Passage of an iron rod though the head. *Boston Medical and Surgical Journal* 39: 389–393.
Harmer CJ & Cowen PJ (2013). 'it's the way that you look at it'–a cognitive neuropsychological account of ssri action in depression. *Philosophical Transactions of the Royal Society of London B Biological Sciences* 368: 20120407.
Hassanpour MS, Simmons WK, Feinstein JS, Luo Q, Lapidus RC, Bodurka J, Paulus MP, & Khalsa SS (2018). The

insular cortex dynamically maps changes in cardiorespiratory interoception. *Neuropsychopharmacology* 43: 426–434.

Hasselmo ME, Rolls ET, & Baylis GC (1989a). The role of expression and identity in the face-selective responses of neurons in the temporal visual cortex of the monkey. *Behavioural Brain Research* 32: 203–218.

Hasselmo ME, Rolls ET, Baylis GC, & Nalwa V (1989b). Object-centered encoding by face-selective neurons in the cortex in the superior temporal sulcus of the monkey. *Experimental Brain Research* 75: 417–429.

Hayden BY, Nair AC, McCoy AN, & Platt ML (2008). Posterior cingulate cortex mediates outcome-contingent allocation of behavior. *Neuron* 60: 19–25.

Hayden BY, Pearson JM, & Platt ML (2011). Neuronal basis of sequential foraging decisions in a patchy environment. *Nature Neuroscience* 14: 933–939.

Heberlein AS, Padon AA, Gillihan SJ, Farah MJ, & Fellows LK (2008). Ventromedial frontal lobe plays a critical role in facial emotion recognition. *Journal of Cognitive Neuroscience* 20: 721–733.

Heilbronner SR, Rodriguez-Romaguera J, Quirk GJ, Groenewegen HJ, & Haber SN (2016). Circuit-based corticostriatal homologies between rat and primate. *Biol Psychiatry* 80: 509–21.

Heilbronner SR, Meyer MAA, Choi EY, & Haber SN (2018). How do cortico-striatal projections impact on downstream pallidal circuitry? *Brain Struct Funct* 223: 2809–2821.

Heims HC, Critchley HD, Dolan R, Mathias CJ, & Cipolotti L (2004). Social and motivational functioning is not critically dependent on feedback of autonomic responses: neuropsychological evidence from patients with pure autonomic failure. *Neuropsychologia* 42: 1979–1988.

Hein G & Knight RT (2008). Superior temporal sulcus–it's my area: or is it? *J Cogn Neurosci* 20: 2125–36.

Helm K, Viol K, Weiger TM, Tass PA, Grefkes C, Del Monte D, & Schiepek G (2018). Neuronal connectivity in major depressive disorder: a systematic review. *Neuropsychiatr Dis Treat* 14: 2715–2737.

Henssen A, Zilles K, Palomero-Gallagher N, Schleicher A, Mohlberg H, Gerboga F, Eickhoff SB, Bludau S, & Amunts K (2016). Cytoarchitecture and probability maps of the human medial orbitofrontal cortex. *Cortex* 75: 87–112.

Hernadi I, Grabenhorst F, & Schultz W (2015). Planning activity for internally generated reward goals in monkey amygdala neurons. *Nat Neurosci* 18: 461–9.

Hertz JA, Krogh A, & Palmer RG (1991). *Introduction to the Theory of Neural Computation*. Addison-Wesley, Wokingham, UK.

Herz RS & von Clef J (2001). The influence of verbal labeling on the perception of odors: evidence for olfactory illusions? *Perception* 30: 381–391.

Hikosaka K & Watanabe M (2000). Delay activity of orbital and lateral prefrontal neurons of the monkey varying with different rewards. *Cerebral Cortex* 10: 263–271.

Hladik CM (1978). Adaptive strategies of primates in relation to leaf-eating. In Montgomery GG, editor, *The Ecology of Arboreal Folivores*, 373–395. Smithsonian Institute Press, Washington, DC.

Hodges JR & Piguet O (2018). Progress and challenges in frontotemporal dementia research: A 20-year review. *J Alzheimers Dis* 62: 1467–1480.

Holland PC & Gallagher M (1999). Amygdala circuitry in attentional and representational processes. *Trends in Cognitive Sciences* 3: 65–73.

Holtzheimer PE, Husain MM, Lisanby SH, Taylor SF, Whitworth LA, McClintock S, Slavin KV, Berman J, McKhann GM, Patil PG, Rittberg BR, Abosch A, Pandurangi AK, Holloway KL, Lam RW, Honey CR, Neimat JS, Henderson JM, DeBattista C, Rothschild AJ, Pilitsis JG, Espinoza RT, Petrides G, Mogilner AY, Matthews K, Peichel D, Gross RE, Hamani C, Lozano AM, & Mayberg HS (2017). Subcallosal cingulate deep brain stimulation for treatment-resistant depression: a multisite, randomised, sham-controlled trial. *Lancet Psychiatry* 4: 839–849.

Hopfield JJ (1982). Neural networks and physical systems with emergent collective computational abilities. *Proceedings of the National Academy of Sciences USA* 79: 2554–2558.

Hornak J, Rolls ET, & Wade D (1996). Face and voice expression identification in patients with emotional and behavioural changes following ventral frontal lobe damage. *Neuropsychologia* 34: 247–261.

Hornak J, Bramham J, Rolls ET, Morris RG, O'Doherty J, Bullock PR, & Polkey CE (2003). Changes in emotion after circumscribed surgical lesions of the orbitofrontal and cingulate cortices. *Brain* 126: 1691–1712.

Hornak J, O'Doherty J, Bramham J, Rolls ET, Morris RG, Bullock PR, & Polkey CE (2004). Reward-related reversal learning after surgical excisions in orbitofrontal and dorsolateral prefrontal cortex in humans. *Journal of Cognitive Neuroscience* 16: 463–478.

Horowitz LF, Saraiva LR, Kuang D, Yoon KH, & Buck LB (2014). Olfactory receptor patterning in a higher primate. *J Neurosci* 34: 12241–52.

Howard JD & Gottfried JA (2014). Configural and elemental coding of natural odor mixture components in the human brain. *Neuron* 84: 857–69.

Howard JD, Gottfried JA, Tobler PN, & Kahnt T (2015). Identity-specific coding of future rewards in the human orbitofrontal cortex. *Proc Natl Acad Sci U S A* 112: 5195–200.

Howard JD, Kahnt T, & Gottfried JA (2016). Converging prefrontal pathways support associative and perceptual features of conditioned stimuli. *Nat Commun* 7: 11546.

Iadarola ND, Niciu MJ, Richards EM, Vande Voort JL, Ballard ED, Lundin NB, Nugent AC, Machado-Vieira R, & Zarate J C A (2015). Ketamine and other n-methyl-d-aspartate receptor antagonists in the treatment of depression: a perspective review. *Therapetic Advances in Chronic Disease* 6: 97–114.

Ikeda K (1909). On a new seasoning. *Journal of the Tokyo Chemistry Society* 30: 820–836.

Imamura K, Mataga N, & Mori K (1992). Coding of odor molecules by mitral/tufted cells in rabbit olfactory bulb. I. Aliphatic compounds. *Journal of Neurophysiology* 68: 1986–2002.

Insabato A, Pannunzi M, Rolls ET, & Deco G (2010). Confidence-related decision-making. *Journal of Neurophysiology* 104: 539–547.

Insausti R, Amaral DG, & Cowan WM (1987). The entorhinal cortex of the monkey. II. Cortical afferents. *Journal of Comparative Neurology* 264: 356–395.

Ishai A, Ungerleider LG, Martin A, & Haxby JV (2000). The representation of objects in the human occipital and temporal cortex. *Journal of Cognitive Neuroscience* 12: 35–51.

Isik L, Koldewyn K, Beeler D, & Kanwisher N (2017). Perceiving social interactions in the posterior superior temporal sulcus. *Proc Natl Acad Sci U S A* 114: E9145–E9152.

Ito M (1976). Mapping unit responses to rewarding stimulation. In Wauquier A & Rolls ET, editors, *Brain-Stimulation Reward*, 89–96. North-Holland, Amsterdam.

Iversen SD & Mishkin M (1970). Perseverative interference in monkey following selective lesions of the inferior prefrontal convexity. *Experimental Brain Research* 11: 376–386.

Izquierdo A (2017). Functional heterogeneity within rat orbitofrontal cortex in reward learning and decision making. *J Neurosci* 37: 10529–10540.

Izquierdo A, Brigman JL, Radke AK, Rudebeck PH, & Holmes A (2017). The neural basis of reversal learning: An updated perspective. *Neuroscience* 345: 12–26.

Jacobsen CF (1936). The functions of the frontal association areas in monkeys. *Comparative Psychology Monographs* 13: 1–60.

Jarvis CD & Mishkin M (1977). Responses of cells in the inferior temporal cortex of monkeys during visual discrimination reversals. *Society for Neuroscience Abstracts* 3: 1794.

Jennings JH, Kim CK, Marshel JH, Raffiee M, Ye L, Quirin S, Pak S, Ramakrishnan C, & Deisseroth K (2019). Interacting neural ensembles in orbitofrontal cortex for social and feeding behaviour. *Nature* .

Johansen-Berg H, Gutman DA, Behrens TE, Matthews PM, Rushworth MF, Katz E, Lozano AM, & Mayberg HS (2008). Anatomical connectivity of the subgenual cingulate region targeted with deep brain stimulation for treatment-resistant depression. *Cerebral Cortex* 18: 1374–1383.

Johns T & Duquette M (1991). Detoxification and mineral supplementation as functions of geophagy. *American Journal of Clinical Nutrition* 53: 448–456.

Johnson SC, Baxter LC, Wilder LS, Pipe JG, Heiserman JE, & Prigatano GP (2002). Neural correlates of self-reflection. *Brain* 125: 1808–14.

Johnstone S & Rolls ET (1990). Delay, discriminatory, and modality specific neurons in striatum and pallidum during short-term memory tasks. *Brain Research* 522: 147–151.

Jones B & Mishkin M (1972). Limbic lesions and the problem of stimulus–reinforcement associations. *Experimental Neurology* 36: 362–377.

Jones EG & Powell TPS (1970). An anatomical study of converging sensory pathways within the cerebral cortex of the monkey. *Brain* 93: 793–820.

Jones-Gotman M & Zatorre RJ (1988). Olfactory identification in patients with focal cerebral excision. *Neuropsychologia* 26: 387–400.

Jouandet M & Gazzaniga MS (1979). The frontal lobes. In Gazzaniga MS, editor, *Handbook of Behavioural Neurobiology*, vol. 2, Neuropsychology, 25–59. Plenum, New York.

Julian JB, Keinath AT, Frazzetta G, & Epstein RA (2018). Human entorhinal cortex represents visual space using a boundary-anchored grid. *Nat Neurosci* 21: 191–194.

Kable JW & Glimcher PW (2007). The neural correlates of subjective value during intertemporal choice. *Nature Neuroscience* 10: 1625–1633.

Kable JW & Glimcher PW (2009). The neurobiology of decision: consensus and controversy. *Neuron* 63: 733–745.

Kadohisa M, Rolls ET, & Verhagen JV (2004). Orbitofrontal cortex neuronal representation of temperature and capsaicin in the mouth. *Neuroscience* 127: 207–221.

Kadohisa M, Rolls ET, & Verhagen JV (2005a). The primate amygdala: neuronal representations of the viscosity, fat texture, grittiness and taste of foods. *Neuroscience* 132: 33–48.

Kadohisa M, Rolls ET, & Verhagen JV (2005b). Neuronal representations of stimuli in the mouth: the primate insular taste cortex, orbitofrontal cortex, and amygdala. *Chemical Senses* 30: 401–419.

Kagan J (1966). Reflection-impulsivity: the generality of dynamics of conceptual tempo. *Journal of Abnormal Psychology* 1: 917–924.

Kagel JH, Battalio RC, & Green L (1995). *Economic Choice Theory: An Experimental Analysis of Animal Behaviour*. Cambridge University Press, Cambridge.

Kahneman D & Tversky A (1979). Prospect theory: An analysis of decision under risk. *Econometrica* 47: 263–292.

Kahneman D & Tversky A (1984). Choices, values, and frames. *American Psychologist* 4: 341–350.

Kanter I & Sompolinsky H (1987). Associative recall of memories without errors. *Physical Review A* 35: 380–392.
Kanwisher N, McDermott J, & Chun MM (1997). The fusiform face area: a module in human extrastriate cortex specialized for face perception. *Journal of Neuroscience* 17: 4301–4311.
Karadi Z, Oomura Y, Nishino H, Scott TR, Lenard L, & Aou S (1990). Complex attributes of lateral hypothalamic neurons in the regulation of feeding of alert monkeys. *Brain Research Bulletin* 25: 933–939.
Karadi Z, Oomura Y, Nishino H, Scott TR, Lenard L, & Aou S (1992). Responses of lateral hypothalamic glucose-sensitive and glucose-insensitive neurons to chemical stimuli in behaving rhesus monkeys. *Journal of Neurophysiology* 67: 389–400.
Kaskan PM, Costa VD, Eaton HP, Zemskova JA, Mitz AR, Leopold DA, Ungerleider LG, & Murray EA (2017). Learned value shapes responses to objects in frontal and ventral stream networks in macaque monkeys. *Cereb Cortex* 27: 2739–2757.
Kawamura Y & Kare MR, editors (1992). *Umami: a Basic Taste*. Dekker, New York.
Kemp JM & Powell TPS (1970). The cortico-striate projections in the monkey. *Brain* 93: 525–546.
Kenet T, Orekhova EV, Bharadwaj H, Shetty NR, Israeli E, Lee AK, Agam Y, Elam M, Joseph RM, Hamalainen MS, & Manoach DS (2012). Disconnectivity of the cortical ocular motor control network in autism spectrum disorders. *Neuroimage* 61: 1226–34.
Kennedy DP & Adolphs R (2011). Reprint of: Impaired fixation to eyes following amygdala damage arises from abnormal bottom-up attention. *Neuropsychologia* 49: 589–595.
Kennedy DP & Adolphs R (2012). The social brain in psychiatric and neurological disorders. *Trends Cogn Sci* 16: 559–72.
Kennerley SW & Wallis JD (2009). Encoding of reward and space during a working memory task in the orbitofrontal cortex and anterior cingulate sulcus. *Journal of Neurophysiology* 102: 3352–3364.
Kennerley SW, Walton ME, Behrens TE, Buckley MJ, & Rushworth MF (2006). Optimal decision making and the anterior cingulate cortex. *Nature Neuroscience* 9: 940–947.
Kennerley SW, Dahmubed AF, Lara AH, & Wallis JD (2009). Neurons in the frontal lobe encode the value of multiple decision variables. *Journal of Cognitive Neuroscience* 21: 1162–1178.
Kennerley SW, Behrens TE, & Wallis JD (2011). Double dissociation of value computations in orbitofrontal and anterior cingulate neurons. *Nature Neuroscience* 14: 1581–1589.
Kennis M, Rademaker AR, & Geuze E (2013). Neural correlates of personality: an integrative review. *Neuroscience and Biobehavioural Reviews* 37: 73–95.
Kepecs A, Uchida N, Zariwala HA, & Mainen ZF (2008). Neural correlates, computation and behavioural impact of decision confidence. *Nature* 455: 227–231.
Kesner RP & Rolls ET (2015). A computational theory of hippocampal function, and tests of the theory: New developments. *Neuroscience and Biobehavioral Reviews* 48: 92–147.
Killcross S & Coutureau E (2003a). Coordination of actions and habits in the medial prefrontal cortex of rats. *Cerebral Cortex* 13: 400–408.
Killcross S & Coutureau E (2003b). Coordination of actions and habits in the medial prefrontal cortex of rats. *Cereb Cortex* 13: 400–8.
Kim HF, Ghazizadeh A, & Hikosaka O (2015). Dopamine neurons encoding long-term memory of object value for habitual behavior. *Cell* 163: 1165–1175.
Kim YS, Leventhal BL, Koh YJ, Fombonne E, Laska E, Lim EC, Cheon KA, Kim SJ, Kim YK, Lee H, Song DH, & Grinker RR (2011). Prevalence of autism spectrum disorders in a total population sample. *Am J Psychiatry* 168: 904–12.
Kircher TT, Senior C, Phillips ML, Benson PJ, Bullmore ET, Brammer M, Simmons A, Williams SC, Bartels M, & David AS (2000). Towards a functional neuroanatomy of self processing: effects of faces and words. *Brain Res Cogn Brain Res* 10: 133–44.
Kircher TT, Brammer M, Bullmore E, Simmons A, Bartels M, & David AS (2002). The neural correlates of intentional and incidental self processing. *Neuropsychologia* 40: 683–92.
Kluver H & Bucy PC (1939). Preliminary analysis of functions of the temporal lobe in monkeys. *Archives of Neurology and Psychiatry* 42: 979–1000.
Kobayashi S, Pinto de Carvalho O, & Schultz W (2010). Adaptation of reward sensitivity in orbitofrontal neurons. *Journal of Neuroscience* 30: 534–544.
Kobayashi Y & Amaral DG (2003). Macaque monkey retrosplenial cortex: Ii. cortical afferents. *J Comp Neurol* 466: 48–79.
Kobayashi Y & Amaral DG (2007). Macaque monkey retrosplenial cortex: Iii. cortical efferents. *J Comp Neurol* 502: 810–33.
Kohonen T (1977). *Associative Memory: A System Theoretical Approach*. Springer, New York.
Kohonen T (1989). *Self-Organization and Associative Memory*. Springer-Verlag, Berlin, 3rd edn.
Kohonen T, Oja E, & Lehtio P (1981). Storage and processing of information in distributed memory systems. In Hinton GE & Anderson JA, editors, *Parallel Models of Associative Memory*, chap. 4, 105–143. Erlbaum, Hillsdale, NJ.
Kolb B & Whishaw IQ (2015). *Fundamentals of Human Neuropsychology*. Macmillan, New York, 7th edn.

Kolling N, Wittmann MK, Behrens TE, Boorman ED, Mars RB, & Rushworth MF (2016). Value, search, persistence and model updating in anterior cingulate cortex. *Nat Neurosci* 19: 1280–5.
Koob GF & Volkow ND (2016). Neurobiology of addiction: a neurocircuitry analysis. *Lancet Psychiatry* 3: 760–73.
Kosar E, Grill HJ, & Norgren R (1986). Gustatory cortex in the rat. II. Thalamocortical projections. *Brain Research* 379: 342–352.
Koski L & Paus T (2000). Functional connectivity of anterior cingulate cortex within human frontal lobe: a brain mapping meta-analysis. *Experimental Brain Research* 133: 55–65.
Kowalska DM, Bachevalier J, & Mishkin M (1991). The role of the inferior prefrontal convexity in performance of delayed nonmatching-to-sample. *Neuropsychologia* 29: 583–600.
Kreps DM (1990). *A Course in Microeconomic Theory*. Princeton University Press, Princeton, N.J.
Krettek JE & Price JL (1974). A direct input from the amygdala to the thalamus and the cerebral cortex. *Brain Research* 67: 169–174.
Krettek JE & Price JL (1977). The cortical projections of the mediodorsal nucleus and adjacent thalamic nuclei in the rat. *Journal of Comparative Neurology* 171: 157–192.
Kringelbach ML & Rolls ET (2003). Neural correlates of rapid reversal learning in a simple model of human social interaction. *Neuroimage* 20: 1371–1383.
Kringelbach ML & Rolls ET (2004). The functional neuroanatomy of the human orbitofrontal cortex: evidence from neuroimaging and neuropsychology. *Progress in Neurobiology* 72: 341–372.
Kringelbach ML, O'Doherty J, Rolls ET, & Andrews C (2003). Activation of the human orbitofrontal cortex to a liquid food stimulus is correlated with its subjective pleasantness. *Cerebral Cortex* 13: 1064–1071.
Kroes MC, Schiller D, LeDoux JE, & Phelps EA (2016). Translational approaches targeting reconsolidation. *Curr Top Behav Neurosci* 28: 197–230.
Krystal JH, Abdallah CG, Sanacora G, Charney DS, & Duman RS (2019). Ketamine: A paradigm shift for depression research and treatment. *Neuron* 101: 774–778.
Kuehner C (2017). Why is depression more common among women than among men? *Lancet Psychiatry* 4: 146–158.
Kumar V, Croxson PL, & Simonyan K (2016). Structural organization of the laryngeal motor cortical network and its implication for evolution of speech production. *J Neurosci* 36: 4170–81.
Kurihara K (2015). Umami the fifth basic taste: History of studies on receptor mechanisms and role as a food flavor. *Biomed Res Int* 2015: 189402.
Lai MC, Lombardo MV, & Baron-Cohen S (2014). Autism. *Lancet* 383: 896–910.
Laibson D (1997). Golden eggs and hyperbolic discounting. *Quarterly Journal of Economics* 112: 443–477.
Lally N, Nugent AC, Luckenbaugh DA, Niciu MJ, Roiser JP, & Zarate J C A (2015). Neural correlates of change in major depressive disorder anhedonia following open-label ketamine. *Journal of Psychopharmacology* 29: 596–607.
Lane RD, Reiman EM, Ahern GL, Schwartz GE, & Davidson RJ (1997a). Neuroanatomical correlates of happiness, sadness, and disgust. *American Journal of Psychiatry* 154: 926–933.
Lane RD, Reiman EM, Bradley MM, Lang PJ, Ahern GL, Davidson RJ, & Schwartz GE (1997b). Neuroanatomical correlates of pleasant and unpleasant emotion. *Neuropsychologia* 35: 1437–1444.
Lane RD, Reiman E, Axelrod B, Yun LS, Holmes AH, & Schwartz G (1998). Neural correlates of levels of emotional awareness. Evidence of an interaction between emotion and attention in the anterior cingulate cortex. *Journal of Cognitive Neuroscience* 10: 525–535.
Laxton AW, Neimat JS, Davis KD, Womelsdorf T, Hutchison WD, Dostrovsky JO, Hamani C, Mayberg HS, & Lozano AM (2013a). Neuronal coding of implicit emotion categories in the subcallosal cortex in patients with depression. *Biological Psychiatry* 74: 714–719.
Laxton AW, Neimat JS, Davis KD, Womelsdorf T, Hutchison WD, Dostrovsky JO, Hamani C, Mayberg HS, & Lozano AM (2013b). Neuronal coding of implicit emotion categories in the subcallosal cortex in patients with depression. *Biological Psychiatry* 74: 714–719.
LeDoux JE (1992). Emotion and the amygdala. In Aggleton JP, editor, *The Amygdala*, chap. 12, 339–351. Wiley-Liss, New York.
LeDoux JE (1994). Emotion, memory and the brain. *Scientific American* 220 (June): 50–57.
LeDoux JE (2008). Emotional coloration of consciousness: how feelings come about. In Weiskrantz L & Davies M, editors, *Frontiers of Consciousness*, 69–130. Oxford University Press, Oxford.
LeDoux JE (2012). Rethinking the emotional brain. *Neuron* 73: 653–676.
LeDoux JE & Pine DS (2016). Using neuroscience to help understand fear and anxiety: A two-system framework. *Am J Psychiatry* 173: 1083–1093.
LeDoux JE, Brown R, Pine DS, & Hofmann SG (2018). Know thyself: Well-being and subjective experience. *Cerebrum* https://www.dana.org/Cerebrum/2018 .
Leech R & Sharp DJ (2014). The role of the posterior cingulate cortex in cognition and disease. *Brain* 137: 12–32.
Leonard CM, Rolls ET, Wilson FAW, & Baylis GC (1985). Neurons in the amygdala of the monkey with responses selective for faces. *Behavioural Brain Research* 15: 159–176.
Lesschaeve I & Noble AC (2005). Polyphenols: factors influencing their sensory properties and their effects on food and beverage preferences. *American Journal of Clinical Nutrition* 81: 330S–335S.

Levy DJ & Glimcher PW (2012). The root of all value: a neural common currency for choice. *Current Opinion in Neurobiology* 22: 1027–1038.
Levy I, Snell J, Nelson AJ, Rustichini A, & Glimcher PW (2010). Neural representation of subjective value under risk and ambiguity. *J Neurophysiol* 103: 1036–1047.
Li CS & Cho YK (2006). Efferent projection from the bed nucleus of the stria terminalis suppresses activity of taste-responsive neurons in the hamster parabrachial nuclei. *American Journal of Physiology Regul Integr Comp Physiol* 291: R914–R926.
Li CS, Cho YK, & Smith DV (2002). Taste responses of neurons in the hamster solitary nucleus are modulated by the central nucleus of the amygdala. *Journal of Neurophysiology* 88: 2979–2992.
Lieberman DA, editor (2000). *Learning: Behavior and Cognition*. Wadsworth, Belmont, CA.
Lin W, Ogura T, & Kinnamon SC (2003). Responses to di-sodium guanosine 5′-monophosphate and monosodium L-glutamate in taste receptor cells of rat fungiform papillae. *Journal of Neurophysiology* 89: 1434–1439.
Liu Z, Ma N, Rolls ET, Wei D, Zhang J, Chen Q, Meng J, Qiu J, & Feng J (2019). Integrating multi-modal data to explore the neural, genetic and behavioral correlates of happiness.
Loh M, Rolls ET, & Deco G (2007). A dynamical systems hypothesis of schizophrenia. *PLoS Computational Biology* 3: e228. doi:10.1371/journal.pcbi.0030228.
Lombardo MV, Chakrabarti B, Bullmore ET, Sadek SA, Pasco G, Wheelwright SJ, Suckling J, Consortium MA, & Baron-Cohen S (2010). Atypical neural self-representation in autism. *Brain* 133: 611–24.
Loonen AJ & Ivanova SA (2016). Circuits regulating pleasure and happiness: the evolution of the amygdalar-hippocampal-habenular connectivity in vertebrates. *Front Neurosci* 10: 539.
Lopatina N, Sadacca BF, McDannald MA, Styer CV, Peterson JF, Cheer JF, & Schoenbaum G (2017). Ensembles in medial and lateral orbitofrontal cortex construct cognitive maps emphasizing different features of the behavioral landscape. *Behav Neurosci* 131: 201–12.
Lozano AM, Giacobbe P, Hamani C, Rizvi SJ, Kennedy SH, Kolivakis TT, Debonnel G, Sadikot AF, Lam RW, Howard AK, Ilcewicz-Klimek M, Honey CR, & Mayberg HS (2012). A multicenter pilot study of subcallosal cingulate area deep brain stimulation for treatment-resistant depression. *Journal of Neurosurgery* 116: 315–322.
Lujan JL, Chaturvedi A, Choi KS, Holtzheimer PE, Gross RE, Mayberg HS, & McIntyre CC (2013). Tractography-activation models applied to subcallosal cingulate deep brain stimulation. *Brain Stimulation* 6: 737–739.
Luk CH & Wallis JD (2009). Dynamic encoding of responses and outcomes by neurons in medial prefrontal cortex. *Journal of Neuroscience* 29: 7526–7539.
Luk CH & Wallis JD (2013). Choice coding in frontal cortex during stimulus-guided or action-guided decision-making. *Journal of Neuroscience* 33: 1864–1871.
Lundqvist M, Herman P, & Miller EK (2018). Working memory: Delay activity, yes! persistent activity? maybe not. *J Neurosci* 38: 7013–7019.
Lundy J R F & Norgren R (2004). Activity in the hypothalamus, amygdala, and cortex generates bilateral and convergent modulation of pontine gustatory neurons. *Journal of Neurophysiology* 91: 1143–1157.
Luo Q, Ge T, Grabenhorst F, Feng J, & Rolls ET (2013). Attention-dependent modulation of cortical taste circuits revealed by Granger causality with signal-dependent noise. *PLoS Computational Biology* 9: e1003265.
Lynch CJ, Uddin LQ, Supekar K, Khouzam A, Phillips J, & Menon V (2013). Default mode network in childhood autism: posteromedial cortex heterogeneity and relationship with social deficits. *Biol Psychiatry* 74: 212–9.
Ma Y (2015). Neuropsychological mechanism underlying antidepressant effect: a systematic meta-analysis. *Molecular Psychiatry* 20: 311–319.
Mackey S & Petrides M (2010). Quantitative demonstration of comparable architectonic areas within the ventromedial and lateral orbital frontal cortex in the human and the macaque monkey brains. *European Journal of Neuroscience* 32: 1940–1950.
Mackey S & Petrides M (2014). Architecture and morphology of the human ventromedial prefrontal cortex. *Eur J Neurosci* 40: 2777–96.
Mackintosh NJ (1983). *Conditioning and Associative Learning*. Oxford University Press, Oxford.
Maltbie EA, Kaundinya GS, & Howell LL (2017). Ketamine and pharmacological imaging: use of functional magnetic resonance imaging to evaluate mechanisms of action. *Behav Pharmacol* 28: 610–622.
Marr D (1971). Simple memory: a theory for archicortex. *Philosophical Transactions of The Royal Society of London, Series B* 262: 23–81.
Martinez-Garcia M, Rolls ET, Deco G, & Romo R (2011). Neural and computational mechanisms of postponed decisions. *Proceedings of the National Academy of Sciences* 108: 11626–11631.
Matrix (2013). Economic analysis of workplace mental health promotion and mental disorder prevention programmes and of their potential contribution to eu health, social and economic policy objectives. *Executive Agency for Health and Consumers, Specific Request EAHC/2011/Health/19 for the Implementation of Framework Contract EAHC/2010/Health/01 /Lot 2* .
Matsumoto K, Suzuki W, & Tanaka K (2003). Neuronal correlates of goal-based motor selection in the prefrontal cortex. *Science* 301: 229–232.
Matsumoto M & Hikosaka O (2007). Lateral habenula as a source of negative reward signals in dopamine neurons. *Nature* 447: 1111–5.

Matsumoto M & Hikosaka O (2009a). Two types of dopamine neuron distinctly convey positive and negative motivational signals. *Nature* 459: 837–841.
Matsumoto M & Hikosaka O (2009b). Representation of negative motivational value in the primate lateral habenula. *Nat Neurosci* 12: 77–84.
Matsumoto M, Matsumoto K, Abe H, & Tanaka K (2007). Medial prefrontal selectivity signalling prediction errors of action values. *Nature Neuroscience* 10: 647–656.
Maximo JO, Cadena EJ, & Kana RK (2014). The implications of brain connectivity in the neuropsychology of autism. *Neuropsychol Rev* 24: 16–31.
Mayberg HS (2003). Positron emission tomography imaging in depression: a neural systems perspective. *Neuroimaging Clinics of North America* 13: 805–815.
Mazur JE (2012). *Learning and Behavior*. Pearson, Boston, MA, 7th edn.
McCabe C & Rolls ET (2007). Umami: a delicious flavor formed by convergence of taste and olfactory pathways in the human brain. *European Journal of Neuroscience* 25: 1855–1864.
McCabe C, Rolls ET, Bilderbeck A, & McGlone F (2008). Cognitive influences on the affective representation of touch and the sight of touch in the human brain. *Social, Cognitive and Affective Neuroscience* 3: 97–108.
McClure SM, Laibson DI, Loewenstein G, & Cohen JD (2004). Separate neural systems value immediate and delayed monetary rewards. *Science* 306: 503–507.
McCormick C, Ciaramelli E, De Luca F, & Maguire EA (2018). Comparing and contrasting the cognitive effects of hippocampal and ventromedial prefrontal cortex damage: A review of human lesion studies. *Neuroscience* 374: 295–318.
McCoy AN & Platt ML (2005a). Expectations and outcomes: decision-making in the primate brain. *Journal of Comparative Physiology A* 191: 201–211.
McCoy AN & Platt ML (2005b). Risk-sensitive neurons in macaque posterior cingulate cortex. *Nature Neuroscience* 8: 1220–1227.
McEwen BS, Gray JD, & Nasca C (2015). 60 years of neuroendocrinology: Redefining neuroendocrinology: stress, sex and cognitive and emotional regulation. *J Endocrinol* 226: T67–83.
McFarland DJ & Sibly RM (1975). The behavioural final common path. *Philosophical Transactions of the Royal Society of London B Biological Science* 270: 265–293.
McQuaid RJ, McInnis OA, Abizaid A, & Anisman H (2014). Making room for oxytocin in understanding depression. *Neurosci Biobehav Rev* 45: 305–22.
Melzack R & Wall PD (1996). *The Challenge of Pain*. Penguin, Harmondsworth, UK.
Mendez MF (2009). The neurobiology of moral behavior: review and neuropsychiatric implications. *CNS Spectrums* 14: 608–620.
Mesulam MM & Mufson EJ (1982a). Insula of the Old World monkey. I: Architectonics in the insulo-orbito-temporal component of the paralimbic brain. *Journal of Comparative Neurology* 212: 1–22.
Mesulam MM & Mufson EJ (1982b). Insula of the Old World monkey. III. Efferent cortical output and comments on function. *Journal of Comparative Neurology* 212: 38–52.
Metcalfe J & Mischel W (1999). A hot/cool-system analysis of delay of gratification: dynamics of willpower. *Psychological Review* 106: 3–19.
Meunier M, Bachevalier J, & Mishkin M (1997). Effects of orbital frontal and anterior cingulate lesions on object and spatial memory in rhesus monkeys. *Neuropsychologia* 35: 999–1015.
Milad MR & Rauch SL (2012). Obsessive-compulsive disorder: beyond segregated cortico-striatal pathways. *Trends Cogn Sci* 16: 43–51.
Miller EK (2013). The "working" of working memory. *Dialogues Clin Neurosci* 15: 411–8.
Miller EK & Cohen JD (2001). An integrative theory of prefrontal cortex function. *Annual Review of Neuroscience* 24: 167–202.
Milner A (2008). Conscious and unconscious visual processing in the human brain. In Weiskrantz L & Davies M, editors, *Frontiers of Consciousness*, chap. 5, 169–214. Oxford University Press, Oxford.
Milner AD & Goodale MA (1995). *The Visual Brain in Action*. Oxford University Press, Oxford.
Milner B (1963). Effects of different brain lesions on card sorting. *Archives of Neurology* 9: 90–100.
Milner B (1982). Some cognitive effects of frontal-lobe lesions in man. *Philosophical Transactions of the Royal Society B* 298: 211–226.
Milton AL, Lee JL, Butler VJ, Gardner R, & Everitt BJ (2008). Intra-amygdala and systemic antagonism of NMDA receptors prevents the reconsolidation of drug-associated memory and impairs subsequently both novel and previously acquired drug-seeking behaviors. *Journal of Neuroscience* 28: 8230–8237.
Minshew NJ & Keller TA (2010). The nature of brain dysfunction in autism: functional brain imaging studies. *Curr Opin Neurol* 23: 124–30.
Mishkin M & Manning FJ (1978). Non-spatial memory after selective prefrontal lesions in monkeys. *Brain Research* 143: 313–324.
Müller RA, Shih P, Keehn B, Deyoe JR, Leyden KM, & Shukla DK (2011). Underconnected, but how? a survey of functional connectivity mri studies in autism spectrum disorders. *Cerebral Cortex* 21: 2233–2243.
Mombaerts P (2006). Axonal wiring in the mouse olfactory system. *Annual Review of Cell and Developmental*

Biology 22: 713–737.
Moniz E (1936). *Tentatives Operatoires dans le Traitment de Certaines Psychoses*. Masson, Paris.
Montague PR & Berns GS (2002). Neural economics and the biological substrates of valuation. *Neuron* 36: 265–284.
Mora F, Mogenson GJ, & Rolls ET (1977). Activity of neurones in the region of the substantia nigra during feeding. *Brain Research* 133: 267–276.
Mora F, Avrith DB, Phillips AG, & Rolls ET (1979). Effects of satiety on self-stimulation of the orbitofrontal cortex in the monkey. *Neuroscience Letters* 13: 141–145.
Mora F, Avrith DB, & Rolls ET (1980). An electrophysiological and behavioural study of self-stimulation in the orbitofrontal cortex of the rhesus monkey. *Brain Research Bulletin* 5: 111–115.
Morecraft RJ & Tanji J (2009). Cingulofrontal interactions and the cingulate motor areas. In Vogt B, editor, *Cingulate Neurobiology and Disease*, chap. 5, 113–144. Oxford University Press, Oxford.
Morecraft RJ, Geula C, & Mesulam MM (1992). Cytoarchitecture and neural afferents of orbitofrontal cortex in the brain of the monkey. *Journal of Comparative Neurology* 323: 341–358.
Morecraft RJ, McNeal DW, Stilwell-Morecraft KS, Gedney M, Ge J, Schroeder CM, & van Hoesen GW (2007). Amygdala interconnections with the cingulate motor cortex in the rhesus monkey. *J Comp Neurol* 500: 134–65.
Mori K & Sakano H (2011). How is the olfactory map formed and interpreted in the mammalian brain? *Annual Reviews of Neuroscience* 34: 467–499.
Mori K, Mataga N, & Imamura K (1992). Differential specificities of single mitral cells in rabbit olfactory bulb for a homologous series of fatty acid odor molecules. *Journal of Neurophysiology* 67: 786–789.
Mori K, Nagao H, & Yoshihara Y (1999). The olfactory bulb: coding and processing of odor molecule information. *Science* 286: 711–715.
Morrison SE, Saez A, Lau B, & Salzman CD (2011). Different time courses for learning-related changes in amygdala and orbitofrontal cortex. *Neuron* 71: 1127–40.
Morrot G, Brochet F, & Dubourdieu D (2001). The color of odors. *Brain and Language* 79: 309–320.
Mufson EJ & Mesulam MM (1982). Insula of the Old World monkey II: Afferent cortical input and comments on the claustrum. *Journal of Comparative Neurology* 212: 23–37.
Munuera J, Rigotti M, & Salzman CD (2018). Shared neural coding for social hierarchy and reward value in primate amygdala. *Nat Neurosci* 21: 415–423.
Murray EA & Izquierdo A (2007). Orbitofrontal cortex and amygdala contributions to affect and action in primates. *Annals of the New York Academy of Sciences* 1121: 273–296.
Murray EA & Rudebeck PH (2018). Specializations for reward-guided decision-making in the primate ventral prefrontal cortex. *Nat Rev Neurosci* 19: 404–417.
Murray EA, Wise SP, & Rhodes SEV (2011). What can different brains do with reward? In Gottfried JA, editor, *Neurobiology of Sensation and Reward*, chap. 4. CRC Press, Boca Raton (FL).
Murray EA, Moylan EJ, Saleem KS, Basile BM, & Turchi J (2015). Specialized areas for value updating and goal selection in the primate orbitofrontal cortex. *Elife* 4: e11695.
Nagai Y, Critchley HD, Featherstone E, Trimble MR, & Dolan RJ (2004). Activity in ventromedial prefrontal cortex covaries with sympathetic skin conductance level: a physiological account of a "default mode" of brain function. *Neuroimage* 22: 243–251.
Nakazawa K, Quirk MC, Chitwood RA, Watanabe M, Yeckel MF, Sun LD, Kato A, Carr CA, Johnston D, Wilson MA, & Tonegawa S (2002). Requirement for hippocampal CA3 NMDA receptors in associative memory recall. *Science* 297: 211–218.
Nakazawa K, Sun LD, Quirk MC, Rondi-Reig L, Wilson MA, & Tonegawa S (2003). Hippocampal CA3 NMDA receptors are crucial for memory acquisition of one-time experience. *Neuron* 38: 305–315.
Nakazawa K, McHugh TJ, Wilson MA, & Tonegawa S (2004). NMDA receptors, place cells and hippocampal spatial memory. *Nature Reviews Neuroscience* 5: 361–372.
Nauta WJH (1972). Neural associations of the frontal cortex. *Acta Neurobiologica Experimentalis* 32: 125–140.
Nesse RM & Lloyd AT (1992). The evolution of psychodynamic mechanisms. In Barkow JH, Cosmides L, & Tooby J, editors, *The Adapted Mind*, 601–624. Oxford University Press, New York.
Niki H & Watanabe M (1979). Prefrontal and cingulate unit activity during timing behavior in the monkey. *Brain Research* 171: 213–224.
Noonan MP, Walton ME, Behrens TE, Sallet J, Buckley MJ, & Rushworth MF (2010). Separate value comparison and learning mechanisms in macaque medial and lateral orbitofrontal cortex. *Proc Natl Acad Sci U S A* 107: 20547–52.
Noonan MP, Kolling N, Walton ME, & Rushworth MF (2012). Re-evaluating the role of the orbitofrontal cortex in reward and reinforcement. *Eur J Neurosci* 35: 997–1010.
Noonan MP, Chau BKH, Rushworth MFS, & Fellows LK (2017). Contrasting effects of medial and lateral orbitofrontal cortex lesions on credit assignment and decision-making in humans. *J Neurosci* 37: 7023–7035.
Norgren R (1974). Gustatory afferents to ventral forebrain. *Brain Research* 81: 285–295.
Norgren R (1976). Taste pathways to hypothalamus and amygdala. *Journal of Comparative Neurology* 166: 17–30.
Norgren R (1990). Gustatory system. In Paxinos G, editor, *The Human Nervous System*, 845–861. Academic Press,

San Diego.
Norgren R & Leonard CM (1971). Taste pathways in rat brainstem. *Science* 173: 1136–1139.
Norgren R & Leonard CM (1973). Ascending central gustatory pathways. *Journal of Comparative Neurology* 150: 217–238.
Nugent AC, Milham MP, Bain EE, Mah L, Cannon DM, Marrett S, Zarate CA, Pine DS, Price JL, & Drevets WC (2006). Cortical abnormalities in bipolar disorder investigated with mri and voxel-based morphometry. *Neuroimage* 30: 485–497.
Nusslock R, Young CB, & Damme KS (2014). Elevated reward-related neural activation as a unique biological marker of bipolar disorder: assessment and treatment implications. *Behaviour Research and Therapy* 62: 74–87.
Nutt DJ, Lingford-Hughes A, Erritzoe D, & Stokes PR (2015). The dopamine theory of addiction: 40 years of highs and lows. *Nat Rev Neurosci* 16: 305–12.
Nymberg C, Jia T, Lubbe S, Ruggeri B, Desrivieres S, Barker G, Buchel C, Fauth-Buehler M, Cattrell A, Conrod P, Flor H, Gallinat J, Garavan H, Heinz A, Ittermann B, Lawrence C, Mann K, Nees F, Salatino-Oliveira A, Paillere Martinot ML, Paus T, Rietschel M, Robbins T, Smolka M, Banaschewski T, Rubia K, Loth E, Schumann G, & Consortium I (2013). Neural mechanisms of attention-deficit/hyperactivity disorder symptoms are stratified by maoa genotype. *Biol Psychiatry* 74: 607–14.
O'Doherty J, Rolls ET, Francis S, Bowtell R, McGlone F, Kobal G, Renner B, & Ahne G (2000). Sensory-specific satiety related olfactory activation of the human orbitofrontal cortex. *NeuroReport* 11: 893–897.
O'Doherty J, Kringelbach ML, Rolls ET, Hornak J, & Andrews C (2001a). Abstract reward and punishment representations in the human orbitofrontal cortex. *Nature Neuroscience* 4: 95–102.
O'Doherty J, Rolls ET, Francis S, Bowtell R, & McGlone F (2001b). The representation of pleasant and aversive taste in the human brain. *Journal of Neurophysiology* 85: 1315–1321.
O'Doherty J, Deichmann R, Critchley HD, & Dolan RJ (2002). Neural response during anticipation of a primary taste reward. *Neuron* 33: 815–826.
O'Doherty J, Winston J, Critchley HD, Perrett DI, Burt DM, & Dolan RJ (2003). Beauty in a smile: the role of the medial orbitofrontal cortex in facial attractiveness. *Neuropsychologia* 41: 147–155.
O'Donoghue T & Rabin M (1999). Doing it now or later. *American Economic Review* 89: 103–124.
Olausson H, Wessberg J, & McGlone F (2016). *Affective touch and the neurophysiology of CT afferents*. Springer.
Olds J (1977). *Drives and Reinforcements: Behavioral Studies of Hypothalamic Functions*. Raven Press, New York.
Olds J & Milner P (1954). Positive reinforcement produced by electrical stimulation of septal area and other regions of the rat brain. *Journal of Comparative and Physiological Psychology* 47: 419–427.
Olds J & Olds M (1965). Drives, rewards, and the brain. In Barron F & Dement WC, editors, *New Directions in Psychology*, vol. 2. Holt, Rinehart and Winston, New York.
O'Neill M & Schultz W (2018). Predictive coding of the statistical parameters of uncertain rewards by orbitofrontal neurons. *Behav Brain Res* 355: 90–94.
Ongur D & Price JL (2000). The organisation of networks within the orbital and medial prefrontal cortex of rats, monkeys and humans. *Cerebral Cortex* 10: 206–219.
Ongur D, Ferry AT, & Price JL (2003). Architectonic subdivision of the human orbital and medial prefrontal cortex. *Journal of Comparative Neurology* 460: 425–449.
Oomura Y, Nishino H, Karadi Z, Aou S, & Scott TR (1991). Taste and olfactory modulation of feeding related neurons in the behaving monkey. *Physiology and Behavior* 49: 943–950.
Orban GA (2011). The extraction of 3D shape in the visual system of human and nonhuman primates. *Annual Reviews of Neuroscience* 34: 361–388.
O'Scalaidhe SP, Wilson FA, & Goldman-Rakic PS (1997). Areal segregation of face-processing neurons in prefrontal cortex. *Science* 278: 1135–1138.
Padoa-Schioppa C (2009). Range-adapting representation of economic value in the orbitofrontal cortex. *Journal of Neuroscience* 29: 14004–14014.
Padoa-Schioppa C (2011). Neurobiology of economic choice: a good-based model. *Annual Review of Neuroscience* 34: 333–359.
Padoa-Schioppa C & Assad JA (2006). Neurons in the orbitofrontal cortex encode economic value. *Nature* 441: 223–226.
Padoa-Schioppa C & Assad JA (2008). The representation of economic value in the orbitofrontal cortex is invariant for changes of menu. *Nature Neuroscience* 11: 95–102.
Padoa-Schioppa C & Conen KE (2017). Orbitofrontal cortex: A neural circuit for economic decisions. *Neuron* 96: 736–754.
Palomero-Gallagher N & Zilles K (2004). Isocortex. In Paxinos G, editor, *The Rat Nervous System*, 729–757. Elsevier Academic Press, San Diego.
Pandya DN (1996). Comparison of prefrontal architecture and connections. *Philosophical Transactions of the Royal Society B* 351: 1423–1432.
Pandya DN, Seltzer B, Petrides M, & Cipolloni PB (2015). *Cerebral Cortex: Architecture, Connections, and the Dual Origin Concept*. Oxford University Press, Oxford.

Panzeri S, Rolls ET, Battaglia F, & Lavis R (2001). Speed of feedforward and recurrent processing in multilayer networks of integrate-and-fire neurons. *Network: Computation in Neural Systems* 12: 423–440.

Passingham R (1975). Delayed matching after selective prefrontal lesions in monkeys (Macaca mulatta). *Brain Research* 92: 89–102.

Passingham REP & Wise SP (2012). *The Neurobiology of the Prefrontal Cortex*. Oxford University Press, Oxford.

Paton JJ, Belova MA, Morrison SE, & Salzman CD (2006). The primate amygdala represents the positive and negative value of visual stimuli during learning. *Nature* 439: 865–870.

Patton JH, Stanford MS, & Barratt ES (1995). Factor structure of the Barratt impulsiveness scale. *Journal of Clinical Psychology* 51: 768–774.

Percheron G, Yelnik J, & François C (1984a). A Golgi analysis of the primate globus pallidus. III. Spatial organization of the striato-pallidal complex. *Journal of Comparative Neurology* 227: 214–227.

Percheron G, Yelnik J, & François C (1984b). The primate striato-pallido-nigral system: an integrative system for cortical information. In McKenzie JS, Kemm RE, & Wilcox LN, editors, *The Basal Ganglia: Structure and Function*, 87–105. Plenum, New York.

Percheron G, Yelnik J, François C, Fenelon G, & Talbi B (1994). Informational neurology of the basal ganglia related system. *Revue Neurologique (Paris)* 150: 614–626.

Perrett DI, Rolls ET, & Caan W (1982). Visual neurons responsive to faces in the monkey temporal cortex. *Experimental Brain Research* 47: 329–342.

Perrett DI, Smith PAJ, Potter DD, Mistlin AJ, Head AS, Milner D, & Jeeves MA (1985). Visual cells in temporal cortex sensitive to face view and gaze direction. *Proceedings of the Royal Society of London, Series B* 223: 293–317.

Perry G, Rolls ET, & Stringer SM (2006). Spatial vs temporal continuity in view invariant visual object recognition learning. *Vision Research* 46: 3994–4006.

Perry G, Rolls ET, & Stringer SM (2010). Continuous transformation learning of translation invariant representations. *Experimental Brain Research* 204: 255–270.

Personnaz L, Guyon I, & Dreyfus G (1985). Information storage and retrieval in spin-glass-like neural networks. *Journal de Physique Lettres (Paris)* 46: 359–365.

Pessoa L & Adolphs R (2010). Emotion processing and the amygdala: from a 'low road' to 'many roads' of evaluating biological significance. *Nature Reviews Neuroscience* 11: 773–783.

Peters J & Buchel C (2009). Overlapping and distinct neural systems code for subjective value during intertemporal and risky decision making. *Journal of Neuroscience* 29: 15727–15734.

Petrides M (1996). Specialized systems for the processing of mnemonic information within the primate frontal cortex. *Philosophical Transactions of the Royal Society of London B* 351: 1455–1462.

Petrides M (2007). The orbitofrontal cortex: novelty, deviation from expectation, and memory. *Ann N Y Acad Sci* 1121: 33–53.

Petrides M & Pandya DN (1988). Association fiber pathways to the frontal cortex from the superior temporal region in the rhesus monkey. *Journal of Comparative Neurology* 273: 52–66.

Petrides M & Pandya DN (1994). Comparative architectonic analysis of the human and macaque frontal cortex. In Grafman J & Boller F, editors, *Handbook of Neuropsychology*, vol. 9, 17–58. Elsevier, Amsterdam.

Petrides M, Tomaiuolo F, Yeterian EH, & Pandya DN (2012). The prefrontal cortex: comparative architectonic organization in the human and the macaque monkey brains. *Cortex* 48: 46–57.

Phelps E, O'Connor KJ, Gatenby JC, Gore JC, Grillon C, & Davis M (2001). Activation of the left amygdala to a cognitive representation of fear. *Nature Neuroscience* 4: 437–441.

Phelps EA (2004). Human emotion and memory: interactions of the amygdala and hippocampal complex. *Current Opinion in Neurobiology* 14: 198–202.

Phelps EA (2006). Emotion and cognition: insights from studies of the human amygdala. *Annual Review of Psychology* 57: 27–53.

Phelps EA & LeDoux JE (2005). Contributions of the amygdala to emotion processing: from animal models to human behavior. *Neuron* 48: 175–187.

Phillips AG & Fibiger HC (1990). Role of reward and enhancement of conditioned reward in persistence of responding for cocaine. *Behavioral Pharmacology* 1: 269–282.

Phillips AG, Mora F, & Rolls ET (1979). Intracranial self-stimulation in the orbitofrontal cortex and caudate nucleus of the alert monkey: effects of apomorphine, pimozide and spiroperidol. *Psychopharmacology* 62: 79–82.

Phillips AG, Mora F, & Rolls ET (1981). Intra-cerebral self-administration of amphetamine by rhesus monkeys. *Neuroscience Letters* 24: 81–86.

Phillips AG, Blaha CD, & Fibiger HC (1989). Neurochemical correlates of brain-stimulation reward measured by ex vivo and in vivo analyses. *Neuroscience and Biobehavioral Reviews* 13: 99–104.

Phillips AG, Pfaus JG, & Blaha CD (1991). Dopamine and motivated behavior: insights provided by in vivo analysis. In Willner P & Scheel-Kruger J, editors, *The Mesolimbic Dopamine System: From Motivation to Action*, chap. 8, 199–224. Wiley, New York.

Phillips AG, Vacca G, & Ahn S (2008). A top-down perspective on dopamine, motivation and memory. *Pharmacol Biochem Behav* 90: 236–49.

Phillips ML, Drevets WC, Rauch SL, & Lane R (2003). Neurobiology of emotion perception II: Implications for major psychiatric disorders. *Biological Psychiatry* 54: 515–528.

Piguet O (2011). Eating disturbance in behavioural-variant frontotemporal dementia. *Journal of Molecuar Neuroscience* 45: 589–593.

Plakke B & Romanski LM (2014). Auditory connections and functions of prefrontal cortex. *Front Neurosci* 8: 199.

Plakke B, Diltz MD, & Romanski LM (2013). Coding of vocalizations by single neurons in ventrolateral prefrontal cortex. *Hear Res* 305: 135–43.

Plassmann H, O'Doherty J, & Rangel A (2007). Orbitofrontal cortex encodes willingness to pay in everyday economic transactions. *Journal of Neuroscience* 27: 9984–9988.

Platt M & Padoa-Schioppa C (2009). Neuronal representations of value. In Glimcher PW, Camerer CF, Fehr E, & Poldrack RA, editors, *Neuroeconomics. Decision Making and the Brain*, chap. 29, 441–462. Academic Press, London.

Platt ML & Glimcher PW (1999). Neural correlates of decision variables in parietal cortex. *Nature* 400: 233–238.

Preuss TM (1995). Do rats have prefrontal cortex? The Rose-Woolsey-Akert program reconsidered. *Journal of Cognitive Neuroscience* 7: 1–24.

Preuss TM & Goldman-Rakic PS (1989). Connections of the ventral granular frontal cortex of macaques with perisylvian premotor and somatosensory areas: anatomical evidence for somatic representation in primate frontal association cortex. *Journal of Comparative Neurology* 282: 293–316.

Price J (2006). Connections of orbital cortex. In Zald DH & Rauch SL, editors, *The Orbitofrontal Cortex*, chap. 3, 39–55. Oxford University Press, Oxford.

Price JL (2007). Definition of the orbital cortex in relation to specific connections with limbic and visceral structures and other cortical regions. *Ann N Y Acad Sci* 1121: 54–71.

Price JL & Drevets WC (2012). Neural circuits underlying the pathophysiology of mood disorders. *Trends in Cognitive Science* 16: 61–71.

Price JL, Carmichael ST, Carnes KM, Clugnet MC, & Kuroda M (1991). Olfactory input to the prefrontal cortex. In Davis JL & Eichenbaum H, editors, *Olfaction: A Model System for Computational Neuroscience*, 101–120. MIT Press, Cambridge, MA.

Pritchard TC, Hamilton RB, Morse JR, & Norgren R (1986). Projections of thalamic gustatory and lingual areas in the monkey. *Journal of Comparative Neurology* 244: 213–228.

Pritchard TC, Hamilton RB, & Norgren R (1989). Neural coding of gustatory information in the thalamus of Macaca mulatta. *Journal of Neurophysiology* 61: 1–14.

Pritchard TC, Schwartz GJ, & Scott TR (2007). Taste in the medial orbitofrontal cortex of the macaque. *Annals of the New York Academy of Sciences* 1121: 121–135.

Procyk E, Wilson CR, Stoll FM, Faraut MC, Petrides M, & Amiez C (2016). Midcingulate motor map and feedback detection: Converging data from humans and monkeys. *Cereb Cortex* 26: 467–76.

Proulx CD, Hikosaka O, & Malinow R (2014). Reward processing by the lateral habenula in normal and depressive behaviors. *Nat Neurosci* 17: 1146–52.

Pryce CR, Azzinnari D, Spinelli S, Seifritz E, Tegethoff M, & Meinlschmidt G (2011). Helplessness: a systematic translational review of theory and evidence for its relevance to understanding and treating depression. *Pharmacol Ther* 132: 242–267.

Quadt L, Critchley HD, & Garfinkel SN (2018). The neurobiology of interoception in health and disease. *Ann N Y Acad Sci* 1428: 112–128.

Quiroga RQ, Kreiman G, Koch C, & Fried I (2008). Sparse but not 'grandmother-cell' coding in the medial temporal lobe. *Trends in Cognitive Sciences* 12: 87–91.

Rachlin H (1989). *Judgement, Decision, and Choice: A Cognitive/Behavioural Synthesis*. Freeman, New York.

Rachlin H (2000). *The Science of Self-Control*. Harvard Univeristy Press, Cambridge, MA.

Rada P, Mark GP, & Hoebel BG (1998). Dopamine in the nucleus accumbens released by hypothalamic stimulation-escape behavior. *Brain Research* 782: 228–234.

Rahman S, Sahakian BJ, Hodges JR, Rogers RD, & Robbins TW (1999). Specific cognitive deficits in mild frontal variant frontotemporal dementia. *Brain* 122: 1469–1493.

Rantala MJ, Luoto S, Krams I, & Karlsson H (2018). Depression subtyping based on evolutionary psychiatry: Proximate mechanisms and ultimate functions. *Brain Behav Immun* 69: 603–617.

Rao VR, Sellers KK, Wallace DL, Lee MB, Bijanzadeh M, Sani OG, Yang Y, Shanechi MM, Dawes HE, & Chang EF (2018). Direct electrical stimulation of lateral orbitofrontal cortex acutely improves mood in individuals with symptoms of depression. *Curr Biol* 28: 3893–3902 e4.

Ratcliff R & Rouder JF (1998). Modeling response times for two-choice decisions. *Psychological Science* 9: 347–356.

Ratcliff R, Zandt TV, & McKoon G (1999). Connectionist and diffusion models of reaction time. *Psychological Reviews* 106: 261–300.

Rauschecker JP & Scott SK (2009). Maps and streams in the auditory cortex: nonhuman primates illuminate human speech processing. *Nat Neurosci* 12: 718–24.

Reber J, Feinstein JS, O'Doherty JP, Liljeholm M, Adolphs R, & Tranel D (2017). Selective impairment of goal-directed decision-making following lesions to the human ventromedial prefrontal cortex. *Brain* 140: 1743–1756.

Rempel-Clower NL (2007). Role of orbitofrontal cortex connections in emotion. *Ann N Y Acad Sci* 1121: 72–86.

Rempel-Clower NL & Barbas H (1998). Topographic organization of connections between the hypothalamus and prefrontal cortex in the rhesus monkey. *Journal of Comparative Neurology* 398: 393–419.

Renart A, Parga N, & Rolls ET (1999a). Backprojections in the cerebral cortex: implications for memory storage. *Neural Computation* 11: 1349–1388.

Renart A, Parga N, & Rolls ET (1999b). Associative memory properties of multiple cortical modules. *Network* 10: 237–255.

Renart A, Moreno R, Rocha J, Parga N, & Rolls ET (2001). A model of the IT–PF network in object working memory which includes balanced persistent activity and tuned inhibition. *Neurocomputing* 38–40: 1525–1531.

Revah-Levy A, Birmaher B, Gasquet I, & Falissard B (2007). The adolescent depression rating scale (adrs): a validation study. *BMC Psychiatry* 7: 2.

Revah-Levy A, Speranza M, Barry C, Hassler C, Gasquet I, Moro MR, & Falissard B (2011). Association between body mass index and depression: the "fat and jolly" hypothesis for adolescents girls. *BMC Public Health* 11: 649.

Riceberg JS & Shapiro ML (2017). Orbitofrontal cortex signals expected outcomes with predictive codes when stable contingencies promote the integration of reward history. *J Neurosci* 37: 2010–2021.

Ridley M (1993). *The Red Queen: Sex and the Evolution of Human Nature*. Penguin, London.

Ridley RM, Hester NS, & Ettlinger G (1977). Stimulus- and response-dependent units from the occipital and temporal lobes of the unanaesthetized monkey performing learnt visual tasks. *Experimental Brain Research* 27: 539–552.

Robbins TW, Vaghi MM, & Banca P (2019). Obsessive-compulsive disorder: Puzzles and prospects. *Neuron* 102: 27–47.

Robertson RG, Rolls ET, & Georges-François P (1998). Spatial view cells in the primate hippocampus: Effects of removal of view details. *Journal of Neurophysiology* 79: 1145–1156.

Robinson L & Rolls ET (2015). Invariant visual object recognition: biologically plausibile approaches. *Biological Cybernetics* 109: 505–535.

Rodriguez S, Warren CS, Moreno S, Cepeda-Benito A, Gleaves DH, Del Carmen Fernandez M, & Vila J (2007). Adaptation of the food-craving questionnaire trait for the assessment of chocolate cravings: Validation across british and spanish women. *Appetite* 49: 245–250.

Roesch MR & Olson CR (2005). Neuronal activity in primate orbitofrontal cortex reflects the value of time. *Journal of Neurophysiology* 94: 2457–2471.

Roesch MR, Taylor AR, & Schoenbaum G (2006). Encoding of time-discounted rewards in orbitofrontal cortex is independent of value representation. *Neuron* 51: 509–520.

Rolls BJ, Rolls ET, Rowe EA, & Sweeney K (1981a). Sensory specific satiety in man. *Physiology and Behavior* 27: 137–142.

Rolls BJ, Rowe EA, Rolls ET, Kingston B, Megson A, & Gunary R (1981b). Variety in a meal enhances food intake in man. *Physiology and Behavior* 26: 215–221.

Rolls BJ, Rowe EA, & Rolls ET (1982a). How sensory properties of foods affect human feeding behavior. *Physiology and Behavior* 29: 409–417.

Rolls BJ, Rowe EA, & Rolls ET (1982b). How flavour and appearance affect human feeding. *Proceedings of the Nutrition Society* 41: 109–117.

Rolls ET (1971). Involvement of brainstem units in medial forebrain bundle self-stimulation. *Physiology and Behavior* 7: 297–310.

Rolls ET (1974). The neural basis of brain-stimulation reward. *Progress in Neurobiology* 3: 71–160.

Rolls ET (1975). *The Brain and Reward*. Pergamon Press, Oxford.

Rolls ET (1976). The neurophysiological basis of brain-stimulation reward. In Wauquier A & Rolls ET, editors, *Brain-Stimulation Reward*, 65–87. North Holland, Amsterdam.

Rolls ET (1981a). Processing beyond the inferior temporal visual cortex related to feeding, learning, and striatal function. In Katsuki Y, Norgren R, & Sato M, editors, *Brain Mechanisms of Sensation*, chap. 16, 241–269. Wiley, New York.

Rolls ET (1981b). Central nervous mechanisms related to feeding and appetite. *British Medical Bulletin* 37: 131–134.

Rolls ET (1981c). Responses of amygdaloid neurons in the primate. In Ben-Ari Y, editor, *The Amygdaloid Complex*, 383–393. Elsevier, Amsterdam.

Rolls ET (1984). Neurons in the cortex of the temporal lobe and in the amygdala of the monkey with responses selective for faces. *Human Neurobiology* 3: 209–222.

Rolls ET (1986a). A theory of emotion, and its application to understanding the neural basis of emotion. In Oomura Y, editor, *Emotions. Neural and Chemical Control*, 325–344. Japan Scientific Societies Press; and Karger, Tokyo; and Basel.

Rolls ET (1986b). Neural systems involved in emotion in primates. In Plutchik R & Kellerman H, editors, *Emotion: Theory, Research, and Experience*, vol. 3: Biological Foundations of Emotion, chap. 5, 125–143. Academic

Press, New York.
Rolls ET (1989a). Functions of neuronal networks in the hippocampus and neocortex in memory. In Byrne JH & Berry WO, editors, *Neural Models of Plasticity: Experimental and Theoretical Approaches*, chap. 13, 240–265. Academic Press, San Diego, CA.
Rolls ET (1989b). Parallel distributed processing in the brain: implications of the functional architecture of neuronal networks in the hippocampus. In Morris RGM, editor, *Parallel Distributed Processing: Implications for Psychology and Neurobiology*, chap. 12, 286–308. Oxford University Press, Oxford.
Rolls ET (1990a). A theory of emotion, and its application to understanding the neural basis of emotion. *Cognition and Emotion* 4: 161–190.
Rolls ET (1990b). Theoretical and neurophysiological analysis of the functions of the primate hippocampus in memory. *Cold Spring Harbor Symposia in Quantitative Biology* 55: 995–1006.
Rolls ET (1992a). Neurophysiology and functions of the primate amygdala. In Aggleton JP, editor, *The Amygdala*, chap. 5, 143–165. Wiley-Liss, New York.
Rolls ET (1992b). Neurophysiological mechanisms underlying face processing within and beyond the temporal cortical visual areas. *Philosophical Transactions of the Royal Society* 335: 11–21.
Rolls ET (1994). Neurophysiology and cognitive functions of the striatum. *Revue Neurologique (Paris)* 150: 648–660.
Rolls ET (1996a). A theory of hippocampal function in memory. *Hippocampus* 6: 601–620.
Rolls ET (1996b). The orbitofrontal cortex. *Philosophical Transactions of the Royal Society B* 351: 1433–1444.
Rolls ET (1999a). *The Brain and Emotion*. Oxford University Press, Oxford.
Rolls ET (1999b). The functions of the orbitofrontal cortex. *Neurocase* 5: 301–312.
Rolls ET (2000a). The orbitofrontal cortex and reward. *Cerebral Cortex* 10: 284–294.
Rolls ET (2000b). Functions of the primate temporal lobe cortical visual areas in invariant visual object and face recognition. *Neuron* 27: 205–218.
Rolls ET (2000c). Neurophysiology and functions of the primate amygdala, and the neural basis of emotion. In Aggleton JP, editor, *The Amygdala: Second Edition. A Functional Analysis*, chap. 13, 447–478. Oxford University Press, Oxford.
Rolls ET (2001a). The representation of umami taste in the human and macaque cortex. *Sensory Neuron* 3: 227–242.
Rolls ET (2001b). The rules of formation of the olfactory representations found in the orbitofrontal cortex olfactory areas in primates. *Chemical Senses* 26: 595–604.
Rolls ET (2003). Consciousness absent and present: a neurophysiological exploration. *Progress in Brain Research* 144: 95–106.
Rolls ET (2004a). Invariant object and face recognition. In Chalupa LM & Werner JS, editors, *The Visual Neurosciences*, 1165–1178. MIT Press, Cambridge, Mass.
Rolls ET (2004b). The functions of the orbitofrontal cortex. *Brain and Cognition* 55: 11–29.
Rolls ET (2004c). A higher order syntactic thought (HOST) theory of consciousness. In Gennaro RJ, editor, *Higher Order Theories of Consciousness*, chap. 7, 137–172. John Benjamins, Amsterdam.
Rolls ET (2005). *Emotion Explained*. Oxford University Press, Oxford.
Rolls ET (2006a). The neurophysiology and functions of the orbitofrontal cortex. In Zald DH & Rauch SL, editors, *The Orbitofrontal Cortex*, chap. 5, 95–124. Oxford University Press, Oxford.
Rolls ET (2006b). Brain mechanisms underlying flavour and appetite. *Philosophical Transactions of the Royal Society B* 361: 1123–1136.
Rolls ET (2007a). The representation of information about faces in the temporal and frontal lobes of primates including humans. *Neuropsychologia* 45: 124–143.
Rolls ET (2007b). Invariant representations of objects in natural scenes in the temporal cortex visual areas. In Funahashi S, editor, *Representation and Brain*, chap. 3, 47–102. Springer, Tokyo.
Rolls ET (2008a). The representation of flavor in the brain. In Basbaum A, Keneko A, Shepherd GM, & Westheimer G, editors, *The Senses - A Comprehensive Reference. Vol. 4 Olfaction and Taste. Eds. Firestein, S. and Beauchamp, G. K.*, chap. 4.26, 469–478. Elsevier, Oxford.
Rolls ET (2008b). *Memory, Attention, and Decision-Making. A Unifying Computational Neuroscience Approach*. Oxford University Press, Oxford.
Rolls ET (2008c). Face representations in different brain areas, and critical band masking. *Journal of Neuropsychology* 2: 325–360.
Rolls ET (2008d). Functions of the orbitofrontal and pregenual cingulate cortex in taste, olfaction, appetite and emotion. *Acta Physiologica Hungarica* 95: 131–164.
Rolls ET (2009a). From reward value to decision-making: neuronal and computational principles. In Dreher JC & Tremblay L, editors, *Handbook of Reward and Decision-Making*, chap. 5, 95–130. Academic Press, New York.
Rolls ET (2009b). Functional neuroimaging of umami taste: what makes umami pleasant. *American Journal of Clinical Nutrition* 90: 803S–814S.
Rolls ET (2009c). The anterior and midcingulate cortices and reward. In Vogt B, editor, *Cingulate Neurobiology and Disease*, chap. 8, 191–206. Oxford University Press, Oxford.
Rolls ET (2010a). A computational theory of episodic memory formation in the hippocampus. *Behavioural Brain*

Research 215: 180–196.

Rolls ET (2010b). The affective and cognitive processing of touch, oral texture, and temperature in the brain. *Neuroscience and Biobehavioral Reviews* 34: 237–245.

Rolls ET (2011a). Face neurons. In Calder AJ, Rhodes G, Johnson MH, & Haxby JV, editors, *The Oxford Handbook of Face Perception*, chap. 4, 51–75. Oxford University Press, Oxford.

Rolls ET (2011b). The neural representation of oral texture including fat texture. *Journal of Texture Studies* 42: 137–156.

Rolls ET (2011c). Chemosensory learning in the cortex. *Frontiers in Systems Neuroscience* 5: 78 (1–13).

Rolls ET (2012a). Glutamate, obsessive-compulsive disorder, schizophrenia, and the stability of cortical attractor neuronal networks. *Pharmacology, Biochemistry and Behavior* 100: 736–751.

Rolls ET (2012b). Taste, olfactory, and food texture reward processing in the brain and the control of appetite. *Proceedings of the Nutrition Society* 71: 488–501.

Rolls ET (2012c). *Neuroculture: On the Implications of Brain Science*. Oxford University Press, Oxford.

Rolls ET (2012d). Invariant visual object and face recognition: neural and computational bases, and a model, VisNet. *Frontiers in Computational Neuroscience* 6: 1–70.

Rolls ET (2012e). Advantages of dilution in the connectivity of attractor networks in the brain. *Biologically Inspired Cognitive Architectures* 1: 44–54.

Rolls ET (2013a). A biased activation theory of the cognitive and attentional modulation of emotion. *Frontiers in Human Neuroscience* 7: 74.

Rolls ET (2013b). A quantitative theory of the functions of the hippocampal CA3 network in memory. *Frontiers in Cellular Neuroscience* 7: 98.

Rolls ET (2013c). What are emotional states, and why do we have them? *Emotion Review* 5: 241–247.

Rolls ET (2014a). *Emotion and Decision-Making Explained*. Oxford University Press, Oxford.

Rolls ET (2014b). Emotion and decision-making explained: Precis. *Cortex* 59: 185–193.

Rolls ET (2015a). Limbic systems for emotion and for memory, but no single limbic system. *Cortex* 62: 119–157.

Rolls ET (2015b). Neural integration of taste, smell, oral texture, and visual modalities. In Doty R, editor, *Handbook of Olfaction and Gustation*, chap. 46, 1027–1047. Wiley, Hoboken, New Jersey, 3rd edn.

Rolls ET (2015c). Taste, olfactory, and food reward value processing in the brain. *Progress in Neurobiology* 127–128: 64–90.

Rolls ET (2015d). Limbic systems for emotion and for memory, but no single limbic system. *Cortex* 62: 119–157.

Rolls ET (2016a). Brain processing of reward for touch, temperature, and oral texture. In Olausson H, Wessberg J, Morrison I, & McGlone F, editors, *Affective Touch and the Neurophysiology of CT Afferents*, chap. 13, 209–225. Springer, Berlin.

Rolls ET (2016b). Functions of the anterior insula in taste, autonomic, and related functions. *Brain and Cognition* 110: 4–19.

Rolls ET (2016c). *Cerebral Cortex: Principles of Operation*. Oxford University Press, Oxford.

Rolls ET (2016d). Pattern separation, completion, and categorisation in the hippocampus and neocortex. *Neurobiology of Learning and Memory* 129: 4–28.

Rolls ET (2016e). A non-reward attractor theory of depression. *Neuroscience and Biobehavioral Reviews* 68: 47–58.

Rolls ET (2016f). Reward systems in the brain and nutrition. *Annual Review of Nutrition* 36: 435–470.

Rolls ET (2017a). The roles of the orbitofrontal cortex via the habenula in non-reward and depression, and in the responses of serotonin and dopamine neurons. *Neuroscience and Biobehavioral Reviews* 75: 331–334.

Rolls ET (2017b). Evolution of the emotional brain. In Watanabe S, Hofman MA, & Shimizu T, editors, *Evolution of Brain, Cognition, and Emotion in Vertebrates*, chap. 12, 251–272. Springer, Tokyo.

Rolls ET (2017c). The orbitofrontal cortex and emotion in health and disease, including depression. *Neuropsychologia* doi: 10.1016/j.neuropsychologia.2017.09.021.

Rolls ET (2018a). The storage and recall of memories in the hippocampo-cortical system. *Cell and Tissue Research* 373: 577–604.

Rolls ET (2018b). *The Brain, Emotion, and Depression*. Oxford University Press, Oxford.

Rolls ET (2019a). The cingulate cortex and limbic systems for action, emotion, and memory. In Vogt BA, editor, *Handbook of Clinical Neurology: Cingulate Cortex*, chap. 2. Elsevier, New York.

Rolls ET (2019b). Emotion and reasoning in human decision-making. *Economics ejournal* http://www.economics-ejournal.org/economics/discussionpapers/2019-8.

Rolls ET (2019c). The representation of oral food texture including fat texture in the brain. *Journal of Texture Studies*

Rolls ET (2019d). The cingulate cortex and limbic systems for emotion, action, and memory .

Rolls ET & Baylis GC (1986). Size and contrast have only small effects on the responses to faces of neurons in the cortex of the superior temporal sulcus of the monkey. *Experimental Brain Research* 65: 38–48.

Rolls ET & Baylis LL (1994). Gustatory, olfactory and visual convergence within the primate orbitofrontal cortex. *Journal of Neuroscience* 14: 5437–5452.

Rolls ET & Cooper SJ (1974). Connection between the prefrontal cortex and pontine brain-stimulation reward sites in the rat. *Experimental Neurology* 42: 687–699.

Rolls ET & de Waal AWL (1985). Long-term sensory-specific satiety: evidence from an Ethiopian refugee camp. *Physiology and Behavior* 34: 1017–1020.

Rolls ET & Deco G (2002). *Computational Neuroscience of Vision*. Oxford University Press, Oxford.

Rolls ET & Deco G (2006). Attention in natural scenes: neurophysiological and computational bases. *Neural Networks* 19: 1383–1394.

Rolls ET & Deco G (2010). *The Noisy Brain: Stochastic Dynamics as a Principle of Brain Function*. Oxford University Press, Oxford.

Rolls ET & Deco G (2011). Prediction of decisions from noise in the brain before the evidence is provided. *Frontiers in Neuroscience* 5: 33.

Rolls ET & Deco G (2015a). A stochastic neurodynamics approach to the changes in cognition and memory in aging. *Neurobiology of Learning and Memory* 118: 150–161.

Rolls ET & Deco G (2015b). Networks for memory, perception, and decision-making, and beyond to how the syntax for language might be implemented in the brain. *Brain Research* 1621: 316–334.

Rolls ET & Deco G (2016). Non-reward neural mechanisms in the orbitofrontal cortex. *Cortex* 83: 27–38.

Rolls ET & Grabenhorst F (2008). The orbitofrontal cortex and beyond: from affect to decision-making. *Progress in Neurobiology* 86: 216–244.

Rolls ET & Johnstone S (1992). Neurophysiological analysis of striatal function. In Vallar G, Cappa S, & Wallesch C, editors, *Neuropsychological Disorders Associated with Subcortical Lesions*, chap. 3, 61–97. Oxford University Press, Oxford.

Rolls ET & McCabe C (2007). Enhanced affective brain representations of chocolate in cravers vs non-cravers. *European Journal of Neuroscience* 26: 1067–1076.

Rolls ET & Mills WPC (2018). Non-accidental properties, metric invariance, and encoding by neurons in a model of ventral stream visual object recognition, visnet. *Neurobiology of Learning and Memory* 152: 20–31.

Rolls ET & Mills WPC (2019). The generation of time in the hippocampal memory system .

Rolls ET & Milward T (2000). A model of invariant object recognition in the visual system: learning rules, activation functions, lateral inhibition, and information-based performance measures. *Neural Computation* 12: 2547–2572.

Rolls ET & Rolls BJ (1982). Brain mechanisms involved in feeding. In Barker L, editor, *Psychobiology of Human Food Selection*, chap. 3, 33–62. AVI Publishing Company, Westport, Connecticut.

Rolls ET & Rolls JH (1997). Olfactory sensory-specific satiety in humans. *Physiology and Behavior* 61: 461–473.

Rolls ET & Scott TR (2003). Central taste anatomy and neurophysiology. In Doty R, editor, *Handbook of Olfaction and Gustation*, chap. 33, 679–705. Dekker, New York, 2nd edn.

Rolls ET & Stringer SM (2001a). Invariant object recognition in the visual system with error correction and temporal difference learning. *Network: Computation in Neural Systems* 12: 111–129.

Rolls ET & Stringer SM (2001b). A model of the interaction between mood and memory. *Network: Computation in Neural Systems* 12: 89–109.

Rolls ET & Stringer SM (2005). Spatial view cells in the hippocampus, and their idiothetic update based on place and head direction. *Neural Networks* 18: 1229–1241.

Rolls ET & Stringer SM (2006). Invariant visual object recognition: a model, with lighting invariance. *Journal of Physiology – Paris* 100: 43–62.

Rolls ET & Stringer SM (2007). Invariant global motion recognition in the dorsal visual system: a unifying theory. *Neural Computation* 19: 139–169.

Rolls ET & Tovee MJ (1994). Processing speed in the cerebral cortex and the neurophysiology of visual masking. *Proceedings of the Royal Society, B* 257: 9–15.

Rolls ET & Tovee MJ (1995). Sparseness of the neuronal representation of stimuli in the primate temporal visual cortex. *Journal of Neurophysiology* 73: 713–726.

Rolls ET & Treves A (1990). The relative advantages of sparse versus distributed encoding for associative neuronal networks in the brain. *Network* 1: 407–421.

Rolls ET & Treves A (1998). *Neural Networks and Brain Function*. Oxford University Press, Oxford.

Rolls ET & Treves A (2011). The neuronal encoding of information in the brain. *Progress in Neurobiology* 95: 448–490.

Rolls ET & Webb TJ (2012). Cortical attractor network dynamics with diluted connectivity. *Brain Research* 1434: 212–225.

Rolls ET & Webb TJ (2014). Finding and recognising objects in natural scenes: complementary computations in the dorsal and ventral visual systems. *Frontiers in Computational Neuroscience* 8: 85.

Rolls ET & Williams GV (1987). Neuronal activity in the ventral striatum of the primate. In Carpenter MB & Jayaraman A, editors, *The Basal Ganglia II – Structure and Function – Current Concepts*, 349–356. Plenum, New York.

Rolls ET & Wirth S (2018). Spatial representations in the primate hippocampus, and their functions in memory and navigation. *Progress in Neurobiology* 171: 90–113.

Rolls ET & Xiang JZ (2005). Reward–spatial view representations and learning in the primate hippocampus. *Journal of Neuroscience* 25: 6167–6174.

Rolls ET & Xiang JZ (2006). Spatial view cells in the primate hippocampus, and memory recall. *Reviews in the Neurosciences* 17: 175–200.

Rolls ET, Judge SJ, & Sanghera M (1977). Activity of neurones in the inferotemporal cortex of the alert monkey. *Brain Research* 130: 229–238.

Rolls ET, Burton MJ, & Mora F (1980). Neurophysiological analysis of brain-stimulation reward in the monkey. *Brain Research* 194: 339–357.

Rolls ET, Rolls BJ, & Rowe EA (1983a). Sensory-specific and motivation-specific satiety for the sight and taste of food and water in man. *Physiology and Behavior* 30: 185–192.

Rolls ET, Thorpe SJ, & Maddison SP (1983b). Responses of striatal neurons in the behaving monkey. 1. Head of the caudate nucleus. *Behavioural Brain Research* 7: 179–210.

Rolls ET, Thorpe SJ, Boytim M, Szabo I, & Perrett DI (1984). Responses of striatal neurons in the behaving monkey. 3. Effects of iontophoretically applied dopamine on normal responsiveness. *Neuroscience* 12: 1201–1212.

Rolls ET, Baylis GC, & Leonard CM (1985). Role of low and high spatial frequencies in the face-selective responses of neurons in the cortex in the superior temporal sulcus. *Vision Research* 25: 1021–1035.

Rolls ET, Murzi E, Yaxley S, Thorpe SJ, & Simpson SJ (1986). Sensory-specific satiety: food-specific reduction in responsiveness of ventral forebrain neurons after feeding in the monkey. *Brain Research* 368: 79–86.

Rolls ET, Scott TR, Sienkiewicz ZJ, & Yaxley S (1988). The responsiveness of neurones in the frontal opercular gustatory cortex of the macaque monkey is independent of hunger. *Journal of Physiology* 397: 1–12.

Rolls ET, Sienkiewicz ZJ, & Yaxley S (1989). Hunger modulates the responses to gustatory stimuli of single neurons in the caudolateral orbitofrontal cortex of the macaque monkey. *European Journal of Neuroscience* 1: 53–60.

Rolls ET, Yaxley S, & Sienkiewicz ZJ (1990). Gustatory responses of single neurons in the orbitofrontal cortex of the macaque monkey. *Journal of Neurophysiology* 64: 1055–1066.

Rolls ET, Hornak J, Wade D, & McGrath J (1994a). Emotion-related learning in patients with social and emotional changes associated with frontal lobe damage. *Journal of Neurology, Neurosurgery and Psychiatry* 57: 1518–1524.

Rolls ET, Tovee MJ, Purcell DG, Stewart AL, & Azzopardi P (1994b). The responses of neurons in the temporal cortex of primates, and face identification and detection. *Experimental Brain Research* 101: 474–484.

Rolls ET, Critchley HD, Mason R, & Wakeman EA (1996a). Orbitofrontal cortex neurons: role in olfactory and visual association learning. *Journal of Neurophysiology* 75: 1970–1981.

Rolls ET, Critchley HD, & Treves A (1996b). The representation of olfactory information in the primate orbitofrontal cortex. *Journal of Neurophysiology* 75: 1982–1996.

Rolls ET, Critchley HD, Wakeman EA, & Mason R (1996c). Responses of neurons in the primate taste cortex to the glutamate ion and to inosine 5'-monophosphate. *Physiology and Behavior* 59: 991–1000.

Rolls ET, Robertson RG, & Georges-François P (1997a). Spatial view cells in the primate hippocampus. *European Journal of Neuroscience* 9: 1789–1794.

Rolls ET, Treves A, Tovee M, & Panzeri S (1997b). Information in the neuronal representation of individual stimuli in the primate temporal visual cortex. *Journal of Computational Neuroscience* 4: 309–333.

Rolls ET, Treves A, & Tovee MJ (1997c). The representational capacity of the distributed encoding of information provided by populations of neurons in the primate temporal visual cortex. *Experimental Brain Research* 114: 149–162.

Rolls ET, Critchley HD, Browning A, & Hernadi I (1998a). The neurophysiology of taste and olfaction in primates, and umami flavor. *Annals of the New York Academy of Sciences* 855: 426–437.

Rolls ET, Treves A, Robertson RG, Georges-François P, & Panzeri S (1998b). Information about spatial view in an ensemble of primate hippocampal cells. *Journal of Neurophysiology* 79: 1797–1813.

Rolls ET, Critchley HD, Browning AS, Hernadi A, & Lenard L (1999). Responses to the sensory properties of fat of neurons in the primate orbitofrontal cortex. *Journal of Neuroscience* 19: 1532–1540.

Rolls ET, Aggelopoulos NC, & Zheng F (2003a). The receptive fields of inferior temporal cortex neurons in natural scenes. *Journal of Neuroscience* 23: 339–348.

Rolls ET, Franco L, Aggelopoulos NC, & Reece S (2003b). An information theoretic approach to the contributions of the firing rates and the correlations between the firing of neurons. *Journal of Neurophysiology* 89: 2810–2822.

Rolls ET, Kringelbach ML, & De Araujo IET (2003c). Different representations of pleasant and unpleasant odours in the human brain. *European Journal of Neuroscience* 18: 695–703.

Rolls ET, O'Doherty J, Kringelbach ML, Francis S, Bowtell R, & McGlone F (2003d). Representations of pleasant and painful touch in the human orbitofrontal and cingulate cortices. *Cerebral Cortex* 13: 308–317.

Rolls ET, Verhagen JV, & Kadohisa M (2003e). Representations of the texture of food in the primate orbitofrontal cortex: neurons responding to viscosity, grittiness, and capsaicin. *Journal of Neurophysiology* 90: 3711–3724.

Rolls ET, Aggelopoulos NC, Franco L, & Treves A (2004). Information encoding in the inferior temporal visual cortex: contributions of the firing rates and the correlations between the firing of neurons. *Biological Cybernetics* 90: 19–32.

Rolls ET, Browning AS, Inoue K, & Hernadi S (2005a). Novel visual stimuli activate a population of neurons in the primate orbitofrontal cortex. *Neurobiology of Learning and Memory* 84: 111–123.

Rolls ET, Xiang JZ, & Franco L (2005b). Object, space and object-space representations in the primate hippocampus. *Journal of Neurophysiology* 94: 833–844.
Rolls ET, Critchley HD, Browning AS, & Inoue K (2006a). Face-selective and auditory neurons in the primate orbitofrontal cortex. *Experimental Brain Research* 170: 74–87.
Rolls ET, Franco L, Aggelopoulos NC, & Jerez JM (2006b). Information in the first spike, the order of spikes, and the number of spikes provided by neurons in the inferior temporal visual cortex. *Vision Research* 46: 4193–4205.
Rolls ET, Grabenhorst F, Margot C, da Silva M, & Velazco MI (2008a). Selective attention to affective value alters how the brain processes olfactory stimuli. *Journal of Cognitive Neuroscience* 20: 1815–1826.
Rolls ET, Grabenhorst F, & Parris B (2008b). Warm pleasant feelings in the brain. *Neuroimage* 41: 1504–1513.
Rolls ET, Loh M, & Deco G (2008c). An attractor hypothesis of obsessive-compulsive disorder. *European Journal of Neuroscience* 28: 782–793.
Rolls ET, Loh M, Deco G, & Winterer G (2008d). Computational models of schizophrenia and dopamine modulation in the prefrontal cortex. *Nature Reviews Neuroscience* 9: 696–709.
Rolls ET, McCabe C, & Redoute J (2008e). Expected value, reward outcome, and temporal difference error representations in a probabilistic decision task. *Cerebral Cortex* 18: 652–663.
Rolls ET, Grabenhorst F, & Franco L (2009). Prediction of subjective affective state from brain activations. *Journal of Neurophysiology* 101: 1294–1308.
Rolls ET, Critchley H, Verhagen JV, & Kadohisa M (2010a). The representation of information about taste and odor in the primate orbitofrontal cortex. *Chemosensory Perception* 3: 16–33.
Rolls ET, Grabenhorst F, & Deco G (2010b). Choice, difficulty, and confidence in the brain. *Neuroimage* 53: 694–706.
Rolls ET, Grabenhorst F, & Deco G (2010c). Decision-making, errors, and confidence in the brain. *Journal of Neurophysiology* 104: 2359–2374.
Rolls ET, Grabenhorst F, & Parris BA (2010d). Neural systems underlying decisions about affective odors. *Journal of Cognitive Neuroscience* 10: 1068–1082.
Rolls ET, Webb TJ, & Deco G (2012). Communication before coherence. *European Journal of Neuroscience* 36: 2689–2709.
Rolls ET, Dempere-Marco L, & Deco G (2013). Holding multiple items in short term memory: a neural mechanism. *PLoS One* 8: e61078.
Rolls ET, Joliot M, & Tzourio-Mazoyer N (2015a). Implementation of a new parcellation of the orbitofrontal cortex in the automated anatomical labeling atlas. *Neuroimage* 122: 1–5.
Rolls ET, Kellerhals MB, & Nichols TE (2015b). Age differences in the brain mechanisms of good taste. *Neuroimage* 113: 298–309.
Rolls ET, Lu W, Wan L, Yan H, Wang C, Yang F, Tan YL, Li L, Group CSC, Yu H, Liddle PF, Palaniyappan L, Zhang D, Yue W, & Feng J (2017). Individual differences in schizophrenia. *British Journal of Psychiatry Open* 3: 265–273.
Rolls ET, Cheng W, Gilson M, Qiu J, Hu Z, Li Y, Huang CC, Yang AC, Tsai SJ, Zhang X, Zhuang K, Lin CP, Deco G, Xie P, & Feng J (2018a). Effective connectivity in depression. *Biological Psychiatry: Cognitive Neuroscience and Neuroimaging* 3: 187–197.
Rolls ET, Cheng W, Gilson M, Qiu J, Hu Z, Ruan H, Li Y, Huang CC, Yang AC, Tsai SJ, Zhang X, Zhuang K, Lin CP, Deco G, Xie P, & Feng J (2018b). Effective connectivity in depression. *Biol Psychiatry Cogn Neurosci Neuroimaging* 3: 187–197.
Rolls ET, Cheng W, Gong W, Qiu J, Zhou C, Zhang J, Lv W, Ruan H, Wei D, Cheng K, Meng J, Xie P, & Feng J (2018c). Functional connectivity of the anterior cingulate cortex in depression and in health. *Cereb Cortex* doi: 10.1093/cercor/bhy236.
Rolls ET, Mills T, Norton A, Lazidis A, & Norton IT (2018d). Neuronal encoding of fat using the coefficient of sliding friction in the cerebral cortex and amygdala. *Cerebral Cortex* 28: 4080–4089.
Rolls ET, Cheng W, Du J, Wei D, Qiu J, Dai D, Zhou Q, Xie P, & Feng J (2019a). Functional connectivity of the right inferior frontal gyrus and orbitofrontal cortex in depression .
Rolls ET, Cheng W, & Feng J (2019b). The orbitofrontal cortex: a key brain region in depression .
Romanski LM & Diehl MM (2011). Neurons responsive to face-view in the primate ventrolateral prefrontal cortex. *Neuroscience* 189: 223–35.
Roper SD & Chaudhari N (2017). Taste buds: cells, signals and synapses. *Nat Rev Neurosci* 18: 485–497.
Rosati AG (2017). The evolution of primate executive function: From response control to strategic decision-making. In Kaas JH, editor, *Evolution of Nervous Systems, 2nd edition, Volume 3*, vol. 3, chap. 23, 423–437. Elsevier, Amsterdam, 2nd edn.
Rosenkilde CE (1979). Functional heterogeneity of the prefrontal cortex in the monkey: a review. *Behavioral and Neural Biology* 25: 301–345.
Rosenkilde CE, Bauer RH, & Fuster JM (1981). Single unit activity in ventral prefrontal cortex in behaving monkeys. *Brain Research* 209: 375–394.
Rosenthal DM (2005). *Consciousness and Mind*. Oxford University Press, Oxford.

Rossi MA, Sukharnikova T, Hayrapetyan VY, Yang L, & Yin HH (2013). Operant self-stimulation of dopamine neurons in the substantia nigra. *PLoS One* 8: e65799.

Rothkirch M, Tonn J, Kohler S, & Sterzer P (2017). Neural mechanisms of reinforcement learning in unmedicated patients with major depressive disorder. *Brain* 140: 1147–1157.

Royet JP, Zald D, Versace R, Costes N, Lavenne F, Koenig O, Gervais R, Routtenberg A, Gardner EI, & Huang YH (2000). Emotional responses to pleasant and unpleasant olfactory, visual, and auditory stimuli: a positron emission tomography study. *Journal of Neuroscience* 20: 7752–7759.

Rubia K, Alegria AA, Cubillo AI, Smith AB, Brammer MJ, & Radua J (2014). Effects of stimulants on brain function in attention-deficit/hyperactivity disorder: a systematic review and meta-analysis. *Biol Psychiatry* 76: 616–28.

Rudebeck PH & Murray EA (2011). Dissociable effects of subtotal lesions within the macaque orbital prefrontal cortex on reward-guided behavior. *Journal of Neuroscience* 31: 10569–10578.

Rudebeck PH & Murray EA (2014). The orbitofrontal oracle: cortical mechanisms for the prediction and evaluation of specific behavioral outcomes. *Neuron* 84: 1143–56.

Rudebeck PH, Behrens TE, Kennerley SW, Baxter MG, Buckley MJ, Walton ME, & Rushworth MF (2008). Frontal cortex subregions play distinct roles in choices between actions and stimuli. *Journal of Neuroscience* 28: 13775–13785.

Rudebeck PH, Saunders RC, Lundgren DA, & Murray EA (2017). Specialized representations of value in the orbital and ventrolateral prefrontal cortex: Desirability versus availability of outcomes. *Neuron* 95: 1208–1220 e5.

Rushworth MF, Noonan MP, Boorman ED, Walton ME, & Behrens TE (2011). Frontal cortex and reward-guided learning and decision-making. *Neuron* 70: 1054–1069.

Rushworth MF, Kolling N, Sallet J, & Mars RB (2012). Valuation and decision-making in frontal cortex: one or many serial or parallel systems? *Current Opinion in Neurobiology* 22: 946–955.

Rushworth MFS, Hadland KA, Paus T, & Sipila PK (2002). Role of the human medial frontal cortex in task-switching: a combined fMRI and TMS study. *Journal of Neurophysiology* 87: 2577–2592.

Rushworth MFS, Walton ME, Kennerley SW, & Bannerman DM (2004). Action sets and decisions in the medial frontal cortex. *Trends in Cognitive Sciences* 8: 410–417.

Rushworth MFS, Buckley MJ, Behrens TE, Walton ME, & Bannerman DM (2007). Functional organization of the medial frontal cortex. *Current Opinion in Neurobiology* 17: 220–227.

Rutishauser U, Tudusciuc O, Neumann D, Mamelak AN, Heller AC, Ross IB, Philpott L, Sutherling WW, & Adolphs R (2011). Single-unit responses selective for whole faces in the human amygdala. *Current Biology* 21: 1654–1660.

Rutishauser U, Mamelak AN, & Adolphs R (2015). The primate amygdala in social perception - insights from electrophysiological recordings and stimulation. *Trends Neurosci* 38: 295–306.

Rylander G (1948). Personality analysis before and after frontal lobotomy. *Association for Research into Nervous and Mental Disorders* 27 (The Frontal Lobes): 691–705.

Saez RA, Saez A, Paton JJ, Lau B, & Salzman CD (2017). Distinct roles for the amygdala and orbitofrontal cortex in representing the relative amount of expected reward. *Neuron* 95: 70–77 e3.

Saint-Cyr JA, Ungerleider LG, & Desimone R (1990). Organization of visual cortical inputs to the striatum and subsequent outputs to the pallido-nigral complex in the monkey. *Journal of Comparative Neurology* 298: 129–156.

Saleem KS, Kondo H, & Price JL (2008). Complementary circuits connecting the orbital and medial prefrontal networks with the temporal, insular, and opercular cortex in the macaque monkey. *Journal of Comparative Neurology* 506: 659–693.

Saleem KS, Miller B, & Price JL (2014a). Subdivisions and connectional networks of the lateral prefrontal cortex in the macaque monkey. *J Comp Neurol* 522: 1641–90.

Saleem KS, Miller B, & Price JL (2014b). Subdivisions and connectional networks of the lateral prefrontal cortex in the macaque monkey. *Journal of Comparative Neurology* 522: 1641–1690.

Sandman N, Merikanto I, Maattanen H, Valli K, Kronholm E, Laatikainen T, Partonen T, & Paunio T (2016). Winter is coming: nightmares and sleep problems during seasonal affective disorder. *J Sleep Res* 25: 612–619.

Sanghera MK, Rolls ET, & Roper-Hall A (1979). Visual responses of neurons in the dorsolateral amygdala of the alert monkey. *Experimental Neurology* 63: 610–626.

Sato T, Kawamura T, & Iwai E (1980). Responsiveness of inferotemporal single units to visual pattern stimuli in monkeys performing discrimination. *Experimental Brain Research* 38: 313–319.

Schiller D, Monfils MH, Raio CM, Johnson DC, LeDoux JE, & Phelps EA (2010). Preventing the return of fear in humans using reconsolidation update mechanisms. *Nature* 463: 49–53.

Schoenbaum G & Eichenbaum H (1995). Information encoding in the rodent prefrontal cortex. I. Single-neuron activity in orbitofrontal cortex compared with that in pyriform cortex. *Journal of Neurophysiology* 74: 733–750.

Schoenbaum G, Chiba AA, & Gallagher M (2000). Changes in functional connectivity in orbitofrontal cortex and basolateral amygdala during learning and reversal training. *J Neurosci* 20: 5179–89.

Schoenbaum G, Roesch MR, Stalnaker TA, & Takahashi YK (2009). A new perspective on the role of the orbitofrontal

cortex in adaptive behaviour. *Nature Reviews Neuroscience* 10: 885–892.
Schultz W (2013). Updating dopamine reward signals. *Current Opinion in Neurobiology* 23: 229–238.
Schultz W (2016a). Dopamine reward prediction-error signalling: a two-component response. *Nat Rev Neurosci* 17: 183–95.
Schultz W (2016b). Reward functions of the basal ganglia. *J Neural Transm (Vienna)* 123: 679–693.
Schultz W, Apicella P, Scarnati E, & Ljungberg T (1992). Neuronal activity in the ventral striatum related to the expectation of reward. *Journal of Neuroscience* 12: 4595–4610.
Schultz W, Romo R, Ljunberg T, Mirenowicz J, Hollerman JR, & Dickinson A (1995). Reward-related signals carried by dopamine neurons. In Houk JC, Davis JL, & Beiser DG, editors, *Models of Information Processing in the Basal Ganglia*, chap. 12, 233–248. MIT Press, Cambridge, MA.
Scott SK, Young AW, Calder AJ, Hellawell DJ, Aggleton JP, & Johnson M (1997). Impaired auditory recognition of fear and anger following bilateral amygdala lesions. *Nature* 385: 254–257.
Scott TR (2011). Learning through the taste system. *Frontiers in Systems Neuroscience* 5: 87.
Scott TR & Giza BK (1987). A measure of taste intensity discrimination in the rat through conditioned taste aversions. *Physiology and Behaviour* 41: 315–320.
Scott TR & Plata-Salaman CR (1999). Taste in the monkey cortex. *Physiology and Behavior* 67: 489–511.
Scott TR & Small DM (2009). The role of the parabrachial nucleus in taste processing and feeding. *Annals of the New York Academy of Sciences* 1170: 372–377.
Scott TR, Yaxley S, Sienkiewicz ZJ, & Rolls ET (1986). Gustatory responses in the frontal opercular cortex of the alert cynomolgus monkey. *Journal of Neurophysiology* 56: 876–890.
Scott TR, Yan J, & Rolls ET (1995). Brain mechanisms of satiety and taste in macaques. *Neurobiology* 3: 281–292.
Seleman LD & Goldman-Rakic PS (1985). Longitudinal topography and interdigitation of corticostriatal projections in the rhesus monkey. *Journal of Neuroscience* 5: 776–794.
Seligman ME (1978). Learned helplessness as a model of depression. Comment and integration. *Journal of Abnormal Psychology* 87: 165–179.
Seltzer B & Pandya DN (1978). Afferent cortical connections and architectonics of the superior temporal sulcus and surrounding cortex in the rhesus monkey. *Brain Research* 149: 1–24.
Seltzer B & Pandya DN (1989). Frontal lobe connections of the superior temporal sulcus in the rhesus monkey. *Journal of Comparative Neurology* 281: 97–113.
Sescousse G, Li Y, & Dreher JC (2015). A common currency for the computation of motivational values in the human striatum. *Soc Cogn Affect Neurosci* 10: 467–73.
Setogawa T, Mizuhiki T, Matsumoto N, Akizawa F, Kuboki R, Richmond BJ, & Shidara M (2019). Neurons in the monkey orbitofrontal cortex mediate reward value computation and decision-making. *Commun Biol* 2: 126.
Shallice T & Cipolotti L (2018). The prefrontal cortex and neurological impairments of active thought. *Annu Rev Psychol* 69: 157–180.
Sharpe MJ, Stalnaker T, Schuck NW, Killcross S, Schoenbaum G, & Niv Y (2019). An integrated model of action selection: Distinct modes of cortical control of striatal decision making. *Annu Rev Psychol* 70: 53–76.
Sheinberg DL & Logothetis NK (2001). Noticing familiar objects in real world scenes: The role of temporal cortical neurons in natural vision. *Journal of Neuroscience* 21: 1340–1350.
Shen X, Tokoglu F, Papademetris X, & Constable RT (2013). Groupwise whole-brain parcellation from resting-state fmri data for network node identification. *Neuroimage* 82: 403–15.
Shepherd SV & Freiwald WA (2018). Functional networks for social communication in the macaque monkey. *Neuron* 99: 413–420 e3.
Shih P, Shen M, Ottl B, Keehn B, Gaffrey MS, & Muller RA (2010). Atypical network connectivity for imitation in autism spectrum disorder. *Neuropsychologia* 48: 2931–9.
Shima K & Tanji J (1998). Role for cingulate motor area cells in voluntary movement selection based on reward. *Science* 13: 1335–1338.
Simmons JM, Minamimoto T, Murray EA, & Richmond BJ (2010). Selective ablations reveal that orbital and lateral prefrontal cortex play different roles in estimating predicted reward value. *Journal of Neuroscience* 30: 15878–15887.
Small DM (2010). Taste representation in the human insula. *Brain Structre and Function* 214: 551–561.
Small DM & Scott TR (2009). Symposium overview: What happens to the pontine processing? Repercussions of interspecies differences in pontine taste representation for tasting and feeding. *Annals of the New York Academy of Science* 1170: 343–346.
Small DM, Zald DH, Jones-Gotman M, Zatorre RJ, Petrides M, & Evans AC (1999). Human cortical gustatory areas: a review of functional neuroimaing data. *NeuroReport* 8: 3913–3917.
Small DM, Bender G, Veldhuizen MG, Rudenga K, Nachtigal D, & Felsted J (2007). The role of the human orbitofrontal cortex in taste and flavor processing. *Annals of the New York Academy of Sciences* 1121: 136–151.
Smerieri A, Rolls ET, & Feng J (2010). Decision time, slow inhibition, and theta rhythm. *Journal of Neuroscience* 30: 14173–14181.
Soares JC & Young AH (2016). *Bipolar Disorder: basic mechanisms and therapeutic implications*. Cambridge

University Press, Cambridge, 3rd edn.
Solanto MV, Abikoff H, Sonuga-Barke E, Schachar R, Logan GD, Wigal T, Hechtman L, Hinshaw S, & Turkel E (2001). The ecological validity of delay aversion and response inhibition as measures of impulsivity in ad/hd: a supplement to the nimh multimodal treatment study of ad/hd. *J Abnorm Child Psychol* 29: 215–28.
Somerville LH, Hare T, & Casey BJ (2011). Frontostriatal maturation predicts cognitive control failure to appetitive cues in adolescents. *Journal of Cognitive Neuroscience* 23: 2123–2134.
Sompolinsky H (1987). The theory of neural networks: the Hebb rule and beyond. In van Hemmen L & Morgenstern I, editors, *Heidelberg Colloquium on Glassy Dynamics*, vol. 275, 485–527. Springer, New York.
Spatz H (1966). Gehirnentwicklung (introversion-promination) und endocranialausguß. In R H & H S, editors, *Evolution of the Forebrain*, 136–152. Springer, Boston, MA.
Spiridon M, Fischl B, & Kanwisher N (2006). Location and spatial profile of category-specific regions in human extrastriate cortex. *Human Brain Mapping* 27: 77–89.
Stalnaker TA, Cooch NK, & Schoenbaum G (2015). What the orbitofrontal cortex does not do. *Nat Neurosci* 18: 620–7.
Stalnaker TA, Liu TL, Takahashi YK, & Schoenbaum G (2018). Orbitofrontal neurons signal reward predictions, not reward prediction errors. *Neurobiol Learn Mem* 153: 137–143.
Steiner AP & Redish AD (2012). The road not taken: neural correlates of decision making in orbitofrontal cortex. *Front Neurosci* 6: 131.
Steiner AP & Redish AD (2014). Behavioral and neurophysiological correlates of regret in rat decision-making on a neuroeconomic task. *Nat Neurosci* 17: 995–1002.
Stephan KE, Weiskopf N, Drysdale PM, Robinson PA, & Friston KJ (2007). Comparing hemodynamic models with DCM. *Neuroimage* 38: 387–401.
Stephenson-Jones M, Yu K, Ahrens S, Tucciarone JM, van Huijstee AN, Mejia LA, Penzo MA, Tai LH, Wilbrecht L, & Li B (2016). A basal ganglia circuit for evaluating action outcomes. *Nature* 539: 289–293.
Strait CE, Blanchard TC, & Hayden BY (2014). Reward value comparison via mutual inhibition in ventromedial prefrontal cortex. *Neuron* 82: 1357–66.
Stringer SM & Rolls ET (2000). Position invariant recognition in the visual system with cluttered environments. *Neural Networks* 13: 305–315.
Stringer SM & Rolls ET (2002). Invariant object recognition in the visual system with novel views of 3D objects. *Neural Computation* 14: 2585–2596.
Stringer SM & Rolls ET (2008). Learning transform invariant object recognition in the visual system with multiple stimuli present during training. *Neural Networks* 21: 888–903.
Stringer SM, Perry G, Rolls ET, & Proske JH (2006). Learning invariant object recognition in the visual system with continuous transformations. *Biological Cybernetics* 94: 128–142.
Stringer SM, Rolls ET, & Tromans JM (2007). Invariant object recognition with trace learning and multiple stimuli present during training. *Network: Computation in Neural Systems* 18: 161–187.
Sugiura M, Watanabe J, Maeda Y, Matsue Y, Fukuda H, & Kawashima R (2005). Cortical mechanisms of visual self-recognition. *Neuroimage* 24: 143–9.
Swann AC (2009). Impulsivity in mania. *Current Psychiatry Reports* 11: 481–487.
Szabo M, Almeida R, Deco G, & Stetter M (2004). Cooperation and biased competition model can explain attentional filtering in the prefrontal cortex. *European Journal of Neuroscience* 19: 1969–1977.
Takagi SF (1991). Olfactory frontal cortex and multiple olfactory processing in primates. In Peters A & Jones EG, editors, *Cerebral Cortex*, vol. 9, 133–152. Plenum Press, New York.
Tamietto M, Pullens P, de Gelder B, Weiskrantz L, & Goebel R (2012). Subcortical connections to human amygdala and changes following destruction of the visual cortex. *Current Biology* 22: 1449–55.
Tanaka K, Saito C, Fukada Y, & Moriya M (1990). Integration of form, texture, and color information in the inferotemporal cortex of the macaque. In Iwai E & Mishkin M, editors, *Vision, Memory and the Temporal Lobe*, chap. 10, 101–109. Elsevier, New York.
Tegelbeckers J, Kanowski M, Krauel K, Haynes JD, Breitling C, Flechtner HH, & Kahnt T (2018). Orbitofrontal signaling of future reward is associated with hyperactivity in attention-deficit/hyperactivity disorder. *J Neurosci* 38: 6779–6786.
Tellez LA, Han W, Zhang X, Ferreira TL, Perez IO, Shammah-Lagnado SJ, van den Pol AN, & de Araujo IE (2016). Separate circuitries encode the hedonic and nutritional values of sugar. *Nat Neurosci* 19: 465–70.
Thapar A, Cooper M, Eyre O, & Langley K (2013). What have we learnt about the causes of adhd? *J Child Psychol Psychiatry* 54: 3–16.
Thorpe SJ, Maddison S, & Rolls ET (1979). Single unit activity in the orbitofrontal cortex of the behaving monkey. *Neuroscience Letters* S3: S77.
Thorpe SJ, Rolls ET, & Maddison S (1983). Neuronal activity in the orbitofrontal cortex of the behaving monkey. *Experimental Brain Research* 49: 93–115.
Tobler PN, Dickinson A, & Schultz W (2003). Coding of predicted reward omission by dopamine neurons in a conditioned inhibition paradigm. *Journal of Neuroscience* 23: 10402–10410.
Tonegawa S, Nakazawa K, & Wilson MA (2003). Genetic neuroscience of mammalian learning and memory.

Philosophical Transactions of the Royal Society of London B Biological Sciences 358: 787–795.
Tovee MJ & Rolls ET (1995). Information encoding in short firing rate epochs by single neurons in the primate temporal visual cortex. *Visual Cognition* 2: 35–58.
Tovee MJ, Rolls ET, Treves A, & Bellis RP (1993). Information encoding and the responses of single neurons in the primate temporal visual cortex. *Journal of Neurophysiology* 70: 640–654.
Tovee MJ, Rolls ET, & Azzopardi P (1994). Translation invariance and the responses of neurons in the temporal visual cortical areas of primates. *Journal of Neurophysiology* 72: 1049–1060.
Tovee MJ, Rolls ET, & Ramachandran VS (1996). Rapid visual learning in neurones of the primate temporal visual cortex. *NeuroReport* 7: 2757–2760.
Trappenberg TP, Rolls ET, & Stringer SM (2002). Effective size of receptive fields of inferior temporal visual cortex neurons in natural scenes. In Dietterich TG, Becker S, & Gharamani Z, editors, *Advances in Neural Information Processing Systems*, vol. 14, 293–300. MIT Press, Cambridge, MA.
Tremblay L & Schultz W (1999). Relative reward preference in primate orbitofrontal cortex. *Nature* 398: 704–708.
Tremblay L & Schultz W (2000). Modifications of reward expectation-related neuronal activity during learning in primate orbitofrontal cortex. *Journal of Neurophysiology* 83: 1877–1885.
Treves A (1993). Mean-field analysis of neuronal spike dynamics. *Network* 4: 259–284.
Treves A & Rolls ET (1991). What determines the capacity of autoassociative memories in the brain? *Network* 2: 371–397.
Treves A & Rolls ET (1994). A computational analysis of the role of the hippocampus in memory. *Hippocampus* 4: 374–391.
Treves A, Panzeri S, Rolls ET, Booth M, & Wakeman EA (1999). Firing rate distributions and efficiency of information transmission of inferior temporal cortex neurons to natural visual stimuli. *Neural Computation* 11: 601–631.
Trivers RL (1985). *Social Evolution*. Benjamin, Cummings, CA.
Tsao DY & Livingstone MS (2008). Mechanisms of face perception. *Annual Reviews of Neuroscience* 31: 411–437.
Tsao DY, Freiwald WA, Tootell RB, & Livingstone MS (2006). A cortical region consisting entirely of face-selective cells. *Science* 311: 617–618.
Tsuchida A & Fellows LK (2012). Are you upset? distinct roles for orbitofrontal and lateral prefrontal cortex in detecting and distinguishing facial expressions of emotion. *Cereb Cortex* 22: 2904–12.
Tversky A & Kahneman D (1992). Advances in prospect theory – cumulative representation of uncertainty. *Journal of Risk and Uncertainty* 5: 297–323.
Uddin LQ, Supekar K, Lynch CJ, Khouzam A, Phillips J, Feinstein C, Ryali S, & Menon V (2013). Salience network{based classification and prediction of symptom severity in children with autism. *JAMA psychiatry* 70: 869–879.
Ullsperger M & von Cramon DY (2001). Subprocesses of performance monitoring: a dissociation of error processing and response competition revealed by event-related fMRI and ERPs. *Neuroimage* 14: 1387–1401.
Uma-Pradeep K, Geervani P, & Eggum BO (1993). Common Indian spices: nutrient composition, consumption and contribution to dietary value. *Plant Foods and Human Nutrition* 44: 138–148.
Ungerstedt U (1971). Adipsia and aphagia after 6-hydroxydopamine induced degeneration of the nigrostriatal dopamine system. *Acta Physiologia Scandinavica* 81 (Suppl. 367): 95–122.
Usher M & McClelland J (2001). On the time course of perceptual choice: the leaky competing accumulator model. *Psychological Reviews* 108: 550–592.
Valenstein ES (1974). *Brain Control. A Critical Examination of Brain Stimulation and Psychosurgery*. Wiley, New York.
van den Heuvel OA, van Wingen G, Soriano-Mas C, Alonso P, Chamberlain SR, Nakamae T, Denys D, Goudriaan AE, & Veltman DJ (2016). Brain circuitry of compulsivity. *Eur Neuropsychopharmacol* 26: 810–27.
Van der Kooy D, Koda LY, McGinty JF, Gerfen CR, & Bloom FE (1984). The organization of projections from the cortex, amygdala, and hypothalamus to the nucleus of the solitary tract in rat. *Journal of Comparative Neurology* 224: 1–24.
Van Hoesen GW (1981). The differential distribution, diversity and sprouting of cortical projections to the amygdala in the rhesus monkey. In Ben-Ari Y, editor, *The Amygdaloid Complex*, 77–90. Elsevier, Amsterdam.
Van Hoesen GW, Yeterian EH, & Lavizzo-Mourey R (1981). Widespread corticostriate projections from temporal cortex of the rhesus monkey. *Journal of Comparative Neurology* 199: 205–219.
van Veen V, Cohen JD, Botvinick MM, Stenger AV, & Carter CS (2001). Anterior cingulate cortex, conflict monitoring, and levels of processing. *Neuroimage* 14: 1302–1308.
Verhagen JV, Rolls ET, & Kadohisa M (2003). Neurons in the primate orbitofrontal cortex respond to fat texture independently of viscosity. *Journal of Neurophysiology* 90: 1514–1525.
Verhagen JV, Kadohisa M, & Rolls ET (2004). The primate insular taste cortex: neuronal representations of the viscosity, fat texture, grittiness, and the taste of foods in the mouth. *Journal of Neurophysiology* 92: 1685–1699.
Vickers D (1979). *Decision Processes in Visual Perception*. Academic Press, New York.
Vickers D & Packer J (1982). Effects of alternating set for speed or accuracy on response time, accuracy and

confidence in a unidimensional discrimination task. *Acta Psychologica* 50: 179–197.
Voellm BA, De Araujo IET, Cowen PJ, Rolls ET, Kringelbach ML, Smith KA, Jezzard P, Heal RJ, & Matthews PM (2004). Methamphetamine activates reward circuitry in drug naive human subjects. *Neuropsychopharmacology* 29: 1715–1722.
Vogt BA, editor (2009). *Cingulate Neurobiology and Disease*. Oxford University Press, Oxford.
Vogt BA (2016). Midcingulate cortex: Structure, connections, homologies, functions and diseases. *J Chem Neuroanat* 74: 28–46.
Vogt BA (2019). *Cingulate Cortex*. Handbook of Clinical Neurology. Elsevier, New York, 3rd edn.
Vogt BA & Laureys S (2009). The primate posterior cingulate gyrus: connections, sensorimotor orientation, gateway to limbic processing. In Vogt BA, editor, *Cingulate Neurobiology and Disease*, chap. 13, 275–308. Oxford University Press, Oxford.
Vogt BA & Pandya DN (1987). Cingulate cortex of the rhesus monkey: II. Cortical afferents. *Journal of Comparative Neurology* 262: 271–289.
Vogt BA & Sikes RW (2000). The medial pain system, cingulate cortex, and parallel processing of nociceptive information. *Progress in Brain Research* 122: 223–235.
Vogt BA, Derbyshire S, & Jones AKP (1996). Pain processing in four regions of human cingulate cortex localized with co-registered PET and MR imaging. *European Journal of Neuroscience* 8: 1461–1473.
Vogt BA, Berger GR, & Derbyshire SWG (2003). Structural and functional dichotomy of human midcingulate cortex. *European Journal of Neuroscience* 18: 3134–3144.
Volkow ND, Wang GJ, Tomasi D, & Baler RD (2013). Obesity and addiction: neurobiological overlaps. *Obesity Reviews* 14: 2–18.
Vul E, Lashkari D, Hsieh PJ, Golland P, & Kanwisher N (2012). Data-driven functional clustering reveals dominance of face, place, and body selectivity in the ventral visual pathway. *J Neurophysiol* 108: 2306–22.
Waelti P, Dickinson A, & Schultz W (2001). Dopamine responses comply with basic assumptions of formal learning theory. *Nature* 412: 43–48.
Wallis G & Rolls ET (1997). Invariant face and object recognition in the visual system. *Progress in Neurobiology* 51: 167–194.
Wallis JD & Miller EK (2003). Neuronal activity in primate dorsolateral and orbital prefrontal cortex during performance of a reward preference task. *European Journal of Neuroscience* 18: 2069–2081.
Wallis JD, Anderson KC, & Miller EK (2001). Single neurons in prefrontal cortex encode abstract rules. *Nature* 411: 953–956.
Walton ME, Bannerman DM, & Rushworth MFS (2002). The role of rat medial frontal cortex in effort-based decision making. *Journal of Neuroscience* 22: 10996–11003.
Walton ME, Bannerman DM, Alterescu K, & Rushworth MFS (2003). Functional specialization within medial frontal cortex of the anterior cingulate for evaluating effort-related decisions. *Journal of Neuroscience* 23: 6475–6479.
Walton ME, Devlin JT, & Rushworth MF (2004). Interactions between decision making and performance monitoring within prefrontal cortex. *Nature Neuroscience* 7: 1259–1265.
Walton ME, Behrens TE, Buckley MJ, Rudebeck PH, & Rushworth MF (2010). Separable learning systems in the macaque brain and the role of orbitofrontal cortex in contingent learning. *Neuron* 65: 927–39.
Wan Z, Rolls ET, Cheng W, & Feng J (2019). Prediction of sensation-seeking from functional connectivities of the medial orbitofrontal cortex. *Organisation for Human Brain Mapping* 3017.
Wang XJ (1999). Synaptic basis of cortical persistent activity: the importance of NMDA receptors to working memory. *Journal of Neuroscience* 19: 9587–9603.
Wang XJ (2002). Probabilistic decision making by slow reverberation in cortical circuits. *Neuron* 36: 955–968.
Wang XJ (2008). Decision making in recurrent neuronal circuits. *Neuron* 60: 215–234.
Wang XJ (2010). Neurophysiological and computational principles of cortical rhythms in cognition. *Physiological Reviews* 90: 1195–1268.
Webb TJ & Rolls ET (2014). Deformation-specific and deformation-invariant visual object recognition: pose vs identity recognition of people and deforming objects. *Frontiers in Computational Neuroscience* 8: 37.
Webb TJ, Rolls ET, Deco G, & Feng J (2011). Noise in attractor networks in the brain produced by graded firing rate representations. *PLoS One* 6: e23620.
Weiner KS & Grill-Spector K (2013). Neural representations of faces and limbs neighbor in human high-level visual cortex: evidence for a new organization principle. *Psychological Research* 77: 74–97.
Weiner KS & Grill-Spector K (2015). The evolution of face processing networks. *Trends Cogn Sci* 19: 240–1.
Weiskrantz L (1956). Behavioral changes associated with ablation of the amygdaloid complex in monkeys. *Journal of Comparative and Physiological Psychology* 49: 381–391.
Weiskrantz L (1997). *Consciousness Lost and Found*. Oxford University Press, Oxford.
Weiskrantz L (1998). *Blindsight*. Oxford University Press, Oxford, 2nd edn.
Weiskrantz L (2009). Is blindsight just degraded normal vision? *Experimental Brain Research* 192: 413–416.
Weitzenhoffer A & Hilgard E (1962). *Stanford Hypnotic Susceptibility Scale: Form C*. Consulting Psychologists Press, Palo Alto, Ca.

Wessa M, Kanske P, & Linke J (2014). Bipolar disorder: a neural network perspective on a disorder of emotion and motivation. *Restorative Neurology and Neuroscience* 32: 51–62.

Whalen PJ & Phelps EA (2009). *The Human Amygdala*. Guilford, New York.

Wheeler EZ & Fellows LK (2008). The human ventromedial frontal lobe is critical for learning from negative feedback. *Brain* 131: 1323–1331.

Whelan R, Conrod PJ, Poline JB, Lourdusamy A, Banaschewski T, Barker GJ, Bellgrove MA, Buchel C, Byrne M, Cummins TD, Fauth-Buhler M, Flor H, Gallinat J, Heinz A, Ittermann B, Mann K, Martinot JL, Lalor EC, Lathrop M, Loth E, Nees F, Paus T, Rietschel M, Smolka MN, Spanagel R, Stephens DN, Struve M, Thyreau B, Vollstaedt-Klein S, Robbins TW, Schumann G, Garavan H, & Consortium I (2012). Adolescent impulsivity phenotypes characterized by distinct brain networks. *Nat Neurosci* 15: 920–5.

Whitlock JR (2017). Posterior parietal cortex. *Curr Biol* 27: R691–R695.

Williams GV, Rolls ET, Leonard CM, & Stern C (1993). Neuronal responses in the ventral striatum of the behaving macaque. *Behavioural Brain Research* 55: 243–252.

Wilson DA & Sullivan RM (2011). Cortical processing of odor objects. *Neuron* 72: 506–519.

Wilson FAW & Rolls ET (1993). The effects of stimulus novelty and familiarity on neuronal activity in the amygdala of monkeys performing recognition memory tasks. *Experimental Brain Research* 93: 367–382.

Wilson FAW & Rolls ET (2005). The primate amygdala and reinforcement: a dissociation between rule-based and associatively-mediated memory revealed in amygdala neuronal activity. *Neuroscience* 133: 1061–1072.

Wilson FAW, O'Scalidhe SP, & Goldman-Rakic PS (1993). Dissociation of object and spatial processing domains in primate prefrontal cortex. *Science* 260: 1955–1958.

Wilson RC, Takahashi YK, Schoenbaum G, & Niv Y (2014). Orbitofrontal cortex as a cognitive map of task space. *Neuron* 81: 267–279.

Wise SP (2008). Forward frontal fields: phylogeny and fundamental function. *Trends in Neuroscience* 31: 599–608.

Xie C, Jia T, Rolls ET, Liu Z, Banaschewski T, Barker G, Bodke A, Bromberg U, C B, Quinlan EB, Desrivieres S, Flor H, Grigis A, Garavan H, Gowland P, Heinz A, Hohmann S, Ittermann B, Martinot JL, Martinot MLP, Nees F, Papadopoulos Orfanos D, Paus T, Poustka L, Frohner JH, Smolka MN, Walter H, Whelan R, Schumann G, Feng J, & IMAGEN C (2019). Reward vs non-reward sensitivity of the medial vs lateral orbitofrontal cortex related to the risk of depression .

Yan J & Scott TR (1996). The effect of satiety on responses of gustatory neurons in the amygdala of alert cynomolgus macaques. *Brain Research* 740: 193–200.

Yaxley S, Rolls ET, & Sienkiewicz ZJ (1988). The responsiveness of neurones in the insular gustatory cortex of the macaque monkey is independent of hunger. *Physiology and Behavior* 42: 223–229.

Yaxley S, Rolls ET, & Sienkiewicz ZJ (1990). Gustatory responses of single neurons in the insula of the macaque monkey. *Journal of Neurophysiology* 63: 689–700.

Yelnik J (2002). Functional anatomy of the basal ganglia. *Movement Disorders* 17 Suppl 3: S15–S21.

Yeterian EH, Pandya DN, Tomaiuolo F, & Petrides M (2012). The cortical connectivity of the prefrontal cortex in the monkey brain. *Cortex* 48: 58–81.

Yih J, Beam DE, Fox KCR, & Parvizi J (2019). Intensity of affective experience is modulated by magnitude of intracranial electrical stimulation in human orbitofrontal, cingulate, and insular cortex. *Soc Cogn Affect Neurosci* .

Yohn CN, Gergues MM, & Samuels BA (2017). The role of 5-ht receptors in depression. *Mol Brain* 10: 28.

Young AW, Aggleton JP, Hellawell DJ, Johnson M, Broks P, & Hanley JR (1995). Face processing impairments after amygdalotomy. *Brain* 118: 15–24.

Young AW, Hellawell DJ, Van de Wal C, & Johnson M (1996). Facial expression processing after amygdalotomy. *Neuropsychologia* 34: 31–39.

Zald DH & Rauch SL, editors (2006). *The Orbitofrontal Cortex*. Oxford University Press, Oxford.

Zanos P & Gould TD (2018). Mechanisms of ketamine action as an antidepressant. *Mol Psychiatry* 23: 801–811.

Zanos P, Moaddel R, Morris PJ, Georgiou P, Fischell J, Elmer GI, Alkondon M, Yuan P, Pribut HJ, Singh NS, Dossou KS, Fang Y, Huang XP, Mayo CL, Wainer IW, Albuquerque EX, Thompson SM, Thomas CJ, Zarate J C A, & Gould TD (2016). Nmdar inhibition-independent antidepressant actions of ketamine metabolites. *Nature* 533: 481–6.

Zapiec B & Mombaerts P (2015). Multiplex assessment of the positions of odorant receptor-specific glomeruli in the mouse olfactory bulb by serial two-photon tomography. *Proc Natl Acad Sci U S A* 112: E5873–82.

Zatorre RJ & Jones-Gotman M (1991). Human olfactory discrimination after unilateral frontal or temporal lobectomy. *Brain* 114: 71–84.

Zatorre RJ, Jones-Gotman M, Evans AC, & Meyer E (1992). Functional localization of human olfactory cortex. *Nature* 360: 339–340.

Zatorre RJ, Jones-Gotman M, & Rouby C (2000). Neural mechanisms involved in odor pleasantness and intensity judgments. *NeuroReport* 11: 2711–2716.

Zhao GQ, Zhang Y, Hoon MA, Chandrashekar J, Erlenbach I, Ryba NJ, & Zucker CS (2003). The receptors for mammalian sweet and umami taste. *Cell* 115: 255–266.

Zorumski CF, Izumi Y, & Mennerick S (2016). Ketamine: Nmda receptors and beyond. *J Neurosci* 36: 11158–11164.

Index

ΔI, 113–123
5HT, 14–16, 220, 224

absolute reward value, 95
absolute value, 101–106
action–outcome learning, 153–154
actions
    cost, 51
activation function, 242
active avoidance, 266
addiction, 128, 157–158
ADHD, 226
ageing, 245
ambiguity, 93, 105
amphetamine, 128
amygdala, 80–83, 179–190
    and reversal, 254
    lesions, 182
    not involved in conscious feelings, 189
    novel stimuli, 187
amygdala neuronal responses, 184–188
antidepressant, 220, 224
associative learning, 237–248
associative processes, 181
astringency, 31–32
attention, 81, 82
attention and emotion, 83–87
attention-deficit hyperactivity disorder, 226
attractor network, 109–123, 240–250, 265
autism, 225
autoassociation network, 240–248
autobiographical memory, 123
autocorrelation memory, 243
autonomic responses, 152, 181, 184
avoidance, 167, 169, 181, 266

backprojections, 251
basal ganglia, 160–164
binding, 62
binge eating, 158
bipolar disorder, 222–225
blindsight, 59, 174
BOLD signal, 25, 265
Borderline Personality Disorder, 143
brain systems and depression, 199
bulimia, 158

capacity
    autoassociator, 246–248
caudate nucleus
    head, 163
choice ambiguity, 105
cingulate cortex, 80–87, 141, 145–155
    midcingulate, 153
    posterior, 154

    subgenual, 152
    taste, 34
cingulate motor area, 153
clamped inputs, 244
classical conditioning, 171, 184, 267
coding, 20, 65–72
coefficient of sliding friction, 30
cognition and emotion, 80–83
cold, 44
common currency, 98–101
common scale of value, 98–101, 150
completion, 243, 244
compulsivity, 226
conditional expected value neurons, 48
conditional reward neurons, 48, 252
conditioned appetite and conditioned satiety, 100
conditioned response, 181, 267
conditioned stimulus, 181, 267
conditioned taste aversion, 100
conditioning, 169–171, 181, 237–240
confabulation, 179
confidence, 113–123
conflict, 178
content addressability, 240
cortex, 109
    rodents, 230–231
cortical design, 228
cortical structure, 228
cost of actions, 51
cost–benefit analysis, 106, 178
costs, 93

deception, 178, 179
decision
    under ambiguity, 93
    under risk, 93
decision times, 116–123
decision under ambiguity, 105
decision under risk, 105
decision under uncertainty, 105
decision-making, 108–123
    medial prefrontal cortex, 113–123
    probabilistic, 108–123
    ventromedial prefrontal cortex, 132, 139
decision-making under risk, 106
decisions, 108–123
decoding, 65
definition
    lateral orbitofrontal cortex, 3
    medial orbitofrontal cortex, 3
    lateral orbitofrontal cortex, 3
    medial orbitofrontal cortex, 3
delay of reward, 106
delayed match to sample, 134, 163, 255
depression, 151, 191–225

behavioural therapy, 218
brain systems, 199
cognitive therapy, 218
effective connectivity, 213
genetics, 193
ketamine, 198
orbitofrontal cortex, 203
pharmacological treatment, 220–222
subtypes, 216
theory of, 191–225
treatments, 217–222
depression and sleep, 215
desire vs pleasure, 184
devaluation, 24, 27, 39, 50, 145, 151
difficult vs easy decisions, 113–123
distributed representation, 65–72
dopamine, 14–16, 155–160
and reward, 155–164
dopamine neurons
error signal, 159–160
reward, 159–160
drinking, 128
drive, 268

Effective connectivity, 265
emotion, 265, 267
and attention, 83–87
and cognition, 80–83
emotion-related learning, 181
emotional memory, 123
empathy, 139
encoding, 20, 65
endocrine responses, 171
energy
in an autoassociator, 243
energy landscape, 116, 243
episodic memory, 123, 248
error
prediction, 266
error neurons, 75–79, 159–160, 194, 195, 251
escape, 167, 169, 181, 266
evolution of emotion, 179
executive function, 91, 107, 175
expected reward value, 50, 105
expected utility, 159–160
expected value, 36–75, 266
expression
face, 52, 70, 78, 141, 187, 189–190
voice, 141
extinction, 75–79, 130, 170, 267
extraversion, 143, 190

face attractiveness, 52, 54
face expression, 52, 70, 78, 141
amygdala, 189–190
face identity, 52, 59–70
fat, 29, 150, 184
fat texture, 29
fault tolerance, 240, 245
fear, 189
firing rate distribution, 248
fitness, 265

flavour, 20–44, 80–91
fMRI, 25, 265
food texture, 28–32, 90, 150, 184–186
Functional connectivity, 265
Functional magnetic resonance imaging, 265
Functional neuroimaging, 266

GABA, gamma-amino-butyric acid, 242
Gage, Phineas, 1
gambling, 138
gambling task, 137
gamma oscillations, 112
generalization, 240, 244
glossary, 265–268
glucose, 20–35, 184
Go/NoGo task, 130, 186, 252
graceful degradation, 240, 245
grandmother cell, 65

habenula, 14–16, 155–160, 220
habit learning, 153, 184
Hebb rule, 237, 239, 241, 245
hedonic assessment, 184
heuristics, 100, 101
hierarchy, 179
hippocampus, 123
homeostasis, 39
Hopfield, 243

implicit responses, 19, 106
impulsive behaviour, 106
impulsiveness, 78, 130, 139, 143–144, 204
impulsivity, 226
individual differences, 172
inferior frontal gyrus, 78, 203
inferior temporal visual cortex, 57–72, 91
information theory, 68
inhibitory neurons, 89, 242, 251
instrumental learning, 153, 169–172, 181, 266
instrumental reinforcers, 17, 169–172, 181, 186, 251, 266
insula, 44
taste, 32
interests, 176
gene-defined, 176
of the individual defined by the reasoning system, 176
introversion, 190
invariance, 58–65
invariant representations, 59–65, 72
Iowa Gambling Task, 137–138

ketamine and depression, 198
ketamine as an antidepressant, 221

lateral hypothalamus, 184
learning
action–outcome, 153–154
associative, 45–75, 181, 237–256
habit, 153
instrumental, 153, 169–172, 181, 251, 266
of emotional responses, 181

of emotional states, 181
stimulus–response, 153
learning rule
local, 245
learning set, 130, 251–256
lithium, 224
local learning rule, 245
long-term depression (LTD), 48, 251, 254, 268
long-term potentiation (LTP), 239, 268

Machiavellian intelligence, 179
mania, 222–225
medial prefrontal cortex, 113–123, 151
memory, 109, 123, 134, 163, 175, 187, 237, 255
model of reversal learning, 251–256
monetary reward, 73, 87, 88, 136, 150
mood, 150
mood stabilizer, 224
morality, 140
motivation, 167, 171, 268
multiple decision-making systems, 179
music, 54

negative reinforcement, 170, 266
negative reinforcer, 266
net value, 92
neural encoding, 65–72
neuroeconomics, 92–107
neuroimaging, 117
  task difficulty, 118–123
neuroticism, 143, 190
NMDA receptors, 184, 254
non-reward, 87, 130, 266
non-reward and depression, 195–218
non-reward neurons, 75–79, 153, 191–194, 251
novel stimuli, 123
novelty, 187
nucleus accumbens, 157–158, 162–164

obesity, 144
object representations, 56–72
obsessive-compulsive disorder, 226
odour, 31, 36–44, 80–87
olfaction, 35–44, 150
  attentional influences, 83–87
  cognitive influences, 80–83
olfactory reward, 37–44
operant response, 157, 169
opiates, 184
oral texture, 27
orbitofrontal cortex, 107
  anatomy, 10–16
  auditory responses, 54
  cognitive influences on, 80–83
  connections, 10–16
  depression, 203
  evolution, 228–231
  face expression processing, 141
  face representations, 52–55, 77–79
  human, 134–144
  influences of attention, 83–87
  lateral, 226

lesions, 130, 134–144
neuroimaging, 17–144
neurophysiology, 17–91
non-reward learning, 132
olfaction, 35–44
relative preference, 90
reversal learning, 132
rodent, 5–7
rule-based learning, 132
taste, 20–35
topology, 87–91
visual inputs, 45–55
voice expression processing, 141
outcome value, 266
output systems for emotion, 152–154, 160–164, 184
oxytocin, 193

pain, 1, 148–153, 170
passive avoidance, 170, 267
pattern association memory, 237–240
pattern association network, 266
Pavlovian conditioning, 171, 181, 267
percent correct, 116
personality, 78, 100, 106, 135, 139, 143, 172, 190, 193, 219
PET, 36
pleasant touch, 150
pleasantness of olfactory stimuli, 37–44, 80–83
pleasure map, 88
pleasure scaling, 150
population code, 20
positive reinforcement, 170, 266
positive reinforcer, 170, 266
positron emission tomography, 36
posterior cingulate cortex, 154
predicted reward value, 73
prediction error, 14, 266
prediction error hypothesis, 105, 159–160, 164
preference
  relative, 45, 47, 73, 90
prefrontal cortex, 5
  medial, 113–123, 151
prefrontal leucotomy, 1
primary reinforcers, 17, 91, 142, 170, 181, 184, 185
Prospect theory, 101
psychiatric symptoms, 143–144
punisher, 17–105, 169–170, 267
punishment, 169–170, 267
pyriform cortex, 39, 83

rational choice, 179
rationality, 176
reaction times, 116–123
reasoning, 176
recall, 81, 237, 239, 242
  in autoassociation memories, 243
reconsolidation, 184
recurrent collateral connections, 109
reinforcement, 170
reinforcers, 134, 169–172, 178, 181, 186, 251, 266
  potential secondary, 36–72
  primary, 170

secondary, 17–79, 158, 169, 170
relative preference, 45, 47, 73, 90
relative reward value, 95
relative value, 101–106
retrieval
  of memory, 123
reversal learning, 45–79, 130, 132, 194
reversal learning set, 130, 251–256
reversal learning, model of, 251–256
reward, 17–129, 159–160, 169, 266
  monetary, 73
reward devaluation, 39, 50
reward predicting neuron, 47
reward prediction error, 75–79, 153, 159–160, 206, 251, 263
reward value, 24, 73, 159–164
risk, 93, 106
risk-taking, 204
Rolls' theory of depression, 191–225

salience, 163, 184
satiety, 20, 25, 228–231
secondary reinforcers, 17–72, 169, 170, 183
self-harming patients, 143
selfish gene, 176–177
selfish individual, 176–177
selfish phene, 176–177
selfish phenotype, 176–177
sensation-seeking, 78
sensory-specific satiety, 25–27, 50
serotonin, 14–16, 220, 224
sexual behaviour, 183
short-term memory, 134, 163, 237, 241, 248, 251
size constancy, 63
size invariance, 63
sleep and depression, 215
smell, 35–44, 80–87
smoking, 128
SNRI, 220, 224
sociopathy, 140
somatosensory insula, 44
sparse distributed encoding, 20
sparseness, 68
speed of processing, 245
spin glass, 243
spontaneous firing
  principles, 245
SSRI, 220, 224
state space, 234
statistical mechanics, 243
stimulus–reinforcer association learning, 37, 45–52, 75–79, 130, 135–140, 169–172, 182–184, 186–187, 237–240
stimulus–reinforcer reversal learning, model of, 251–256
stop inhibition, 139
stop-signal task, 78
striatal neuronal activity, 162
striatum, 162–164
  ventral, 14–16, 155–164
subgenual cingulate cortex, 145, 148, 151, 152
symmetric synaptic weights, 241

synaptic modification, 237–251, 254
synaptic weight vector, 237–240

taste, 20–35, 43–44, 77, 150, 184–186
  insula, 32
taste aversion learning, 100
taste reward, 228–231
temperature, 44
temporal difference (TD) error, 160
temporal discounting, 95
temporal discounting of value, 106
temporal lobes, 231
texture, 28–32, 150, 184–186
  fat, 29
  viscosity, 28
theory of mind, 175
time out, 170, 267
touch, 44, 89, 150, 181
tricyclic antidepressant, 220, 224

umami taste, 20–24, 91
uncertainty, 105, 106, 159–160
unclamped inputs, 244
unconditioned response, 181, 267
unconditioned stimulus, 48, 171, 181, 237–240, 267

valence, 58, 163
valproate, 224
value, 58, 266
  absolute, 101–106
  expected, 36–75
  outcome, 20–35
  relative, 101–106
  scaling, 98–101
value scaling
  an 'ultimate' account, 100
vector, 237–240
ventral striatum, 71, 107, 157–158, 162–164, 183, 184
ventral visual system, 57–72
ventromedial prefrontal cortex, 113–123, 132, 139, 147, 151
viscosity, 28, 29, 150, 184
vision, 59–72
  association learning, 45–55
visual stimuli
  as primary reinforcers, 142
VMPFC, 113–123, 132, 139, 147
voice expression, 141–143

warmth, 44
Weber's law, 108

The manufacturer's authorised representative in the EU for product safety is
Oxford University Press España S.A. of el Parque Empresarial San Fernando de
Henares, Avenida de Castilla, 2 – 28830 Madrid (www.oup.es/en or product.
safety@oup.com). OUP España S.A. also acts as importer into Spain of products
made by the manufacturer.

www.ingramcontent.com/pod-product-compliance
Ingram Content Group UK Ltd.
Pitfield, Milton Keynes, MK11 3LW, UK
UKHW052118190426
11946UKWH00024B/107

9 780198 845997